Nutrition and Human Oral Health

Nutrition and Human Oral Health

Editors

Kirstin Vach
Johan Peter Woelber

MDPI • Basel • Beijing • Wuhan • Barcelona • Belgrade • Manchester • Tokyo • Cluj • Tianjin

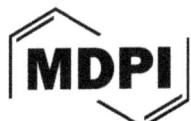

Editors

Kirstin Vach
Institute of Medical Biometry
and Statistics
University of Freiburg
Freiburg
Germany

Johan Peter Woelber
Department of Operative
Dentistry and Periodontology
University of Freiburg
Freiburg
Germany

Editorial Office
MDPI
St. Alban-Anlage 66
4052 Basel, Switzerland

This is a reprint of articles from the Special Issue published online in the open access journal *Nutrients* (ISSN 2072-6643) (available at: www.mdpi.com/journal/nutrients/special_issues/Nutrition_Oral_Health).

For citation purposes, cite each article independently as indicated on the article page online and as indicated below:

LastName, A.A.; LastName, B.B.; LastName, C.C. Article Title. *Journal Name* **Year**, *Volume Number*, Page Range.

ISBN 978-3-0365-4550-9 (Hbk)
ISBN 978-3-0365-4549-3 (PDF)

Contents

About the Editors

Kirstin Vach

Kirstin Vach studied mathematics in Freiburg and has since been working on statistical problems in the evaluation of medical data. She has worked at the Institute of General Medicine, Odense (Denmark), Institute of Medical Biometry and Statistics, Freiburg (Germany), and Centre for Dental Medicine, Medical Centre - University of Freiburg. She is also interested in the interaction between different scientific disciplines.

Johan Peter Woelber

Johan Peter Woelber graduated in dentistry at the University of Freiburg, Germany, and undergone a specialization in nutritional medicine. He is Associate Professor at the Department of Operative Dentistry and Periodontology at the Medical Center from the University of Freiburg, Germany. His interests are the prevention and supportive therapy of dental and periodontal diseases by nutritional and lifestyle dentistry.

Preface to "Nutrition and Human Oral Health"

Dear Readers,

We are proud to present the *Nutrients* Special Issue "Nutrition and Human Oral Health", now in a book form. It contains 18 wonderful publications that provide an outline of current scientific work in the field of nutritional dentistry. The topic is not only of interest to other scientists, but also offers every person in everyday life the opportunity to use nutrition to make teeth and gums healthier or to keep them healthy.

We would like to thank Ms. Alva Wu of MDPI Publishing for her consistent support in running the Special Issue and this book.

Kirstin Vach and Johan Peter Woelber
Editors

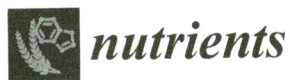

MDPI

Editorial

The Emerging Field of Nutritional Dentistry

Johan Peter Woelber [1,*] and Kirstin Vach [1,2,*]

1 Department of Operative Dentistry and Periodontology, Faculty of Medicine, University of Freiburg, Hugstetter Str. 55, 79106 Freiburg, Germany
2 Faculty of Medicine, Institute of Medical Biometry and Statistics, University of Freiburg, Zinkmattenstr. 6A, 79108 Freiburg, Germany
* Correspondence: johan.woelber@uniklinik-freiburg.de (J.P.W.); kv@imbi.uni-freiburg.de (K.V.)

Citation: Woelber, J.P.; Vach, K. The Emerging Field of Nutritional Dentistry. *Nutrients* 2022, 14, 2076. https://doi.org/10.3390/nu14102076

Received: 3 May 2022
Accepted: 6 May 2022
Published: 16 May 2022

Publisher's Note: MDPI stays neutral with regard to jurisdictional claims in published maps and institutional affiliations.

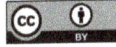

Nutrition is, like oxygen, one of the basic requirements for animals and, accordingly, Homo sapiens to live. The entire evolution of Homo sapiens was consistently influenced by the nutritional environment, which also included the microbial coevolution. While the most common oral diseases in the form of caries and periodontal diseases were very rare in prehistoric hominins and are still very rare in wild-living animals [1–3], today, caries and periodontitis taken together are the most common diseases of mankind [4,5]. Reasons for this dramatic increase can be found in the successive appearance of disease-promoting risk factors in the course of cultural evolution from the Neolithic era to the Industrial Revolution, especially regarding the dietary patterns [6]. This change from a whole-food natural diet towards a Western diet, rich in macronutrients and salt, but poor in fibers and micronutrients, has not only increased the prevalence of oral diseases, but also caused a dramatic increase in non-communicable diseases [7]. Today, diet has even become the strongest risk factor for premature death [8]. On the other hand, these widespread and harmful conditions of a Western diet explains why dietary interventions for oral diseases are so efficient [7,9–12].

Accordingly, a cause-related prevention and therapy in dentistry must consider these dietary changes in human evolution, which is a fundamental call for the field of nutritional dentistry. This field does not exclude modern symptomatic approaches like plaque control and the use of fluorides [13,14]. It rather aims to build a preventive basis in order to address both oral and other non-communicable diseases in one approach. This strategy is in line with the so-called common risk factor approach [15], which aims to address up-stream risk factors to heighten the efficacy of prevention on an individual and public health level.

Research on this topic demands adequate methods for collecting or generating relevant data as well as for analyzing these data. More and more apps are now being used in addition to the previously widespread paper-based food diaries [16]. In order to achieve comparability of the results, of course, validated survey instruments in several languages are necessary to capture information at different stages across countries and cultures [17]. The statistical analysis of the data also has to meet requirements that go beyond purely descriptive analyses, in order to be able to take the overall complexity into account. In nutritional dentistry, different study types are used, whereas randomized trials of dietary interventions have several limitations and are often unfeasible for ethical or practical reasons, at least as long-term studies. Similar to nutritional epidemiology, there is a broad field of outcomes and exposures.

Against this background, we are honored to add important pieces of evidence for nutritional dentistry by presenting this Special Issue on "Nutrition and Human Oral Health". It includes twelve studies, two systematic reviews and two narrative reviews. Please let us introduce the articles with a short summary:

Renggli et al. [18] further analyzed data of the Cambodian Health and Nutrition Monitoring Study (CAHENMS) on sociodemographic characteristics, feeding practices and clinical measures for the anthropometric measures and dental status of related Cambodian toddlers. Based on the results, they concluded that severe caries experience was associated with poorer childhood growth and, as such, could be an underinvestigated contributor to stunting.

Components of foods often have special properties, like anti-inflammatory or anti-bacterial effects. Chrubasik-Hausmann et al. [19] investigated the antimicrobial effects of antimicrobial photodynamic therapy (aPDT) with pure juices against typical cariogenic oral Streptococcus pathogens in their planktonic form and its eradication potential on total human salivary bacteria. This pilot study has shown that pure pomegranate juice is superior to the berry juices as a multicomponent PS for killing pathogenic oral bacteria with aPDT.

In nutritional dentistry research, a basic challenge is to understand the influence of nutrition on the oral microbiota and on the interaction between the oral bacteria, which is also statistically challenging. Thus, Vach et al. [20] investigated log-transformed ratios of two bacteria concentrations as the basic analytic tool. The framework was illustrated by application in an experimental study exposing eleven participants to different nutrition schemes in five consecutive phases. The methods presented made it possible to become independent of the behaviour of other bacteria, which is an advantage compared to common analysis methods of compositions.

Dental patients are often interested in the topic of oil pulling as an additional tool in oral hygiene. In this Special Issue, Kensche et al. [21] investigated the effects of linseed oil on the composition and ultrastructure of the in situ pellicle. They found that linolenic acid was an excellent marker for the investigation of fatty acid accumulation in the pellicle. New preventive strategies could benefit from the accumulation of lipid components in the pellicle.

Dodington et al. [22] determined whether a relationship between periodontal healing and protein intake existed in patients undergoing non-surgical treatment for periodontitis. Dietary protein intake was assessed using the 2005 Block food frequency questionnaire in patients with chronic generalized periodontitis undergoing scaling and root planing. The researchers concluded consuming ≥ 1 g protein/kg body weight/day was associated with reductions in periodontal disease burdens, following scaling and root planing in patients who were nonsmokers.

In order to identify natural diet-based mouthwashes, Kurz et al. [23] examined the antimicrobial effect of Inula viscosa extract on the initial microbial adhesion in the oral cavity in situ. For the first time, significant antimicrobial effects on the initial microbial adhesion in in situ oral biofilms were reported for an I. viscosa extract.

Since healthy diets and their associations might not only rely on one dietary factor, it is important to investigate their association with regard to complete dietary patterns. Within this context, Altun et al. [24] investigated the relationship between specific known dietary patterns and the prevalence of periodontal disease in a northern population-based cohort study. They evaluated data from 6209 participants of the Hamburg City Health Study (HCHS). The current cross-sectional study identified a significant association between higher adherence to the DASH and Mediterranean diets and lower odds of being affected by periodontal diseases (irrespective of disease severity).

Ketogenic diets are dietary patterns, which almost completely exclude carbohydrates. They're used for a variety of diseases and corresponding dietary therapies like epilepsy, forms of cancer, obesity, or diabetes. Woelber et al. [25] investigated the safety and the effect of a ketogenic diet on oral parameters. They found that the ketogenic diet did not lead to clinical changes in periodontal parameters in healthy participants under continued oral hygiene, but it did lead to a significant weight loss.

Since the relationship between low-density lipoprotein cholesterol (LDL-C) or levels of 25-hydroxyvitamin D (25OHD) with periodontal diseases is frequently discussed in the literature, Thim et al. [26] investigated the association between these serum parameters and radiographic levels of bone loss in 163 dental patients. They found that radiographic bone loss (RBL) was associated with known patient-specific markers, particularly with age and

Nutrients **2022**, *14*, 2076

high LDL-C levels. Patients with high 25OHD levels ($\geq$40 ng/mL) exhibited significantly less RBL.

A further important topic in this area is the assessment of dietary behavior in relation to oral health. Schlenz et al. [27] investigated whether traditional dietary questionnaires are suitable for assessing the relationship between tooth wear and diet. They found that none of the assessed dietary parameters showed a significant relationship with tooth wear and concluded that the suitability of dietary questionnaires to assess tooth-relevant dietary behavior seems to be limited. Bartha et al. [28] analyzed data of a randomized clinical trial to assess the usefulness of the Mediterranean Diet Adherence Screener (MEDAS) with regard to periodontal parameters. They found that MEDAS was a sufficient diet correlating with oral inflammatory parameters. Due to this, the MEDAS might also be useful in dental practice.

Nicklisch et al. [29] performed a bioarchaeological study on caries and stable isotope data obtained from prehistoric individuals (n = 101) 17 from three Early Neolithic sites (c. 5500-4800 BCE) in central Germany. The combined evidence from caries and isotope analysis suggested a prevalence of starchy foods, such as cereals, in the diet of these early farmers.

Even though these studies represent a rather small sample, one can already gain an impression of the efficacy and power of nutritional dentistry. Furthermore, this field is still quite uninvestigated, with a lot of unknown helpful knowledge which could empower everyone's lives in regard to oral and overall health. This also applies to the pathogenicity of oral biofilms (dental plaque) and the corresponding host resistance, whereby initial nutritional studies no longer see any or only a very weak correlation between plaque and oral diseases, like caries and periodontal inflammation, in natural or optimized dietary environments [9–11]. Future studies will also have to consider the application and development of new statistical methods in order to deliver a sufficient picture of the connections [20,30].

Based on the impressive studies of this Special Issue, we hope to have made a small contribution to the emerging field of nutritional dentistry.

Author Contributions: Conceptualization, J.P.W. and K.V.; writing—review and editing, J.P.W. and K.V. All authors have read and agreed to the published version of the manuscript.

Funding: This research received no external funding.

Acknowledgments: The editors would like to thank all participating authors.

Conflicts of Interest: The authors declare no conflict of interest.

References

1. Oxilia, G.; Peresani, M.; Romandini, M.; Matteucci, C.; Spiteri, C.D.; Henry, A.G.; Schulz, D.; Archer, W.; Crezzini, J.; Boschin, F. Earliest Evidence of Dental Caries Manipulation in the Late Upper Palaeolithic. *Sci. Rep.* **2015**, *5*, 12150. [CrossRef]
2. Bailey, S.E.; Hublin, J.-J. *Dental Perspectives on Human Evolution: State of the Art Research in Dental Paleoanthropology*; Springer: Berlin/Heidelberg, Germany, 2007.
3. Wang, Q.; Turnquist, J.E.; Kessler, M.J. Free-Ranging Cayo Santiago Rhesus Monkeys (Macaca Mulatta): III. Dental Eruption Patterns and Dental Pathology. *Am. J. Primatol.* **2016**, *78*, 127–142. [CrossRef]
4. Marcenes, W.; Kassebaum, N.J.; Bernabé, E.; Flaxman, A.; Naghavi, M.; Lopez, A.; Murray, C.J.L. Global Burden of Oral Conditions in 1990–2010: A Systematic Analysis. *J. Dent. Res.* **2013**, *92*, 592–597. [CrossRef]
5. Kassebaum, N.J.; Bernabé, E.; Dahiya, M.; Bhandari, B.; Murray, C.J.L.; Marcenes, W. Global Burden of Severe Periodontitis in 1990–2010: A Systematic Review and Meta-Regression. *J. Dent. Res.* **2014**, *93*, 1045–1053. [CrossRef]
6. Konner, M.; Eaton, S.B. Paleolithic Nutrition: Twenty-Five Years Later. *Nutr. Clin. Pr.* **2010**, *25*, 594–602. [CrossRef]
7. Woelber, J.P.; Tennert, C. Chapter 13: Diet and Periodontal Diseases. *Monogr. Oral Sci.* **2020**, *28*, 125–133. [CrossRef]
8. Murray, C.J.; Abraham, J.; Ali, M.K.; Alvarado, M.; Atkinson, C.; Baddour, L.M.; Bartels, D.H.; Benjamin, E.J.; Bhalla, K.; Birbeck, G. The State of US Health, 1990–2010: Burden of Diseases, Injuries, and Risk Factors. *JAMA* **2013**, *310*, 591–606. [CrossRef] [PubMed]
9. Baumgartner, S.; Imfeld, T.; Schicht, O.; Rath, C.; Persson, R.E.; Persson, G.R. The Impact of the Stone Age Diet on Gingival Conditions in the Absence of Oral Hygiene. *J. Periodontol.* **2009**, *80*, 759–768. [CrossRef] [PubMed]

10. Woelber, J.P.; Bremer, K.; Vach, K.; König, D.; Hellwig, E.; Ratka-Krüger, P.; Al-Ahmad, A.; Tennert, C. An Oral Health Optimized Diet Can Reduce Gingival and Periodontal Inflammation in Humans—A Randomized Controlled Pilot Study. *BMC Oral Health* **2016**, *17*, 28. [CrossRef] [PubMed]

11. Woelber, J.P.; Gärtner, M.; Breuninger, L.; Anderson, A.; König, D.; Hellwig, E.; Al-Ahmad, A.; Vach, K.; Dötsch, A.; Ratka-Krüger, P.; et al. The Influence of an Anti-Inflammatory Diet on Gingivitis. A Randomized Controlled Trial. *J. Clin. Periodontol.* **2019**, *46*, 481–490. [CrossRef] [PubMed]

12. Bartha, V.; Exner, L.; Schweikert, D.; Peter Woelber, J.; Vach, K.; Meyer, A.-L.; Basrai, M.; Bischoff, S.C.; Meller, C.; Wolff, D. Effect of the Mediterranean Diet on Gingivitis: A Randomized Controlled Trial. *J. Clin. Periodontol.* **2021**, *49*, 111–122. [CrossRef] [PubMed]

13. Axelsson, P.; Nyström, B.; Lindhe, J. The Long-Term Effect of a Plaque Control Program on Tooth Mortality, Caries and Periodontal Disease in Adults. Results after 30 Years of Maintenance. *J. Clin. Periodontol.* **2004**, *31*, 749–757. [CrossRef] [PubMed]

14. Bernabé, E.; Vehkalahti, M.M.; Sheiham, A.; Lundqvist, A.; Suominen, A.L. The Shape of the Dose-Response Relationship between Sugars and Caries in Adults. *J. Dent. Res.* **2016**, *95*, 167–172. [CrossRef] [PubMed]

15. Sheiham, A.; Watt, R.G. The Common Risk Factor Approach: A Rational Basis for Promoting Oral Health. *Community Dent. Oral Epidemiol.* **2000**, *28*, 399–406. [CrossRef] [PubMed]

16. Maringer, M.; van't Veer, P.; Klepacz, N.; Verain, M.C.D.; Normann, A.; Ekman, S.; Timotijevic, L.; Raats, M.M.; Geelen, A. User-Documented Food Consumption Data from Publicly Available Apps: An Analysis of Opportunities and Challenges for Nutrition Research. *Nutr. J.* **2018**, *17*, 59. [CrossRef]

17. Lövestam, E.; Vivanti, A.; Steiber, A.; Boström, A.-M.; Devine, A.; Haughey, O.; Kiss, C.M.; Lang, N.R.; Lieffers, J.; Lloyd, L.; et al. The International Nutrition Care Process and Terminology Implementation Survey: Towards a Global Evaluation Tool to Assess Individual Practitioner Implementation in Multiple Countries and Languages. *J. Acad. Nutr. Diet.* **2019**, *119*, 242–260. [CrossRef]

18. Renggli, E.P.; Turton, B.; Sokal-Gutierrez, K.; Hondru, G.; Chher, T.; Hak, S.; Poirot, E.; Laillou, A. Stunting Malnutrition Associated with Severe Tooth Decay in Cambodian Toddlers. *Nutrients* **2021**, *13*, 290. [CrossRef]

19. Chrubasik-Hausmann, S.; Hellwig, E.; Müller, M.; Al-Ahmad, A. Antimicrobial Photodynamic Treatment with Mother Juices and Their Single Compounds as Photosensitizers. *Nutrients* **2021**, *13*, 710. [CrossRef]

20. Vach, K.; Al-Ahmad, A.; Anderson, A.; Woelber, J.P.; Karygianni, L.; Wittmer, A.; Hellwig, E. A Log Ratio-Based Analysis of Individual Changes in the Composition of the Oral Microbiota in Different Dietary Phases. *Nutrients* **2021**, *13*, 793. [CrossRef]

21. Kensche, A.; Reich, M.; Hannig, C.; Kümmerer, K.; Hannig, M. Modification of the Lipid Profile of the Initial Oral Biofilm In Situ Using Linseed Oil as Mouthwash. *Nutrients* **2021**, *13*, 989. [CrossRef]

22. Dodington, D.W.; Young, H.E.; Beaudette, J.R.; Fritz, P.C.; Ward, W.E. Improved Healing after Non-Surgical Periodontal Therapy Is Associated with Higher Protein Intake in Patients Who Are Non-Smokers. *Nutrients* **2021**, *13*, 3722. [CrossRef] [PubMed]

23. Kurz, H.; Karygianni, L.; Argyropoulou, A.; Hellwig, E.; Skaltsounis, A.L.; Wittmer, A.; Vach, K.; Al-Ahmad, A. Antimicrobial Effects of Inula Viscosa Extract on the In Situ Initial Oral Biofilm. *Nutrients* **2021**, *13*, 4029. [CrossRef] [PubMed]

24. Altun, E.; Walther, C.; Borof, K.; Petersen, E.; Lieske, B.; Kasapoudis, D.; Jalilvand, N.; Beikler, T.; Jagemann, B.; Zyriax, B.-C.; et al. Association between Dietary Pattern and Periodontitis—A Cross-Sectional Study. *Nutrients* **2021**, *13*, 4167. [CrossRef] [PubMed]

25. Woelber, J.P.; Tennert, C.; Ernst, S.F.; Vach, K.; Ratka-Krüger, P.; Bertz, H.; Urbain, P. Effects of a Non-Energy-Restricted Ketogenic Diet on Clinical Oral Parameters. An Exploratory Pilot Trial. *Nutrients* **2021**, *13*, 4229. [CrossRef] [PubMed]

26. Thim, T.; Scholz, K.J.; Hiller, K.-A.; Buchalla, W.; Kirschneck, C.; Fleiner, J.; Woelber, J.P.; Cieplik, F. Radiographic Bone Loss and Its Relation to Patient-Specific Risk Factors, LDL Cholesterol, and Vitamin D: A Cross-Sectional Study. *Nutrients* **2022**, *14*, 864. [CrossRef]

27. Schlenz, M.A.; Schlenz, M.B.; Wöstmann, B.; Jungert, A.; Glatt, A.S.; Ganss, C. The Suitability of Questionnaires for Exploring Relations of Dietary Behavior and Tooth Wear. *Nutrients* **2022**, *14*, 1165. [CrossRef]

28. Bartha, V.; Exner, L.; Meyer, A.-L.; Basrai, M.; Schweikert, D.; Adolph, M.; Bruckner, T.; Meller, C.; Woelber, J.P.; Wolff, D. How to Measure Adherence to a Mediterranean Diet in Dental Studies: Is a Short Adherence Screener Enough? A Comparative Analysis. *Nutrients* **2022**, *14*, 1300. [CrossRef]

29. Nicklisch, N.; Oelze, V.M.; Schierz, O.; Meller, H.; Alt, K.W. A Healthier Smile in the Past? Dental Caries and Diet in Early Neolithic Farming Communities from Central Germany. *Nutrients* **2022**, *14*, 1831. [CrossRef]

30. Vach, K.; Al-Ahmad, A.; Anderson, A.; Woelber, J.P.; Karygianni, L.; Wittmer, A.; Hellwig, E. Analysing the Relationship between Nutrition and the Microbial Composition of the Oral Biofilm-Insights from the Analysis of Individual Variability. *Antibiotics* **2020**, *9*, 479. [CrossRef]

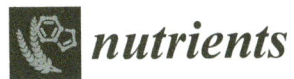 *nutrients*

Article

Stunting Malnutrition Associated with Severe Tooth Decay in Cambodian Toddlers

Eva Peris Renggli [1,*], Bathsheba Turton [2], Karen Sokal-Gutierrez [3], Gabriela Hondru [4], Tepirou Chher [5], Sithan Hak [6], Etienne Poirot [7] and Arnaud Laillou [8]

1   Centre for International Health Protection, Robert Koch Institute, 13353 Berlin, Germany
2   Department of Dentistry, University Puthisistra, 12211 Phnom Penh, Cambodia; bethy.turton@gmail.com
3   School of Public Health, University of California, Berkeley, CA 94720, USA; ksokalg@berkeley.edu
4   UNICEF Cambodia, 12100 Phnom Penh, Cambodia; gabriela.hondru@gmail.com
5   Oral Health Bureau, Department of Preventive Medicine, Ministry of Health, 12211 Phnom Penh, Cambodia; tepirou@yahoo.com
6   Department of Preventive Medicine, Ministry of Health, 12211 Phnom Penh, Cambodia; sithan_hak@yahoo.com
7   UNICEF Chad, 1146 N'Djamena, Chad; epoirot@unicef.org
8   UNICEF Ethiopia, 1169, Addis Ababa, Ethiopia; alaillou@unicef.org
*   Correspondence: evaperisrenggli@gmail.com

Abstract: Background: The persistently high prevalence of undernutrition in Cambodia, in particular stunting or chronic malnutrition, calls for innovative investigation into the risk factors that affect children's growth during critical phases of development. Methods: Secondary data analysis was performed on a subgroup of children who were present at two time points within the Cambodian Health and Nutrition Monitoring Study (CAHENMS) and who were less than 24 months of age at the nominated baseline. Data consisted of parent interviews on sociodemographic characteristics and feeding practices, and clinical measures for anthropometric measures and dental status. Logistic regression modelling was used to examine the associations between severe dental caries (tooth decay)—as indicated by the Significant Caries Index—and the presence of new cases of stunting malnutrition at follow-up. Results: There were 1595 children who met the inclusion criteria and 1307 (81.9%) were followed after one year. At baseline, 14.4% of the children had severe dental caries, 25.6% presented with stunted growth. 17.6% of the children transitioned from healthy status to a low height-for-age over the observation period. Children with severe dental caries had nearly double the risk (OR = 1.8; CI 1.0–3.0) of making that transition. Conclusion: Severe caries experience was associated with poorer childhood growth and, as such, could be an underinvestigated contributor to stunting.

Keywords: severe caries; tooth decay; dental; early childhood; early childhood caries; malnutrition; undernutrition; stunting; growth and development

Citation: Renggli, E.P.; Turton, B.; Sokal-Gutierrez, K.; Hondru, G.; Chher, T.; Hak, S.; Poirot, E.; Laillou, A. Stunting Malnutrition Associated with Severe Tooth Decay in Cambodian Toddlers. *Nutrients* **2021**, *13*, 290. https://doi.org/10.3390/nu13020290

Academic Editor: Kirstin Vach
Received: 9 December 2020
Accepted: 15 January 2021
Published: 20 January 2021

Publisher's Note: MDPI stays neutral with regard to jurisdictional claims in published maps and institutional affiliations.

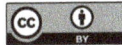
1. Introduction

Over recent decades, early childhood undernutrition has been declining globally. However, high rates of stunting have persisted, while the rates of obesity have increased [1–3]. The modern challenge of the "double burden" of undernutrition and obesity calls for an examination of the neglected risk factors that may contribute to the high prevalence of child malnutrition. Globalization and urbanization have led to a global nutrition transition, dramatically increasing young children's consumption of sugary drinks and snacks, contributing to both child obesity and tooth decay (dental caries) [4].

Dental caries is a process which leads to the destruction of tooth tissue. Dental cavities result when net demineralization occurs at the surface of the tooth in response to pH changes in the microbial biofilm (plaque). When the biofilm is exposed to free sugars, then acid is produced, and in the absence of protective factors such as tooth brushing with fluoride toothpaste, then the tooth surface will break down and carious lesions will progress [5,6]. When a carious lesion is present among children less than 6 years of age, it is commonly referred to in the literature as early childhood caries (ECC) [7]. Globally, dental caries is the most prevalent chronic disease, affecting 60–90% of schoolchildren [8]. Among the youngest age groups, most carious lesions (dental cavities) remain untreated due to limited access to dental care, particularly among low- and middle-income populations and socioeconomically disadvantaged groups [9–11]. Severe and uncontrolled dental caries can lead to oral infection and inflammation (abscesses), which can cause mouth pain, decreased appetite, inability to chew food, inadequate sleep, and chronic inflammation if persistent over time [12–14]. These factors, added to well-known aspects such as child nutrition, breastfeeding, infectious diseases, mother's health, and psychosocial stimulation, could all contribute to undernutrition [15].

In Cambodia, the current rates of both early childhood undernutrition and dental caries are among the highest in the world. Contributors include Cambodia´s long period of war and humanitarian crises followed by rapid economic growth since the late 1990s, involving the introduction of ultraprocessed foods and beverages, and a dramatic increase in childhood sugar consumption [16,17]. Among Cambodian children under age 5, 32% experience stunting and 10% wasting malnutrition [18], and the prevalence of dental caries exceeds 90% [19]. Among 3–5-year-olds, 16.1% had one or more severe, deep caries infecting the surrounding soft tissues and commonly causing mouth pain, and the prevalence of this type of dental infection increases to 86% among 6-year-old children [20–22]. In Cambodia, the high prevalence of severe caries experience by age 2, within the first 1000 days of life, elevates the concern about the potential for adverse effects on children's short-term and long-term growth and development. In fact, stunting, an indicator for chronic malnutrition, has been described to peak between 1 and 2 years of age [23]. Nevertheless, recent studies have proposed that the prevalence of stunting can increase beyond 24 months of age in suboptimal environments [24–27].

Given the high rates of chronic malnutrition and dental caries among Cambodian children, there is a pressing need to explore the potential relationship between these two conditions. This could help to better understand the role of severe dental caries as an under-recognized contributor to stunting. This longitudinal study examines the relationship between severe dental caries and anthropometric changes over a one-year period, in children under 2 years of age at baseline.

2. Materials and Methods

This is a secondary analysis of a longitudinal cohort study, the Cambodian Health and Nutrition Monitoring Study (CAHENMS), and an added oral health component (Figure A1). Data were collected from three Cambodian provinces: two predominantly rural northeastern provinces, Ratanakiri and Kratie; and an urban area, the capital Phnom Penh. Data were collected in 2017 (baseline) and 2018 (follow-up) using 8 trained teams specialized in conducting questionnaires, anthropometric measurements, and intraoral examinations.

The original protocol for the CAHENMS was reviewed by the National Ethics Committee for Health Research, Ministry of Health, Cambodia, prior to collecting data (117/NECHR). Written consent was obtained from the parents of the participants before the baseline data collection, and verbal consent was obtained at each subsequent contact. A data-sharing agreement was made prior to the transfer of de-identified data. This is a secondary analysis of a de-identified dataset and was considered research on nonhuman subjects. Information about the original CAHENMS study is provided in the supplement.

The study population consists of a final sub-sample of 1307 children <24 months of age at baseline and approximately one year older at follow-up, as presented in Figure 1. Children lost to attrition ($N = 12.5\%$), older than 23.9 months at baseline ($N = 30.5\%$) and with missing anthropometric measurements were not considered in the present analysis ($N = 0.5\%$).

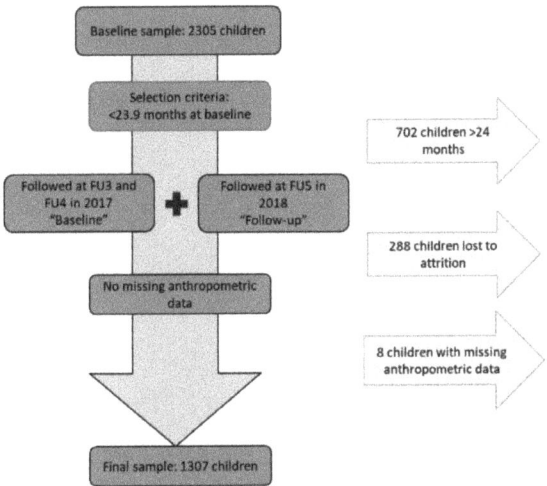

Figure 1. Flow chart depicting selection criteria of individuals included in the final sample size.

G*power (version 3.9.1.2) was used to calculate implied power using Chi-squared tests given a sample size of 1307 participants and the intention to observe a clinically significant 5% difference in new cases of stunting (Height-for-age Z-score, HAZ < −2) from 30% down to 25%. The present sample size implies a 98.6% chance of detecting a 5% difference in the incidence of stunting.

2.1. Questionnaires

The 2 sets of questionnaires for sociodemographic characteristics and child feeding practices were administered at baseline by trained Cambodian interviewers in Khmer, or translated into the local indigenous language for some minority populations in northeastern provinces. Dietary intake was assessed using a 24-h recall period, based on WHO guidelines and described in published articles on child feeding practices status [28–30]. Parents/caregivers were asked to recall and report on breastfeeding frequency, consumed food groups, frequency of meals, and amount of food given during meals using as unit of measure context relevant utensils: spoons and Chan Chang Koeh, a traditional bowl in Southeast Asia.

To assess socioeconomic status (SES), questions were asked about assets, employment, and household characteristics to further calculate the wealth index using Principal Component Analysis (PCA) based on the validated tool performed by Filmer and Pritchett without expenditure data [31].

2.2. Clinical Examinations

Separate teams performed anthropometric measurements, and intraoral examinations and data were recorded on separate devices to ensure that examiners were blinded to the participants' status. Anthropometric measures were assessed in duplicates according to the WHO guidelines, and the mean value was further used [32]. Recumbent length was recorded in children under 2 years of age or unable to stand up, and in children above the age of 2 years height was recorded. Weight was measured with a calibrated precise scale for mother and child.

Intraoral examinations were performed by one of 8 calibrated examiners with the help of a trained assistant. All examiners achieved a kappa score of >0.9, indicating near-perfect agreement. The examination was done in supine position with a handheld torch and mouth mirror. The decayed, missing, and filled teeth (dmft) index as defined by WHO was used to measure dental caries experience [33].

2.3. Data Analysis

Data were delivered through Microsoft Excel and entered into IBM SPSS 25. Statistical significance was considered for p-values below 0.05, and no imputation method was used. Data were cleaned and each variable was divided into relevant categories for age groups, socioeconomic status (SES), feeding practices, anthropometric measurements, and dental caries measurements. The Wealth index scores were broken down into quintiles to categorize participants by SES. Age data were based on months at baseline, and children were categorised into one of four age groups (<6 months, 6–12 months, 12–18 months, >18 months).

The Minimum Acceptable Diet (MAD) was calculated using the WHO Guidelines and is a composite index of breastfeeding or milk feedings, Minimum Diet Diversity and Minimum Meal Frequency; indicators being available for children aged 6 to 23.9 months at baseline. The Minimum Diet Diversity, after the 2010 guidelines, was based on whether or not the child consumed in the past 24 h a minimum 4 out of a list of 7 food groups. These food groups included: (1) Grains, roots and tubers; (2) Legumes and nuts; (3) Dairy products; (4) Flesh foods; (5) Eggs; (6) Vitamin A-rich fruits and vegetables; and (7) Other fruits and vegetables. The Minimum Meal Frequency was calculated on the minimum amount of times that the child received solid, semisolid or soft foods the previous day according to their age group and breastfeeding status [34,35].

As a Cambodian specific diet indicator, The Cambodian Complementary Feeding (CCF) variable was calculated based on the Nutrition Handbook for the family, prepared and adapted by the National Cambodian Nutrition Program [36]. It was based on the number of spoons of Chan Chang Koeh and determined according to age and breastfeeding status [29,30].

Anthropometric measurements were converted to sex-specific height/length-for-age Z-scores using the WHO Child Growth Standards 2016 [32], and identified as stunting at <−2SDs. The low proportion of obese children in the sample (<2%), identified at >+2SDs for weight-for-age, was insufficient in number to establish a comparison group. New cases of stunting were identified, i.e., children who had optimal HAZ at baseline, while at 1-year follow-up were identified with HAZ below −2 SDs. To assess caries experience, the Significant Caries Index (ScI) was calculated at baseline and follow-up by ranking individuals within age groups according to the number of teeth with carious lesions (based on the dmft index: decayed, missing or filled teeth). Subsequently, the mean of the most severe one-third of the population was calculated [37]. That value was then used to create an age-adjusted dichotomous variable to indicate the presence or absence of ScI. This index represents a more "severe" disease experience, as children with a high dmft score and presenting ScI would be more likely to develop lesions that might create mouth pain or infection, which are acknowledged consequences of carious lesions [12–14].

After cleaning and categorising the data, descriptive and multivariate analyses were performed. The Chi-squared test was used to examine differences in proportions among sociodemographic subgroups for stunting, caries, and diet indicators. Multivariate logistic regression was performed to explore the relationship between severe caries experience (by ScI) at baseline and follow-up with the onset of new cases of stunting over the observation period. Gender, province, age, SES, and the MAD and CCF variables for diet indicators were included in the multivariate modelling.

3. Results

3.1. Descriptive Statistics

3.1.1. Demographic Profile and Clinical Characteristics at Baseline

Baseline participants' characteristics are shown in Table 1. Three out of four participants came from the northeastern provinces of Kratie and Ratanakiri and one quarter from Phnom Penh. There was an even gender distribution. Two-thirds of participants were 1 to 2 years of age at baseline; and over one-third of participants belonged to the lowest two wealth index quintiles. Stunted growth was present in 25.6% of the children.

Males, children from Ratanakiri province, those from the older age groups, and those from the second quintile, "low", presented a significantly higher prevalence of stunting. Overall, 51.9% of the children presented with "any caries" at baseline and there was no statistically significant difference by gender. Those in Ratanakiri and in older age groups had a significantly higher prevalence of any caries and severe caries (by baseline ScI). When looking at SES, those in the medium quintile presented the lowest caries experience, and the lowest wealth index quintile had the higher proportion of children who had ScI at baseline compared to the other quintiles (21% vs. 12–14%, $p = 0.040$; χ^2 test).

Table 1. Sociodemographic and clinical characteristics at baseline.

	Total	Stunting Baseline		Any Caries Baseline		ScI [1] Baseline	
	N (Row %)	N (Row %)		N (Row %)		N (Row %)	
		Yes	No	Yes	No	Yes	No
Total	1307 (100)	332 (25.4)	975 (74.6)	629 (51.9)	678 (48.1)	188 (14.4)	1119 (85.6)
Gender							
Male	631 (48.3)	179 (28.4)	452 (71.6)	316 (50.1)	315 (49.9)	100 (15.8)	531 (84.2)
Female	676 (51.7)	153 (22.6)	523 (77.4)	313 (46.3)	363 (53.7)	88 (13.0)	588 (87.0)
p-value [2]			0.017		0.172		0.145
Province							
Phnom Penh	319 (24.4)	39 (12.2)	280 (87.8)	153 (48.0)	166 (52.0)	39 (12.2)	280 (87.8)
Kratie	551 (42.2)	136 (24.7)	415 (75.3)	235 (42.6)	316 (57.4)	66 (12.0)	485 (88.0)
Ratanakiri	437 (33.4)	157 (35.9)	280 (64.1)	241 (55.1)	196 (44.9)	83 (19.0)	354 (81.0)
p-value [2]			<0.001		<0.001		0.003
Age at baseline							
<6 months	143 (10.9)	17 (11.9)	126 (88.1)	15 (10.5)	128 (89.5)	15 (10.5)	128 (89.5)
6–12 months	278 (21.3)	53 (19.1)	225 (80.9)	71 (25.5)	207 (74.5)	45 (16.2)	233 (83.8)
12–18 months	438 (33.5)	116 (26.5)	322 (73.5)	246 (56.2)	192 (43.8)	65 (14.8)	373 (85.2)
18–24 months	448 (34.3)	146 (32.6)	302 (67.4)	297 (66.3)	151 (33.7)	63 (14.1)	385 (85.9)
p-value [2]			<0.001		<0.001		0.456
SES							
Lowest	220 (16.8)	71 (32.3)	149 (67.7)	118 (53.6)	102 (46.4)	46 (20.9)	174 (79.1)
Low	265 (20.3)	83 (31.3)	182 (68.7)	135 (50.9)	130 (49.1)	34 (12.8)	231 (87.2)
Medium	393 (30.1)	91 (23.2)	302 (76.8)	171 (43.5)	222 (56.5)	56 (14.2)	337 (85.8)
High	215 (16.4)	34 (15.8)	181 (84.2)	115 (53.5)	100 (46.5)	25 (11.6)	190 (88.4)
Highest	214 (16.4)	53 (24.8)	161 (75.2)	90 (42.1)	124 (57.9)	27 (12.6)	187 (87.4)
p-value [2]			<0.001		0.014		0.040
Caries							
Dmft mean (SD)		2.7 (3.5)	2.3 (3.6)	5.1 (3.6)		8.8 (4.1)	1.4 (2.0)
p-value [2]			0.053				0.001

[1] ScI: Significant Caries Index. [2] χ^2 test for differences among groups within the same columns or ANOVA. SES: socioeconomic status.

The mean (SD) dmft for children with caries at baseline was 5.1 (3.6). The mean cutoff of ScI by age groups at baseline was 4.7; with a mean dmft of 8.8 (4.1) for children with ScI and 1.4 (2.0) in children without. Children with stunting presented a dmft of 2.7 (3.5) and children without stunting 2.3 (3.6) ($p = 0.053$).

3.1.2. Clinical Characteristics at Follow-Up

The participants' characteristics at follow-up are shown in Table 2. Stunted growth was present in 39.9% of the children. In contrast to baseline, females had a significantly higher chance of presenting with stunting at follow-up (42.2% vs. 36.1%, $p = 0.026$ χ^2 test). Children from Ratanakiri province, approximately >12 months of age, and from the "low" SES quintile, continued to present the highest prevalence of stunting.

Table 2. Sociodemographic and clinical characteristics at follow-up.

	Stunting Follow-Up		Any Caries Follow-Up		Sci [1] Follow-Up	
	N (Row %)		N (Row %)		N (Row %)	
	Yes	No	Yes	No	Yes	No
Total	513 (39.3)	794 (60.7)	831 (63.6)	476 (36.4)	193 (14.8)	1114 (85.2)
Gender						
Male (631)	228 (36.1)	403 (63.9)	401 (63.5)	230 (36.5)	111 (17.6)	520 (82.4)
Female (676)	285 (42.2)	391 (57.8)	430 (63.6)	246 (36.4)	82 (12.1)	594 (87.9)
p-value [3]		0.026		0.982		0.005
Province						
Phnom Penh (319)	74 (23.2)	245 (76.8)	255 (79.9)	64 (20.1)	60 (18.8)	259 (81.2)
Kratie (551)	206 (37.4)	345 (62.6)	318 (57.7)	233 (42.3)	79 (14.3)	472 (85.7)
Ratanakiri (437)	233 (53.3)	204 (46.7)	258 (59.9)	179 (41.0)	54 (12.4)	383 (87.6)
p-value [3]		<0.001		<0.001		0.044
Approx. age follow-up [2]						
<12 months (143)	74 (51.7)	69 (48.3)	52 (36.4)	91 (63.6)	32 (22.4)	111 (77.6)
12–18 months (278)	109 (39.2)	169 (60.8)	148 (53.2)	130 (46.8)	15 (5.4)	263 (94.6)
18–24 months (438)	160 (36.5)	278 (63.5)	283 (64.6)	155 (35.4)	68 (15.5)	370 (84.5)
24–36 months (448)	170 (37.9)	278 (62.1)	348 (77.7)	100 (22.3)	78 (17.4)	370 (82.6)
p-value [3]		0.011		<0.001		<0.001
SES						
Lowest (220)	99 (45.0)	121 (55.0)	107 (48.6)	113 (51.4)	21 (9.5)	199 (90.5)
Low (265)	147 (55.5)	118 (44.5)	168 (63.4)	97 (36.6)	37 (14.0)	228 (86.0)
Medium (393)	130 (33.1)	263 (66.9)	259 (65.9)	134 (34.1)	67 (17.0)	326 (83.0)
High (215)	58 (27.0)	157 (73.0)	136 (63.3)	79 (36.7)	34 (15.8)	181 (84.2)
Highest (214)	79 (36.9)	135 (63.1)	161 (75.2)	53 (24.8)	34 (15.9)	180 (84.1)
p-value [3]		<0.001		<0.001		0.140
Caries						
Dmft mean (SD)	3.2 (3.9)	3.3 (4.1)	5.1 (3.9)		10.6 (4.0)	2.0 (2.2)
p-value [3]		0.800				<0.001

[1] ScI: Significant Caries Index. [2] Approximate age mean (SD) at follow-up: 30.79 (6.52). [3] χ^2 test for differences among groups within the same columns or ANOVA.

Overall, 63.6% of the children at follow-up presented dental caries. A higher proportion of males than females presented with ScI at follow-up (17.6 vs. 12.1%, $p = 0.005$; χ^2 test). Children living in Phnom Penh experienced a greater increase in caries and demonstrated higher overall caries experience at follow-up compared to other provinces. Differences in caries experience were seen among the five SES groups, whereby the highest SES group had a greater proportion of children with any caries (75% vs. 49–66%) and higher mean dmft ($p < 0.001$; χ^2 test, ANOVA). A higher prevalence of ScI among the lowest SES was no longer significant at follow-up.

The mean (SD) dmft for children with caries at follow-up was 5.1 (3.9). The mean cutoff of ScI by age groups at follow-up was 7.2, with a mean dmft of 10.6 (4.0) for children with ScI and 2.0 (2.2) in children without. The mean dmft in stunted children was 3.2 (3.9) and in non-stunted children 3.3 (4.1) ($p = 0.800$).

3.1.3. New Cases of Stunting, Significant Caries, and Dietary Adequacy by Sociodemographic Characteristics

Overall, 17.6% of children transitioned from normal values at baseline to suboptimal level of length/height-for-age at follow-up. Children who presented stunted malnutrition at baseline were excluded from the analysis (n = 332). Females were significantly more likely to transition to a suboptimal level of height-for-age at follow-up; one out of four females and one out of five males presented new cases of stunting (p = 0.001; χ^2 test). Children in Ratanakiri had a higher proportion of new cases of stunting when compared to other provinces (p-value $\leq$ 0.001; χ^2 test). Children from the youngest age group, at approximately 18 months at follow-up, presented the highest frequency of new cases of stunting (p-value < 0.001, χ^2 test). Regarding SES, the children from the second wealth index quintile (low) presented the highest prevalence of new cases of stunted malnutrition (p-value $\leq$ 0.001; χ^2 test).

Measures of dietary adequacy by sociodemographic characteristics are presented in Table 3. Males were more likely than females to have adequate dietary intake, including a significantly higher likelihood of achieving CCF (62.6% vs. 51.3%, p < 0.001; χ^2 test). Phnom Penh had the highest proportion, and Ratanakiri the lowest proportion of children who met the criteria for MAD and CCF. Children 0–6 months of age presented the highest proportion of acceptable CCF intake (p < 0.001; χ^2 test). Children 12 months and over were more likely than children age 6–12 months to have received MAD (p < 0.001; χ^2 test). Children in the first 4 SES quintiles demonstrated a progressively higher chance of meeting dietary criteria by MAD and CCF; however, those in the highest quintile appeared to have a lower dietary quality than those in the high quintile (p < 0.001; χ^2 test).

Table 3. Sociodemographic characteristics of new cases of stunting, severe caries and dietary adequacy.

	New Cases Stunting		ScI Baseline		ScI Follow-Up		CCF [1]		MAD [2]	
	Valid: 975 Missing: 332 N (Row %)		Valid: 1307 Missing: 0 N (Row %)		Valid: 1307 Missing: 0 N (Row %)		Valid: 1127 Missing: 180 N (Row %)		Valid: 1017 Missing: 290 N (Row %)	
	Yes	No	Yes	No	Yes	No	Yes	No	Yes	No
Total	230 (17.6)	745 (57.0)	188 (14.4)	1119 (85.6)	193 (14.8)	1114 (85.2)	201 (15.4)	816 (62.4)	640 (49.0)	487 (37.3)
Gender										
Male (631)	85 (18.8)	367 (81.2)	100(15.8)	531 (84.2)	111 (17.6)	520 (82.4)	113 (22.1)	398 (77.9)	343 (62.6)	205 (37.4)
Female (676)	145 (27.7)	378 (72.3)	88 (13.0)	588 (87.0)	82 (12.1)	594 (87.9)	88 (17.4)	418 (82.6)	297 (51.3)	282 (48.7)
p-value [3]		0.001		0.145		0.005		0.059		<0.001
Province										
Phnom Penh (319)	42 (15.0)	238 (85.0)	39 (12.2)	280 (87.8)	60 (18.8)	259 (81.2)	94 (38.5)	150 (61.5)	201 (71.3)	81 (28.7)
Kratie (551)	97 (23.4)	317 (76.6)	66 (12.0)	485 (88.0)	79 (14.3)	472 (85.7)	77 (17.9)	357 (82.1)	257 (53.3)	225 (46.7)
Ratanakiri (437)	91 (32.5)	189 (67.5)	83 (19.0)	354 (81.0)	54 (12.4)	383 (87.6)	30 (8.7)	313 (91.3)	182 (50.1)	181 (49.9)
p-value [3]		<0.001		0.003		0.044		<0.001		<0.001
Approx. age follow-up										
<12 months (143)	58 (46.0)	68 (54.0)	15 (10.5)	128 (89.5)	32 (22.4)	111 (77.6)	/	/	106 (89.1)	13 (10.9)
12–18 months (278)	63 (28.0)	162 (72.0)	45 (16.2)	233 (83.8)	15 (5.4)	263 (94.6)	28 (10.9)	228 (89.1)	122 (67.8)	58 (32.2)

Table 3. Cont.

	New Cases Stunting		ScI Baseline		ScI Follow-Up		CCF [1]		MAD [2]	
	Valid: 975 Missing: 332 N (Row %)		**Valid: 1307 Missing: 0 N (Row %)**		**Valid: 1307 Missing: 0 N (Row %)**		**Valid: 1127 Missing: 180 N (Row %)**		**Valid: 1017 Missing: 290 N (Row %)**	
	Yes	**No**	**Yes**	**No**	**Yes**	**No**	**Yes**	**No**	**Yes**	**No**
18–24 months (438)	55 (17.1)	267 (82.9)	65 (14.8)	373 (85.2)	68 (15.5)	370 (84.5)	92 (23.3)	303 (76.7)	167 (40.0)	251 (60.0)
24–36 months (448)	54 (17.9)	248 (82.1)	63 (14.1)	385 (85.9)	78 (17.4)	370 (82.6)	81 (22.1)	225 (77.9)	245 (59.8)	165 (40.2)
p-value [3]		<0.001		0.456		<0.001		<0.001		<0.001
SES										
Lowest (220)	35 (23.5)	114 (76.5)	46 (20.9)	174 (79.1)	21 (9.5)	199 (90.5)	23 (12.3)	164 (87.7)	79 (43.6)	102 (56.4)
Low (265)	77 (42.3)	105 (57.5)	34 (12.8)	231 (7.2)	37 (14.0)	228 (86.0)	22 (11.2)	175 (88.8)	139 (61.2)	88 (38.8)
Medium (393)	57 (18.9)	245 (81.1)	56 (14.2)	337 (85.8)	67 (17.0)	326 (83.0)	57 (20.0)	228 (80.0)	196 (59.9)	131 (40.1)
High (215)	28 (15.5)	153 (84.5)	25 (11.6)	190 (88.4)	34 (15.8)	181 (84.2)	60 (34.9)	112 (65.1)	139 (69.5)	61 (30.5)
Highest (214)	33 (20.5)	128 (79.5)	27 (12.6)	187 (87.4)	34 (15.9)	180 (84.1)	39 (22.2)	137 (77.8)	87 (45.3)	105 (54.7)
p-value [3]		<0.001		0.040		0.140		<0.001		<0.001

[1] CCF: Cambodian complementary feeding. [2] MAD: Minimum acceptable diet. [3] χ^2 test for differences among groups within the same columns or ANOVA.

3.2. Multivariate Analysis: Logistic Regression

Results of multivariate logistic regression on odds ratios for new cases of stunting based on severe dental caries by ScI at baseline and follow-up are presented in Table 4 (Models 1 and 2).

Table 4. Logistic regression models for the risk of stunting by caries experience, sociodemographic and diet indicators.

	New Cases Stunting			
	Based on ScI at Baseline MODEL 1		**Based on ScI at Follow-Up MODEL 2**	
	OR (95% CI)	**p-Value**	**OR (95% CI)**	**p-Value**
Caries experience				
No ScI [1]				
Had ScI	0.8 (0.5–1.5)	0.524	1.8 (1.0–3.0)	0.039
Gender				
Male [1]				
Female	1.7 (1.1–2.5)	0.012	1.7 (1.2–2.6)	0.009
Province				
Phnom Penh [1]				
Kratie	2.3 (1.3–4.0)	0.003	2.5 (1.4–4.3)	0.002
Ratanakiri	3.1 (1.7–5.6)	<0.001	3.3 (1.8–6.0)	<0.001
Age at baseline				
6–12 months [1]				
12–18 months	0.5 (0.3–0.8)	0.009	0.4 (0.3–0.8)	0.004
18–24 months	0.6 (0.4–1.0)	0.068	0.5 (0.3–0.9)	0.027
SES				

Table 4. *Cont.*

	Based on ScI at Baseline MODEL 1		Based on ScI at Follow-Up MODEL 2	
	OR (95% CI)	*p*-Value	OR (95% CI)	*p*-Value
Lowest [1]				
Low	2.0 (1.0–3.7)	0.040	2.0 (1.0–3.8)	0.038
Medium	0.7 (0.3–1.3)	0.211	0.7 (0.3–1.2)	0.195
High	1.0 (0.5–2.0)	0.964	1.0 (0.5–2.0)	0.978
Highest	1.3 (0.6–2.5)	0.512	1.3 (0.7–2.6)	0.422
Diet indicators				
No CCF [1]				
CCF	1.2 (0.8–1.9)	0.333	1.2 (0.8–1.9)	0.367
No MAD [1]				
MAD	1.9 (1.2–3.2)	0.011	1.9 (1.1–3.1)	0.014

(New Cases Stunting)

[1] Reference value.

Having severe caries by ScI at baseline was not associated with developing new-onset stunting, although children with ScI at follow-up had approximately twice the risk with an odds ratio of 1.8 (95% CI = 1.0–3.0, p = 0.039; χ^2 test) after controlling for gender, province, age, SES, and diet indicators. The highest risk for developing new cases of stunting was seen in females (OR 1.7; CI 1.2, 2.6) from rural areas (OR 2.5–3.3; CI 1.4, 6.0), at the age of approximately 1–2 years at follow-up (<12 months at baseline) (OR 0.4–0.5; CI 0.3, 0.9), and coming from the second lowest SES quintile (OR 2.0; CI 1.0, 3.8), even in the presence of MAD (OR 1.9; CI 1.1, 3.1).

Collinearity between MAD and CCF is taken into consideration and ruled out because both variables capture different aspects of the feeding practices.

4. Discussion

This secondary analysis of longitudinal data on Cambodian children under age 2 at baseline and 1 year later at follow-up showed that children with severe dental caries (as indicated by the ScI) had almost twice the odds of developing chronic malnutrition. This suggests that dental caries experience could be an important contributor to child growth restriction at a critical stage of child development. The results of the present analysis align with some cross-sectional and longitudinal studies that reported a positive association between severe dental caries and different forms of undernutrition [38–41]. The present study is unique in that it uses a longitudinal study design, controlled for the children's dietary intake, and included children under 2 years of age at baseline from a population with severe caries experience.

A number of systematic reviews have examined the relationship between dental caries and malnutrition; some studies show association of caries with undernutrition, others with obesity, and others show no association [42–47]. The differences in child age, country's socioeconomic standing, and socioeconomic and behavioural disparities within the countries may explain the disparate findings in the literature. Moreover, the caries–malnutrition relationship appears to play out differently in urban and rural areas, different SES groups, and different countries and regions based on their stage in the nutrition transition [48–52]. The data from this study suggested that children in predominantly rural northeastern provinces had worse baseline dietary, anthropometric, and caries experience. However, children in the predominantly urban Phnom Penh presented with worse caries experience over the observation period, which may be explained by higher sugar consumption.

Suboptimal dietary, anthropometric, and caries indicators were seen in the low/lowest SES population; however, the highest SES population did not present the best outcomes—the wealthiest SES group demonstrated lower rates of dietary adequacy and higher rates of dental caries and undernutrition compared to the adjacent lower SES strata. Furthermore, some children in the higher SES strata may be vulnerable to overnutrition [53], but the limited number of obese participants in the sample precluded analysis of the relationship of severe dental caries and overnutrition. There is consensus that frequent consumption of high-calorie and sugary foods and drinks contributes to dental caries and overweight [6,54]. On the other hand, consuming sugary foods and drinks may also displace the intake of nutritious foods and drinks, and contribute to dental caries and undernutrition [55,56]. This suggests that, in low-middle-income countries, there may be a "u-shaped" association between SES and dietary adequacy, caries and nutritional status, rather than the linear relationship between SES and good nutrition and oral health generally described in higher-income countries [53,57,58]. Nonetheless, there is a paucity of research about the role of sugary diets in undernutrition, including the comorbidity with dental caries. This may be explained by the lack of oral health awareness among non-dental medical and public health professionals [59], and the economic power of the food and beverage companies that sell sugary snacks and beverages as well as oral health care products, and sponsor caries research that focuses on dental care products rather than on the cause of caries: sugar [60].

In addition, a growing body of research highlights gender inequalities in child nutrition and health [61,62]. In this sample, females showed worse diet and anthropometric outcomes, and males presented more severe caries experience at follow-up. However, Cambodian national data show no substantial difference in nutritional outcomes by gender in children under 5 [18,63]. The findings also support the understanding that both dental caries and chronic undernutrition are socially driven phenomena with complex and poorly studied interrelationships with each other and with sociocultural, economic and behavioural factors. In this study sample, it appears that male infants/toddlers, and those in the higher SES strata may have consumed larger quantities of food as implied by the CCF data, which may protect first against growth faltering; however, the same subgroups may also have greater consumption of sugary foods and drinks, thereby contributing to the finding of more severe caries experience, and associated long-term growth faltering. This highlights the need to address the structural drivers of early childhood caries and undernutrition from early infancy onward to reduce the long-term adverse impacts of dental caries on children's nutrition, health, and development [13].

Several limitations should be recognized in this study. The CAHENMS and the oral health survey were not specifically intended to examine the impact of tooth decay on malnutrition, and lacked detailed data on maternal health, education, and comorbidities that might contribute to the higher risk for stunting in the presence of severe caries. The dietary surveys were subject to recall bias and the diet indicators of this secondary analysis presented some constraints. The WHO indicator, Minimal Acceptable Diet (MAD) is not country-specific, and many Cambodian food items were missed. Moreover, the Minimal Diet Diversity (MDD) does not include breast milk as it has been recently proposed in the most recent guidelines. The Cambodian Complementary Feeding (CCF) indicator includes the quantity of complementary feeding and breastfeeding but not the frequency of meals per day. Thereby, the diet indicators may not have fully captured children's diet in Cambodia and data were not collected on daily child consumption of non-nutritious food and drinks (junk food). Those food groups contain high amounts of sugar, and are hypothesized to be primary causes of caries and associated stunted growth. Finally, as malnutrition and dental caries are multifactorial diseases that evolve over time [64], this one-year follow-up does not capture the cumulative impact of disease, the mitigating effect of oral hygiene and dental treatment, and a longer follow-up considering these factors is warranted. This would also allow for change modelling of trends in growth and development for which binary logistic regression may not be sensitive.

In order to use human and financial resources wisely, it is important to work closely with programmes focused on the prevention of non-communicable diseases (NCDs) that share common risk factors with tooth decay [65]. Although many countries have introduced school-based caries-prevention programmes with successful outcomes [66,67], most caries risk factors and adverse outcomes begin in early childhood, before the child attends school and before the child sees a dentist. Thus, there is an evidence-based opportunity to integrate caries prevention into existing primary care maternal-child health programmes from birth onwards [68].

The findings of this study suggest that reducing the severity of dental caries could, in turn, reduce the long-term adverse impact on linear growth among young children. Therefore, it could be justified to incorporate caries prevention initiatives with general child nutrition and health promotion initiatives. Such interventions might include supporting adequate infant breast- and complementary feeding [69,70], babyWASH and consumption of safe water [71], and healthy environments with restricted access to sugar [72]. This should go along with an improvement of oral hygiene practices—toothbrushing two times a day with fluoride toothpaste [73]—and oral health initiatives such as population-based fluoride [74,75], and preventing caries lesions through application of sealants [76], fluoride varnishes [73,77], and topical silver and fluoride agents [78]. Finally, particularly relevant to the Cambodian context of widespread food insecurity is the need for political will to limit the global marketing of low-cost, ultra-processed junk food and sugar-sweetened drinks to improve child nutritional status, decrease the incidence of dental caries, and ultimately support children's growth and development.

5. Conclusions

This is the first longitudinal study to examine the association between dental caries and stunted growth in children under 2 years in Cambodia, and to demonstrate that severe tooth decay is associated with developing stunting malnutrition. The study highlights the need to prevent and treat early childhood tooth decay as an important part of programmes to prevent child undernutrition as well as NCDs, and to promote children's optimal growth and development during a critical stage of life.

Author Contributions: Conceptualization, B.T., E.P., A.L.; methodology, B.T., E.P., A.L., T.C., S.H.; software, B.T.; validation, B.T.; formal analysis, E.P.R.; investigation, E.P.R., B.T., K.S.-G., S.H., T.C., G.H., E.P., A.L.; resources, B.T., T.C., S.H., A.L., E.P.; data curation, B.T., G.H.; writing—original draft preparation, E.P.R., K.S.-G., B.T.; writing—review and editing, G.H., E.P., A.L., T.C., S.H.; visualization, E.P.R.; supervision, B.T., K.S.-G., G.H.; project administration, G.H., T.C., S.H.; funding acquisition B.T., T.C., S.H., A.L., E.P. All authors have read and agreed to the published version of the manuscript.

Funding: Grant from The Borrow Foundation.

Institutional Review Board Statement: The study was conducted according to the guidelines of the Declaration of Helsinki, and approved by the National Ethics Committee for Health Research, Cambodia (117 NECHR January 2016).

Informed Consent Statement: Informed consent was obtained from all subjects involved in the study.

Data Availability Statement: Restrictions apply to the availability of these data. Data was obtained from the Health and Nutrition Monitoring Study (CAHENMS) in the North East of Cambodia 2016-2019 and are available with the permission of the principal investigator.

Acknowledgments: UNICEF and the Cambodian Oral Health Bureau.

Conflicts of Interest: The authors declare no conflict of interest.

Appendix A. Overview of the CAHENMS Study

The study monitored health and nutrition indicators for children between birth and 4 years of age and collected individual information about dietary intake, anthropometric measures, cognitive development, the prevalence of diarrhoea and acute respiratory infections as well as information in the household level: SES, handwashing and sanitation. Cases of severe acute malnutrition were referred to the hospital and cases of moderate malnutrition were treated with Numtrey. The wider study included questions about water and hand sanitation, stool, borbor (rice porridge) consumption, and Oral-Health-Related Quality of Life which, were not analysed as part of the present investigation.

Baseline data were collected in December 2015 and the enrolled children were followed until June 2019; the 6th follow-up (FU6). Data collection and follow-ups were performed every month and every two months after FU5 (Figure A1).

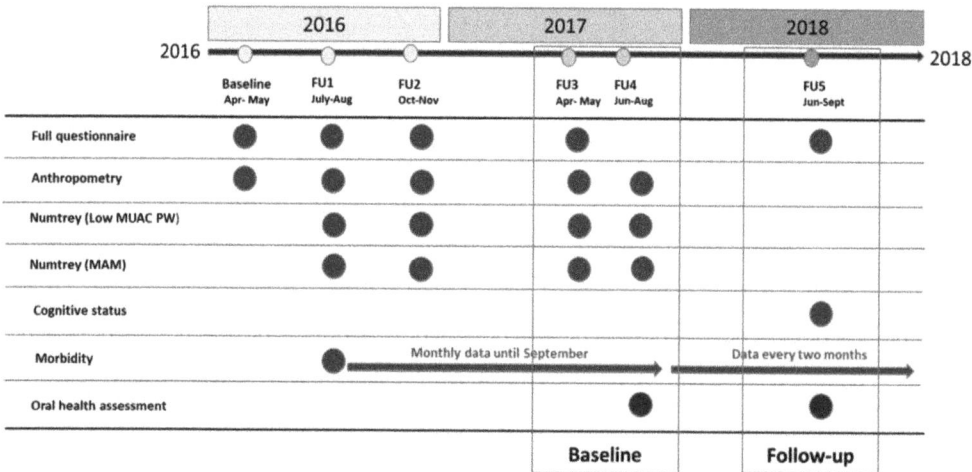

Figure A1. Overview of the CAHENMS study.

The present study used data from follow-up 3 (FU3), follow-up 4 (FU4), and follow-up 5 (FU5), as well as data from children who received an oral examination at CAHENMS FU4 and who were followed a year later at FU5. Parents/caregivers of children who were identified as having carious lesions were informed and instructed to seek further care through a dentist of their choice or through the primary healthcare setting. For the purpose of this analysis, FU3 and FU4 occurring 3 months apart in 2017 were merged as "Baseline"; and FU5 occurring approximately one year later in 2018 was considered as "Follow-up" (FU).

Appendix B. Attrition Analysis

Table A1 presents the attrition sociodemographic profile of the original sample with 2305 children. There was a statistically significant variation in attrition among age group and province between followed and not-followed children, whereby older children presented higher attrition rate ($p < 0.001$; χ^2 test), although the age group included in the study sample, younger than 23.9 months at baseline, presented similar attrition rates (7–9%). The province of Ratanakiri presented a higher proportion of children who were lost to follow-up (11.1% vs. 7.0–7.2%, $p = 0.003$; χ^2 test).

Table A1. Attrition analysis of the original sample with sociodemographic profile.

	Followed N (Row %)	Lost N (Row %)	Total N (Column %)	*p*-Value [1]
	2107 (91.4)	198 (8.6)	2305 (100.0)	
Gender				0.512
Male	1057 (91.4)	99 (8.6)	1156 (50.2)	
Female	1050 (91.4)	99 (8.6)	1149 (49.8)	
Age group				<0.001
<6 months	143 (92.3)	12 (7.7)	155 (6.7)	
6–11 months	280 (92.7)	22 (7.3)	302 (13.1)	
12–17 months	441 (91.5)	41 (8.5)	482 (20.9)	

Table A1. *Cont.*

	Followed N (Row %)	Lost N (Row %)	Total N (Column %)	p-Value [1]
18–23 months	451 (91.3)	43 (8.7)	494 (21.4)	
24–29 months	454 (95.4)	22 (4.6)	476 (20.7)	
30–35 months	288 (90.0)	32 (10.0)	320 (13.9)	
36–41 months	50 (65.8)	26 (34.2)	76 (3.3)	
Province				0.003
Phnom Penh	493 (92.8)	38 (7.2)	531 (23.0)	
Kratie	840 (93.0)	63 (7.0)	903 (39.2)	
Ratanakiri	774 (88.9)	97 (11.1)	871 (37.8)	
SES				0.277
Lowest	347 (90.6)	36 (9.4)	383 (17.4)	
Low	528 (92.1)	45 (7.9)	573 (26.1)	
Medium	445 (89.2)	54 (10.8)	499 (22.7)	
High	352 (92.6)	28 (7.4)	380 (17.3)	
Highest	333 (92.5)	27 (7.5)	260 (16.4) 260 260 (16.4)	

[1] χ^2 test for differences among groups within the same column.

References

1. UNICEF; WHO; World Bank Group Joint. *Malnutrition in Children*; UNICEF: New York, NY, USA, 2020. Available online: https://data.unicef.org/topic/nutrition/malnutrition/ (accessed on 29 August 2020).
2. Roser, M.; Ritchie, H. *Hunger and Undernourishment*; Our World Data: Oxford, UK, 2013. Available online: https://ourworldindata.org/hunger-and-undernourishment (accessed on 17 February 2020).
3. Roser, M.; Ritchie, H. *Obesity*; Our World Data: Oxford, UK, 2017. Available online: https://ourworldindata.org/obesity (accessed on 30 August 2020).
4. Bleich, S.N.; Vercammen, K.A. The negative impact of sugar-sweetened beverages on children's health: An update of the literature. *BMC Obes.* **2018**, *5*, 1–27. [CrossRef]
5. Featherstone, J.D.B. Caries prevention and reversal based on the caries balance. *Pediatr. Dent.* **2006**, *28*, 128–132.
6. Sheiham, A.; James, W. Diet and Dental Caries. *J. Dent. Res.* **2015**, *94*, 1341–1347. [CrossRef]
7. World Health Organization. *Ending Childhood Dental Caries*; World Health Organization: Geneva, Switzerland, 2019.
8. FDI World Dental Federation. *Facts, Figures and Stats*; FDI World Dental Federation: Geneva, Switzerland, 25 April 2019. Available online: https://www.fdiworlddental.org/oral-health/ask-the-dentist/facts-figures-and-stats (accessed on 26 June 2020).
9. Anil, S.; Anand, P.S. Early childhood caries: Prevalence, risk factors, and prevention. *Front. Pediatr.* **2017**, *5*, 157. [CrossRef] [PubMed]
10. Lagerweij, M.D.; Van Loveren, C. Declining caries trends: Are we satisfied? *Curr. Oral Heath. Rep.* **2015**, *2*, 212–217. [CrossRef] [PubMed]
11. Verlinden, D.A.; Reijneveld, S.A.; Lanting, C.I.; Van Wouwe, J.P.; Schuller, A.A. Socio-economic inequality in oral health in childhood to young adulthood, despite full dental coverage. *Eur. J. Oral Sci.* **2019**, *127*, 248–253. [CrossRef] [PubMed]
12. Alkarimi, H.A.; Watt, R.G.; Pikhart, H.; Jawadi, A.H.; Sheiham, A.; Tsakos, G. Impact of treating dental caries on schoolchildren's anthropometric, dental, satisfaction and appetite outcomes: A randomized controlled trial. *BMC Public Health* **2012**, *12*, 706. [CrossRef]
13. Khanh, L.N.; Ivey, S.L.; Sokal-Gutierrez, K.; Barkan, H.; Ngo, K.M.; Hoang, H.T.; Vuong, I.; Thai, N. Early childhood caries, mouth pain, and nutritional threats in vietnam. *Am. J. Public Health* **2015**, *105*, 2510–2517. [CrossRef]
14. So, M.; Ellenikiotis, Y.A.; Husby, H.M.; Paz, C.L.; Seymour, B.; Sokal-Gutierrez, K. Early childhood dental caries, mouth pain, and malnutrition in the ecuadorian amazon region. *Int. J. Environ. Res. Public Health* **2017**, *14*, 550. [CrossRef]
15. World Health Organization. *Essential Nutrition Actions: Improving Maternal, Newborn, Infant and Young Child Health and Nutrition*; WTO: Geneva, Switzerland, 2013.
16. Cambodia Centrifugal Sugar Human Domestic Consumption by Year (1000 MT). 2020. Available online: https://www.indexmundi.com/agriculture/?country=kh&commodity=centrifugal-sugar&graph=human-domestic-consumption (accessed on 20 August 2020).
17. World Health Organization. *Who's Oral Health Country/Area Profile Programme (Capp) Database*; WTO: Geneva, Switzerland, 2013. Available online: https://capp.mau.se/country-areas/ (accessed on 30 August 2020).
18. National Institute of Statistics. *Cambodia Health and Demographic Survey 2014*; ICF Macro: Calverton, MD, USA, 2014.
19. Duangthip, D.; Gao, S.S.; Lo, E.C.M.; Chu, C.H. Early childhood caries among 5- to 6-year-old children in Southeast Asia. *Int. Dent. J.* **2017**, *67*, 98–106. [CrossRef]

20. Chher, T.; Turton, B.J.; Hak, S.; Beltran, E.; Courtel, F.; Durward, C.; Hobdell, M. Dental caries experience in Cambodia: Findings from the 2011 Cambodia national oral health survey. *J. Int. Oral Health* **2016**, *8*, 1.
21. Oral Health Office; Preventive Medicine Department Cambodia. *Cambodia National Oral Health Survey 2011*; Preventive Medicine Department Cambodia: Phnom Penh, Cambodia, 2011.
22. Turton, B.; Chher, T.; Sabbah, W.; Durward, C.; Sithan, H.; Laillou, A. Epidemiological survey of early childhood caries in Cambodia. *BMC Oral Health* **2019**, *19*, 107. [CrossRef] [PubMed]
23. Victora, C.G.; De Onis, M.; Hallal, P.C.; Blössner, M.; Shrimpton, R. Worldwide timing of growth faltering: Revisiting implications for interventions. *Pediatrics* **2010**, *125*, e473–e480. [CrossRef] [PubMed]
24. De Onis, M.; Branca, F. Childhood stunting: A global perspective. *Matern. Child Nutr.* **2016**, *12*, 12–26. [CrossRef]
25. Yang, Y.Y.; Kaddu, G.; Ngendahimana, D.; Barkoukis, H.; Freedman, D.; Lubaale, Y.A.; Mupere, E.; Bakaki, P.M. Trends and determinants of stunting among under-5s: Evidence from the 1995, 2001, 2006 and 2011 Uganda Demographic and Health Surveys. *Public Health Nutr.* **2018**, *21*, 2915–2928. [CrossRef]
26. Sultana, P.; Rahman, M.; Akter, J. Correlates of stunting among under-five children in Bangladesh: A multilevel approach. *BMC Nutr.* **2019**, *5*, 1–12. [CrossRef]
27. Ikeda, N.; Irie, Y.; Shibuya, K. Determinants of reduced child stunting in Cambodia: Analysis of pooled data from three Demographic and Health Surveys. *Bull. World Health Organ.* **2013**, *91*, 341–349. [CrossRef]
28. Dewey, R.J.; Arimond, C.M.; Ruel, M.T. *Developing and Validating Simple Indicators of Complementary Food Intake and Nutri-Ent Density for Breastfed Children in Developing Countries*; Academy for Educational Development: Washington, DC, USA, 2006. Available online: https://pdf.usaid.gov/pdf_docs/Pnadj223.pdf (accessed on 20 October 2020).
29. Hondru, G.; Laillou, A.; Wieringa, F.T.; Poirot, E.; Berger, J.; Christensen, D.; Roos, N. Age-appropriate feeding practices in cambodia and the possible influence on the growth of the children: A longitudinal study. *Nutrients* **2019**, *12*, 12. [CrossRef]
30. Som, S.V.; Van Der Hoeven, M.; Laillou, A.; Poirot, E.; Chan, T.; Polman, K.; Ponce, M.C.; Wieringa, F.T. Adherence to child feeding practices and child growth: A retrospective cohort analysis in cambodia. *Nutrients* **2020**, *13*, 137. [CrossRef]
31. Filmer, D.; Pritchett, L.H. Estimating wealth effects without expenditure data—or tears: An application to educational enrollments in states of India. *Demography* **2001**, *38*, 115–132. [CrossRef]
32. World Health Organization. *Who Child Growth Standards: Training Course on Child Growth Assessment*; WTO: Geneva, Switzerland, 2008.
33. Petersen, P.E.; Baez, R. *World Health Organization. Oral Health Surveys: Basic Methods*, 5th ed; World Health Organization: Paris, France, 2013.
34. World Health Organisation. *Data Sources and Inclusion Criteria*; WHO: Geneva, Switzerland, 2020. Available online: https://www.who.int/nutrition/databases/infantfeeding/data_source_inclusion_criteria/en/ (accessed on 10 October 2020).
35. World Health Organization. 2010. *Indicators for Assessing Infant and Young Child Feeding Practices: Part 2: Measurement*; WTO: Geneva, Switzerland, 2020.
36. National Nutrition Program. *Nutrition Handbook for the Family*; FAO: Rome, Italy, 2011.
37. Bratthall, D. Introducing the significant caries index together with a proposal for a new global oral health goal for 12-year-olds. *Int. Dent. J.* **2000**, *50*, 378–384. [CrossRef] [PubMed]
38. Benzian, H.; Monse, B.; Heinrich-Weltzien, R.; Hobdell, M.; Mulder, J.; Helderman, W.V.P. Untreated severe dental decay: A neglected determinant of low body mass index in 12-year-old Filipino children. *BMC Public Health* **2011**, *11*, 558. [CrossRef] [PubMed]
39. Shen, A.; Bernabé, E.; Sabbah, W. The bidirectional relationship between weight, height and dental caries among preschool children in China. *PLoS ONE* **2019**, *14*, e0216227. [CrossRef] [PubMed]
40. Mishu, M.P.; Hobdell, M.; Khan, M.H.; Hubbard, R.M.; Sabbah, W. Relationship between Untreated dental caries and weight and height of 6- to 12-year-old primary school children in Bangladesh. *Int. J. Dent.* **2013**, *2013*, 1–5. [CrossRef] [PubMed]
41. Tsang, C.; Sokal-Gutierrez, K.; Patel, P.; Lewis, B.; Huang, D.; Ronsin, K.; Baral, A.; Bhatta, A.; Khadka, N.; Barkan, H.; et al. Early childhood oral health and nutrition in urban and rural Nepal. *Int. J. Environ. Res. Public Health* **2019**, *16*, 2456. [CrossRef]
42. Alshihri, A.A.; Rogers, H.J.; Alqahtani, M.A.; Aldossary, M.S. Association between dental caries and obesity in children and young people: A narrative review. *Int. J. Dent.* **2019**, *2019*, 1–8. [CrossRef]
43. Chen, D.; Zhi, Q.; Zhou, Y.; Tao, Y.; Wu, L.; Lin, H.-C. Association between dental caries and BMI in children: A systematic review and meta-analysis. *Caries Res.* **2018**, *52*, 230–245. [CrossRef]
44. Hayden, C.; Bowler, J.O.; Chambers, S.; Freeman, R.; Humphris, G.M.; Richards, D.; Cecil, J.E. Obesity and dental caries in children: A systematic review and meta-analysis. *Community Dent. Oral Epidemiol.* **2013**, *41*, 289–308. [CrossRef]
45. Hooley, M.; Skouteris, H.; Boganin, C.; Satur, J.; Kilpatrick, N. Body mass index and dental caries in children and adolescents: A systematic review of literature published 2004 to 2011. *Syst. Rev.* **2012**, *1*, 57. [CrossRef]
46. Paisi, M.; Kay, E.J.; Bennett, C.; Kaimi, I.; Witton, R.; Nelder, R.; Lapthorne, D. Body mass index and dental caries in young people: A systematic review. *BMC Pediatr.* **2019**, *19*, 1–9. [CrossRef]
47. Shivakumar, S.; Shivakumar, G.C.; Srivastava, A. Body mass index and dental caries: A systematic review. *Int. J. Clin. Pediatr. Dent.* **2018**, *11*, 228–232. [CrossRef] [PubMed]

48. Anik, A.I.; Rahman, M.M.; Rahman, M.M.; Tareque, M.I.; Khan, M.N.; Alam, M.M. Double burden of malnutrition at household level: A comparative study among Bangladesh, Nepal, Pakistan, and Myanmar. *PLoS ONE* **2019**, *14*, e0221274. [CrossRef] [PubMed]

49. Benefice, E.; Lévi, P.; Banouvong, P. Progressive growth deterioration in a context of nutritional transition: A case study from Vientiane (Lao PDR). *Ann. Hum. Biol.* **2012**, *39*, 239–246. [CrossRef] [PubMed]

50. Cordero, M.L.; Cesani, M.F. Nutritional transition in schoolchildren from Tucumán, Argentina: A cross-sectional analysis of nutritional status and body composition. *Am. J. Hum. Biol.* **2019**, *31*, e23257. [CrossRef] [PubMed]

51. Ghattas, H.; Acharya, Y.; Jamaluddine, Z.; Assi, M.; El Asmar, K.; Jones, A.D. Child-level double burden of malnutrition in the MENA and LAC regions: Prevalence and social determinants. *Matern. Child Nutr.* **2020**, *16*, e12923. [CrossRef]

52. De Mola, C.L.; Quispe, R.; Valle, G.A.; Poterico, J.A. Nutritional Transition in children under five years and women of reproductive age: A 15-years trend analysis in Peru. *PLoS ONE* **2014**, *9*, e92550. [CrossRef]

53. Vazquez, C.E.; Cubbin, C. Socioeconomic status and childhood obesity: A review of literature from the past decade to inform intervention research. *Curr. Obes. Rep.* **2020**, *2020*, 1–9. [CrossRef]

54. World Health Organization. *Guideline: Sugars Intake for Adults and Children*; WTO: Geneva, Switzerland, 2015.

55. Mühlendahl, K.E.V.; Kromburg, S. A clumsy 3-year-old who liked junk food. *Lancet* **1996**, *348*, 1705. [CrossRef]

56. Smith, M.M.; Lifshitz, F. Excess fruit juice consumption as a contributing factor in nonorganic failure to thrive. *Pediatrics* **1994**, *93*, 438–443.

57. Peres, A.M.; MacPherson, L.M.D.; Weyant, R.J.; Daly, B.; Venturelli, R.; Mathur, M.R.; Listl, S.; Celeste, R.K.; Guarnizo-Herreño, C.C.; Kearns, C.; et al. Oral diseases: A global public health challenge. *Lancet* **2019**, *394*, 249–260. [CrossRef]

58. Bommer, C.; Vollmer, S.; Subramanian, S.V. How socioeconomic status moderates the stunting-age relationship in low-income and middle-income countries. *BMJ Glob. Health* **2019**, *4*, e001175. [CrossRef] [PubMed]

59. Gambhir, R.S.; Batth, J.S.; Arora, G.; Anand, S.; Bhardwaj, A.; Kaur, H. Family physicians' knowledge and awareness regarding oral health: A survey. *J. Educ. Health Promot.* **2019**, *8*, 45. [CrossRef] [PubMed]

60. Kearns, C.E.; Bero, L.A. Conflicts of interest between the sugary food and beverage industry and dental research organisations: Time for reform. *Lancet* **2019**, *394*, 194–196. [CrossRef]

61. Abassi, M.M.; Sassi, S.; El Ati, J.; Ben Gharbia, H.; Delpeuch, F.; Traissac, P. Gender inequalities in diet quality and their socioeconomic patterning in a nutrition transition context in the Middle East and North Africa: A cross-sectional study in Tunisia. *Nutr. J.* **2019**, *18*, 18. [CrossRef]

62. Richards, E.; Theobald, S.; George, A.; Kim, J.C.; Rudert, C.; Jehan, K.; Tolhurst, R. Going beyond the surface: Gendered intra-household bargaining as a social determinant of child health and nutrition in low and middle income countries. *Soc. Sci. Med.* **2013**, *95*, 24–33. [CrossRef]

63. Miller, J.E.; Rodgers, Y. Mother's education and children's nutritional status: New evidence from Cambodia. *Asian Dev. Rev.* **2009**, *26*, 131–165.

64. Bell, L.K.; Schammer, C.; Devenish, G.; Ha, D.; Thomson, M.W.; Spencer, A.J.; Do, L.G.; Scott, J.A.; Golley, R.K. Dietary patterns and risk of obesity and early childhood caries in australian toddlers: Findings from an australian cohort study. *Nutrients* **2019**, *11*, 2828. [CrossRef]

65. Watt, R.G.; Listl, S.; Peres, M.; Heilmann, A. *Social Inequalities in Oral Health: From Evidence to Action*; UCL: London, UK, 2015.

66. Petersen, E.P.; Hunsrisakhun, J.; Thearmontree, A.; Pithpornchaiyakul, S.; Hintao, J.; Jürgensen, N.; Ellwood, R.P. School-based intervention for improving the oral health of children in southern Thailand. *Community Dent Health* **2015**, *32*, 44–50.

67. Jürgensen, N.; Petersen, P.E. Promoting oral health of children through schools—results from a WHO global survey. *Community Dent Health* **2013**, *30*, 204–218.

68. Phantumvanit, P.; Makino, Y.; Ogawa, H.; Rugg-Gunn, A.; Moynihan, P.; Petersen, P.E.; Evans, R.W.; Feldens, C.A.; Lo, E.; Khoshnevisan, M.H.; et al. WHO global consultation on public health intervention against early childhood caries. *Community Dent. Oral Epidemiol.* **2018**, *46*, 280–287. [CrossRef]

69. World Health Organisation. *Exclusive Breastfeeding for Optimal Growth, Development and Health of Infants*; WHO: Geneva, Switzerland, 2020. Available online: http://www.who.int/elena/titles/exclusive_breastfeeding/en/ (accessed on 20 August 2020).

70. World Health Organization. *Complementary Feeding: Report of The Global Consultation, and Summary of Guiding Principles For Com-Plementary Feeding of The Breastfed Child*; WHO: Geneva, Switzerland, 2003. Available online: https://apps.who.int/iris/handle/10665/42739 (accessed on 20 August 2020).

71. Dominguez, E.I. *Baby WASH and the 1000 Days—A Practical Package for Stunting Reduction*; Action Against Hunger: Madrid, Spain, 2017. Available online: https://www.actionagainsthunger.org/sites/default/files/publications/2017_BabyWASH_EN.pdf (accessed on 20 August 2020).

72. World Health Organization. *Guidance on Ending the Inappropriate Promotion of Foods for Infants and Young Children: Implementa-Tion Manual*; WTO: Geneva, Switzerland, 2017.

73. Turton, B.; Durward, C.; Crombie, F.; Sokal-Gutierrez, K.; Soeurn, S.; Manton, D.J. Evaluation of a community-based early childhood caries (ECC) intervention in Cambodia. *Community Dent. Oral Epidemiol.* **2020**. [CrossRef] [PubMed]

74. Petersen, P.E.; Ogawa, H. Prevention of dental caries through the use of fluoride—the WHO approach. *Community Dent. Health* **2016**, *33*, 66–68. [PubMed]

75. Yeung, C.A. A systematic review of the efficacy and safety of fluoridation. *Evid. Based Dent.* **2008**, *9*, 39–43. [CrossRef] [PubMed]

76. Wright, J.T.; Tampi, M.; Graham, L.; Estrich, C.; Crall, J.J.; Fontana, M.; Gillette, E.J.; Nový, B.B.; Dhar, V.; Donly, K.; et al. Sealants for preventing and arresting pit-and-fissure occlusal caries in primary and permanent Molars. *Pediatr. Dent.* **2016**, *38*, 282–308. [CrossRef] [PubMed]

77. Lenzi, T.L.; Montagner, A.F.; Soares, F.; Rocha, R.D.O. Are topical fluorides effective for treating incipient carious lesions? *J. Am. Dent. Assoc.* **2016**, *147*, 84–91.e1. [CrossRef] [PubMed]

78. Duangthip, D.; Chen, K.J.; Gao, S.S.; Lo, E.C.M.; Chu, C.H. Managing early childhood caries with atraumatic restorative treatment and topical silver and fluoride agents. *Int. J. Environ. Res. Public Health* **2017**, *14*, 1204. [CrossRef]

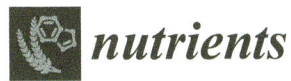

Article

Antimicrobial Photodynamic Treatment with Mother Juices and Their Single Compounds as Photosensitizers

Sigrun Chrubasik-Hausmann [1]**, Elmar Hellwig** [2]**, Michael Müller** [3] **and Ali Al-Ahmad** [2,*]

1   Institute of Forensic Medicine, Faculty of Medicine, University of Freiburg, 79104 Freiburg, Germany;
    sigrun.chrubasik@klinikum.uni-freiburg.de
2   Department of Operative Dentistry and Periodontology, Medical Center, Faculty of Medicine,
    University of Freiburg, 79106 Freiburg, Germany; elmar.hellwig@uniklinik-freiburg.de
3   Institute of Pharmaceutical Sciences, Pharmaceutical and Medicinal Chemistry, University of Freiburg,
    79104 Freiburg, Germany; michael.mueller@pharmazie.uni-freiburg.de
*   Correspondence: ali.al-ahmad@uniklinik-freiburg.de; Tel.: +49-761-270-48940

Citation: Chrubasik-Hausmann, S.; Hellwig, E.; Müller, M.; Al-Ahmad, A. Antimicrobial Photodynamic Treatment with Mother Juices and Their Single Compounds as Photosensitizers. *Nutrients* **2021**, *13*, 710. https://doi.org/10.3390/nu13030710

Academic Editor: Paola Roggero

Received: 20 January 2021
Accepted: 19 February 2021
Published: 24 February 2021

Publisher's Note: MDPI stays neutral with regard to jurisdictional claims in published maps and institutional affiliations.

Abstract: The potent antimicrobial effects of antimicrobial photodynamic therapy (aPDT) with visible light plus water-filtered infrared-A irradiation and natural compounds as photosensitizers (PSs) have recently been demonstrated. The aim of this study was to obtain information on the antimicrobial effects of aPDT with mother juices against typical cariogenic oral *Streptococcus* pathogens in their planktonic form and determine its eradication potential on total human salivary bacteria from volunteers. Mother juices of pomegranate, bilberry, and chokeberry at different concentrations were used as PSs. The unweighted (absolute) irradiance was 200 mW cm^{-2}, applied five minutes. Planktonic cultures of *Streptococcus mutans* and *Streptococcus sobrinus* and total mixed bacteria from pooled saliva of volunteers were treated with aPDT. Up to more than 5 $\log_{10}$ of *S. mutans* and *S. sobrinus* were killed by aPDT with 0.4% and 0.8% pomegranate juice, 3% and 50% chokeberry juice, and 12.5% bilberry juice (both strains). Concentrations of at least 25% (pomegranate) and >50% (chokeberry and bilberry) eradicated the mixed bacteria in saliva samples. This pilot study has shown that pomegranate mother juice is superior to the berry juices as a multicomponent PS for killing pathogenic oral bacteria with aPDT.

Keywords: *Punica granatum*; *Vaccinium myrtillus*; *Aronia melanocarpa*; punicalagin; cyanidin 3-glucoside and hyperoside; *Streptococcus mutans*; *Streptococcus sobrinus*; photosensitizer; antimicrobial photodynamic treatment

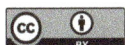
1. Introduction

Caries and chronic inflammation of the periodontal tissues are related to the accumulation of bacterial plaque. Mechanical methods are insufficient to improve periodontitis and often the administration of antibiotics is required following mechanical debridement. However, due to microbial resistance towards most antibiotics as well as disinfectants such as chlorhexidine digluconate and patient allergies, alternative methods are needed. Antimicrobial photodynamic therapy (aPDT) is one such method, being well studied since its discovery around 1900 [1]. The technique requires a visible light source, a non-toxic photosensitizer (PS), and tissue oxygen. The wavelength of the light source needs to be appropriate to excite the PS to produce radicals (singlet oxygen) and/or reactive oxygen species. The latter cause irreversible damage to bacteria, fungi, and viruses [2].

As PSs, tetrapyrrole structures and synthetic dyes are in current use, as well as natural compounds such as the red colors hypericin and riboflavin (vitamin B2), yellow curcumin [1], quercetin (a flavonol) [3], and psoralens [4]. Our group has successfully introduced aPDT with visible light (VIS) plus water-filtered infrared-A (wIRA) irradiation and toluidine blue, chlorine e6 [5–7], indocyanine green [8], and hypericum perforatum ethanolic extract [9] as PSs. The results from the aforementioned studies were encouraging for the use of aPDT with VIS + wIRA to treat oral diseases such as periodontitis and peri-implantitis. However, this requires a photosensitizing agent that can be used in the oral cavity without any toxic effects for oral mucous membranes and human cells. Mother juices are freshly squeezed juices from harvested fruit that do not contain any added colorings, preservatives, or sugar. After squeezing, they are pasteurized and immediately bottled. Hence, the aim of this pilot study was to (i) evaluate the phototoxic effects of aPDT with mother juices against typical cariogenic oral *Streptococcus* pathogens in their planktonic form and (ii) determine its eradication potential on total human salivary bacteria from volunteers.

2. Materials and Methods

2.1. Radiation Source and Photosensitizers

A broadband visible light (VIS) and water-filtered infrared-A (wIRA) radiator (Hydrosun 750 FS, Hydrosun Medizintechnik GmbH, Müllheim, Germany) containing a 7 mm water cuvette was used as described elsewhere in detail [6,9,10]. The radiator comprised a halogen lamp with an accessory water filter (dimensions: length: 28 cm, width: 27 cm, height: 28 cm) using 750 W (voltage: 230 V, 50–60 Hz), which was inserted into the light path for absorbing the infrared-B and -C wavelengths. Additionally, the radiator also included an orange filter (BTE 31, 10 cm in diameter and 200 mW/cm^2 efficiency). More than doubled-weighted efficient integral illumination with reference to the absorption spectrum of protoporphyrin IX was enabled by using a BTE 31 filter. The 944 and 1180 nm absorption bands were also filtered to prevent superficial overheating. The water-filtered absorption revealed a total spectrum in the range of 570 to 1400 nm, with local minima at around 970, 1200, and 1430 nm. The amount of unweighted radiation applied to the microbial samples was 48 mW cm^{-2} VIS and 152 mW cm^{-2} wIRA (200 mW cm^{-2} in total). All samples were irradiated for 5 min.

As PSs, we used mother juices of pomegranate (*Punica granatum*, L6349), chokeberry (*Aronia melanocarpa*, L6294), and bilberry (*Vaccinium myrtillus*, L7074) from Biotta AG CH-8274 Tägerwilen, with expiry dates of 7 June 2018, 13 April 2019, and 6 September 2018, respectively (Table 1). The absorbance spectra of all juices were measured using a Tecan Infinite 200 reader (Tecan, Crailsheim, Germany).

Table 1. Polyphenol content (Folin–Ciocalteu method, mg/100 mL) of the mother juices. The analyses were carried out by Pharma Bellavista GmbH, CH 9404 Rorschacherberg, using established methods defined in the European Pharmacopeia.

	Pomegranate	Bilberry	Chokeberry
Total polyphenols calculated as pyrogallols *	384	693	697
Tannins calculated as pyrogallols *	218	371	446
Procyanidins calculated as cyanidin chloride **	100		836
Ellagic acid ***	8.6		

* PhEur 2.8.14, ** PhEur 2.2.25, *** PhEur 2.2.29.

In addition, we investigated the compounds punicalagin (PHL80524, Sigma Aldrich, Traufkirchen, Germany), cyanidin 3-glucoside (PHL89616, Merck, Darmstadt, Germany), and hyperoside (0018-05-85, Planegg/Martinsried, Germany).

2.2. Bacterial Strains and Total Human Salivary Bacteria

Two bacterial strains belonging to the mutans streptococci that have been considered as main oral cariogenic bacteria were tested in this study: *Streptococcus mutans* DSM20523, and *Streptococcus sobrinus* DSM 203815. Long-term storage of both bacterial strains was at $-80\ ^\circ$C in brain heart infusion containing 15% (*v/v*) glycerol as described by Jones et al. [11] and Al-Ahmad et al. [12]. Maintenance with weekly subculturing was conducted on Columbia blood agar (CBA) at 37 $^\circ$C in an aerobic atmosphere including 5–10% CO$_2$. Overnight cultures of the bacterial strains were prepared in tryptic soy broth (TSB, Merck, Darmstadt, Germany) at 37 $^\circ$C in an aerobic atmosphere including 5–10% CO$_2$.

Three healthy volunteers gave written consent after the ethics committee of the Albert-Ludwigs-University of Freiburg had approved the study protocol (Nr. 91/13). Exclusion criteria included the use of antibacterial mouth rinses or antibiotics in the three-month period prior to the start of the experiment, pregnancy or lactation, smoking, severe systemic diseases, or participation in another clinical study during the previous three months. The volunteers donated unstimulated human saliva, which was pooled to gain total salivary bacteria. All total salivary samples were taken on the same day, directly before conducting the experiments, to avoid alteration of the total salivary microbiota.

2.3. Application Protocol of aPDT

The bacterial samples and pooled human salivary bacteria were incubated for two minutes in different concentrations of the mother juices prior to irradiation. All dilutions of the mother juices were conducted in 0.95% NaCl solution. The samples were then irradiated by VIS + wIRA for five minutes at 37 °C. Samples treated with chlorhexidine (CHX) served as a positive control. Samples treated with 0.95% NaCl solution, with the mother juices, or solely with irradiation were used as negative controls. The negative controls were incubated in the dark to exclude any accessory effects of day light. The colony-forming units (CFUs) of treated and untreated bacterial strains were determined on CBA at 37 °C and with 5–10% CO_2 atmosphere for two days and depicted as log10 values.

Human salivary samples were vortexed for 30 s before determining the CFUs on CBA aerobically at 37 °C and with 5–10% CO_2 atmosphere for five days. The killing rate in terms of CFU reduction after aPDT was calculated by comparison with the negative control. A statistical analysis was not required if a reduction rate higher than two log10 steps was achieved.

The activity of the PSs remained stable for six months of storage at low temperature (3 °C) in the dark using a light-tight bottle.

3. Results

All three mother juices showed light absorption at a wide wavelength range (Figure 1) close to the emission spectrum of the light source [13].

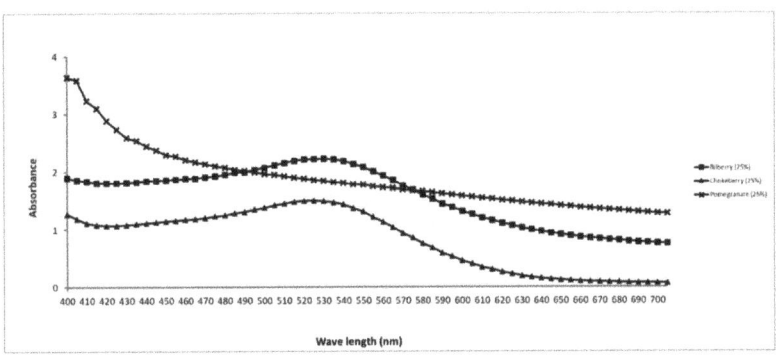

Figure 1. Absorbance spectrum of the mother juices employed in this study.

The high killing effects of aPDT with pomegranate mother juice on *S. mutans* and *S. sobrinus* are shown in Figure 2 and Table 2. Approximately all bacterial cells were eradicated at PS concentrations ranging between 6% and 0.8%. Even the low concentration of 0.4% showed a high killing rate of one Log_{10} on the planktonic culture of both species. No killing effect of aPDT was shown with 0.2% pomegranate mother juice. The aPDT effects of pomegranate juice on total salivary bacteria (Figure 2) revealed an eradication range between one (12.5%) and 4 Log_{10} (50%). A pomegranate juice concentration lower than 6%

showed no antimicrobial effects as a PS with aPDT. The treatment of both pathogens as well as total salivary bacteria with CHX resulted in a total killing effect of 100%.

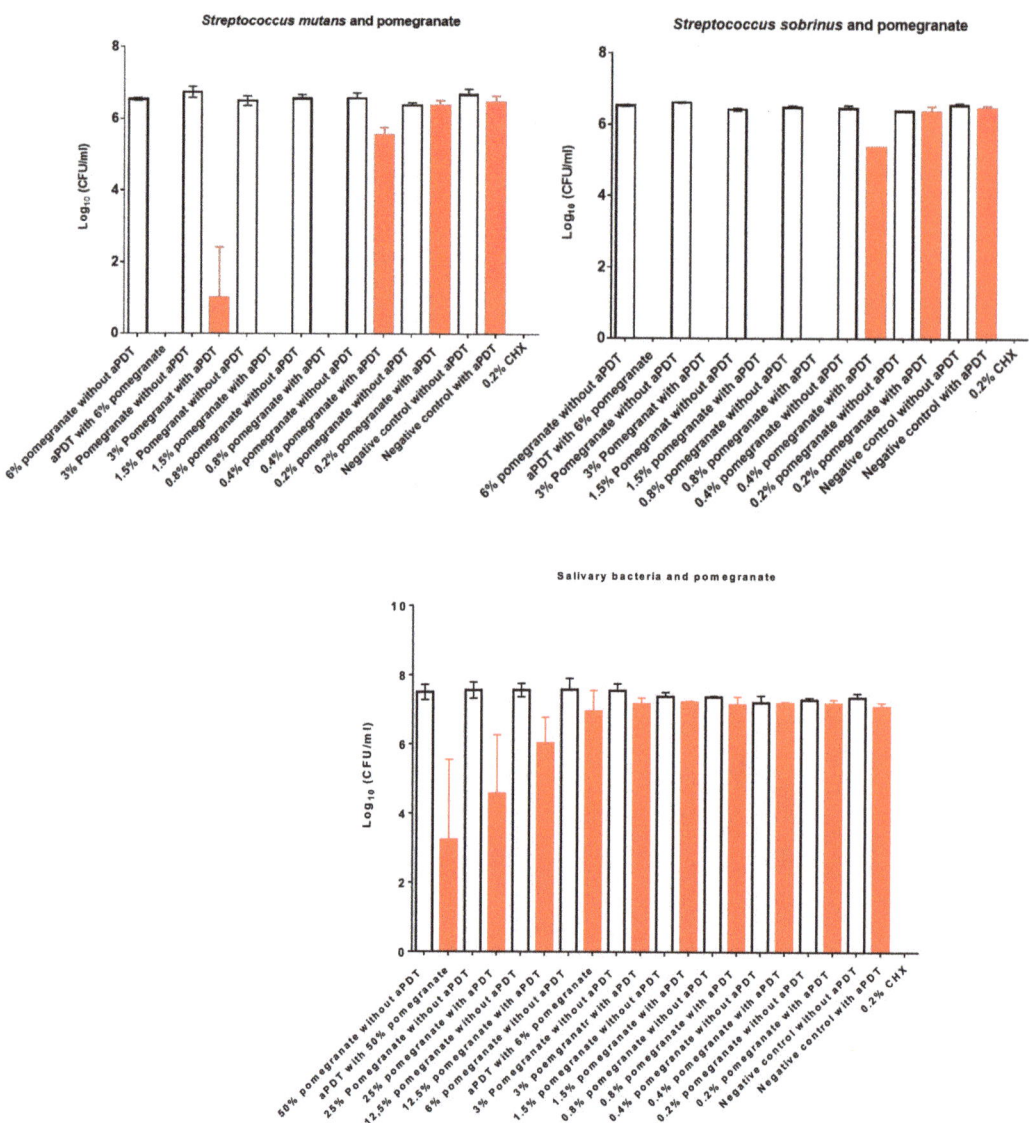

Figure 2. The effects of antimicrobial photodynamic therapy (aPDT) using visible light and water-filtered infrared-A (VIS + wIRA) in combination with pomegranate mother juice as a photosensitizer (PS) against *S. mutans*, *S. sobrinus*, and total salivary bacteria. Untreated and mother juice-treated negative controls are added. Additionally, aPDT without mother juices was conducted as a negative control. Treatment with 0.2% CHX served as a positive control. Red bars depict values with photodynamic treatment; white bars represent values without photodynamic treatment. CHX, chlorhexidine.

Table 2. Killing effects of aPDT using pomegranate mother juice as a photosensitizer.

Target	Concentration of the Photosensitizer	Killing Effects
S. mutans	0.8–6%	≥3 Log10
	0.2–0.4%	≤1 Log10
S. sobrinus	0.8–6%	≥3 Log10
	0.2–0.4%	≤1 Log10
Total salivary bacteria	25–50%	≥3 Log10
	12.5%	≤1 Log10

The killing effect of aPDT with chokeberry mother juice on S. mutans (Figure 3, Table 3) was dependent on the concentration of the PS and it ranged from 0.8 (0.2% chokeberry juice) to 4.2 Log10 (50% chokeberry juice). Even the low concentration of 3% showed a high killing rate of 2.4 Log_{10}. Similar concentration-dependent antimicrobial effects were shown for S. sobrinus (Figure 3, Table 3). The killing of S. sobrinus ranged from 0.4 to 2.1 Log_{10} with chokeberry juice concentrations of 0.4% and 50%, respectively. The 6% chokeberry juice showed a killing effect of 1.1 Log_{10} on planktonic S. sobrinus.

Table 3. Killing effects of aPDT using chokeberry mother juice as a photosensitizer.

Target	Concentration of the Photosensitizer	Killing Effects
S. mutans	6–50%	≥3 Log10
	1.5–3%	≤2.4 Log10
	0.2–0.8%	≤1 Log10
S. sobrinus	50%	2.1 Log10
	6–25%	1–1.4 Log10
Total salivary bacteria	50%	1.3 Log10
	0.3–25%	≤0.8 Log10

The aPDT effects of chokeberry juice on total salivary bacteria (Figure 3, Table 3) revealed an eradication range between 0.8 and 1.3 Log10. The treatment of both pathogens as well as the salivary bacteria with CHX resulted in a total killing effect of 100%.

The aPDT with 50%, 25%, and 12.5% bilberry mother juices on S. mutans resulted in total killing of all bacteria (Figure 4, Table 4). The aPDT with 6% bilberry juice killed S. mutans by two Log_{10} (99%). All negative controls including treatment with pure bilberry juice without irradiation (8.3–8.4 Log10) as well as bacteria incubated solely in 0.95% NaCl solution (with and without irradiation; 7.2–7.4 Log_{10}) revealed no antimicrobial effects. The combination of aPDT with 25% and 12.5% bilberry juices also killed all S. sobrinus pathogens, whereas the 6% juice reduced the CFUs from 8.3 to 7.6 Log_{10}. Treatment with pure juice without irradiation showed no antimicrobial effects (Figure 4, Table 4). Treatment with 0.2% CHX killed all planktonic cells of S. mutans and S. sobrinus as well as all salivary bacteria. The aPDT with 50% bilberry juice reduced the CFUs of total salivary bacteria from 7.7 to 6.0 Log_{10} (Figure 4, Table 4), reflecting a high killing rate of >90%. A killing effect of one and 0.5 Log_{10} was shown for aPDT with 25% and 12.5% bilberry juices, respectively.

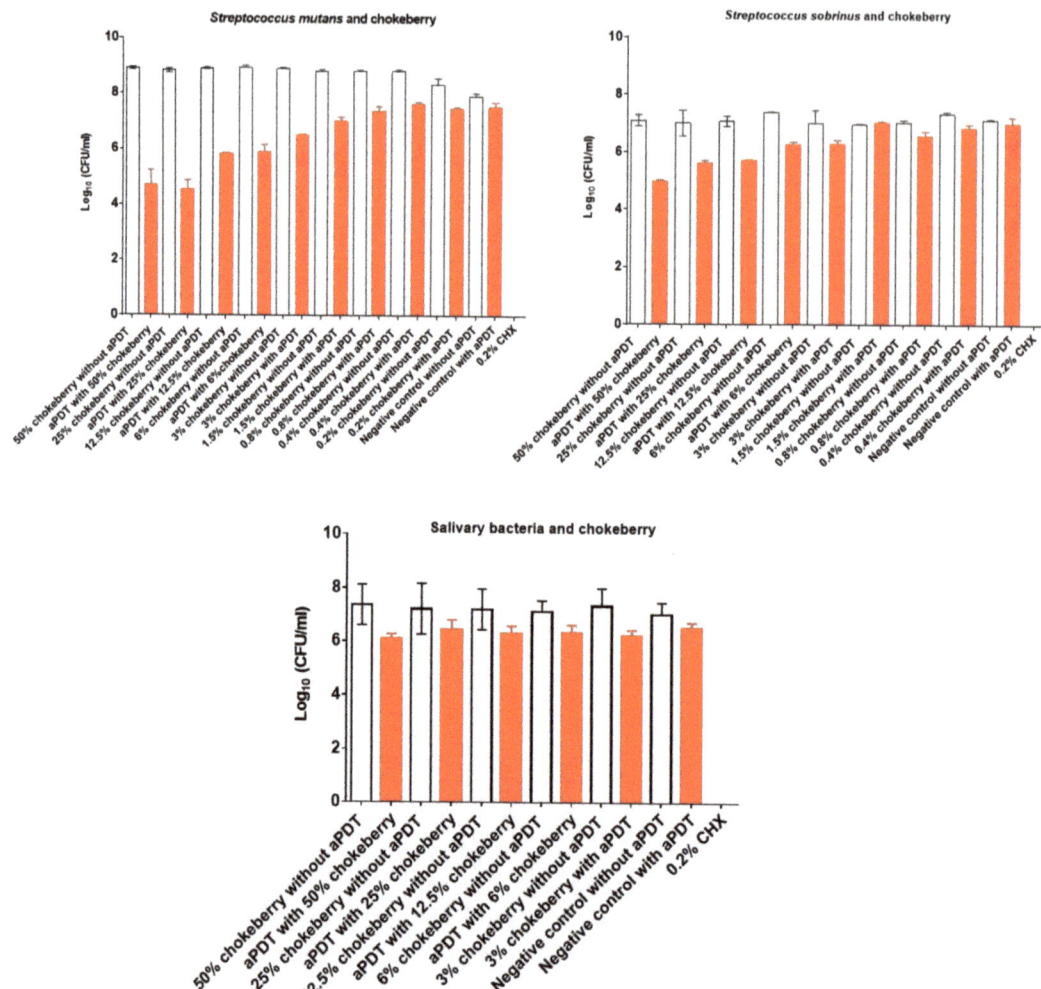

Figure 3. The effects of aPDT using VIS + wIRA in combination with chokeberry mother juice as a PS against *S. mutans*, *S. sobrinus*, and total salivary bacteria. Untreated and mother juice-treated negative controls are added. Additionally, aPDT without mother juices was conducted as a negative control. Treatment with 0.2% CHX served as a positive control. Red bars depict values with photodynamic treatment; white bars represent values without photodynamic treatment. CHX, chlorhexidine; aPDT, antimicrobial photodynamic therapy.

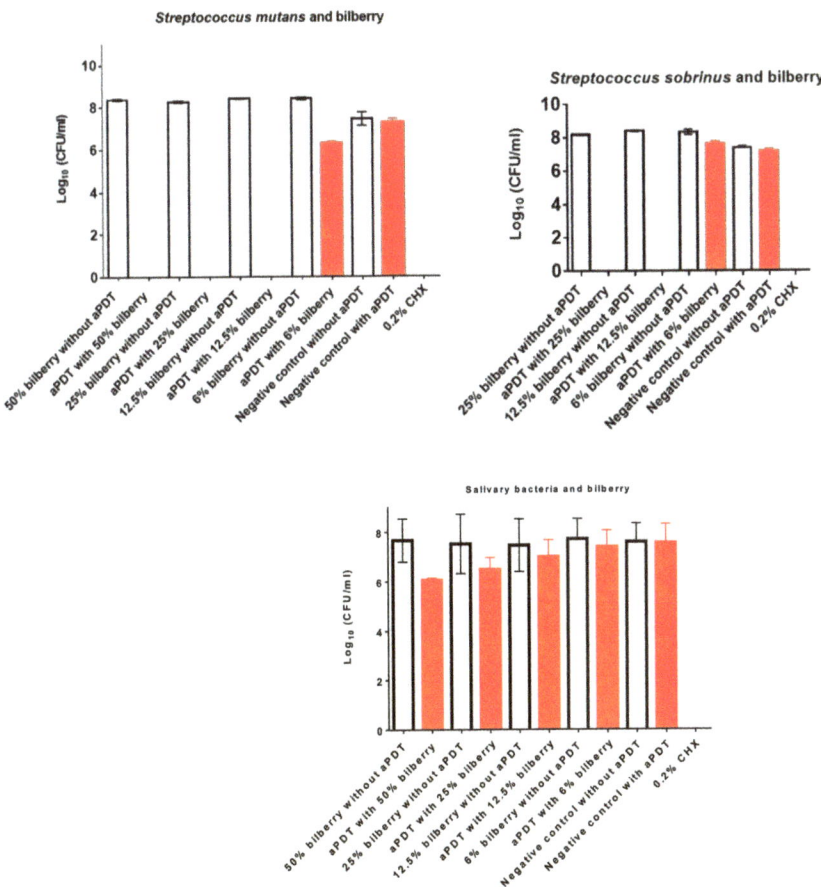

Figure 4. The effects of aPDT using VIS + wIRA in combination with bilberry mother juice as a PS against *S. mutans*, *S. sobrinus*, and total human salivary bacteria. Untreated and mother juice-treated negative controls are added. Additionally, aPDT without mother juices was conducted as a negative control. Treatment with 0.2% CHX served as a positive control. Red bars depict values with photodynamic treatment; white bars represent values without photodynamic treatment. CHX, chlorhexidine; aPDT, antimicrobial photodynamic therapy.

Table 4. Killing effects of aPDT using bilberry mother juice as a photosensitizer.

Target	Concentration of the Photosensitizer	Killing Effects
S. mutans	12.5–50%	$\geq$3 Log10
	6%	2 Log10
	0.2–0.8%	$\leq$1 Log10
S. sobrinus	12.5–25%	$\geq$3 Log10
	6%	0.9 Log10
Total salivary bacteria	50%	1.7 Log10
	25%	1 Log10
	12.5%	0.5 Log10

The aPDT with 0.5 mg/mL punicalgin and 1 mg/mL hyperoside showed only a minor killing effect on *S. mutans* at a range less than 0.5 Log$_{10}$ (Figure 5, Table 5). All other concentrations demonstrated no antimicrobial effect. The aPDT with cyanidin 3-glucoside chloride did not show any killing effects on *S. mutans* at the concentration range of 1 to 0.03 mg/mL. However, the mixture of the three compounds (equal amount of each compound) had a high photosensitizing potential and killed *S. mutans* by more than 4 $\log_{10}$ at a concentration of 1 mg/mL (Figure 6). Even at 0.5 mg/mL, the mixture killed *S. mutans* at a bactericidal level of more than 3 $\log_{10}$. Treatment only with juices or single compounds without radiation or radiation with VIS + wIRA without PSs showed no antimicrobial effects.

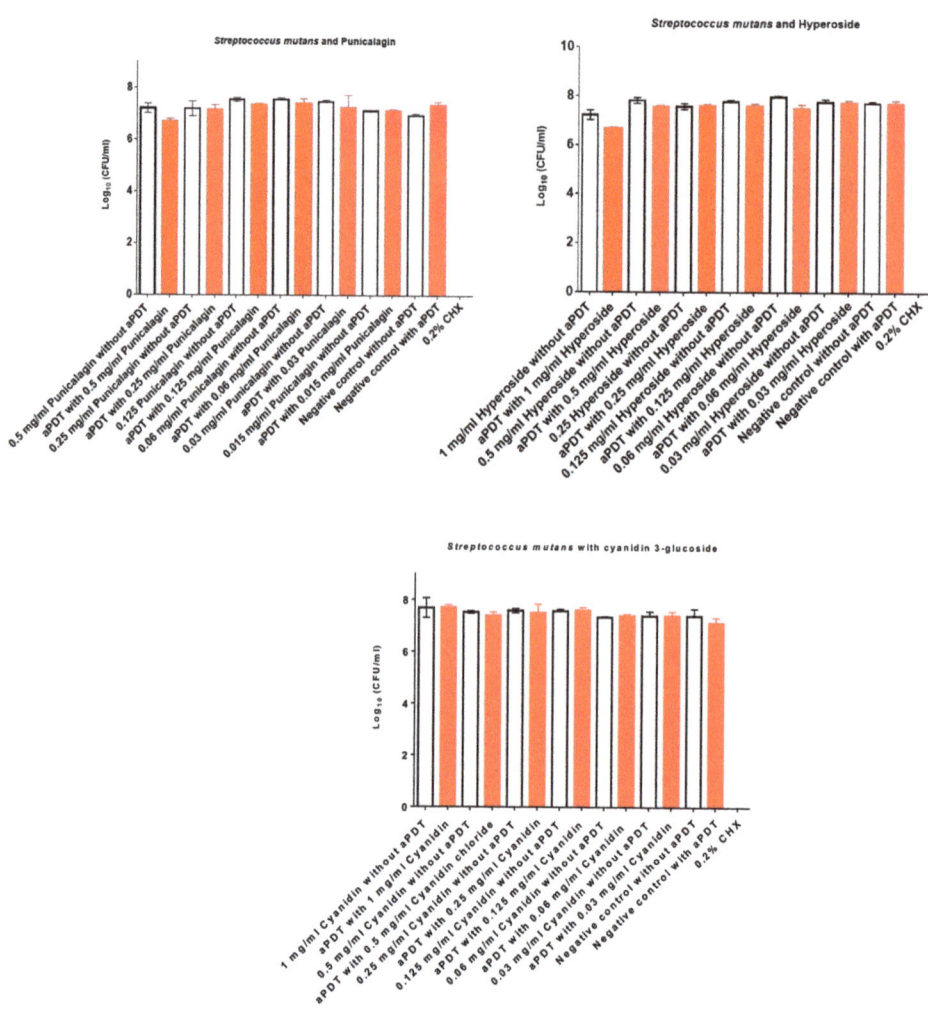

Figure 5. The effects of aPDT using VIS + wIRA in combination with single compounds as PSs against *S. mutans*. Untreated and mother juice-treated negative controls are added. Additionally, aPDT without mother juices was conducted as a negative control. Treatment with 0.2% CHX served as a positive control. Red bars depict values with photodynamic treatment; white bars represent values without photodynamic treatment. CHX, chlorhexidine; aPDT, antimicrobial photodynamic therapy.

Table 5. Effects of aPDT using single compounds as photosensitizers against *Streptococcus mutans*.

Compound	Concentration of the Photosensitizer	Killing Effects
Punicalagin	0.015–0.5 mg/mL 0.015–0.5 mg/mL	0.4 Log10 no effects
Hyperoside	1 mg/mL 0.03–0.5 mg/mL	0.5 Log10 no effects
Cyanidin 3-glucoside chloride	0.03–1 mg/mL	no effects

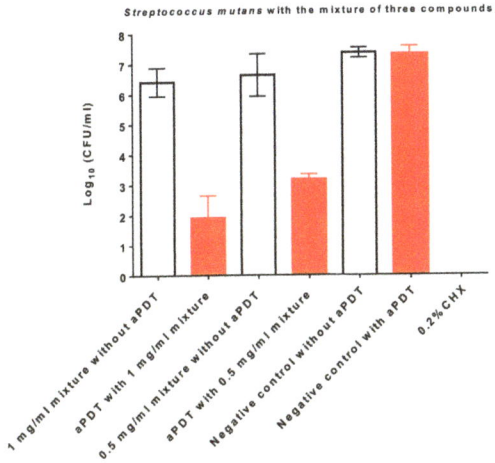

Figure 6. The effects of aPDT using VIS + wIRA in combination with a mixture of all three substances (equal amount of each compound) as a PS against S. mutans. Untreated and mother juice-treated negative controls are added. Additionally, aPDT without a PS was conducted as an additional negative control. Treatment with 0.2% CHX served as a positive control. Red bars depict values with photodynamic treatment; white bars represent values without photodynamic treatment. CHX, chlorhexidine; aPDT, antimicrobial photodynamic therapy.

4. Discussion

The antimicrobial effects of aPDT with VIS + wIRA in combination with mother juices demonstrated that all juices had a photosensitizing potential that could be used to regain oral health in the case of infections. There are three types of PSs: (i) those that stay in close proximity to a bacterial cell wall, (ii) those that bind to the bacterial cell, which may limit the oxidative damage to outer cell structures, and (iii) those that enter bacterial cells and reach the cytoplasm, which results in damage to intracellular components such as cytoplasmic proteins or DNA [14]. Mother juices per se have a potent antimicrobial activity, although when diluted in non-antimicrobial concentrations, they may serve as PSs.

4.1. Pomegranate

A lipophilic extract of *Punica granatum* was antimicrobial to *S. mutans*, *Staphylococcus aureus*, and *Candida albicans* at bactericidal concentrations of 12.5, 25, and 50 mg/mL, respectively [15]. *S. mutans* was more sensitive to pomegranate than the other microorga-nisms including *Porphyromonas gingivalis* [16]. A hydroalcoholic extract of pomegranate juice inhibited the *S. mutans* Clarke ATCC® 25175™ strain (minimum inhibitory concentration (MIC) 25 μg/μL, minimum bactericidal concentration (MBC) 40 μg/μL) and a *Rothia dento-cariosa* clinical isolate (MIC 20 μg/μL, MBC 140 μg/μL) [17]. Pomegranate fruit peel crude extract killed *S. mutans* (MBC 6.25 mg/mL). At sub-bactericidal concentrations, it reduced acid production, biofilm formation, and insoluble extracellular polysaccharide production (EPS) in the biofilm of the planktonic cells of *S. mutans*. The production of soluble EPS was not affected [18].

The antimicrobial activity was attributed to the presence of tannin derivatives including punicalagin [19]. As the mechanism of action, inhibition of extracellular microbial enzymes, deprivation of the substrates required for microbial growth, direct action on microbial metabolism through inhibition of oxidative phosphorylation, and iron deprivation have been suggested [20]. However, other compounds such as phloretin, punigratane, and coutaric acid occurring in trace amounts in the pomegranate showed even higher microbicide effects and may contribute to the overall antibacterial effect [21]. A gel equivalent to 0.234% punicalagin inhibited *S. mutans* and *Streptococcus sanguinis* but not *Lactobacillus casei* within 24 h of incubation in vitro [22].

Topalovic and co-workers [23] identified in pomegranate 97 phenolic compounds, 23 anthocyanins and derivatives, 33 ellagitannins and derivatives of ellagic acid, 12 flavanols, 4 flavonol glycosides (among them quercetin, myricetin, kaempferol [24], and hyperoside [25]), one flavone (according to Zhao et al. [24], two flavones: apigenin and luteolin), 17 hydroxybenzoic acids, and 7 hydroxycinnamic acids and derivatives thereof. Flavanols, ellagitannins, and derivatives of ellagic acid had the highest concentrations in pomegranate juice. While isolated colorless tannins were ineffective as PSs for aPDT in killing *S. mutans* (Figure 5, data for procyanidin A2 not shown), the mixture of characteristic compounds contributes to the photosensitizing effect (Figure 6).

Our results show that pomegranate mother juice in concentrations of 0.8% (*S. mutans*) and 0.4% (*S. sobrinus*) with aPDT was associated with a high killing rate of the streptococci. For a high eradication rate of total human salivary samples, a concentration of at least 25% was required. Such concentrations had no impact on the streptococci without aPDT.

The content of anthocyanins in pomegranate juice of industrial production was on average 1 mg/100 cm^3, and cyanidin 3,5-*O*-diglucoside accounted for about 40% of them [26], while other studies identified cyanidin 3-*O*-glucoside as the predominant anthocyanin (41%), followed by cyanidin 3,5-*O*-diglucoside (27%) [27]. Cyanidin 3-*O*-glucoside was more instable at the storage temperature than delphinidin 3,5-di- and cyanidin 3,5-diglucosides [28]. Our data show that cyanidin 3-*O*-glucoside in combination with punicalagin and hyperoside may contribute to the PS activity (Figure 6), as quercetin certainly did [3]. It remains to be established whether dilutions of the cytotoxic pomegranate extracts prepared from the whole fruit, juice, or peel with the solvents propylene glycol, ethanol, and methanol, respectively, are also useful PSs.

4.2. Chokeberry

Aronia melanocarpa demonstrated potent antimicrobial activity against ten human pathogens [29]. Denev and coworkers investigated crude extract standardized on 20% and 40% anthocyanins on proanthocyanins (PACs), as well as pure compounds (chlorogenic acid, cyanidin 3-*O*-galactoside, epicatechin, rutin, and quercetin). They demonstrated that the antimicrobial effect of chokeberry is mainly due to the action of condensed tannins (PACs), and that quercetin and epicatechin contribute to the antimicrobial activity. By contrast, the anthocyanin fraction was ineffective.

Exposure to 1/10 diluted chokeberry juice for one minute significantly reduced *S. mutans* biofilm formation in vitro without affecting streptococcal growth [30]. One week of oral rinse with diluted chokeberry juice led to significantly fewer salivary streptococcal CFUs than rinsing with water. Lee and coworkers concluded that the juice might inhibit initial biofilm formation by decomposing extracellular RNA [30]. When chokeberry extracts, subfractions, and compounds were tested for their potential to prevent biofilm formation and inhibit bacterial growth of *Escherichia coli* and *Bacillus cereus*, the 50% ethanolic extract was more potent than other extracts. Moreover, epicatechin was the most effective among the compounds tested, while the effects of oligomeric and polymeric PACs were negligible. Interestingly, cyanidin 3-xyloside showed activity against Gram-negative *E. coli* and Gram-positive *B. cereus*, whereas the other anthocyanins were inactive [31].

Chokeberry dry fruit contains up to 7849 mg polyphenols per 100 g. The dark color of the fruit is caused by the high concentration of anthocyanins, which include cyanidin 3-glucoside, 3-galactoside, 3-xyloside, and 3-arabinoside. A small proportion of anthocyanins was attributed to pelargonidine 3-galactoside and 3-arabinoside. Chokeberry flavonols mainly comprise quercetin derivatives and, to a lower degree, isorhamnetin 3-derivatives, myricetin, and kaempherol 3 derivatives. The flavan-3-ols comprise monomeric epicatechin and oligomeric and polymeric PACs. Chlorogenic and neochlorogenic acids are the main phenolic acids [32].

Our results indicate that chokeberry mother juice was less effective in killing *S. mutans* and *S. sobrinus* compared with pomegranate mother juice and required concentrations of 6% and 50%, respectively (Figure 3). The killing rate of the mixed bacteria from salivary samples was similar to that of bilberry juice with a concentration of 50% (Figure 3). It remains to be established whether chokeberry extracts are more effective PSs.

4.3. Bilberry

The MIC of a lipophilic bilberry (*Vaccinium myrtillus*) extract against *P. gingivalis* was 500 μg/mL [33]. A fraction of it showed antibacterial activity against other oral bacteria with MICs against *P. gingivalis*, *Fusobacterium nucleatum*, and *Prevotella intermedia* of 26, 59, and 45 μg/mL, respectively. The MIC against *S. mutans* was >62.5 μg/mL. It seemed likely that the antimicrobial effect was attributed to the predominant non-anthocyanin phenolic compounds, accounting for approximately 80% of the total phenolic content [34].

Bilberry contains at least 42 bioactive substances including 22 phenolic acids, 15 flavonols, and 5 flavan-3-ols [34]. Derivatives of quercetin, myricetin, isorhamnetin, and kaempferol are among the flavonols identified [35]. The major anthocyanin among the fifteen identified is delphinidin 3-O-β-D-glucopyranoside [36]. The group of Liu [37] suggested using cyanidin 3-glucoside as an appropriate marker for bilberry. However, when using several authentic anthocyanin references to quantify anthocyanin contents, a higher anthocyanidin content was revealed, accounting for 1610 mg/L in bilberry juice compared with 417 mg/L in blueberry juice [38]. Thus, anthocyanins predominate in *V. myrtillus*, whereas *Vaccinium angustifolium* contains more hydroxycinnamic acids. The contents of PACs and flavonols are rather similar [39].

Miari and colleagues [40] observed that 25% *V. angustifolium* aqueous extract reduced biofilm formation without affecting the growth of *Pseudomonas aeruginosa*. The decrease in the relative gene expression of exopolysaccharides and quorum sensing encoding genes sheds light on the mechanism of action [40]. Highbush blueberry PACs reduced the growth of *Aggregatibacter actinomycetemcomitans* and prevented biofilm formation at subinhibitory concentrations. PAC treatment of pre-formed biofilms resulted in a loss of bacterial viability, probably due to damage of the bacterial cell membrane. In addition, the PACs protected the oral keratinocytes barrier integrity from damage caused by *A. actinomycetemcomitans* [41]. The same extract with 17% phenolic acids, 13% flavonoids (flavonols, anthocyanins, flavan-3-ols), and almost 3% procyanidins (oligomeric (epi)catechin derivatives) showed antibacterial activity against periodontopathogenic *F. nucleatum* (MIC 1 mg/mL). The authors supposed that the antibacterial activity was caused by the ability of blueberry polyphenols to chelate iron [42]. Blueberry juice also inhibited enzymes such as α-glucosidase dipeptidyl peptidase-4 and tyrosinase dose-dependently. Increased acidity in the biofilms may thus contribute to the antibacterial activity of blueberry preparations [43]. The aforementioned blueberry extract at 62.5 μg/mL inhibited *F. nucleatum* biofilm formation by almost 90%, as well as a number of proinflammatory and cartilage-destructing cytokines (NF-κB, IL-1β, TNF-α, IL-6, MMP-8, and MMP-9). This indicates that blueberry and bilberry extracts have a dual antibacterial and anti-inflammatory action [42]. The latter action is supported by an animal experiment in which a daily oral bilberry extract had a protective effect on oral mucosal damage induced by 5-fluorouracil in hamsters [44], as well as a clinical study in individuals with gingivitis in which the volunteers consumed either 250 or 500 g of bilberries over seven days. The mean reduction in bleeding on probing after consumption of the berries was 41% (250 g) and 59% (500 g) compared with 31% in the placebo group, and 58% in the standard care reference group. Only in the group consuming 500 g of bilberries/day were gingival crevicular fluid cytokines (IL-1ß, IL-6, VEGF) reduced [45].

Our results show that bilberry mother juice is less effective than pomegranate juice as a PS for aPDT. Concentrations of 12.5% and higher were needed to kill the two streptococci species and a concentration of 50% was required to kill total mixed bacteria of pooled human saliva samples. It remains to be established whether bilberry extracts are more effective PSs.

4.4. Multicomponent PSs for aPDT

Our data with isolated compounds indicate that co-administration of an anthocyanin pigment, a flavone (hyperoside), and a tannin (punicalagin) had a photosensitizing effect, although the single compounds had little effect or were ineffective. The flavonol quercetin contained in all mother juices has already been shown to be an appropriate PS [3]. We therefore suggest that the multicomponent cocktail of anthocyanins, flavonols, and tannins contributes to the photosensitizing activity of mother juices. The unique composition of compounds in pomegranate makes this fruit juice superior to berry mother juices. The question of whether to rinse one's mouth with pomegranate mother juice or its anthocyanin-flavonol-tannin fraction prior to aPDT with VIS + wIRA requires further investigations. To date, the evidence between mother juice intake and damaging caries and tooth erosion is not conclusive. Overall, prospective cohort studies in children and adolescents have found no association between the juice intake and tooth erosion or dental caries, although data from randomized controlled trials (RCT) in adults suggests that the intake of mother juices could worsen oral health. However, the RCT data were from small, short-term studies that utilized intra-oral devices generally devoid of normal plaque or saliva action, and they generally employed conditions that were not reflective of normal juice consumption [46].

As oral bacteria exist in the oral biofilm and not in the planktonic state, additional experiments on oral biofilms are required to evaluate the efficiency of this novel aPDT. However, it is important to note that the total salivary bacteria also include flocs of the oral biofilm as has previously been shown by our research group [47]. Hence, the results of the present study give preliminary indications regarding an effect of the applied aPDT on the oral biofilm, which has to be confirmed in future studies.

The lower activity of aPDT against total human salivary bacteria as compared to the effects on *S. mutans* and *S. sobrinus* can be caused by the high heterogeneity of the salivary microbiome that consists of hundreds of different species [48]. More than 700 different species belonging to the Gram-negative and Gram-positive bacteria have been reported as belonging to the oral microbiota [49]. The different structure of the cell wall may lead to a lower sensitivity of Gram-negative bacteria, as the permeability of the photosensitizer could be decreased when compared to the Gram-positive species. Moreover, flocs of oral biofilms have been shown in unstimulated human saliva [47]. Due to the extracellular matrices, these flocs could be less sensitive to the aPDT used as when compared to the planktonic single species cultures of *S. mutans* and *S. sobrinus*.

5. Conclusions

This study has revealed a higher killing effect of pomegranate mother juice in low concentration in comparison with bilberry or chokeberry mother juice. Testing of the single compounds showed that only a mixture of different components has a photosensitizing killing effect in combination with VIS + wIRA. Due to the known healing effects of wIRA on human cells, the aPDT using VIS + wIRA in combination with components of pomegranate fruit juice may be a promising technique for treating oral infections. In order to evaluate the potential of this, novel aPDT future clinical studies should be conducted using different fractions of pomegranate mother juice.

Author Contributions: S.C.-H.: drafted and critically revised the manuscript, data analysis and interpretation. E.H.: contribution to the conception and design of the study. M.M.: contribution to the conception and design of the study, critically revised the manuscript. A.A.-A.: principal investigator and contributed to the conception, design, data analysis and interpretation, drafted and critically revised the manuscript. All authors have read and agreed to the published version of the manuscript.

Funding: This study was supported by the Swiss Dr. Braun Science Foundation and in part by the German Research Foundation (DFG; Grant AL 1179/4-1).

Institutional Review Board Statement: The study was conducted according to the guidelines of the Declaration of Helsinki, and approved by the Ethics Committee of the University of Freiburg (Nr. 91/13).

Informed Consent Statement: Informed consent was obtained from all subjects involved in the study.

Data Availability Statement: Data available on request due to restrictions e.g., privacy or ethical. The data presented in this study are available on request from the corresponding author.

Acknowledgments: Bettina Spitzmüller is acknowledged for skillful technical laboratory assistance during the live/dead assay.

Conflicts of Interest: The authors declare no conflict of interest. The funders had no role in the design of the study; in the collection, analyses, or interpretation of data; in the writing of the manuscript, or in the decision to publish the results.

References

1. Abrahamse, H.; Hamblin, M.R. New photosensitizers for photodynamic therapy. *Biochem. J.* **2016**, *473*, 347–364. [CrossRef]
2. Pérez-Laguna, V.; García-Malinis, A.J.; Aspiroz, C.; Rezusta, A.; Gilaberte, Y. Antimicrobial effects of photodynamic therapy. *G. Ital. Di Dermatol. E Venereol. Organo Uff. Soc. Ital. Di Dermatol. E Sifilogr.* **2018**, *153*, 833–846. [CrossRef] [PubMed]
3. de Paula Rodrigues, R.; Tini, I.R.; Soares, C.P.; da Silva, N.S. Effect of photodynamic therapy supplemented with quercetin in hep-2 cells. *Cell Biol. Int.* **2014**, *38*, 716–722. [CrossRef] [PubMed]
4. Yin, R.; Hamblin, M.R. Antimicrobial photosensitizers: Drug discovery under the spotlight. *Curr. Med. Chem.* **2015**, *22*, 2159–2185. [CrossRef] [PubMed]
5. Al-Ahmad, A.; Bucher, M.; Anderson, A.C.; Tennert, C.; Hellwig, E.; Wittmer, A.; Vach, K.; Karygianni, L. Antimicrobial photoinactivation using visible light plus water-filtered infrared-a (vis + wira) alters in situ oral biofilms. *PLoS ONE* **2015**, *10*, e0132107. [CrossRef] [PubMed]
6. Al-Ahmad, A.; Tennert, C.; Karygianni, L.; Wrbas, K.T.; Hellwig, E.; Altenburger, M.J. Antimicrobial photodynamic therapy using visible light plus water-filtered infrared-a (wira). *J. Med. Microbiol.* **2013**, *62*, 467–473. [CrossRef]
7. Al-Ahmad, A.; Walankiewicz, A.; Hellwig, E.; Follo, M.; Tennert, C.; Wittmer, A.; Karygianni, L. Photoinactivation using visible light plus water-filtered infrared-a (vis+wira) and chlorine e6 (ce6) eradicates planktonic periodontal pathogens and subgingival biofilms. *Front. Microbiol.* **2016**, *7*, 1900. [CrossRef] [PubMed]
8. Burchard, T.; Karygianni, L.; Hellwig, E.; Follo, M.; Wrbas, T.; Wittmer, A.; Vach, K.; Al-Ahmad, A. Inactivation of oral biofilms using visible light and water-filtered infrared a radiation and indocyanine green. *Future Med. Chem.* **2019**, *11*, 1721–1739. [CrossRef] [PubMed]
9. Vollmer, A.; Al-Ahmad, A.; Argyropoulou, A.; Thurnheer, T. Antimicrobial photoinactivation using visible light plus water-filtered infrared-a (vis + wira) and hypericum perforatum modifies in situ oral biofilms. *Sci. Rep.* **2019**, *9*, 20325. [CrossRef] [PubMed]
10. Karygianni, L.; Ruf, S.; Follo, M.; Hellwig, E.; Bucher, M.; Anderson, A.C.; Vach, K.; Al-Ahmad, A. Novel broad-spectrum antimicrobial photoinactivation of in situ oral biofilms by visible light plus water-filtered infrared a. *Appl. Environ. Microbiol.* **2014**, *80*, 7324–7336. [CrossRef]
11. Jones, D.; Pell, P.A.; Sneath, P.H.A. Maintenance of bacteria on glass beads at −60 °C to −76 °C. In *Maintenance of Microorganisms and Cultured Cells A Manual of Laboratory Methods*, 2nd ed.; Kirsop, B.E., Doyle, A.E., Eds.; Academic Press: London, UK, 1991; pp. 45–50.
12. Al-Ahmad, A.; Auschill, T.M.; Braun, G.; Hellwig, E.; Arweiler, N.B. Overestimation of streptococcus mutans prevalence by nested pcr detection of the 16s rrna gene. *J. Med. Microbiol.* **2006**, *55*, 109–113. [CrossRef] [PubMed]
13. Hoffmann, G. Principles and working mechanisms of water-filtered infrared-a (wira) in relation to wound healing. *GMS Krankenh. Interdiszip.* **2007**, *2*, Doc54.
14. Cieplik, F.; Deng, D.; Crielaard, W.; Buchalla, W.; Hellwig, E.; Al-Ahmad, A.; Maisch, T. Antimicrobial photodynamic therapy—What we know and what we don't. *Crit. Rev. Microbiol.* **2018**, *44*, 571–589. [CrossRef] [PubMed]
15. de Oliveira, J.R.; de Castro, V.C.; das Graças Figueiredo Vilela, P.; Camargo, S.E.; Carvalho, C.A.; Jorge, A.O.; de Oliveira, L.D. Cytotoxicity of brazilian plant extracts against oral microorganisms of interest to dentistry. *BMC Complement. Altern. Med.* **2013**, *13*, 208. [CrossRef] [PubMed]

16. Rosas-Piñón, Y.; Mejía, A.; Díaz-Ruiz, G.; Aguilar, M.I.; Sánchez-Nieto, S.; Rivero-Cruz, J.F. Ethnobotanical survey and antibacterial activity of plants used in the altiplane region of mexico for the treatment of oral cavity infections. *J. Ethnopharmacol.* **2012**, *141*, 860–865. [CrossRef] [PubMed]
17. Ferrazzano, G.F.; Scioscia, E.; Sateriale, D.; Pastore, G.; Colicchio, R.; Pagliuca, C.; Cantile, T.; Alcidi, B.; Coda, M.; Ingenito, A.; et al. In vitro antibacterial activity of pomegranate juice and peel extracts on cariogenic bacteria. *BioMed Res. Int.* **2017**, *2017*, 2152749. [CrossRef] [PubMed]
18. Gulube, Z.; Patel, M. Effect of punica granatum on the virulence factors of cariogenic bacteria streptococcus mutans. *Microb. Pathog.* **2016**, *98*, 45–49. [CrossRef]
19. Mphahlele, R.R.; Fawole, O.A.; Makunga, N.P.; Opara, U.L. Effect of drying on the bioactive compounds, antioxidant, antibacterial and antityrosinase activities of pomegranate peel. *BMC Complement. Altern. Med.* **2016**, *16*, 143. [CrossRef]
20. Scalbert, A. Antimicrobial properties of tannins. *Phytochemistry* **1991**, *30*, 3875–3883. [CrossRef]
21. Nazeam, J.A.; Al-Shareef, W.A.; Helmy, M.W.; El-Haddad, A.E. Bioassay-guided isolation of potential bioactive constituents from pomegranate agrifood by-product. *Food Chem.* **2020**, *326*, 126993. [CrossRef]
22. Millo, G.; Juntavee, A.; Ratanathongkam, A.; Nualkaew, N.; Peerapattana, J.; Chatchiwiwattana, S. Antibacterial inhibitory effects of punica granatum gel on cariogenic bacteria: An in vitro study. *Int. J. Clin. Pediatr. Dent.* **2017**, *10*, 152–157. [CrossRef]
23. Topalović, A.; Knežević, M.; Gačnik, S.; Mikulic-Petkovsek, M. Detailed chemical composition of juice from autochthonous pomegranate genotypes (punica granatum l.) grown in different locations in montenegro. *Food Chem.* **2020**, *330*, 127261. [CrossRef] [PubMed]
24. Zhao, X.; Fang, Y.; Yin, Y.; Feng, L. Flavonols and flavones changes in pomegranate (punica granatum l.) fruit peel during fruit development. *J. Agric. Sci. Technol.* **2014**, *16*, 1649–1659.
25. Khanavi, M.; Moghaddam, G.; Oveisi, M.R.; Sadeghi, N.; Jannat, B.; Rostami, M.; Saadat, M.A.; Hajimahmoodi, M. Hyperoside and anthocyanin content of ten different pomegranate cultivars. *Pak. J. Biol. Sci. PJBS* **2013**, *16*, 636–641. [CrossRef]
26. Khomich, L.M.; Perova, I.B.; Eller, K.I. Pomegranate juice nutritional profile. *Vopr. Pitan.* **2019**, *88*, 80–92.
27. Gardeli, C.; Varela, K.; Krokida, E.; Mallouchos, A. Investigation of anthocyanins stability from pomegranate juice (punica granatum l. Cv ermioni) under a simulated digestion process. *Medicines* **2019**, *6*, 90. [CrossRef]
28. Vegara, S.; Mena, P.; Martí, N.; Saura, D.; Valero, M. Approaches to understanding the contribution of anthocyanins to the antioxidant capacity of pasteurized pomegranate juices. *Food Chem.* **2013**, *141*, 1630–1636. [CrossRef] [PubMed]
29. Denev, P.; Číž, M.; Kratchanova, M.; Blazheva, D. Black chokeberry (aronia melanocarpa) polyphenols reveal different antioxidant, antimicrobial and neutrophil-modulating activities. *Food Chem.* **2019**, *284*, 108–117. [CrossRef]
30. Lee, H.J.; Oh, S.Y.; Hong, S.H. Inhibition of streptococcal biofilm formation by aronia by extracellular rna degradation. *J. Sci. Food Agric.* **2020**, *100*, 1806–1811. [CrossRef] [PubMed]
31. Bräunlich, M.; Økstad, O.A.; Slimestad, R.; Wangensteen, H.; Malterud, K.E.; Barsett, H. Effects of aronia melanocarpa constituents on biofilm formation of escherichia coli and bacillus cereus. *Molecules* **2013**, *18*, 14989–14999. [CrossRef] [PubMed]
32. Sidor, A.; Gramza-Michałowska, A. Black chokeberry aronia melanocarpa l.-a qualitative composition, phenolic profile and antioxidant potential. *Molecules* **2019**, *24*, 3710. [CrossRef] [PubMed]
33. Satoh, Y.; Ishihara, K. Investigation of the antimicrobial activity of bilberry (vaccinium myrtillus l.) extract against periodonto-pathic bacteria. *J. Oral Biosci.* **2020**, *62*, 169–174. [CrossRef]
34. Liu, S.; Marsol-Vall, A.; Laaksonen, O.; Kortesniemi, M.; Yang, B. Characterization and quantification of nonanthocyanin phenolic compounds in white and blue bilberry (vaccinium myrtillus) juices and wines using uhplc-dad−esi-qtof-ms and uhplc-dad. *J. Agric. Food Chem.* **2020**, *68*, 7734–7744. [CrossRef] [PubMed]
35. Koponen, J.M.; Happonen, A.M.; Auriola, S.; Kontkanen, H.; Buchert, J.; Poutanen, K.S.; Törrönen, A.R. Characterization and fate of black currant and bilberry flavonols in enzyme-aided processing. *J. Agric. Food Chem.* **2008**, *56*, 3136–3144. [CrossRef] [PubMed]
36. Ichiyanagi, T.; Hatano, Y.; Matsugo, S.; Konishi, T. Structural dependence of hplc separation pattern of anthocyanins from bilberry (vaccinium myrtillus l.). *Chem. Pharm. Bull.* **2004**, *52*, 628–630. [CrossRef]
37. Liu, B.; Hu, T.; Yan, W. Authentication of the bilberry extracts by an hplc fingerprint method combining reference standard extracts. *Molecules* **2020**, *25*, 2514. [CrossRef] [PubMed]
38. Müller, D.; Schantz, M.; Richling, E. High performance liquid chromatography analysis of anthocyanins in bilberries (vaccinium myrtillus l.), blueberries (vaccinium corymbosum l.), and corresponding juices. *J. Food Sci.* **2012**, *77*, C340–C345. [CrossRef]
39. Riihinen, K.; Jaakola, L.; Kärenlampi, S.; Hohtola, A. Organ-specific distribution of phenolic compounds in bilberry (vaccinium myrtillus) and 'northblue' blueberry (vaccinium corymbosum x v. Angustifolium). *Food Chem.* **2008**, *110*, 156–160. [CrossRef] [PubMed]
40. Miari, M.; Rasheed, S.S.; Haidar Ahmad, N.; Itani, D.; Abou Fayad, A.; Matar, G.M. Natural products and polysorbates: Potential inhibitors of biofilm formation in pseudomonas aeruginosa. *J. Infect. Dev. Ctries.* **2020**, *14*, 580–588. [CrossRef]
41. Ben Lagha, A.; LeBel, G.; Grenier, D. Dual action of highbush blueberry proanthocyanidins on aggregatibacter actinomycetem-comitans and the host inflammatory response. *BMC Complement. Altern. Med.* **2018**, *18*, 10. [CrossRef]
42. Ben Lagha, A.; Dudonné, S.; Desjardins, Y.; Grenier, D. Wild blueberry (vaccinium angustifolium ait.) polyphenols target fusobacterium nucleatum and the host inflammatory response: Potential innovative molecules for treating periodontal diseases. *J. Agric. Food Chem.* **2015**, *63*, 6999–7008. [CrossRef]
43. Cásedas, G.; Les, F.; Gómez-Serranillos, M.P.; Smith, C.; López, V. Anthocyanin profile, antioxidant activity and enzyme inhibiting properties of blueberry and cranberry juices: A comparative study. *Food Funct.* **2017**, *8*, 4187–4193. [CrossRef] [PubMed]

44. Davarmanesh, M.; Miri, R.; Haghnegahdar, S.; Tadbir, A.A.; Tanideh, N.; Saghiri, M.A.; Garcia-Godoy, F.; Asatourian, A. Protective effect of bilberry extract as a pretreatment on induced oral mucositis in hamsters. *Oral Surg. Oral Med. Oral Pathol. Oral Radiol.* **2013**, *116*, 702–708. [CrossRef]

45. Widén, C.; Coleman, M.; Critén, S.; Karlgren-Andersson, P.; Renvert, S.; Persson, G.R. Consumption of bilberries controls gingival inflammation. *Int. J. Mol. Sci.* **2015**, *16*, 10665–10673. [CrossRef]

46. Liska, D.; Kelley, M.; Mah, E. 100% fruit juice and dental health: A systematic review of the literature. *Front. Public Health* **2019**, *7*, 190. [CrossRef] [PubMed]

47. Al-Ahmad, A.; Wiedmann-Al-Ahmad, M.; Carvalho, C.; Lang, M.; Follo, M.; Braun, G.; Wittmer, A.; Mülhaupt, R.; Hellwig, E. Bacterial and Candida albicans adhesion on rapid prototyping produced 3D-scaffolds manufactured as bone replacement materials. *J. Biomed. Mater. Res. A* **2008**, *87*, 933–943. [CrossRef]

48. Zaura, E.; Brandt, B.W.; Prodan, A.; Teixeira de Mattos, M.J.; Imangaliyev, S.; Kool, J.; Buijs, M.J.; Jagers, F.L.; Hennequin-Hoenderdos, N.L.; Slot, D.E.; et al. On the ecosystemic network of saliva in healthy young adults. *Int. Soc. Microb. Ecol. J.* **2017**, *11*, 1218–1231. [CrossRef]

49. Mark Welch, J.L.; Rossetti, B.J.; Rieken, C.W.; Dewhirst, F.E.; Borisy, G.G. Biogeography of a human oral microbiome at the micron scale. *Proc. Natl. Acad. Sci. USA* **2016**, *113*, E791–E800. [CrossRef] [PubMed]

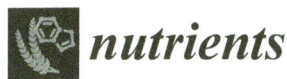

Article

A Log Ratio-Based Analysis of Individual Changes in the Composition of the Oral Microbiota in Different Dietary Phases

Kirstin Vach [1,2,*], Ali Al-Ahmad [2], Annette Anderson [2], Johan Peter Woelber [2], Lamprini Karygianni [3], Annette Wittmer [4] and Elmar Hellwig [2]

[1] Institute of Medical Biometry and Medical Statistics, Faculty of Medicine and Medical Center, University of Freiburg, Stefan-Meier-Str. 26, D-79104 Freiburg, Germany
[2] Center for Dental Medicine, Department of Operative Dentistry and Periodontology, Faculty of Medicine and Medical Center, University of Freiburg, Hugstetter Straße 55, D-79106 Freiburg, Germany; ali.al-ahmad@uniklinik-freiburg.de (A.A.-A.); annette.anderson@uniklinik-freiburg.de (A.A.); johan.woelber@uniklinik-freiburg.de (J.P.W.); elmar.hellwig@uniklinik-freiburg.de (E.H.)
[3] Clinic for Conservative and Preventive Dentistry, Center of Dental Medicine, University of Zurich, Plattenstrasse 11, CH-8032 Zurich, Switzerland; Lamprini.Karygianni@zzm.uzh.ch
[4] Institute of Medical Microbiology and Hygiene, Department of Medical Microbiology and Hygiene, Faculty of Medicine and Medical Center, University of Freiburg, Hermann-Herder-Straße 11, D-79104 Freiburg, Germany; annette.wittmer@uniklinik-freiburg.de
* Correspondence: kv@imbi.uni-freiburg.de; Tel.: +49-761-203-5004

Citation: Vach, K.; Al-Ahmad, A.; Anderson, A.; Woelber, J.P.; Karygianni, L.; Wittmer, A.; Hellwig, E. A Log Ratio-Based Analysis of Individual Changes in the Composition of the Oral Microbiota in Different Dietary Phases. *Nutrients* 2021, 13, 793. https://doi.org/10.3390/nu13030793

Academic Editor: Eva Untersmayr

Received: 1 February 2021
Accepted: 23 February 2021
Published: 28 February 2021

Publisher's Note: MDPI stays neutral with regard to jurisdictional claims in published maps and institutional affiliations.

Abstract: Background: Investigating the influence of nutrition on oral health has a long scientific history. Due to recent technical advances like sequencing techniques for the oral microbiota, this topic has gained scientific interest again. A basic challenge is to understand the influence of nutrition on the oral microbiota and on the interaction between the oral bacteria, which is also statistically challenging. Methods: Log-transformed ratios of two bacteria concentrations are introduced as the basic analytic tool. The framework is illustrated by application in an experimental study exposing eleven participants to different nutrition schemes in five consecutive phases. Results: The method could be sufficiently used to analyse the interrelation between the bacteria and to identify some bacterial groups with the same as well as different reactions to additional dietary components. It was found that the strongest changes in bacterial concentrations were achieved by the additional consumption of dairy products. Conclusion: A log ratio-based analysis offers insights into the relation of different bacteria while taking specific features of compositional data into account. The presented methods allow becoming independent of the behaviour of other bacteria, which is a disadvantage of common analysis methods of compositions. The results indicate that modulations of the oral biofilm microbiota due to nutrition change can be attained.

Keywords: compositional data; ratio fractions; nutrition; microbiome; oral health

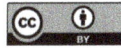
1. Introduction

In recent years, the influence of nutrition on oral biofilm has received increasing attention. Dietary factors have a major influence on the microbiota of the oral biofilm and can lead to disturbances of the homeostasis of the more than 700 bacterial species within its complex network. For example, frequent consumption of simple carbohydrates can favour acidogenic and acidiuric bacterial species, consequently leading to carious lesions [1]. On the other hand, frequent consumption of dairy products, dietary fibre and certain vegetable foods is associated with lower caries incidence [2–4]. The calcium, phosphate and casein phosphopeptides contained in dairy products can counteract acidic demineralisation and promote remineralisation processes, thus having a caries preventive effect. In terms of plant-based foods, different ingredients are concerned with either promoting remineralisation (e.g., phosphates) or reducing bacterial adhesion and growth, thereby reducing the risk of caries development [1,5–7]. It is known that simple carbohydrates can lead to a higher proportion of acidogenic and aciduric species, which can promote the development of carious lesions [8]. Concerning the different bacterial species involved in the caries process, for a long time, mutans streptococci and lactobacilli were thought to be the main species responsible for the acid production and demineralisation of the tooth structure. However, in recent years it has become clear that various additional bacterial species are associated with different stages of caries development: non-mutans streptococci, such as *Streptococcus salivarius* and *Streptococcus parasanguinis*, and species of the genus *Actinomyces* have been associated with the initial stages, while *Veillonella* spp., *Lactobacillus* spp., *Atopobium* spp. and other taxa dominate the more advanced stages [9–11]. The effect of nutrition on the oral microbiota has mostly been investigated with either in vitro experimental approaches, testing individual ingredients, using animal experiments or analysing epidemiological data. In this paper, we consider a study analysing the influence of certain foods on the whole microbiota of the oral biofilm, was tested in situ using splint systems worn by study participants on which the oral biofilm was grown. The bacterial composition of the oral biofilm was then analysed by culture technique [1].

When analysing this type of oral biofilm data, it is common practice to examine the fractions of total concentration rather than the pure concentrations. These fractions sum up to 1, which causes special challenges in terms of the statistical analysis. Data of this kind are called compositional data, and its analysis has attracted strong attention in recent years [12–16]. We present a case study, in which we apply a log ratio-based approach to oral biofilm data. This approach allows analysing changes in the composition when additional standardised dietary intakes are available and the interest lies in comparing with one baseline condition (regular diet).

2. Materials and Methods

2.1. The Data

We consider a study funded by the German Research Foundation (DFG) with eleven participants and data investigating the influence of additional standardised diet components on the microbiota of the oral biofilm over 15 months. The participants underwent five phases, each of which lasted three months. During these phases, standardised dietary components in the form of sucrose, dairy products and vegetables in addition to the regular diet were investigated. Phase I was a lead-in phase without changing the nutrition habits. In phase II, participants consumed an additional 10 g of rock candy per day (Weisser Kandis; Südzucker AG, Mannheim, Germany), sucking small pieces of 2 g five times in between meals. In phase III, additional milk products were consumed (150 g of plain yoghurt 3 times daily and 100 mL of long-life milk twice a day, both 1.5% fat; Schwarzwaldmilch GmbH, Freiburg, Germany). In phase IV, 500 g of vegetable puree (types: white carrot, parsnip, carrot, "jardinière" (carrot, potato, cauliflower and pea), pumpkin and garden vegetables (carrot, potato, spinach, parsnip and leeks), Reine Weiße Karotte, Reine Pastinake, Reine Frühkarotte, and Gemüse-Allerlei (Hipp GmbH, Pfaffenhofen, Germany) and Kürbis pur and Gartengemüse (Alnatura, Darmstadt, Germany)) per day was given, before the participants returned to their individual regular diet in phase V.

An in situ splint system was used to sample the dental plaque. Individual upper jaw rigid acrylic appliances were manufactured for each study participant [17]. The splint system was taken out and stored in saline solution (0.9% NaCl) for regular meals and during oral hygiene only. It was worn while consuming the phase-specific additional foods, which were eaten slowly to expose them to the oral cavity for several minutes. During all phases, the oral biofilm was allowed to grow on embedded enamel slabs over the course of seven days. Subsequently, the splint system was removed for analysis of the oral biofilm, cleaned and after seven days it was reapplied for another seven days. This procedure was repeated three times all together. Participants brushed their teeth with standardised tooth brushes and toothpaste with a sodium fluoride content of 1450 ppm.

The oral biofilm grown in all five phases was analysed using culture techniques averaging over three measurements, which were taken within four weeks per phase.

Twenty-seven groups of bacteria were identified from a total of 93 different cultivated species. Details about the course of the study and data collection can be found in [18,19].

A main focus of this work was to ascertain whether the additional standardised dietary intake leads to changes in oral microbiota. It makes sense to only consider bacteria that are usually above the detection limit. According to the results of [19], only disjunct bacterial groups were chosen, where the percentage of values above the detection limit was greater than 75%. All values below the detection limit were set to the detection limit. The bacterial groups together with the colour scheme that we use in all of our figures can be found in Figure 1. A detailed list can be found in the Appendices A and B.

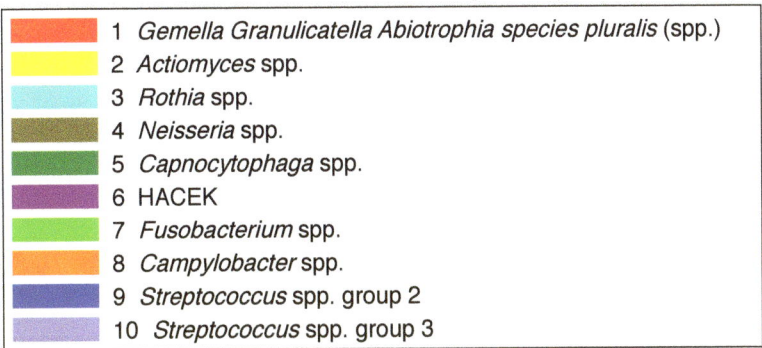

Figure 1. Bacterial groups and colour scheme for all figures.

If the sum of the concentrations of the bacterial groups listed here is used as the total concentration, the fractions of the single bacterial groups sum up to 1 and the data has a compositional character. For each bacterial group, participant and phase, the starting point is considered to be its fraction among the total concentration of the analysed bacterial groups.

2.2. Analytic Strategy

1. For each pair of bacteria, the ratio between the two fractions is built for each participant and phase. Such a pairwise ratio directly depicts the relation between two bacteria. They do not depend on the concentration of the other bacteria or the overall concentration. If a third bacterium has an unusually high or low concentration, this affects the overall concentration and hence the fractions, but it does not affect the ratio. Therefore, in this way we become independent of the behaviour of other bacteria. Ratios also have a simple direct interpretation describing how more frequent one bacterium is compared with the other. Note that a ratio between two fractions can also be interpreted directly as the ratio between two corresponding concentrations.

2. The second step is to consider the logarithm with the base 10 of the ratio. This is useful because ratios tend to have a skewed and unstable distribution, whereas taking logarithms leads to a more symmetric distribution of the values. The basis 10 was chosen due to its strong interpretability: a value of 1 in the log_{10} scale means the tenfold in the real concentration setting. A ratio of 1—i.e., equal concentrations—has a value of 0 in the log_{10} setting. For ratios smaller than 1, the log_{10} transformed value becomes negative. Therefore, a positive (negative) value means that the first bacteria is less (more) frequent than the second one.

3. Logarithmising the ratios leads to one number per participant and phase, which can be analysed just like any other number [15]. In particular, mean values and standard deviations can be calculated. In this step, for each pair of bacteria we consider the mean value of the log ratios across all participants per phase. It is interpretable as the typical relationship between these two bacteria in this phase. Therefore, this

mean value offers the opportunity to check, whether the relationship between two bacteria is similar in different phases or whether it changes due to changes in the nutrition. Accordingly, we can analyse the stability between bacteria between the phases. Similarly as above, a mean value of 1 suggests that typically the first bacterium has ten times the concentration of the second bacterium.

4. We also analyse the corresponding standard deviations, which are a measure of the stability of the relationship between two bacteria within one phase. The closer that the value is to 0, the more homogeneous are the values across participants, i.e., the relation between the two considered bacteria is stable and can thus be assumed as "typical". For example, if we observe a standard deviation of 0.5 and a mean log ratio of 0 for two bacteria, then the application of the 2 sigma rule leads to a 95% range of $(-1, 1)$, i.e., 95% of the observed ratios are between $1/10$ and 10.

5. As the aim is to study the impact of an additional standardised diet on the microbiome, we also depict the changes of the concentrations compared with the first phase. For a given pair of bacteria, for each participant and phase we consider the difference in the log ratio compared with the first phase. A difference above 0 means that the ratio increased, i.e., the first bacterium became more frequent relative to the second one. As a difference in the log ratio is equal to the logarithm of the ratio of ratios, we can also interpret the values themselves. A difference of 1 means, that the ratio has increased by a factor of ten. For example, this may reflect a change from 1.2 to 12, or from 0.3 to 3. Again, we can consider mean values and standard deviations across participants per phase for phases II to V. The mean values inform us about the typical change in the relation between the two bacteria. The standard deviations offer a hint about the stability of these changes across the participants.

6. Finally, we also consider a bacterium-specific summary measure, which is based on averaging the log ratio changes for one bacterium over all other bacteria within a single participant If this way a bacterium has a value greater than 0, this can be interpreted as having increased its fraction on average relative to all other bacteria. The bacterium with the largest positive value is the one with the most distinct increase compared with all other bacteria. We refer to this value for each participant as the average log ratio change.

A detailed mathematical description of the different quantities can be found in the Appendix B. For all means and standard deviations, 95% confidence intervals can be computed using statistical standard methods. We only report them for the most fundamental analyses, focussing on the mean values in pairs and the mean average log ratios. For the analyses, the statistics program STATA (StataCorp LT, College Station, TX, USA, Version 16.1) was used. For graphical presentation, bar and pie charts, scatter plots and forest plots were used.

2.3. Analysing Change or Comparing Phases Directly

In studies using a baseline condition, it is usual to consider the individual changes from the baseline, in order to investigate the impact of the subsequent conditions. However, this is not necessarily the most adequate strategy in the context of this study. It may be the case that the standardised dietary additions imply that all participants exhibit a common composition in each phase, overruling the individual differences at the baseline. In such a scenario, it would be more adequate to compare the composition directly between the conditions instead of investigating the change from the baseline. The standard deviations of the log ratios will inform us about the homogeneity of bacteria spectra in each phase, whereby we will be able to judge whether the scenario is present or not.

3. Results

3.1. A First Look at the Raw Data

In Figure 2, the fractions of the total concentrations for all ten bacterial groups are shown for each participant for each of the five phases. If the nutrition leads to a certain bacteria pattern, the pictures would have to be similar in one line each, while they would differ in the columns. This should at least apply from phase II to phase IV, as a change to a specific additional diet took place from this point onwards. However, instead of uniform patterns in each phase, we observe rather individual pattern across phases, similar to phase I. Here, the different patterns are unsurprising for the different participants, because the nutrition was in no way influenced.

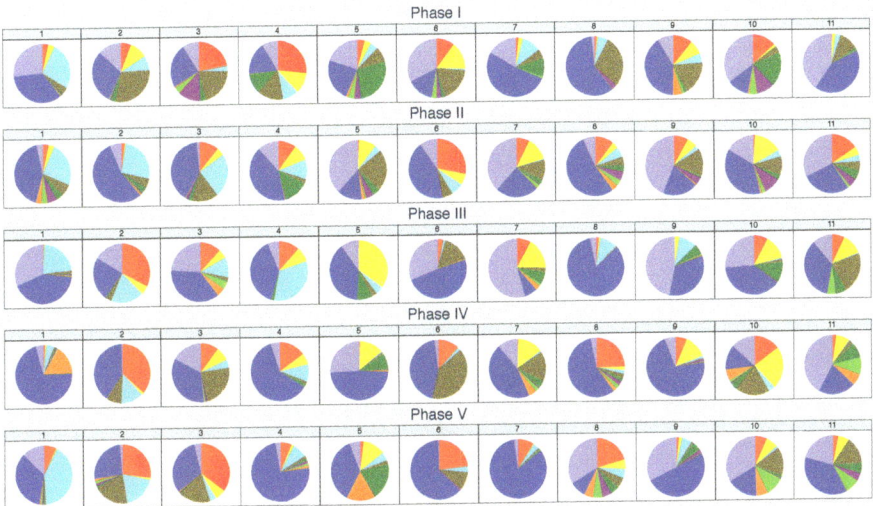

Figure 2. Fractions of the bacterial groups on the total concentration per participant (column) and phase (row) based on mean values per phase.

If we now consider the mean values per phase (Figure 3), we see that specific bacterial groups are actually rather common in all phases. We also observe that the differences between the phases are quite small.

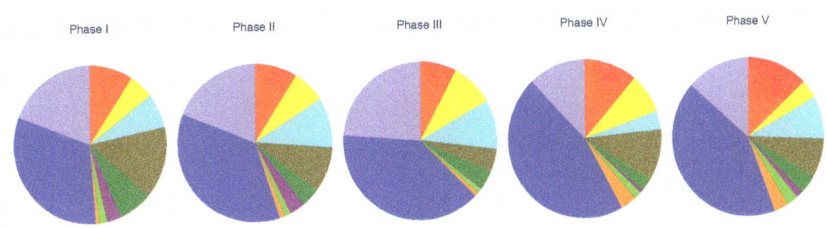

Figure 3. Fractions of the bacterial groups on the total concentration per phase based on mean values per phase.

3.2. Stability of the Relation between Bacterial Groups between Phases

The relation between two bacterial groups may remain stable between the phases, or it may change. Stability may indicate that the relation is minimally affected by changes in nutrition, whereas instability may indicate sensitivity to changes. For each combination of two bacterial groups, we look at the log ratio for each participant in each phase and consider the phase-specific mean value. We can see in Figure 4 that there are differences between the pairs. At the bottom of the picture, we find pairs, where the relation to each other is very similar over all phases. At the top of the picture, we see pairs with distinct differences across the phases. Note that among the pairs with the lowest variation in the mean log ratio, we find bacterial group numbers 1, 3, 5 and 7 several times. In four instances we find bacterial group 1, and twice we find bacterial groups 3, 5 and 7. In particular, all combinations of the bacterial groups 1, 3 and 5 are among the pairs with the lowest variation in the mean log ratio.

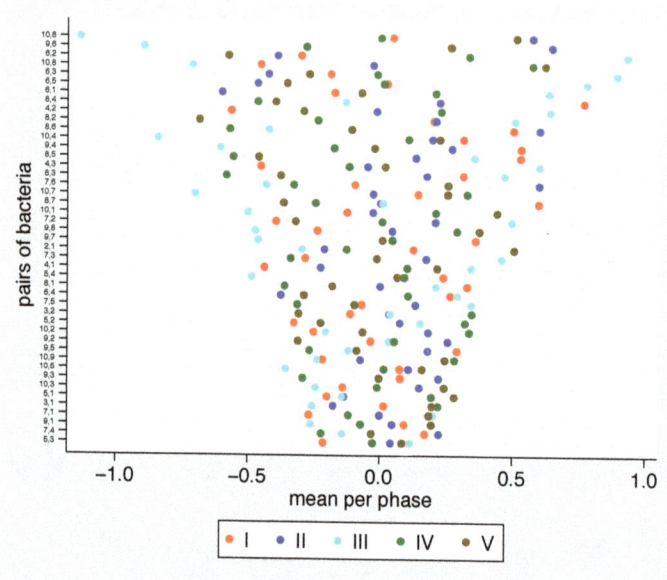

Figure 4. Mean log ratios for all bacterial pairs of bacterial groups and phases. The values are centred around 0 for each bacterial pair. The bacterial pairs are ordered according to the range of the mean values.

Further, the mean log ratio in phase III is often far on the left or far on the right, i.e., in this phase we see the most extreme ratios.

3.3. Stability of the Relation between Bacterial Groups within Phases

The mean values above offer a hint whether the pairwise relation between bacterial groups is common in different phases. Now the question remains how stable the pairwise relation between bacterial groups is within one phase. Therefore, we take a look at the standard deviations of the phase-specific log ratios in Figure 5.

Some bacterial pairs show low values for all phases, such as 9-3, 9-10, 9-1, 5-2, 10-2 and 10-5. This means that the relation between these bacteria is stable within participants within each phase. However, even for these pairs we observe standard deviations in the magnitude of 0.5 or above, indicating rather wide 95% ranges across participants. This corresponds with the high individual variation observed in Figure 2. It is interesting to note that all six of these bacterial pairs also showed a low variation in mean values across the phases. They were all among the fourteen bacterial pairs (out of 45) with lowest range in Figure 4, i.e., these bacterial pairs tend to be stable in their relation across participants *and* phases. The opposite relation does not seem to hold: the bacterial pairs 5-3, 7-1 and 5-1 show little variation in mean values, but nevertheless high standard deviations within each phase. For some bacterial pairs, the stability substantially varies across the phases. For example, the bacterial pairs 8-1 and 7-1 show high stability in phase I and low stability in other phases, suggesting that the specific dietary supplements destroy a rather stable relation seen at the baseline. Another example is the bacterial pair 4-3, where phase III shows a much higher standard deviation than the other phases.

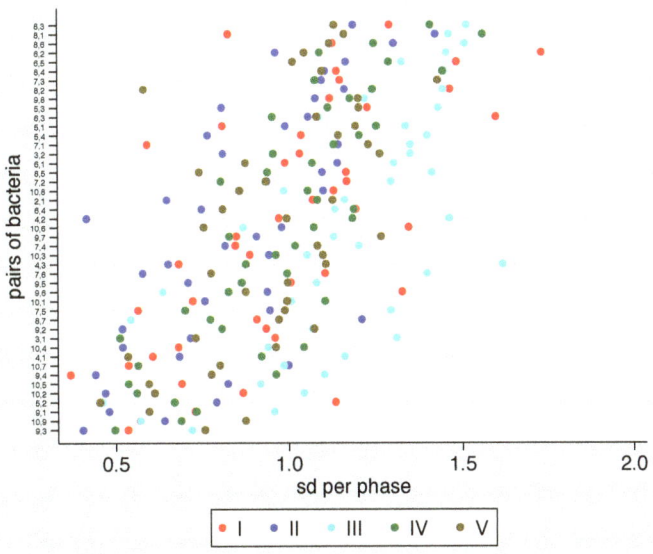

Figure 5. Standard deviations (sd) for phase-specific log ratios for all bacterial pairs of bacterial groups and phases based on empirical estimates. The pairs are sorted by the mean sd value over all phases.

If we compare the phases I–IV (the nutrition in phase V was analogous to phase I by study design), the lowest standard deviation can be found in twelve out of 45 bacterial pairs in phase I, suggesting that there is no tendency towards a more uniform composition after standardised dietary supplementation. Therefore, there is no argument against analysing the changes, i.e., the changes from the baseline.

3.4. Identification of Bacterial Pairs with a Change in Relation in Comparison with the Baseline

In Figure 6, the mean log ratio changes with 95% confidence intervals for all pairs of bacteria are shown. While in phase II the additional diet only leads to few changes, more reactions can be observed in the other phases. The observed patterns are very similar in phases IV and V. Overall, we have to conclude that definitive statements about a "statistically significant" change in the relation in one specific phase are difficult to justify, as only few of the overall 180 confidence intervals do not include 0. However, in phase III eleven, in phase IV seven and in phase V six out of 45 confidence intervals do not include 0, i.e., we observe more than the 2.25 that we should expect under chance level. Consequently, the observed mean log ratio changes do not simply reflect random noise.

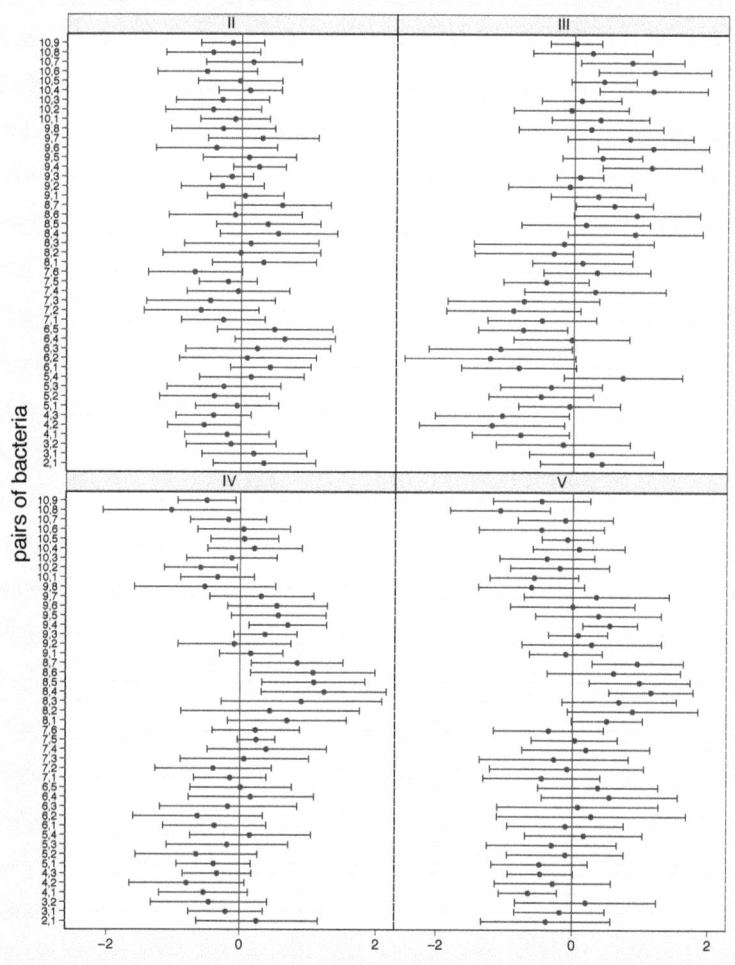

Figure 6. Mean log ratio changes for all bacterial pairs for phases II–V with 95% confidence intervals.

3.5. Stability of Change in Relation between Phases

To gain a better overview of these numbers and in particular the relation to the different phases, in Figure 7 we show the phase-specific mean values for each bacterial pair. We have sorted the pairs of bacteria by (a) their range within the different phases (small ranges on the bottom, larger ranges on the top) and (b) by the mean over the phases. In Figure 7a, we observe that the bacterial pairs 5-3, 7-1, 8-7, 5-1, 7-4, 9-1 and 9-5 show the smallest range, meaning that they show a common reaction on the additional diet in all phases, while the bacterial pairs 10-6, 9-6, 6-2, 10-8, 6-3, 6-5 and 6-1 show a large variation in their reactions in different phases. Additionally, one can see in Figure 7b that the bacterial pairs 4-2, 4-3, 4-1, 7-2, 5-2, 7-1, 10-2, 5-3 and 5-1 (8-4, 8-7, 9-4, 8-5, 9-7, 8-1, 10-4 and 9-5) show a positive (negative) value in all phases, meaning that the second bacterium tends to be more (less) frequent than the first one in each phase. Several bacterial pairs show relation changes into different directions in different phases, which could be a sign that they react differently to the nutrition change.

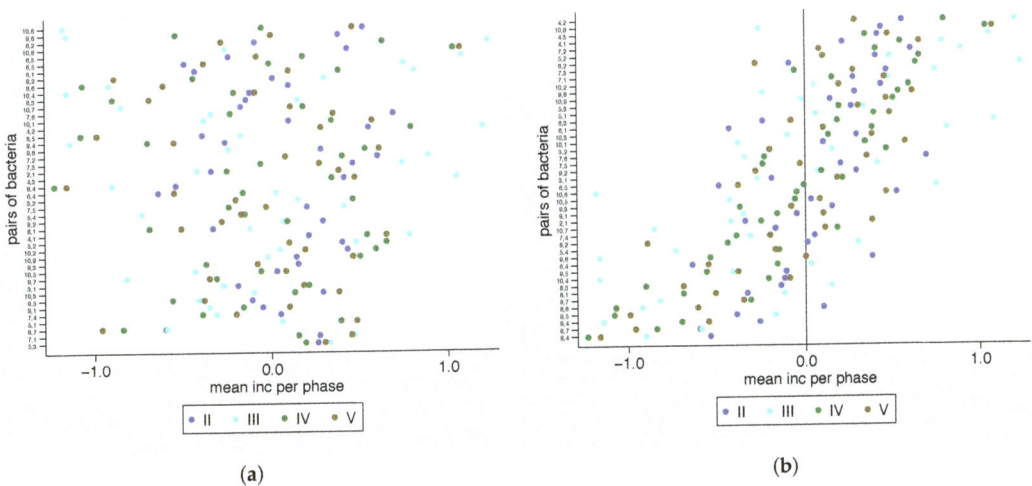

(a)

(b)

Figure 7. Mean values for phase-based log ratios for changes for all pairs of bacteria and phases sorted by range (**a**) and mean (**b**).

3.6. Stability of Change in Relation within Phases

The corresponding estimated standard deviations are shown in Figure 8. We observe some bacterial pairs, where the reaction to the additional diet is rather uniform across participants in all phases. These are nearly the same bacterial pairs such as in Figure 5, namely, 9-3, 7-5, 10-9, 10-5, 9-4, 9-1, 4-1 and 10-1. The bacterial pairs that always show high instability—6-2,8-2, 8-3, 6-3 and 7-3—are also nearly identical to the former observations. Note that only the pairs 9-1, 9-5, 9-4 and 8-7 with low variation in mean values across the phases also show stability within phases. By contrast, we observe lower values in standard deviations for the bacterial pair 10-1, but high variation in mean values. The least uniform reaction often occurs in phase III.

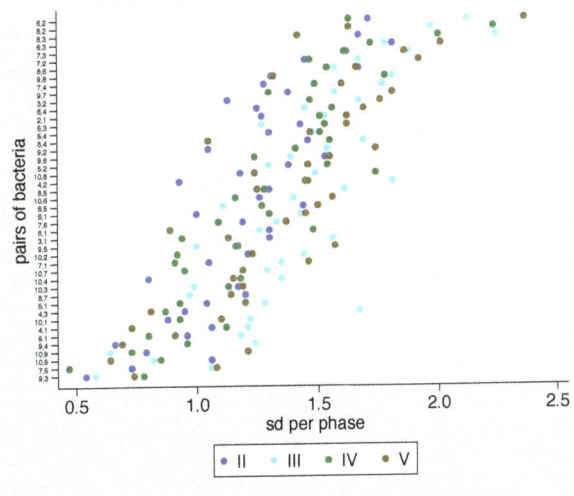

Figure 8. Standard deviation (sd) for phase-based log ratios for changes for all pairs of bacteria and phases estimated empirical and sorted by mean of sd over the phases.

3.7. Interim Summary

In Table 1, we present an overview of the results of the four previous analyses: the bacterial pairs with the lowest or highest stability in the four different analyses are marked with letters differentiating between the analyses performed on the raw values (small letters) and on change values (capital letters) and between analyses within and between phases.

Table 1. Overview of results from the analyses in Sections 3.2–3.6: The ten bacterial pairs with the highest (half-matrix left bottom) and the lowest (half-matrix right top) stability in each analysis are marked with b (between) and w (within) phases and corresponding capital letters for changes in comparison to baseline.

	1	*2*	*3*	*4*	*5*	*6*	*7*	*8*	*9*	*10*
1						*bB*		*w*		
2				*b*		*bwBW*	*W*	*bwBW*		
3	bB				*w*	*bBW*	*wW*	*wW*		
4	wW		W				*W*	*bw*		*B*
5	bBW	w	bB	W		*bwB*				
6								*wBW*	*bB*	*bB*
7	bB		bB	W					*W*	
8							B		*wW*	*bB*
9	bwBW		bwW	w	B		B			
10	W	w	bB	w	bwW		w		bwW	

For example, the bacterial pair 3-1 is among the ten bacterial pairs with the highest stability with respect to the analysis of the pairwise relation between phases and the change in relation between phases, and thus it is marked as bB. The bacterial pair 4-8 is among the ten bacterial pairs with the lowest stability when analysing the pairwise bacterial relation between and within phases, and thus it is marked with *bw*. First of all, we can state that many pairs can be found more than once among those with the highest (or lowest) stability, indicating a rather robust classification as "stable" (or "unstable"). Sub-patterns that we typically observe are bB and wW, indicating that analysing raw values or changes provide similar results. This mainly reflects the fact that high stability in raw values also implies some stability in changes, and that low stability in raw values also makes a low stability in changes likely if the correlation between phases is only moderate.

Conceptually, it is more interesting whether stability within phases coincides with stability between phases, i.e., the bwBW pattern in the lower triangle. We can identify one bacterial pair (1-9) with high stability across all analyses. The bacterial pairs 1-5, 3-9, 5-10 and 9-10 show high stability in at least both a within-phase and between-phase analysis of the same values (bw or BW sub-pattern in the lower triangle). The relation between these pair of bacteria seems to be difficult to modify by dietary supplements or other external factors. On the other hand, we can identify two bacterial pairs with low stability in all analyses: 2-6 and 2-8 (i.e., the *bwBW* pattern in the upper triangle) and the bacterial pairs 3-6, 4-8 and 6-8 with low stability in at least both a within-phase and between-phase analysis (*bw* or *BW* sub-pattern in the upper triangle). The relation between these pairs of bacteria seems to be highly modifiable by diet as well as other external factors.

Pairs with high stability within phases but low stability between phases might hold the strongest interest, as these are the pairs that most distinctly react to the dietary supplements. Indeed, we can find one of such pairs 4-10 (w, W or wW in the lower triangle and *b*, *B* or *bB* in the upper triangle). Interestingly, there are also three pairs with the opposite pattern: 3-5, 4-7 and 7-9 (*w*, *W* or *wW* in the upper triangle and b, B or bB in the lower triangle), i.e., high stability between phases but low stability within phases. Finally, note that bacterial groups 6 and 8 have an entry together with nearly all other bacterial groups in the upper triangle with low stability to other bacterial groups, while the bacterial group 1 is marked with most of the bacterial groups in the lower triangle with high stability. This may reflect the notion that bacterial group 1 is rather stable and bacterial groups 6 and 8 are rather unstable. Bacterial group 10 is striking: while it still showed little variation among the participants, one has a large variation between the phases.

3.8. Average Log Ratio Changes

Figure 9 shows the mean values of the average log ratio changes for each bacterial group in each phase. Definite statements about a specific change in a specific phase are difficult to make, as only few confidence intervals do not include 0. However, we observe that some bacterial groups tend to increase (bacterial group 8) or decrease in frequency (4, 7) for all phases, whereas other bacterial groups tend to differ in the direction of change over phases (e.g., 6, 10). We see the smallest overall changes in phase II. In Figure 10, within each phase we sort the bacterial groups by mean values of the average log changes to focus on the phase-specific pattern in the change of the bacterial spectrum. A striking feature here is the similarity of the pattern between phases IV and V. This is quite astonishing, as in phase V the same nutrition is given as with the baseline. One possible explanation would be that the effect of the nutrition change will last longer.

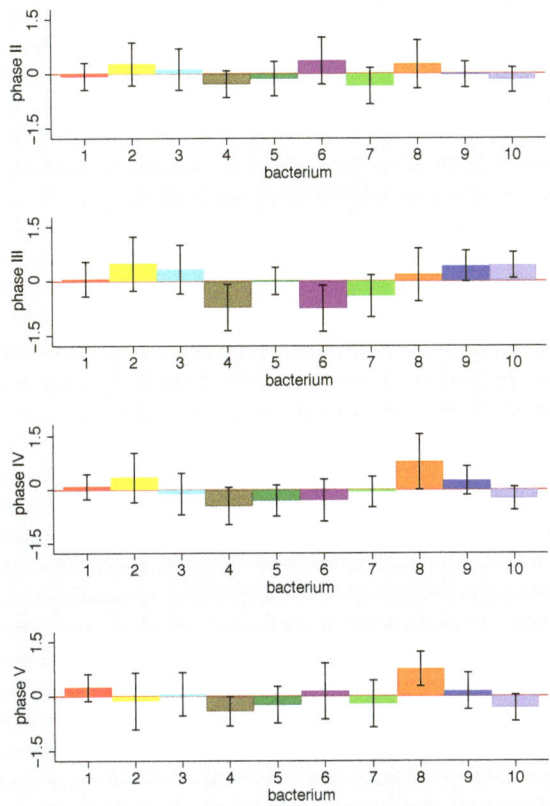

Figure 9. Mean values of average log ratio changes with 95% CI for bacterial groups 1 to 10 for phase II (**top**) to phase V (**bottom**). For colour scheme, see Figure 1.

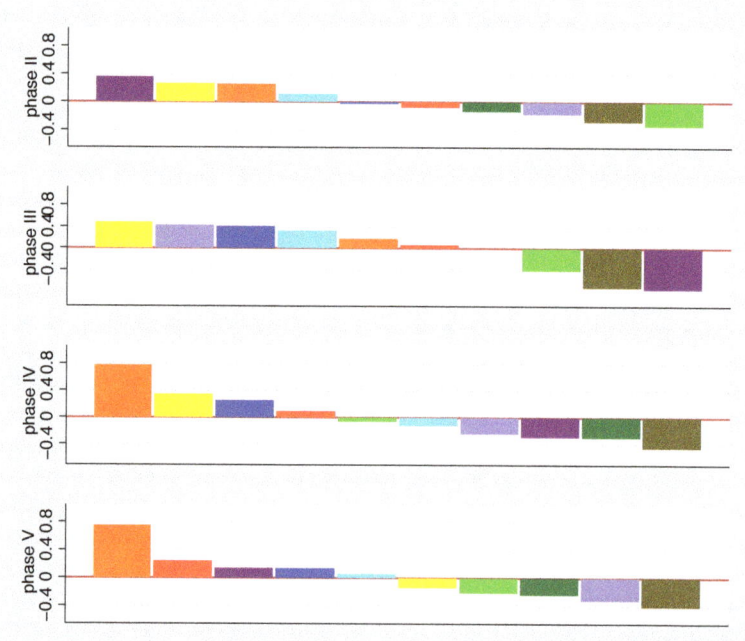

Figure 10. Mean values of average log ratio changes sorted for bacterial groups 1 to 10 for phase II (**top**) to phase V (**bottom**). For colour scheme, see Figure 1.

3.8.1. Global *p*-Value Per Phase

When looking at the single bacterial species, the question remains whether a global effect per phase can be observed, i.e., which additional diet led to a concentration change in nearly all bacterial groups. The global *p*-value (Table 2, the test used is explained in Appendix B.2) only shows a value that comes near to significance ($p = 0.055$) for phase III.

Table 2. Global *p*-value per phase.

	Phase II	Phase III	Phase IV	Phase V
p-value	0.459	0.055	0.096	0.289

3.9. Similarity of Change Pattern Across Bacterial Groups

Figures 6 and 10 indicate some similarity in how bacterial groups react to the additional diet across different phases. We investigate this in more detail in Figure 11. We observe stronger correlations for phase II against phase V and phase IV against V. This impression is strengthened if we look in more detail at the left bottom, where all bacterial combinations are plotted.

The correlation coefficients (Table 3) confirm this impression.

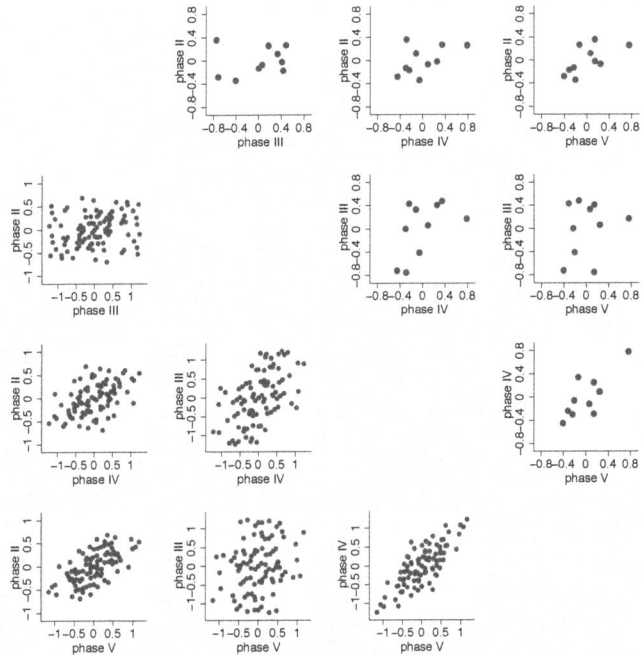

Figure 11. Scatter plots of the mean values of bacterial groups' specific average log ratio changes. Half-matrix right top: mean value for each bacterial group in one phase against the other phases. Half-matrix left bottom: mean value for each bacterial pair in one phase against the other phases.

Table 3. Correlation coefficients for bacterial groups' specific average log ratio changes between phases.

	Phase III	Phase IV	Phase V
Phase II	0.199	0.488	0.628
Phase III		0.528	0.205
Phase IV			0.780

4. Discussion

In this paper, we have presented an advantageous statistical approach to analyse a study investigating the influence of specific additional diets on the bacterial composition in the oral microbiota in an experimental manner. Traditionally, such analyses are focused on the (absolute or relative) concentration of the single bacterial species. Here, we adopt a different approach, looking at all pairs of bacteria and focusing on the quantitative relation of the two bacteria within each pair.

While this approach naturally adds complexity, it has one basic conceptual advantage that is particularly important when analysing a change in the spectrum: if the concentration or fraction of one bacterium increases or decreases distinctly, this does not directly affect the relation between any other pair of bacteria. Indeed, the simultaneous investigation of all bacterial pairs revealed that there are some pairs of bacteria that have a rather stable relation across participants within each phase. Some of them also have a rather stable relation across the phases, while some do not. Similar behaviour can be observed when examining the changes compared with the baseline.

It is rather natural that the simultaneous consideration of all bacterial pairs is not very useful to allow very specific statements for single pairs, in particular if the sample size is limited, as in our study. The general approach is mainly useful to draw an overall picture of bacterial correlation with the diet of the different phases of this longitudinal clinical study. For example, it became rather obvious that the diet of phase II had a lower impact on the composition than the dietary supplement in phases III and IV. Additionally, we could not observe the expected move back to the baseline scenario in phase V.

We could also address the fundamental question of whether an analysis of the study should focus on the individual changes in composition or on a typical composition for each nutrition. We found no evidence for the latter, and thus could stick to the intended analysis of the changes relative to the baseline.

With respect to the concrete insights gained by our analysis, the main results present the following points:

1. The bacterial pair *Gemella Granulicatella A.* spp.–*Streptococcus* spp. group 2 is the one with high stability across all analyses.
2. The bacterial pairs *Actiomyces.* spp.–HACEK and *Actiomyces.* spp.–*Campylobacter* spp. are the bacterial pairs with low stability across all analyses.
3. The bacterial pair *Neisseria* spp.–*Streptococcus* spp. group 3 could be identified as the bacterial pair that most distinctly reacts to the dietary supplements.
4. Bacterial pairs with high stability in at least both a within-phase and between-phase analysis were *Gemella Granulicatella A.* spp.–*Capnocytophaga* spp., *Rothia* spp.–*Streptococcus* spp. group 2, *Capnocytophaga* spp.–*Streptococcus* spp. group 3 and *Streptococcus* spp. group 2–*Streptococcus* spp. group 3.
5. The most distinct changes in the spectrum were observed in phase III, i.e., the phase with additional milk products. In particular, the relation of *Neisseria* spp. to *Streptococcus* spp. group 2 and group 3 changed. When looking at the single bacterial species, the most distinct change was a decrease of *Neisseria* spp. and HACEK.
6. In phases IV and V, when looking at the single bacterial species, the increase of *Campylobacter* spp. should be mentioned. On the other hand, the figures in phases IV and V were very similar, although in phase V the participants returned to their individual nutrition without specific additions.
7. For *Gemella Granulicatella A.* spp., *Rothia* spp. and *Streptococcus* spp. group 3, we observed rather stable relations to other bacterial groups, while for HACEK and *Campylobacter* spp. the relations are rather variable.

At least some of these findings can be explained. As *Gemella Granulicatella A.* spp. and *Streptococcus* spp. groups 2 and 3 are kinds of the *Streptococcus* species or relatives, they can all utilise the same substrate, and consequently a similar reaction is unsurprising. This explains our main result 1 and partly the results 4 and 7. HACEK are fastidious microorganisms, which could be an explanation for the fact that they also react quickly and strongly to changing environmental conditions, which supports the results 2, 5 and 7. The high variability of *Campylobacter* spp. (result 6 and 7) could be explained by the fact that in the presence of *Actiomyces* spp. and *Streptococcs* spp. the formate can be utilised by *Campylobacter* spp., which *Actiomyces* spp. and *Streptococcus* spp. produce in glycolysis.

Note that though different microbial compositions were revealed in the different diet phases and mainly after the additional consumption of dairy products, the detected bacterial species have different potential for fermentation of carbohydrates by glycolysis leading to acids like formate, acetate and propionate. To avoid demineralisation of enamel and subsequently caries development a balanced diet is required which can sustain a balanced microbial composition of the supragingival oral biofilm.

Further Insights

In this type of experimental setup, it cannot be expected that the individual oral biofilm returns to its original composition in a short time when participants are allowed to return to their individual nutrition without studying specific additions. Inspection of the diaries of the participants suggests that they did indeed return to the individual nutrition and did not continue to use higher levels of carbohydrates, fats and proteins. Further research including a combination of different microbiological analysing methods is necessary to understand whether this observation is indeed due to a long-lasting effect of nutrition on the oral biofilm. This would have a direct impact on the design of future studies.

In contrast to the DNA-based molecular determination technique of the microbiome, the culture technique depicts active and viable bacteria [20]. In a comprehensive analysis of the microbiota of endodontic infections, the authors of the aforementioned study even showed that some bacterial species, that could be isolated and identified by the culture technique could not be detected by the culture-independent cloning technique. On the other hand, it has been shown that up to 50% of the oral bacteria could not be detected by the culture technique [21]. Zaura et al. [22] showed that healthy individuals exposed to a single antibiotic treatment undergo considerable microbial shifts of the microbiome of their faeces, while their salivary microbiome composition remains more robust and stable. The minor changes in bacterial composition revealed in the present study deliver another hint regarding the stability of the oral microbiota, including in the supragingival oral biofilm.

5. Conclusions

Systematically considering the log ratio of concentrations between bacterial pairs has offered new insights into the influence of nutrition on the oral biofilm and the relation of specific bacterial groups with each other. The methods make it possible to circumvent some typical problems encountered in the analysis of compositional data.

Author Contributions: A.A.-A., A.A., J.P.W. and E.H. designed the original study. L.K. and A.A. coordinated the sample collection and participated in data analysis. K.V. had the idea for the topic, performed the statistical analysis and designed the figures. All authors edited the manuscript and approved the final article. All authors have read and agreed to the published version of the manuscript.

Funding: This study was supported by the German Research Foundation (DFG, AL-1179/2-1). The article processing charge was funded by the Baden-Württemberg Ministry of Science, Research and Art and the University of Freiburg in the Open Access Publishing funding program. The funding had no influence on the design of the study and collection, analysis and interpretation of data and in writing the manuscript.

Institutional Review Board Statement: The study was conducted according to the guidelines of the Declaration of Helsinki, and approved by the Ethics Committee of the University of Freiburg (Nr. 237/14). All experiments and data collections were performed in accordance with relevant guidelines and regulations.

Informed Consent Statement: A written informed consent was obtained from all participants involved in the study.

Data Availability Statement: The data are available on request from the authors.

Acknowledgments: The authors thank Werner Vach for critical remarks.

Conflicts of Interest: The authors report no conflicts of interest.

Sample Availability: The data are available on request from the authors.

Appendix A. Description of the Bacterial Groups

- *Gemella Granulicatella Abiotrophia* spp.: *Gemella morbillorum, Gemella haemolysans, Gemella sanguinis, Granulicatella adiacens, Granulicatella elegans, Abiotrophia defectiva*
- *Actinomyces* spp.: *Actinomyces oris, Actinomyces odontolyticus, Actinomyces dentalis, Actinomyces georgiae, Actinomyces naeslundii*
- *Rothia* spp.: *Rothia mucilaginosa, Rothia dentocariosa, Rothia aeria, Corynebacterium* spp.

- *Neisseria* spp.: *Neisseria macacae/mucosa, Neisseria oralis, Neisseria subflava, Neisseria bacilliformis, Neisseria elongata, Neisseria flavescens, Neisseria perflava, Neisseria cinerea, Lautrop mirabilis*
- *Capnocytophaga* spp.: *Capnocytophaga granulosa, Capnocytophaga gingivalis, Capnocytophaga ochracea, Capnocytophaga sputigena*
- HACEK: *Haemophilus haemolyticus, Haemophilus parahaemolyticus, Haemophilus parainfluenzae, Haemophilus influenzae, Cardiobacterium hominis, Eikenella corrodens, Kingella* spp.
- *Fusobacterium* spp.: *Fusobacterium nucleatum,Fusobacterium periodontium*
- *Campylobacter* spp.: *Campylobacter rectus, Campylobacter concisus, Campylobacter showae*
- *Streptococcus* spp. group 2: *Streptococcus oralis, Streptococcus mitis, Streptococcus infantis, Streptococcus australis, Streptococcus peroris, Streptococcus salivarius, Streptococcus vestibularis, Streptococcus anginosus* group
- *Streptococcus* spp. group 3: *Streptococcus sanguinis, Streptococcus parasanguinis, Streptococcus gordonii*

Appendix B. Materials and Methods

Appendix B.1. Notation

Let f_{ip}^{b} denote the fraction of bacterium b in participant i and phase p.

Appendix B.1.1. Log Ratio-Based Analysis of Fractions

For each participant i with $1, ..., I$ and phase p, we consider the log ratios l_{ip}^{bc} comparing the fractions of the two bacteria b and c, i.e., $l_{ip}^{bc} = log_{10} \frac{f_{ip}^{b}}{f_{ip}^{c}}$. The mean μ_{p}^{bc} is estimated by $\hat{\mu}_{p}^{bc} = \frac{1}{I} \sum_{i=1}^{I} l_{ip}^{bc}$ and the standard deviation by $\hat{\sigma}_{p}^{bc} = \frac{1}{I-1} \sqrt{\sum_{i=1}^{I} (l_{ip}^{bc} - \hat{\mu}_{p}^{bc})^2}$.

Appendix B.1.2. Pairwise Differences in Log Ratio Changes and Their Characteristics

Let us consider the ratio $\frac{f_{ip}^{b}}{f_{i1}^{b}}$ for a bacterium b, which relates the fractions of phase p to the baseline phase I. Subsequently, we can build ratios for two different bacteria b and c: $\frac{f_{ip}^{b}}{f_{i1}^{b}} / \frac{f_{ip}^{c}}{f_{i1}^{c}}$ to compare the changes of these 2 bacteria. Hence,

$$\Delta_{ip}^{bc} = log_{10} \frac{f_{ip}^{b}}{f_{i1}^{b}} - log_{10} \frac{f_{ip}^{c}}{f_{i1}^{c}} \tag{A1}$$

can be interpreted as a difference in log ratio changes:

$$\text{(A)} \qquad \Delta_{ip}^{bc} = l_{ip}^{b} - l_{ip}^{c} \qquad \text{with} \quad l_{ip}^{b} = log_{10} \frac{f_{ip}^{b}}{f_{i1}^{b}}$$

or as changes in the pairwise log ratios

$$\text{(B)} \qquad \Delta_{ip}^{bc} = l_{ip}^{bc} - l_{i1}^{bc} \qquad \text{with} \quad l_{ip}^{bc} = log_{10} \frac{f_{ip}^{b}}{f_{ip}^{c}}$$

We are interested in the mean value and standard deviation of Δ_{ip}^{bc}, which can be estimated by $\hat{\mu}_{\Delta_p}^{bc} = \frac{1}{I} \sum_{i=1}^{I} \Delta_{ip}^{bc}$ and $\hat{\sigma}_{\Delta_p}^{bc} = \frac{1}{I-1} \sqrt{\sum_{i=1}^{I} (\Delta_{ip}^{bc} - \hat{\mu}_{\Delta_p}^{bc})^2}$. We report t-test-based 95% confidence intervals.

Appendix B.1.3. Average Log Ratio Changes

The expected pairwise log ratio changes also allow us to characterise the location of each bacterium across all bacteria for each participant by looking at the average, i.e., by considering

$$\mu^b_{\Delta_p} = \frac{1}{B} \sum_{c=1}^{B} \mu^{bc}_{\Delta_p} \tag{A2}$$

which we call average log ratio changes.

$\mu^b_{\Delta_p}$ (and its estimate $\hat{\mu}^b_{\Delta_p}$) also have by definition the attractive feature, that its mean value over all bacteria $\bar{\mu}^\bullet$ is equal to 0, because $\mu^{bc} = -\mu^{cb}$. This is useful from a pedagogical perspective, as when presenting the estimates of μ^b for all bacteria $b = 1, \ldots, B$ together all deviations from 0 sum up to 0, which complies with the behaviour of fractions. For the latter, it is natural that changes in one direction for some bacteria are compensated by changes in the opposite direction for the other bacteria. Bar charts of $\hat{\mu}^b$ with 95% confidence intervals over the bacteria are used to visualise the distribution of the changes. Similar charts [23,24] have been used to show the distribution of log ratios in cross-sectional analyses.

Appendix B.2. Evidence of Composition Change

To consider the overall evidence of a change in the composition of the bacteria from baseline to a specific phase, we can consider as a test statistic the sum of the absolute deviations of μ^b form 0 over all bacteria, or the sum of the absolute deviations of μ^{bc} over all bacterial pairs. The test statistic corresponds to the area of a bar chart type presentations of these values, as we use in this paper.

The null hypothesis of interest corresponds to no effect of the change in nutrition to the bacterial spectrum in each individual. Therefore, the spectra observed at baseline and in the specific phase are simply observations of the same true spectrum blurred by some noise. Consequently, the two observations are exchangeable under the null hypothesis, and the distribution of a test statistic under the null hypothesis can be obtained by allowing randomly exchanging the whole spectrum in each individual. An exact approximation is obtained by considering all 2^{11} possibilities to exchange the spectra in a subset of the individuals. The *p*-value can then be determined by counting how often the observed value exceeds the values of the test statistic observed for each possibility.

References

1. Anderson, A.C.; Rothballer, M.; Altenburger, M.J.; Woelber, J.P.; Karygianni, L.; Vach, K.; Hellwig, E.; Al-Ahmad, A. Long-term fluctuation of oral biofilm microbiota following different dietary phases. *Appl. Environ. Microbiol.* **2020**. [CrossRef]
2. Bradshaw, D.J.; Lynch, R.J.M. Diet and the microbial aetiology of dental caries: New paradigms. *Int. Dent. J.* **2013**, *63*, 64–72. [CrossRef]
3. Moynihan, P.; Petersen, P.E. Diet, nutrition and the prevention of dental diseases. *Public Health Nutr.* **2004**, *7*, 201–226. [CrossRef] [PubMed]
4. Petti, S.; Simonetti, R.; Simonetti D'Arca, A. The effect of milk and sucrose consumption on caries in 6-to-11-year-old Italian schoolchildren. *Eur. J. Epidemiol.* **1997**, *13*, 659–664. [CrossRef]
5. Aimutis, W.R. Bioactive Properties of Milk Proteins with Particular Focus on Anticariogenesis. *J. Nutr.* **2004**, *134*, 989S–995S. [CrossRef] [PubMed]
6. Reynolds, E.C.; Cai, F.; Shen, P.; Walker, G.D. Retention in Plaque and Remineralization of Enamel Lesions by Various Forms of Calcium in a Mouthrinse or Sugar-free Chewing Gum. *J. Dent. Res.* **2016**. [CrossRef]
7. Schlafer, S.; Ibsen, C.J.S.; Birkedal, H.; Nyvad, B. Calcium-Phosphate-Osteopontin Particles Reduce Biofilm Formation and pH Drops in in situ Grown Dental Biofilms. *Caries Res.* **2017**, *51*, 26–33. [CrossRef] [PubMed]
8. Takahashi, N.; Nyvad, B. Caries ecology revisited: Microbial dynamics and the caries process. *Caries Res.* **2008**, *42*, 409–418. [CrossRef]
9. Marsh, P.D. In Sickness and in Health—What Does the Oral Microbiome Mean to Us? An Ecological Perspective. *Adv. Dent. Res.* **2018**. [CrossRef] [PubMed]
10. Mira, A. Oral Microbiome Studies: Potential Diagnostic and Therapeutic Implications. *Adv. Dent. Res.* **2018**. [CrossRef] [PubMed]

11. Aas, J.A.; Griffen, A.L.; Dardis, S.R.; Lee, A.M.; Olsen, I.; Dewhirst, F.E.; Leys, E.J.; Paster, B.J. Bacteria of Dental Caries in Primary and Permanent Teeth in Children and Young Adults. *J. Clin. Microbiol.* **2008**, *46*, 1407–1417. [CrossRef] [PubMed]

12. Levy, R.M.; Giannobile, W.V.; Feres, M.; Haffajee, A.D.; Smith, C.; Socransky, S.S. The Effect of Apically Repositioned Flap Surgery on Clinical Parameters and the Composition of the Subgingival Microbiota: 12-Month Data. *Int. J. Periodontics Restor. Dent.* **2002**, *22*, 209–219.

13. Koopman, J.E.; van der Kaaij, N.C.W.; Buijs, M.J.; Elyassi, Y.; van der Veen, M.H.; Crielaard, W.; Ten Cate, J.M.; Zaura, E. The Effect of Fixed Orthodontic Appliances and Fluoride Mouthwash on the Oral Microbiome of Adolescents—A Randomized Controlled Clinical Trial. *PLoS ONE* **2015**, *10*, e0137318. [CrossRef]

14. Velmurugan, S.; Gan, J.M.; Rathod, K.S.; Khambata, R.S.; Ghosh, S.M.; Hartley, A.; Van Eijl, S.; Sagi-Kiss, V.; Chowdhury, T.A.; Curtis, M.; et al. Dietary nitrate improves vascular function in patients with hypercholesterolemia: A randomized, double-blind, placebo-controlled study. *Am. J. Clin. Nutr.* **2016**, *103*, 25–38. [CrossRef]

15. Greenacre, M.J. *Compositional Data Analysis in Practice*; CRC Press: Boca Raton, FL, USA; Taylor & Francis Group: Abingdon, UK, 2019.

16. Lamont, R.J.; Koo, H.; Hajishengallis, G. The oral microbiota: Dynamic communities and host interactions. *Nat. Reviews. Microbiol.* **2018**, *16*, 745–759. [CrossRef] [PubMed]

17. Bernardi, S.; Karygianni, L.; Filippi, A.; Anderson, A.C.; Zürcher, A.; Hellwig, E.; Vach, K.; Macchiarelli, G.; Al-Ahmad, A. Combining culture and culture-independent methods reveals new microbial composition of halitosis patients' tongue biofilm. *MicrobiologyOpen* **2020**, *9*, e958. [CrossRef] [PubMed]

18. Anderson, A.C.; Rothballer, M.; Altenburger, M.J.; Woelber, J.P.; Karygianni, L.; Lagkouvardos, I.; Hellwig, E.; Al-Ahmad, A. In-vivo shift of the microbiota in oral biofilm in response to frequent sucrose consumption. *Sci. Rep.* **2018**, *8*. [CrossRef] [PubMed]

19. Vach, K.; Al-Ahmad, A.; Anderson, A.; Woelber, J.P.; Karygianni, L.; Wittmer, A.; Hellwig, E. Analysing the Relationship between Nutrition and the Microbial Composition of the Oral Biofilm—Insights from the Analysis of Individual Variability. *Antibiotics* **2020**, *9*, 479. [CrossRef] [PubMed]

20. Anderson, A.C.; Hellwig, E.; Vespermann, R.; Wittmer, A.; Schmid, M.; Karygianni, L.; Al-Ahmad, A. Comprehensive Analysis of Secondary Dental Root Canal Infections: A Combination of Culture and Culture-Independent Approaches Reveals New Insights. *PLoS ONE* **2012**, *7*, e49576. [CrossRef]

21. Paster, B.J.; Boches, S.K.; Galvin, J.L.; Ericson, R.E.; Lau, C.N.; Levanos, V.A.; Sahasrabudhe, A.; Dewhirst, F.E. Bacterial Diversity in Human Subgingival Plaque. *J. Bacteriol.* **2001**, *183*, 3770–3783. [CrossRef]

22. Zaura, E.; Brandt, B.W.; Teixeira de Mattos, M.J.; Buijs, M.J.; Caspers, M.P.M.; Rashid, M.U.; Weintraub, A.; Nord, C.E.; Savell, A.; Hu, Y.; Coates, A.R.; Hubank, M.; Spratt, D.A.; Wilson, M.; Keijser, B.J.F.; Crielaard, W. Same Exposure but Two Radically Different Responses to Antibiotics: Resilience of the Salivary Microbiome versus Long-Term Microbial Shifts in Feces. *mBio* **2015**, *6*, e01693-15. [CrossRef] [PubMed]

23. Chastin, S.; Palarea-Albaladejo, J.; Dontje, M.; Skelton, D. Combined Effects of Time Spent in Physical Activity, Sedentary Behaviors and Sleep on Obesity and Cardio-Metabolic Health Markers: A Novel Compositional Data Analysis Approach. *PLoS ONE* **2015**, *10*, e0139984. [CrossRef] [PubMed]

24. Martín Fernández, J.A.; Daunis i Estadella, J.; Mateu i Figueras, G. On the Interpretation of Differences between Groups for Compositional Data. *Sort Stat. Oper. Res. Trans.* **2015**, *39*, 231–252.

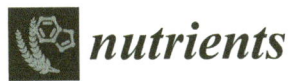 *nutrients*

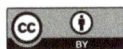 MDPI

Article

Modification of the Lipid Profile of the Initial Oral Biofilm In Situ Using Linseed Oil as Mouthwash

Anna Kensche [1,*,†] , Marco Reich [2,†] , Christian Hannig [1] , Klaus Kümmerer [2] and Matthias Hannig [3]

1   Clinic of Operative and Pediatric Dentistry, Medical Faculty Carl Gustav Carus, TU Dresden, Fetscherstr. 74, D-01307 Dresden, Germany; christian.hannig@uniklinikum-dresden.de
2   Faculty of Sustainability, Institute of Sustainable and Environmental Chemistry, Leuphana University Lueneburg, Universitaetsallee. 1, C13, 21335 Lueneburg, Germany; marco.reich@leuphana.de (M.R.); klaus.kuemmerer@leuphana.de (K.K.)
3   Clinic of Operative Dentistry, Periodontology and Preventive Dentistry, University Hospital, Saarland University, Building 73, D-66421 Homburg, Germany; matthias.hannig@uks.eu
*   Correspondence: Anna.Kensche@uniklinikum-dresden.de; Tel.: +49-(0)351-458-2713; Fax: +49-(0)351-458-5381
†   These authors contributed equally to this work.

Abstract: Lipids are of interest for the targeted modification of oral bioadhesion processes. Therefore, the sustainable effects of linseed oil on the composition and ultrastructure of the in situ pellicle were investigated. Unlike saliva, linseed oil contains linolenic acid (18:3), which served as a marker for lipid accumulation. Individual splints with bovine enamel slabs were worn by five subjects. After 1 min of pellicle formation, rinses were performed with linseed oil for 10 min, and the slabs' oral exposure was continued for up to 2 or 8 h. Gas chromatography coupled with electron impact ionization mass spectrometry (GC-EI/MS) was used to characterize the fatty acid composition of the pellicle samples. Transmission electron microscopy was performed to analyze the ultrastructure. Extensive accumulation of linolenic acid was recorded in the samples of all subjects 2 h after the rinse and considerable amounts persisted after 8 h. The ultrastructure of the 2 h pellicle was less electron-dense and contained lipid vesicles when compared with controls. After 8 h, no apparent ultrastructural effects were visible. Linolenic acid is an excellent marker for the investigation of fatty acid accumulation in the pellicle. New preventive strategies could benefit from the accumulation of lipid components in the pellicle.

Keywords: pellicle; linseed oil; fatty acid; ultrastructure; in situ

Citation: Kensche, A.; Reich, M.; Hannig, C.; Kümmerer, K.; Hannig, M. Modification of the Lipid Profile of the Initial Oral Biofilm In Situ Using Linseed Oil as Mouthwash. *Nutrients* **2021**, *13*, 989. https://doi.org/10.3390/nu13030989

Academic Editor: Kirstin Vach

Received: 22 February 2021
Accepted: 15 March 2021
Published: 19 March 2021

1. Introduction

Bioadhesion and development of pathogenic biofilms on non-shedding solid surfaces are the key features for the initiation of caries, gingivitis, periodontitis as well as the increasing periimplantitis [1–5]. Due to this fact, one approach in developing new prophylactic mouthwashes is the search for agents that allow targeted and sustainable modulation of initial bioadhesion. The first step of bioadsorption in the oral cavity is the formation of the pellicle. This layer is composed of proteins, peptides, glycoproteins but also metabolites and lipids from the oral fluids [6–8]. Over the past decade, several in situ studies have demonstrated a noteworthy correlation between compositional and ultrastructural pellicle modifications and the variation of the pellicles' protective properties at the tooth surface [9–12]. In this context, more and more food components and plant extracts have come into focus. Due to their biocompatibility, substances such as lipids and polyphenolic compounds might get integrated into or interfere with the natural adsorption processes at the tooth surface [12,13].

There are controversial data on the impact of oil mouthrinses on (bacterial) biofilm formation and erosion prevention under in vitro or in situ conditions [10,14–18]. Nevertheless, lipids are still of considerable interest due to their lipophilic character [7]. They account for 20% of the pellicle's dry weight, but the lack of suitable and reliable methods to obtain the biological material in situ and to detect the specific components have in the past been clear limitations in this field of research [7,19,20]. Hydrophobic interactions are suggested to be a significant driving force for pellicle formation. The topical adsorption of lipophilic substances at the tooth surface after different lipid-containing mouthrinses was shown in a few in situ studies [7,10,17,19,21]. However, it remains uncertain whether and how the applied macromolecules are integrated into the in situ pellicle and whether the pellicle's composition, structural pattern and properties can be altered sustainably, for example, by mouthrinses with edible oils. Precise detection of the applied lipid components is a prerequisite for corresponding investigations.

Up to now, there are only a few studies on the lipid and fatty acid composition of the pellicle layer [20–23]. For that reason, we have already investigated the fatty acid content of the in situ pellicle with highly sensitive methods [19,24]. Based on gas chromatography coupled with electron impact ionization mass spectrometry, a pellicle-characteristic fatty acid profile with little interindividual variability was determined. Distinct differences were only detected regarding the total amount of adsorbed fatty acids, which also depended on the pellicles' formation time [19]. Furthermore, the ultrastructure of the in situ pellicle and the initial biofilm had been characterized in detail by transmission electron microscopy [25–27]. Alterations were observed by TEM for a short period after mouthrinses with safflower oil [10]. In comparison to the native control, 2 h in situ pellicles that had been formed after the application of the oil mouthrinse appeared to be less electron-dense with a rather loose protein accumulation. Following this, an accumulation of lipid droplets at the in situ pellicle's surface has only recently been visualized by environmental scanning electron microscopy for up to 9.5 h after rinsing with safflower oil [21].

Based on the knowledge from previous investigations, the present study aimed to clarify if rinses with a specific edible oil can modify the composition and ultrastructure of the pellicle layer sustainably. Linseed oil was selected for this purpose as it contains linolenic acid (18:3), which is not a physiological component of the saliva and accordingly served as a marker molecule. The obtained results will be relevant for the targeted development of new strategies in preventive dentistry that rely on the modulation of native bioadhesion processes. In this context, lipids could also serve as carriers that deliver protective substances to the tooth surface. In addition, valuable information may be gained about the dynamics of biomolecule adsorption at the tooth surface and the turnover of the in situ pellicle in general.

2. Materials and Methods

2.1. Subjects

As a preliminary investigation for this study, native saliva samples were collected from 12 subjects and the fatty acid profile was determined by GC-MS (see below). All volunteers had given their informed written consent about participation in the study. They underwent a clinical oral examination by an experienced dentist to ensure that they had no unrestored carious lesions, periodontal diseases, or an unphysiological salivary flow rate. Due to the high methodical effort, further in situ experiments regarding the effects of mouthrinses with linseed oil on saliva and the in situ pellicle were continued with five participants (aged 21–36). The study design was approved by the Ethics committee of the Medical Faculty, Technische Universität Dresden, Germany (vote: EK 475112016). Individual upper jaw splints were prepared for every participant to enable the exposure of bovine enamel specimens to the oral cavity for intraoral pellicle formation. Enamel slabs were obtained from the incisors of 2-year-old cattle, which are recognized as a suitable substitute for human enamel [28]. For in situ exposure, all enamel slabs were prepared as described in numerous previous publications [10,11,17,24]. The slabs' surfaces were wet-ground and polished according to a standardized protocol with up to 4000 grit abrasive paper, and the resulting smear layer was then removed by ultrasonication in 3% NaOCl for 3 min. Two washing cycles in distilled water for 5 min were followed by disinfection of the specimens in 70% ethanol, all activated by ultrasonication. Finally, the bovine enamel specimens were stored in distilled water at 4 °C for up to 24 h before intraoral exposure.

2.2. Adopted Mouth Rinse and Rinsing Procedure

Different in situ experiments were carried out on separate days allowing a wash-out period of at least 48 h in which the subjects were asked to perform their regular oral hygiene. Two hours before an intraoral test period, the volunteers had to brush their teeth without toothpaste. In the following, no food or drinks other than water were to be consumed until the collection of in situ pellicle/biofilm samples. All participants had to carry their individual splints intraorally for either 120 min or 8 h overnight, with the enamel slabs attached in little cavities in the buccal and palatal region of the premolars and the first molar. Twelve enamel slabs per splint were exposed at a time to obtain sufficient in situ pellicle material necessary for the lipid analyses. TEM was performed on two pellicle samples per time of investigation and volunteer. The in situ rinsing protocol and exposure times were planned on the basis of earlier studies in this field [10,12,15,29], see Figure 1 for an overview of the experimental setup. After 1 min of pellicle formation in situ, mouthrinses were performed for 10 min with 10 mL of linseed oil. This specific edible oil was chosen as it contains linolenic acid (18:3), which under physiological conditions cannot be detected in the fatty acid profile of human saliva or salivary in situ pellicles. The fatty acid composition of the linseed oil used in this study is shown in Table 1.

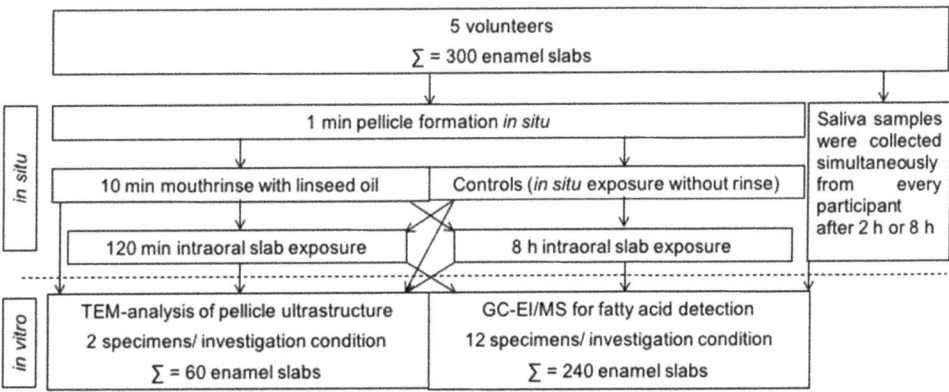

Figure 1. Overview of the experimental setup performed in this study. In situ pellicle and initial biofilm samples were obtained from 5 volunteers, who all underwent the different investigation conditions. In total, 300 enamel slabs were used in this study.

Table 1. Fatty acid composition of major fatty acids (in %, in relation to total fatty acids) in linseed oil with linolenic acid (18:3) being the predominant fatty acid. Comparison of the composition between oil used as a mouthrinse in this study (composition was determined by the GC-MS method described in this paper) and data provided in literature [30,31].

Fatty Acid	Linseed Oil (Used in this Study)	Linseed Oil (Literature Values)
16:0	4–9%	4–6%
18:0	2–9%	2–3%
18:1	12–14%	10–22%
18:2	12–14%	12–18%
18:3	58–66%	56–71%

Finally, all enamel slabs were removed from the splints and subjected to in vitro investigation methods. Simultaneously, unstimulated saliva samples were obtained from every participant. These samples were centrifuged at $6000 \times g$ for 10 min and sterile filtered (0.2 μm) before analysis. The same experimental runs were made without the use of oil. This allowed the collection of enamel slabs, as well as saliva, which had not been exposed to the oil and served as control.

2.3. GC-MS Analysis of the Fatty Acid Composition

The analysis of fatty acids in saliva and pellicle desorbates was performed as described in detail previously [24].

2.4. Sample Preparation

Tridecanoic and nonadecanoic acid were used as internal standards and were added to the desorbed pellicle samples before all sample preparation steps. The pellicle lipids were initially separated from the matrix by liquid/liquid extraction. For this step, an adapted Folch extraction procedure was used, in which the lipids were extracted from the desorbed pellicle sample with a mixture of methanol and chloroform. Rapid transesterification (1 h; 100 °C) of all fatty acids (FAs) containing lipids into fatty acid methyl esters (FAME) was carried out in methanol using concentrated HCl (35%, w/w) as an acidic catalyst. The FAMEs were then extracted by adding hexane and deionized water. The hexane phase was isolated, evaporated under a gentle stream of nitrogen, and the residue was redissolved in 0.1 mL of hexane. For GC-MS analyses, 1 μL of this solution was injected.

2.5. GC-MS (Instrumental Conditions)

GC/EI-MS was performed with an ISQ™ 7000 Single Quadrupole GC-MS system (Thermo Scientific, Dreieich, Germany). The injector was operated in splitless mode at 260 °C. For the separation of the target compounds, a TRACE™ TR FAME fused silica capillary column (30 m × 0.25 mm × 0.25 μm; Thermo Scientific, Dreieich, Germany) and helium as carrier gas was used with a constant flow of 1.5 mL/min. The oven temperature was programmed at 50 °C for 5 min, followed by an increase of 6.5 °C/min until the final temperature of 260 °C was reached and then held for 8 min. The electron energy was 70 eV, and the ion source temperature was set to 270 °C. A mass range of m/z 60–400 was recorded in full scan mode. Additionally, selected ion monitoring (SIM), recording fragment ions including m/z 74, m/z 79, m/z 81, and m/z 87 was performed throughout the run.

In order to visualize the impact of mouthrinses with linseed oil on the ultrastructure of the in situ pellicle over time, transmission electron microscopy was performed on pellicle samples directly after the rinse, after 2 h or after 8 h of oral exposure, respectively. The findings were compared with control images of a characteristic native 3 min, 30 min, 120 min and an 8 h in situ pellicle. After completion of the oral exposure times, the enamel specimens were carefully rinsed with distilled water and fixed in 2.5% glutaraldehyde and 0.1 M cacodylate buffer for 1 h at 4 °C. Five washing cycles were performed in phosphate buffer before 1% osmium tetroxide was applied for 1 h to visualize the organic structures. The samples were then dehydrated in an ascending alcohol series and embedded in Araldite CY212 (Agar Scientific Ltd., Stansted, United Kingdom). All enamel residues were decalcified with 0.1 M HCl, and the remaining pellicle samples were re-embedded in Araldite. Ultrathin sections of the embedded pellicle samples were cut in series with a diamond knife in an ultramicrotome (Ultracut E, Reichert, Bensheim, Germany). The samples were mounted on pioloform coated copper grids (Plano, Wetzlar, Germany), and uranyl acetate and lead citrate were applied to enhance contrasts. TEM-analysis was performed at magnification from 20,000 to 100,000-fold using a TEM TECNAI 12 Biotwin (FEI, Eindhoven, The Netherlands). Representative images were taken during the investigation of the entire pellicle samples.

3. Results

3.1. Modification of the Pellicle's Lipid Profile

Modifications of the pellicle's lipid profile were detected after gas chromatography coupled with electron impact ionization mass spectrometry (GC-EI/MS) was performed on pellicle samples that were collected in situ with or without having been exposed to mouthrinses with linseed oil. Linseed oil contains linolenic acid (18:3) (Table 1), which is not physiologically present in the human oral flora and thus serves as a reliable biomarker. Under consideration of already available data from previous investigations, the results focus on the detection of linolenic acid in comparison to the four major fatty acids palmitic (16:0), stearic (18:0), oleic (18:1) and linoleic acid (18:2), which generally account for approximately 90% of all investigated fatty acids in saliva and the in situ pellicle [19]. The analyzed pellicle samples after linseed oil rinsing showed a shift to a higher percentage of unsaturated fatty acids and a strongly increased proportion of linolenic acid (Figures 2 and 3). Even 8 h after rinsing, the specific fatty acid 18:3 is still clearly detectable, which indicates that the lipids introduced through the mouthwash are sustainably integrated into the pellicle structure.

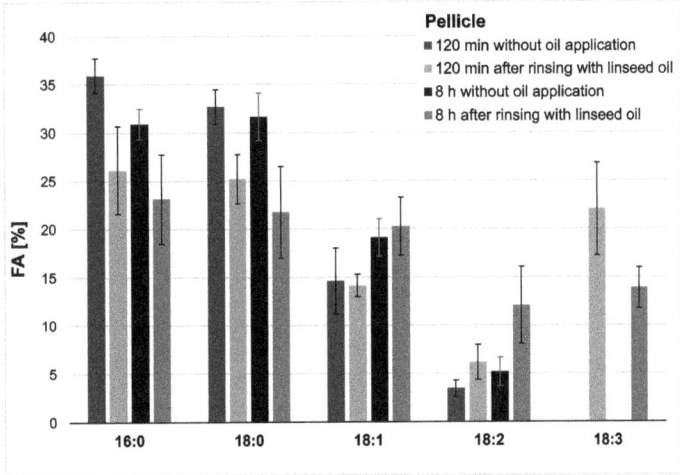

Figure 2. Percentage of the four major fatty acids and linolenic acid (18:3) in the pellicles. Measurements were performed after 2 h or 8 h of pellicle formation, either with or without linseed oil applied as a mouthrinse. Modifications of the in situ pellicle's profile due to the oil application could be seen clearly at both investigation times. While linolenic acid could not be detected in the native controls at any time, it made approximately 22% of the total fatty acid composition after 2 h of pellicle formation and could still be detected in the 8 h biofilm samples (13%). It can be assumed that the fatty acids provided by the linseed oil mouthrinse were sustainably integrated into the in situ pellicle's composition.

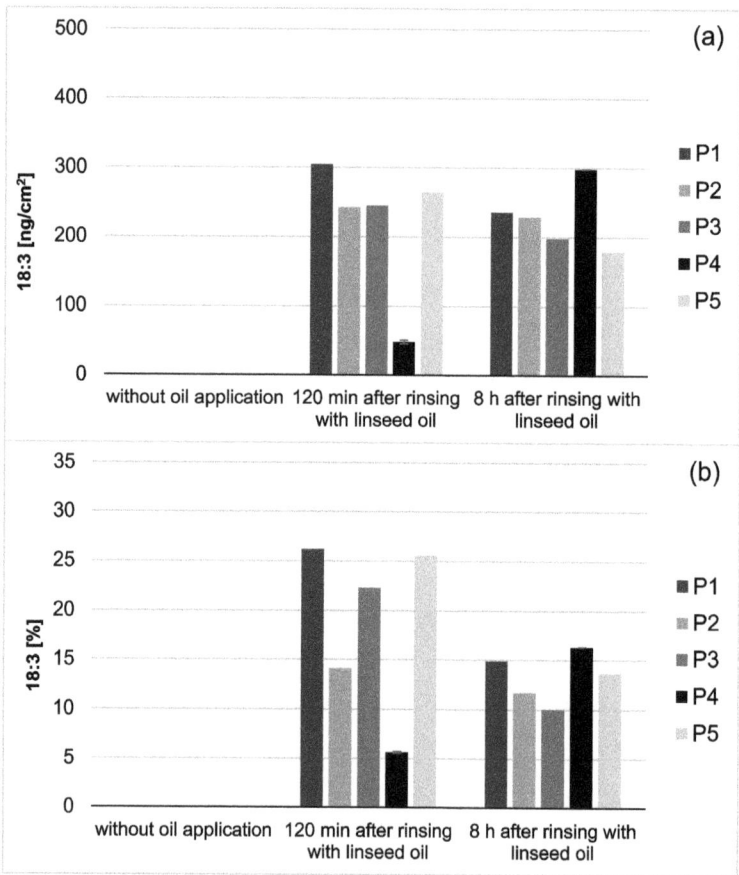

Figure 3. Total amount of 18:3 in the in situ pellicle (**a**) and proportion of 18:3 on the total fatty acid profile (**b**) of the 5 individual subjects (P1-5). In general, 18:3 was only detectable if mouthrinses with linseed oil had been applied. During the investigation period (2–8 h), the adsorbed amount of 18:3 appeared to be relatively consistent. However, after 8 h of biofilm formation, the proportion of 18:3 on the total fatty acid profile has decreased noticeably (**b**). This might be due to the salivary clearance, reduced availability of the specific fatty acid, and the resulting shift towards fatty acids naturally contained in saliva. Notably, smaller amounts of 18:3 were measured for participant 4 (P4) compared to the other subjects. However, the repetition of the measurements with new investigation material ($n = 2$) confirmed the previous results.

In saliva, a high proportion of linolenic acid was found 2 h after the rinse, while the percentages of palmitic (16:0), stearic (18:0), oleic acid (18:1) were obviously reduced. The concentration and content of linolenic acid decreased notably within the examination period of 8 h after oil rinsing (Figures 4 and 5). However, it is remarkable that under the given sampling conditions, even 8 h after oil rinsing, linolenic acid is still detectable in saliva. In the reference saliva samples (without preceding oil rinsing), linolenic acid was not detectable in any of the samples.

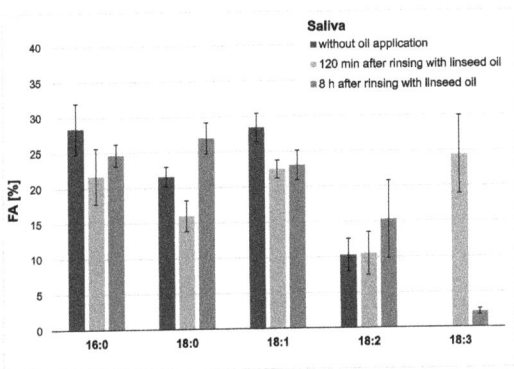

Figure 4. Percentage of the four major fatty acids and 18:3 in the saliva's total fatty acid profile. The mean values and standard deviation are shown based on the data from five participants (*n* = 5). Saliva samples were collected 2 h and 8 h after the mouthrinse with linseed oil. Corresponding native saliva samples without oil application served as controls. The highest concentration of 18:3 was measured 2 h after the mouthrinse (approximately 24% of all fatty acids (FAs)). Even after 8 h, residues of 18:3 were still detectable. Linolenic acid was not found in any of the controls.

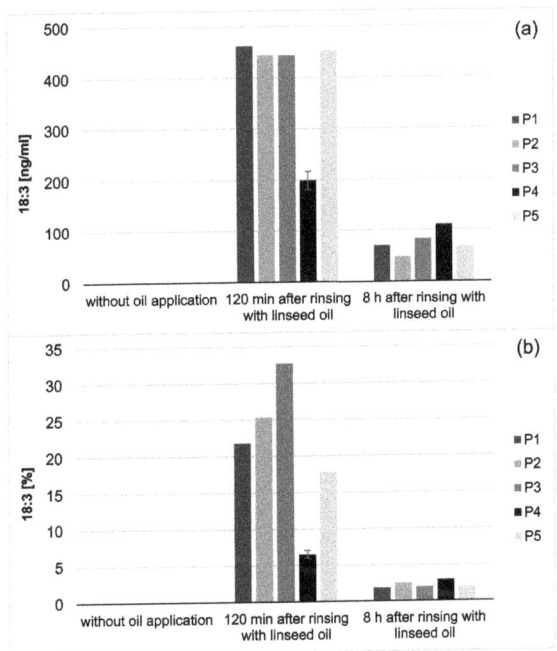

Figure 5. Total concentration of 18:3 in saliva (**a**) and proportion of 18:3 on the total salivary fatty acid profile (**b**) of five individual subjects (P1–5). 18:3 was only detectable if mouthrinses with linseed oil had been applied. Both, the total concentration as well as the proportion of 18:3 on the total fatty acid profile of the investigated saliva samples decreased considerably during the 8 h investigation period. Remarkably, small amounts of 18:3 could still be detected in the saliva samples 8 h after the linseed oil mouthrinse had been performed. Notably, smaller amounts of 18:3 were measured for participant 4 (P4) than for the other subjects. However, the repetition of the measurements with new investigation material (*n* = 2) confirmed the previous results.

In this study, no statistical analysis was performed. For the first time, the accumulation of an applied specific fatty acid (18:3) was transparently determined in the pellicle and in saliva with highly sensitive methods. The investigation focused on the detectability of linolenic acid after oil mouthrinses. Considering the one-to-one correspondence of present or absent linolenic acid in the investigated samples, statistical analyses of any kind were irrelevant.

3.2. Transmission Electron Microscopic Analysis

Alterations of the pellicle's ultrastructure were also temporarily seen by transmission electron microscopic analysis. The early stages of bioadsorption at the tooth surface generally create a characteristic image of a two-layer pellicle ultrastructure, as shown in Figure 6. Almost immediately, the enamel surface is covered by a relative uniform continuous 10–20 nm-thick electron-dense basal layer. As a result of prolonged oral exposure, more granular and globular structures adhere to the pellicle surface forming a second layer of variable thickness.

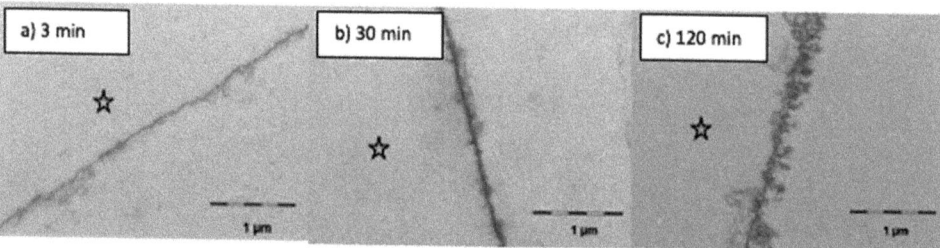

Figure 6. Transmission electron microscopy—control samples. The 3 min pellicle has a continuous electron dense basal layer with few granular structures (**a**). After longer oral exposure for 30 min (**b**) or 120 min (**c**) more granular and globular structures adsorb to the pellicle layer. The enamel was removed during the preparation of the samples; the former enamel side is marked with an asterisk.

It was observed in this study that the formation and the appearance of this second more heterogeneous pellicle layer, to a certain extent, depended on the local accumulation of biological macromolecules at the tooth surface (Figure 7). Initially, rinsing with linseed oil for 10 min appeared to result in a slight dissolution or loosening of the pellicle's ultrastructure, however creating a smooth surface. Oil droplets were randomly detected at the pellicle surface. On the other hand, in some parts, the protein adsorption to the enamel surface appeared to be optimized with proteinaceous structures covering even nano- and micro-pores like a subsurface pellicle. This slightly promoted affinity of proteins to the tooth surface and was still visible after 120 min of pellicle formation where the basal pellicle was thicker and more electron-dense than in the control. During these early stages of biofilm formation at the tooth surface, only a few bacteria were detected at the pellicle surface. Their morphology appeared to be affected by the linseed oil mouthrinse. The cell walls were damaged, and no cell division was observed.

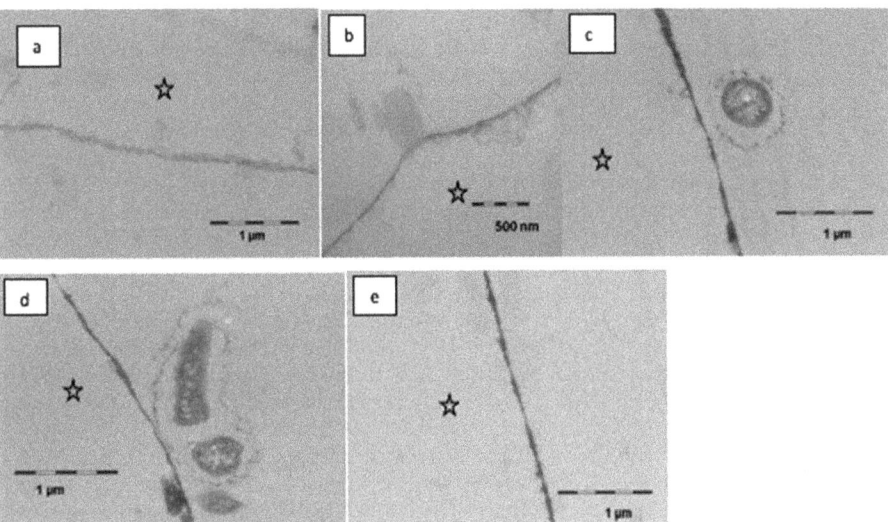

Figure 7. Transmission electron microscopy, in situ application of linseed oil for 10 min after 1 min of pellicle formation. Rinsing with the oil leads to a slight dissolution and thinning of the pellicle, partially the surface is smoother than in controls (**a,b**). Oil droplets were observed seldomly (**b**). In part, there was an optimized wetting of the surface in the sense of a subsurface pellicle. During further oral exposure for up to 120 min, a modified ultrastructure was still visible (**c–e**). The basal pellicle is thicker and more electron dense, sometimes pores in the enamel are filled with proteinaceous structures. Furthermore, first adherent bacteria were detectable; the cell wall of the bacteria is damaged (**c,d**). The enamel was removed during the preparation of the samples; the former enamel side is marked with an asterisk.

However, after 8 h of oral exposure, a considerable attachment of viable bacteria had occurred in several areas of the investigated samples (Figure 8). In comparison to the controls, more bacteria were found in the samples that had been exposed to the linseed oil mouthrinses. The cell walls appeared to be intact, and cell division as a sign of viability was detected. Even though the structure of this bacterial biofilm was still very loose, the bacteria's interactions by bacterial fimbriae could be seen. Regarding protein accumulation or potential persistence of lipid components at this time, no notable ultrastructural differences were observed between the samples that had/ had not been exposed to the linseed oil mouthrinse.

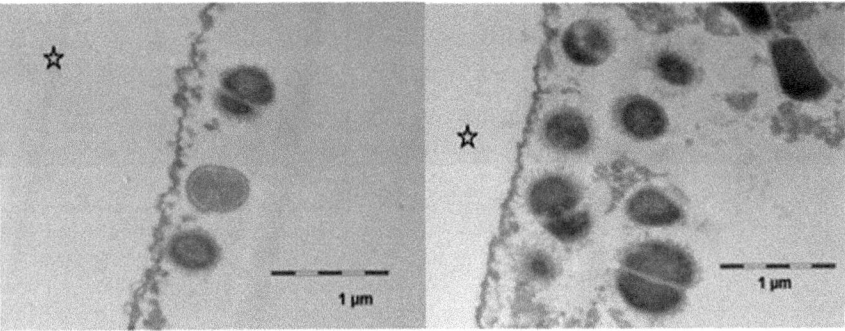

Figure 8. Transmission electron microscopy, in situ application of linseed oil for 10 min after 1 min of initial pellicle formation. The samples were kept in the oral cavity overnight for 8 h. There was a pronounced bacterial colonization, the adherent bacteria showed an intact ultrastructure and cell division was observed. No differences were observed as compared with controls. The enamel was removed during the preparation of the samples; the former enamel side is marked with an asterisk.

4. Discussion

In recent years, few in situ studies have been published that made a scientifically sound contribution to the incomplete knowledge about the involvement of lipids in initial bioadhesion processes at the tooth surface [10,15,19,21,32]. Clearly, as had already been suggested earlier, lipids and lipophilic molecules must be regarded as essential components of the in situ pellicle at various formation times [19,20,33]. At the same time, it appears that a modification of the lipid components provided in the oral cavity may have a detectable effect on the pellicle's composition, structure, and functional properties [10,17,21]. However, only modern and highly sensitive analytical methods will give greater certainty about the actual integration of lipid components into the pellicle layer and their alteration due to remodeling processes.

With this aim in mind, the performed application of gas chromatography coupled with electron impact ionization mass spectrometry (GC–EI/MS) as well as electron microscopic techniques (TEM) were suitable methods to detect and quantify (specific) lipid components in the in situ pellicle samples. At the time the study was conducted, micellar molecule aggregations had already been visualized in pellicle samples shortly after mouthrinses with edible oils and lipids containing food components [10,11]. Similar observations were made in the present investigation. In comparison to the native control, the ultrastructure of the in situ pellicle after mouthrinses with linseed oil showed a slightly more heterogeneous pattern during the first 120 min of pellicle formation (Figures 6–8). It must be assumed that lipid components were adsorbed to the pellicle layer and that the resulting molecular interactions had a notable effect on the adsorption and distribution of proteins at the tooth surface. Most biological lipids (phospholipids, sphingolipids, glycolipids), as well as free fatty acids, are amphiphilic molecules with hydrophilic and lipophilic properties [20]. On the one hand, hydrophobic repellent forces of the long hydrocarbon chains of fatty acids could be the reason for the slightly loosened ultrastructure of the second pellicle layer. On the other hand, in aqueous solution, fatty acids tend to form micellar aggregations (Figure 7b). It is even conceivable that these acted as carrier systems that delivered non-polar proteins to the tooth surface [22]. Two hours after the mouthrinse with linseed oil, a subsurface pellicle was occasionally detected, and parts of the basal pellicle appeared slightly more electron dense. The affinity of lipids to bind amphiphilic molecules or proteins, respectively, and to therefore alter the ultrastructure of the in situ pellicle had been described earlier in case of mouthrinses with bovine milk [17]. However, considering the dynamics of dental biofilm formation and the salivary clearance, it remained uncertain if these pellicle modifications had any sustainable effect for more than 2 h. Furthermore, details on the type of lipids or fatty acids accumulated in the pellicle were preferable to possibly understand their impact on pellicle and initial bacterial biofilm formation.

Characteristic distributions of major fatty acids were detected in both physiological saliva and pellicle samples by GC–EI/MS. A comparatively higher proportion of saturated fatty acids in the pellicle demonstrates the selective adsorption of salivary components on the tooth surface. During maturation of the in situ pellicle overnight, the fatty acid profile appeared to be relatively consistent.

Choosing linseed oil for the mouthrinse allowed the definite detection of oil-associated lipid accumulations in all investigated saliva and pellicle samples by GC–EI/MS. Linolenic acid (18:3) is not included in the physiological fatty acid profile of the oral fluids, and its detection in the pellicle could reliably be correlated with its absorption from the oil mouthrinse. Therefore, this specific fatty acid served as a suitable biological marker for the tracking of bioadhesion processes and their durability at the tooth surface. Based hereon, it was shown that the mouthrinse initially induced a shift of the major fatty acid composition to a higher percentage of unsaturated fatty acids and a remarkable accumulation of linolenic acid in both the saliva and pellicle samples (2 h). As already indicated above, the higher percentage of unsaturated fatty acids and the high reactivity of their double bonds might have influenced the surface wettability and the molecular interactions during pellicle formation. As expected, after 8 h, the mouthrinse alterations of saliva's major fatty acid

Nutrients **2021**, *13*, 989

profile were almost eliminated due to the salivary clearance. The content of linolenic acid decreased by approximately 85% from 2 to 8 h after the rinse, yet linolenic acid was still traceable (Figure 3). Interestingly, pellicle maturation during these hours only depended to a certain extent on the availability of lipid components provided by the saliva. Oil-induced modifications of the pellicle's fatty acid profile appeared to be notably more, continuing with a considerably lower turnover after 8 h of initial biofilm formation (~35% less linolenic acid from 2 to 8 h after the oil-rinse, Figure 2). Simultaneously, augmentation of pellicles' thickness and bacterial adhesion were shown in the electron microscopic analyses. However, the ultrastructural pattern did not differ notably from the native controls.

Concerning a potential modification of functional pellicle properties in terms of erosion prevention or bacterial biofilm formation, so far, there is no undoubted evidence that mouthrinses with edible oils have a convincing health-promoting effect [10,14–16,20]. Nevertheless, the present TEM-images still indicate that components of the linseed oil initially affected the morphology of oral bacteria (Figure 7). Damage to the cell wall integrity of bacteria can be a sign of reduced viability. Taking in vitro studies into account, it can be assumed that certain free fatty acids, possibly also linolenic acid, had an antibacterial effect on salivary bacteria [34,35]. Fatty acids might have affected the integrity of bacteria's cell membranes and interfered in metabolic processes which could explain the deformed morphology of some bacteria shortly after the mouthrinse. However, these effects were only seen in the first 2 h after the mouthrinse. It is also conceivable that bacteria's adhesion on the pellicle was influenced by the distribution pattern of lipid components in the in situ pellicle. Looking at the TEM-images after 8 h of biofilm formation, bacterial adhesion appeared to have proceeded unhampered, if not had even been enhanced by lipid components, respectively. No clear difference could be seen between the controls and the samples that had been exposed to the linseed oil mouthrinse regarding the morphology of the adhering bacteria. This is in line with previous in situ investigations that did not measure a significant effect of edible oil mouthrinses on the adherence or live/dead ratio of bacteria at the tooth surface after 8 h of biofilm formation [15]. Further investigations in this field will be necessary.

5. Conclusions

Using highly sensitive analytical methods, this study clarified for the first time that mouthrinses with edible oil can alter the fatty acid profile of the in situ pellicle and the initial bacterial biofilm sustainably. In this context, linolenic acid was identified as a valuable biological marker as it is not present in the fatty acid profile of native saliva or in situ pellicles. The results obtained from this investigation provide important information about the kinetics of pellicle formation at the tooth surface in general. However, further research should focus on the relevance of lipid components' molecular characteristics and molecular interactions for the accumulation of proteins and bacteria at the tooth surface, respectively. The modification of lipid components in the in situ pellicle remains an interesting approach to alter and possibly improve the physiological functional properties of the in situ pellicle.

Author Contributions: A.K.: main writer of the manuscript, literature research, analysis and interpretation of data; M.R.: co-writer of the manuscript, experimental work (lipid analyses), analysis and interpretation of data; C.H.: conceptualization of study, acquisition of research funding (German Research Foundation), interpretation of data, editing and review of manuscript; K.K.: conceptualization of study, acquisition of research funding (German Research Foundation), interpretation of data (lipid analysis), editing and review of manuscript; M.H.: conceptualization of study, acquisition of research funding (German Research Foundation), expertise in the field of transmission electron microscopic analyses (experimental work and interpretation), editing and review of manuscript. All authors have read and agreed to the published version of the manuscript.

Funding: This study has been funded by the German Research Foundation (HA 2718/14-3, HA 5192/2-3, KU 1271/6-3).

Institutional Review Board Statement: The study was conducted according to the guidelines of the Declaration of Helsinki and approved by the Ethics committee of the Medical Faculty, Technische Universität Dresden, Germany (vote: EK 475112016).

Informed Consent Statement: Informed consent was obtained from all subjects involved in the study.

Data Availability Statement: All relevant data are contained in the article.

Acknowledgments: The authors thank Jens Robertson for technical assistance with the fatty acid analyses. Transmission electron microscopy was kindly prepared and performed by Wiebke Hoth-Hannig.

Conflicts of Interest: All authors declare that there is no conflict of interest regarding the publication of this paper.

Abbreviations

GC-EI/MS	Coupled with electron impact ionization mass spectrometry
TEM	Transmission electron microscopy
18:3	Linolenic acid
16:0	Palmitic acid
18:0	Stearic acid
18:1	Oleic acid
18:2	Linoleic acid
NaOCl	sodium hypochlorite
NaOCl	sodium hypochlorite
FAME	Fatty acid methyl esters
HCl	Hydrochloric acid

References

1. Bowen, W.H. Dental caries—Not just holes in teeth! A perspective. *Mol. Oral Microbiol.* **2016**, *31*, 228–233. [CrossRef]
2. Bowen, W.H.; Burne, R.A.; Wu, H.; Koo, H. Oral Biofilms: Pathogens, Matrix, and Polymicrobial Interactions in Microenvironments. *Trends Microbiol.* **2018**, *26*, 229–242. [CrossRef] [PubMed]
3. Daubert, D.M.; Weinstein, B.F. Biofilm as a risk factor in implant treatment. *Periodontology 2000* **2019**, *81*, 29–40. [CrossRef] [PubMed]
4. Marsh, P.D. Dental plaque as a microbial biofilm. *Caries Res.* **2004**, *38*, 204–211. [CrossRef] [PubMed]
5. Marsh, P.D.; Bradshaw, D.J. Dental plaque as a biofilm. *J. Ind. Microbiol.* **1995**, *15*, 169–175. [CrossRef] [PubMed]
6. Hannig, M.; Joiner, A. The structure, function and properties of the acquired pellicle. *Monogr. Oral Sci.* **2006**, *19*, 29–64. [CrossRef] [PubMed]
7. Kensche, A.; Reich, M.; Kümmerer, K.; Hannig, M.; Hannig, C. Lipids in preventive dentistry. *Clin. Oral Investig.* **2013**, *17*, 669–685. [CrossRef]
8. Siqueira, W.L.; Custodio, W.; McDonald, E.E. New insights into the composition and functions of the acquired enamel pellicle. *J. Dent. Res.* **2012**, *91*, 1110–1118. [CrossRef] [PubMed]
9. Cassiano, L.P.S.; Ventura, T.M.S.; Silva, C.M.S.; Leite, A.L.; Magalhães, A.C.; Pessan, J.P.; Buzalaf, M.A.R. Protein Profile of the Acquired Enamel Pellicle after Rinsing with Whole Milk, Fat-Free Milk, and Water: An in vivo Study. *Caries Res.* **2018**, *52*, 288–296. [CrossRef]
10. Hannig, C.; Wagenschwanz, C.; Pötschke, S.; Kümmerer, K.; Kensche, A.; Hoth-Hannig, W.; Hannig, M. Effect of safflower oil on the protective properties of the in situ formed salivary pellicle. *Caries Res.* **2012**, *46*, 496–506. [CrossRef]
11. Kensche, A.; Buschbeck, E.; König, B.; Koch, M.; Kirsch, J.; Hannig, C.; Hannig, M. Effect of fluoride mouthrinses and stannous ions on the erosion protective properties of the in situ pellicle. *Sci. Rep.* **2019**, *9*, 5336. [CrossRef]
12. Weber, M.-T.; Hannig, M.; Pötschke, S.; Höhne, F.; Hannig, C. Application of Plant Extracts for the Prevention of Dental Erosion: An in situ/in vitro Study. *Caries Res.* **2015**, *49*, 477–487. [CrossRef] [PubMed]
13. Hannig, M.; Hannig, C. The pellicle and erosion. *Monogr. Oral Sci.* **2014**, *25*, 206–214. [CrossRef] [PubMed]
14. Cukkemane, N.; Bikker, F.J.; Nazmi, K.; Brand, H.S.; Sotres, J.; Lindh, L.; Arnebrant, T.; Veerman, E.C.I. Anti-adherence and bactericidal activity of sphingolipids against Streptococcus mutans. *Eur. J. Oral Sci.* **2015**, *123*, 221–227. [CrossRef] [PubMed]
15. Hannig, C.; Kirsch, J.; Al-Ahmad, A.; Kensche, A.; Hannig, M.; Kümmerer, K. Do edible oils reduce bacterial colonization of enamel in situ? *Clin. Oral Investig.* **2013**, *17*, 649–658. [CrossRef]
16. Ionta, F.Q.; de Alencar, C.R.B.; Val, P.P.; Boteon, A.P.; Jordao, M.C.; Honorio, H.M.; Buzalaf, M.A.R.; Rios, D. Effect of vegetable oils applied over acquired enamel pellicle on initial erosion. *J. Appl. Oral Sci.* **2017**, *25*, 420–426. [CrossRef]

17. Kensche, A.; Dürasch, A.; König, B.; Henle, T.; Hannig, C.; Hannig, M. Characterization of the in situ pellicle ultrastructure formed under the influence of bovine milk and milk protein isolates. *Arch. Oral Biol.* **2019**, *104*, 133–140. [CrossRef]
18. Rykke, M.; Rölla, G. Effect of silicone oil on protein adsorption to hydroxyapatite in vitro and on pellicle formation in vivo. *Scand. J. Dent. Res.* **1990**, *98*, 401–411. [CrossRef] [PubMed]
19. Reich, M.; Kümmerer, K.; Al-Ahmad, A.; Hannig, C. Fatty acid profile of the initial oral biofilm (pellicle): An in-situ study. *Lipids* **2013**, *48*, 929–937. [CrossRef]
20. Slomiany, B.L.; Murty, V.L.; Zdebska, E.; Slomiany, A.; Gwozdzinski, K.; Mandel, I.D. Tooth surface-pellicle lipids and their role in the protection of dental enamel against lactic-acid diffusion in man. *Arch. Oral Biol.* **1986**, *31*, 187–191. [CrossRef]
21. Peckys, D.B.; DEJonge, N.; Hannig, M. Oil droplet formation on pellicle covered tooth surfaces studied with environmental scanning electron microscopy. *J. Microsc.* **2019**, *274*, 158–167. [CrossRef]
22. Rawat, M.; Singh, D.; Saraf, S.; Saraf, S. Lipid Carriers: A Versatile Delivery Vehicle for Proteins and Peptides. *Yakugaku Zasshi* **2008**, *128*, 269–280. [CrossRef]
23. Slomiany, B.L.; Zdebska, E.; Murty, V.L.; Slomiany, A.; Mandel, I.D. Lipid composition of human pellicle. *J. Dent. Res.* **1984**, *63*, 271.
24. Reich, M.; Hannig, C.; Al-Ahmad, A.; Bolek, R.; Kümmerer, K. A comprehensive method for determination of fatty acids in the initial oral biofilm (pellicle). *J. Lipid Res.* **2012**, *53*, 2226–2230. [CrossRef] [PubMed]
25. Al-Ahmad, A.; Follo, M.; Selzer, A.-C.; Hellwig, E.; Hannig, M.; Hannig, C. Bacterial colonization of enamel in situ investigated using fluorescence in situ hybridization. *J. Med. Microbiol.* **2009**, *58*, 1359–1366. [CrossRef] [PubMed]
26. Hannig, M. Ultrastructural investigation of pellicle morphogenesis at two different intraoral sites during a 24-h period. *Clin. Oral Investig.* **1999**, *3*, 88–95. [CrossRef]
27. Hannig, M. Transmission electron microscopy of early plaque formation on dental materials in vivo. *Eur. J. Oral Sci.* **1999**, *107*, 55–64. [CrossRef]
28. Pelá, V.T.; Cassiano, L.P.S.; Ventura, T.M.d.S.; Souza-e-Silva, C.M.D.; Gironda, C.C.; Rios, D.; Buzalaf, M.A.R. Proteomic analysis of the acquired enamel pellicle formed on human and bovine tooth: A study using the Bauru in situ pellicle model (BISPM). *J. Appl. Oral Sci.* **2018**, *27*, e20180113. [CrossRef]
29. Kirsch, J.; Jung, A.; Hille, K.; König, B.; Hannig, C.; Kölling-Speer, I.; Speer, K.; Hannig, M. Effect of fragaria vesca, hamamelis and tormentil on the initial bacterial colonization in situ. *Arch. Oral Biol.* **2020**, *118*, 104853. [CrossRef]
30. German Society for Fat Science (DGF). Fatty Acid Composition of Vegetable and Animal Edible Fats and Oils. 2020. Available online: http://www.dgfett.de/material/fszus.php (accessed on 2 May 2020).
31. Patterson, H.B.W. Chapter 8—Hydrogenation Methods. In *Hydrogenation of Fats and Oils*, 2nd ed.; AOCS Press: Urbana, IL, USA, 2011; pp. 189–278.
32. Matczuk, J.; Żendzian-Piotrowska, M.; Maciejczyk, M.; Kurek, K. Salivary lipids: A review. *Adv. Clin. Exp. Med.* **2017**, *26*, 1021–1029. [CrossRef]
33. Slomiany, B.L.; Murty, V.L.; Mandel, I.D.; Sengupta, S.; Slomiany, A. Effect of lipids on the lactic acid retardation capacity of tooth enamel and cementum pellicles formed in vitro from saliva of caries-resistant and caries-susceptible human adults. *Arch. Oral Biol.* **1990**, *35*, 175–180. [CrossRef]
34. Desbois, A.P.; Smith, V.J. Antibacterial free fatty acids: Activities, mechanisms of action and biotechnological potential. *Appl. Microbiol. Biotechnol.* **2010**, *85*, 1629–1642. [CrossRef] [PubMed]
35. Jung, J.-E.; Pandit, S.; Jeon, J.-G. Identification of linoleic acid, a main component of the n-hexane fraction from Dryopteris crassirhizoma, as an anti-Streptococcus mutans biofilm agent. *Biofouling* **2014**, *30*, 789–798. [CrossRef] [PubMed]

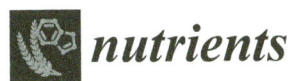 *nutrients*

MDPI

Review

Nutrition Care Practices of Dietitians and Oral Health Professionals for Oral Health Conditions: A Scoping Review

Jessica R. L. Lieffers *, Amanda Gonçalves Troyack Vanzan, Janine Rover de Mello and Allison Cammer

College of Pharmacy and Nutrition, University of Saskatchewan, Saskatoon, SK S7N 5E5, Canada; agv665@usask.ca (A.G.T.V.); jar018@usask.ca (J.R.d.M.); allison.cammer@usask.ca (A.C.)
* Correspondence: jessica.lieffers@usask.ca

Abstract: Background: Oral health conditions, such as dental caries, pose a substantial burden worldwide. Although there are many risk factors for poor oral health, diet is often implicated as a cause of these issues. The purpose of this scoping review was to identify and map studies that have captured information on the "real-world" nutrition care practices of oral health professionals (OHPs) and dietitians to optimize oral health, and specifically the dentition and periodontium. Methods: A search of peer-reviewed articles was conducted using MEDLINE, CINAHL, and Embase. Articles that addressed the review objective and met the following criteria were included: English language, published since 2000, and study conducted in a high-income country. Results: Overall, 70 articles were included. Most articles reported on cross-sectional survey studies and provided self-reported data on OHP practices; few articles reported on dietitians. Most articles reported only general/unspecific information on assessment and intervention practices, such as dietary analysis, nutrition counselling, and diet advice, and lacked specific information about the care provided, such as the dietary assessment tools used, type of information provided, and time spent on these activities. Barriers to the provision of nutrition care by OHPs were common and included time and lack of remuneration. Few studies reported on collaboration between dietitians and OHPs. Conclusions: Several studies have captured self-reported information on nutrition care practices of OHPs related to oral health; however, there is limited information available on the details of the care provided. Few studies have examined the practices of dietitians.

Keywords: oral health; dental caries; diet therapy; dentists; dental auxiliaries; nutritionists; dietitian; surveys and questionnaires; qualitative research; review

Citation: Lieffers, J.R.L.; Vanzan, A.G.T.; Rover de Mello, J.; Cammer, A. Nutrition Care Practices of Dietitians and Oral Health Professionals for Oral Health Conditions: A Scoping Review. *Nutrients* **2021**, *13*, 3588. https://doi.org/10.3390/nu13103588

Academic Editors: Kirstin Vach and Johan Peter Woelber

Received: 15 September 2021
Accepted: 2 October 2021
Published: 13 October 2021

Publisher's Note: MDPI stays neutral with regard to jurisdictional claims in published maps and institutional affiliations.

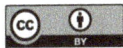

1. Introduction

Worldwide, oral health issues (e.g., dental caries, periodontal disease) affect 3.5 billion people [1], with dental caries being the most common concern [2]. Oral health issues also affect many people in Canada. For example, the 2007–2009 Canadian Health Measures Survey (CHMS) reported that 57%, 59%, and 96% of 6–11-year-olds, 12–19-year-olds, and adults, respectively, had experienced dental caries [3]. Dental caries are also the most common reason for day surgery in children 12–59 months of age in Canada [4]. Periodontal issues are also common in Canada; according to the 2007–2009 CHMS, 21% of adults with teeth were found to have or previously had moderate or severe periodontal issues [3]. Various factors can affect the risk of oral health issues, including fluoride, oral hygiene (e.g., brushing, flossing), tobacco, and diet [5].

More specific to diet, both the physical and chemical properties of the foods we eat, as well as how the foods we eat are consumed (e.g., frequency, delivery) can have protective or detrimental effects on oral health (and specifically the dentition and periodontium) [6]. Fermentable carbohydrates (e.g., sucrose) have a known relationship with dental caries [7]; however, the relationship between oral health and diet is much more extensive [8]. For example, hard cheese; sugar alcohols (e.g., xylitol); diets rich in vegetables, fruits, whole grains, and high-quality proteins; and adequate spacing between eating occasions are thought to be protective against dental caries [6,8,9]. Acidic foods and beverages have also been previously linked with tooth erosion [10,11]. The relationship between diet and oral health has been summarized in several articles [6,8–10,12–17], and some organizations have released statements and guidelines on this topic [8,18–20]. We also know that many people in Canada have diet behaviours associated with poor health (e.g., high intakes of sugar-sweetened beverages [21]). In addition to diet being linked to various oral health issues, poor oral health can also have nutritional implications (e.g., children with early childhood caries can experience difficulties eating [22]). Importantly, the relationship between nutrition and oral health is important throughout the entire human lifespan [8,12].

The provision of nutrition care to optimize oral health is within the scope of practice of different health professions including dietitians and oral health professionals. In addition, healthy eating has been identified as a priority area by the World Health Organization when initiating and strengthening oral health programs [23,24]. To date, information on the current "real-world" practices regarding nutrition care for oral health (and specifically the dentition and periodontium) provided by dietitians and oral health professionals has been captured in different types of studies with different focuses; however, reviews on this topic are limited. A previous review article published in 2014 examined the diet advice practices of oral health professionals, including variables that influence this activity [25]. Since this article has been published, there have been several other relevant studies that have emerged. This article also did not examine the practices of dietitians.

The purpose of this scoping review is to identify and map current studies that have captured information on the "real-world" nutrition care practices of oral health professionals and dietitians to optimize oral health (specifically the dentition and periodontium), in addition to collaboration between the two professions. We wanted to capture information on the scope of the literature addressing this topic and consolidate the wide range of studies to identify gaps in the literature to understand how to move this area of research forward. This project lends itself well to a scoping review because of the diversity of studies and study designs that have investigated this topic. This review did not seek to investigate the impact of different types of nutrition care practices on oral health.

2. Materials and Methods

The scoping review framework outlined by Arksey and O'Malley [26] was used to guide this review. In addition, the article by Levac et al. [27] was also used to help guide this review. The five steps that were followed to conduct this review are outlined below. A review protocol does not exist for this scoping review.

Stage 1: Research Question Development

The first component of conducting a scoping review is to identify the research question that will be investigated. The question that was used to guide the review was as follows: What is reported in the literature about the "real-world" practices of dietitians and oral health professionals regarding nutrition care for oral health (and specifically conditions that affect the dentition and periodontium)? In addition, we were also interested in understanding what has been studied regarding collaboration between the two professions for this purpose. According to the FDI World Dental Federation definition, "oral health is multi-faceted and includes the ability to speak, smile, smell, taste, touch, chew, swallow and convey a range of emotions through facial expressions with confidence and without pain, discomfort and disease of the craniofacial complex (head, face, and oral cavity)" [28]. We were specifically interested in studies focusing on the health of the dentition and periodontium. A scoping review for this research question is suitable as we were interested in understanding the range of the evidence to date, and because there are numerous possible study designs that could address the research question. The purpose of this review is to help to summarize the extent and nature of the research activity in this area. This review will help to identify and clarify research needs to help advance the area of nutrition care and oral health (specifically conditions that affect the dentition and periodontium) to help decrease the burden of oral diseases in Canada and beyond.

Stage 2: Identification of Relevant Studies

A literature search was conducted using the MEDLINE, CINAHL, and Embase databases in May 2020 and repeated in May 2021 (as there were delays completing this review due to the COVID-19 pandemic). Health science academic librarians provided guidance on the database searches. Three categories of concepts that were derived from the research question were used in the literature search. The first category related to oral and dental health, dentistry, and oral health professionals. The second category related to dietitians, nutrition services, dietetics, food, nutrition, and diet. The third category related to professional practices and behaviours. The MEDLINE search strategy is provided in Table 1.

Table 1. MEDLINE search strategy.

Concept Category #1: Oral and Dental Health, Dentistry, Oral Health Professionals	Concept Category #2: Dietitians, Nutrition Services, Dietetics, Food, Nutrition, Diet	Concept Category #3: Professional Practices and Behaviours
Oral Health/OR exp periodontal diseases/OR exp tooth diseases/OR exp Dentition/OR exp Odontogenesis/OR exp dental auxiliaries/OR exp dental staff/OR exp dentists/OR exp faculty, dental/OR exp dentistry/OR exp public health dentistry/OR exp Dental Facilities/OR exp Dental Health Services/OR Dental Records/OR exp societies, dental/OR Licensure, Dental/OR Schools, Dental/OR exp Education, Dental/OR Insurance, Dental/OR exp Economics, Dental/OR dent*.ti,ab,kw. OR tooth.ti,ab,kw. OR teeth.ti,ab,kw.	exp "diet, food, and nutrition"/OR exp Carbohydrates/OR exp sugar alcohols/OR drinking behavior/OR exp feeding behavior/OR exp Feeding Methods/OR Cariogenic Agents/OR Nutritionists/OR exp Nutritional Sciences/OR exp Dietary Services/OR exp Nutrition Therapy/OR nutrition assessment/OR exp Body Weight/OR exp Nutrition Disorders/OR diet*.ti,ab,kw. OR sugar*.ti,ab,kw. OR nutritio*.ti,ab,kw.	"attitude of health personnel"/OR attitude to health/OR health knowledge, attitudes, practice/OR Practice Patterns, Dentists'/OR professional-patient relations/OR professional-family relations/OR interprofessional relations/OR interdisciplinary communication/OR intersectoral collaboration/OR Patient Care Team/OR Professional Practice Gaps/OR exp Professional Practice/OR exp Professional Role/OR practice*.ti,ab,kw. OR interprofessional*.ti,ab,kw. OR interdisciplin*.ti,ab,kw. OR multidisciplin*.ti,ab,kw. OR collaborat*.ti,ab,kw. OR multi-disciplin*.ti,ab,kw. OR inter-disciplin*.ti,ab,kw. OR trans-disciplin*.ti,ab,kw. OR transdisciplin*.ti,ab,kw. OR cross-disciplin*.ti,ab,kw. OR referral*.ti,ab,kw.

In addition to database searches, reference lists from all included articles were examined for additional articles. Moreover, the citations for relevant articles were searched in Google Scholar for any other papers that might have been missed. Relevant review articles in this area were also consulted to capture any additional articles [25,29,30]. Hand searches of journals likely to have articles in this area (Journal of Dental Hygiene, International Journal of Dental Hygiene, Community Dental Health, Canadian Journal of Dental Hygiene) were also conducted. All articles were imported into a reference management system and duplicates were removed.

Stage 3: Article Selection

Article inclusion and exclusion criteria are listed in Table 2. In order to be included, articles had to meet the following criteria: English language, published in year 2000 or later, conducted in a World Bank high-income country, reported information on the "real-world" practices of dietitians/nutritionists and/or oral health professionals (not including students) regarding nutrition care for oral health (and specifically conditions affecting the dentition and periodontium). Articles were included regardless of quality. Clinical trials were not included except for baseline information on current professional practices. The year 2000 was chosen to select articles that were relatively recent. World Bank high-income countries were chosen to provide articles that are most relevant to the Canadian context. Exclusion criteria included information on the practices of students (e.g., nutrition students, dental students, dental hygiene students), where results of dietitians/nutritionists and/or oral health professionals were combined with other professionals (e.g., nurses, physicians) and could not be isolated, information on professional commentary regarding treatment plans for case studies, and when information about nutrition care practices was combined with other dental prevention practices (and cannot be isolated) (e.g., dental preventative activities in general were assessed which could include nutrition interventions amongst other activities such as fluoride application). Studies that were conducted in Special Supplemental Nutrition Program for Women, Infant, and Children (WIC) personnel were included as well. WIC is a federally funded government program in the United States that is available for low-income pregnant women, postpartum breastfeeding and nonbreastfeeding women, and children less than 5 years of age [31]. This program provides healthy foods, nutrition education, and health care referrals. Of note, many WIC staff members are also dietitians. We also included studies that included information on practices related to oral health (e.g., tooth brushing instruction) in dietitians, nutritionists and/or WIC personnel.

Table 2. Inclusion and exclusion criteria.

Inclusion Criteria	Exclusion Criteria
<ul><li>Article published in year 2000 or later</li><li>Peer-reviewed research article</li><li>Article written in English</li><li>Study conducted in humans</li><li>Study conducted in a World Bank high-income country</li><li>Article reported information on the real-world nutrition care practices (e.g., diet advice, nutrition counselling) (including barriers) of dietitians/nutritionists/WIC personnel and/or oral health professionals to optimize oral health (and specifically the dentition and periodontium).<ul><li>Studies describing the nutrition care practices of oral health professionals without reference to a specific oral health condition were included as they were assumed to be referring to oral health, specifically the dentition/periodontium.</li></ul></li><li>Articles that reported practices related to oral health (e.g., tooth brushing counselling) in dietitians/nutritionists/WIC personnel without reference to a specific oral health condition were included as they were assumed to be referring to oral health and specifically dentition/periodontium.</li></ul>	<ul><li>Letters to the editor, commentaries, conference abstracts, thesis documents, grey literature, review articles</li><li>Information about practices and/or barriers of providing nutrition care reported by students (e.g., nutrition students, dental students, dental hygiene students)</li><li>Information about nutrition care practices for dietitians/nutritionists/WIC personnel and/or oral health professionals is combined with other dental prevention activities (and cannot be isolated)</li><li>Information about nutrition care practices of dietitians/nutritionists/WIC personnel and/or oral health professionals is combined with another profession (e.g., nurses, physicians)</li><li>Information on nutrition care practices provided by dietitians/nutritionists/WIC personnel and/or oral health professionals from the patient perspective</li><li>Information about practices regarding fluoride supplements, sugar alcohols, herbal supplements, homeopathy, and alcohol by oral health professionals</li><li>Information about diabetes, obesity, cardiovascular disease, hypertension screening/management by oral health professionals</li><li>Information about body weight and blood glucose screening/monitoring by oral health professionals</li><li>Information about how dietitians/nutritionists/WIC personnel and/or oral health professionals would treat hypothetical patient case scenarios/studies</li></ul>

WIC: Special Supplemental Nutrition Program for Women, Infants, and Children.

Two individuals independently screened the titles and abstracts of all articles from the search conducted in May 2020 using the study inclusion and exclusion criteria with Rayyan [32]; if the abstracts did not provide enough information, the full text of the article was consulted. For the articles from the search conducted in May 2021, the articles were also screened by two individuals using the study inclusion and exclusion criteria. Cases of disagreement were reviewed and discussed by a third member of the research team until consensus was reached.

Stage 4: Charting the Data

The following information was charted from all eligible articles: author(s), year of publication, study location, study dates, study population, sample size, study methodology, oral health issue of focus, and key findings. Only information relevant to the inclusion criteria was extracted; for example, if a study included information about physicians and oral health professionals, only the information about oral health professionals was charted. The source of funding for the included studies was also captured. As with many scoping reviews, a quality assessment was not carried out.

Stage 5: Collating, Summarizing, and Reporting the Results

Following extraction of all data, the results were collapsed into tables to report information on sample size, type of professional studied, patient population and/or concern of focus, and information about the topics investigated in the article. This process was conducted by JRLL, and the content was verified by AGTV or JRdM by looking at the content of the table and cross-checking it with the article. The articles were sorted based on the type of professional studied, the types of outcomes reported, and the study methodology.

3. Results

In total, $n = 70$ articles were included in the scoping review (Figure 1). Most articles describe studies that were conducted in one of the following four regions: United States ($n = 23$), United Kingdom ($n = 17$), Nordic countries (Norway, Finland, Iceland, Sweden, Denmark) ($n = 12$), and Australia ($n = 7$). However, there were also articles from Japan ($n = 3$), Germany ($n = 2$), Saudi Arabia ($n = 2$), Canada ($n = 1$), Hong Kong ($n = 1$), New Zealand ($n = 1$), and Taiwan ($n = 1$). In total, $n = 32$ articles were published in 2010 or earlier and $n = 38$ articles were published in 2011 or later. Almost half of the articles did not report any funding source ($n = 32$); articles reporting funding sources ($n = 38$ articles) reported that their studies were funded by various sources including government/government agency ($n = 25$ articles), university/hospital ($n = 6$), professional association/organization ($n = 3$), and other sources (i.e., foundation, charity, company) ($n = 10$).

Most studies focused on oral health professionals; only six studies provided information on dietitians, nutritionists, and/or WIC personnel (many of whom are dietitians or nutritionists). Most articles did not focus specifically on diet and nutrition but rather had focuses including preventative dentistry, prevention and/or treatment of specific oral health conditions, infant oral health care/examinations, dental practice patterns, and public dental service use. Only $n = 18$ articles referred to something that was obviously related to nutrition and/or diet in their title (e.g., diet, nutrition, sugar-sweetened beverage, dietitian, nutritionist, WIC). Most included articles were cross-sectional survey studies of professionals (sample size range: $n = 9$ to $n = 2294$ professionals); however, other study methods included chart reviews (sample size range: $n = 285$ to >10,000 patients), observation studies (sample size: $n = 3751$ patient visits in 120 general dental practices), and qualitative interviews and/or focus groups of professionals (sample size range: $n = 10$ to 93). In addition, one study captured information on how different types of data compared to one another.

In this review, the articles were organized based on the type of professional studied, the methods used in the study (e.g., survey, qualitative interview), and types of care provided which encompassed either assessment practices (i.e., dietary assessment practices by oral health professionals; assessment practices regarding oral health and nutrition by dietitians, nutritionists, and/or WIC personnel) or intervention practices (e.g., diet counselling, diet advice by oral health professionals; intervention practices regarding oral health and nutrition by dietitians, nutritionists, and/or WIC personnel). Of note, two cross-sectional survey studies included only a combined measure of assessment and intervention practices; these articles are included in both of those sections.

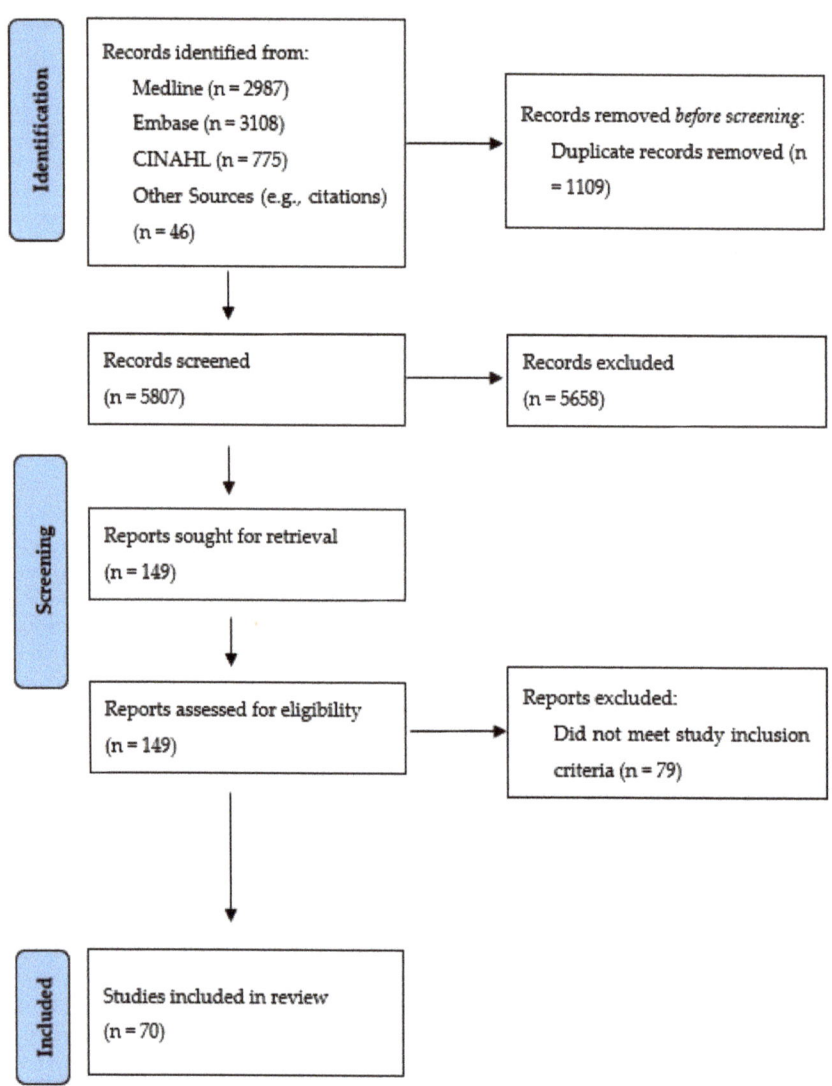

Figure 1. Search results.

3.1. Assessment Practices

3.1.1. Oral Health Professionals

Nineteen articles provided information on the dietary assessment practices of oral health professionals. These studies are described in Table 3. Overall, most of these articles were cross-sectional survey studies usually of dentists; however, other types of studies also captured this information, including chart reviews and a qualitative interview study. Overall, these studies captured information on various dietary assessment practices including general/unspecific assessment practices (e.g., dietary analysis), use of specific diet assessment tools (e.g., food records), and inquiries about specific patient behaviours or concerns (e.g., bottle use, cariogenic food consumption). In addition, two studies examined barriers regarding dietary assessment. A few of these studies examined whether there were differences in these outcomes by professional type, patient type, and various professional and practice factors.

Table 3. Assessment practice information reported in the included articles.

Study Authors, Year, and Country	Sample Size *	Professional Type	Population and/or Concern of Focus	General/Unspecific Assessment Practices (e.g., Dietary Analysis)	Use of Specific Assessment Tools, Strategies, or Practices (e.g., Food Records)	Inquiries about Specific Patient Behaviours or Concerns (e.g., Bottle Use, Cariogenic Food Consumption)	Barriers (or Reasons for Lack of Use) Regarding Assessment Practices
SURVEY STUDIES							
Oral Health Professionals							
Roshan et al., 2003 [33]; UK	687	general dental practitioners; community dental officers	children	(X)^Practice/Prof			
Hawkins and Locker, 2005 [34]; Canada	672	general dentists	older adults		X	X^Practice/Prof	
Sajnani-Oommen et al., 2006 [35]; USA	180	pediatric dentists	children		X		
Bubna et al., 2012 [36]; USA	554	pediatric dentists	infants	(X)			
Clovis et al., 2012 [37]; USA	540	dental hygienists	children; dental caries			X^Practice/Prof	
Mulic et al., 2012 [38]; Norway	705	public dental health service dentists	adults; dental erosive wear	X	X		
Garton and Ford, 2013 [39]; Australia	638	dentists (including specialists)	root caries	X			X^Practice/Prof
Sim et al., 2014 [40]; USA	86	pediatric dentists	infants and toddlers; dental caries			X	
Yusuf et al., 2016 [41]; UK	164	National Health Service general dental practitioners		X^Practice/Prof			
Widström et al., 2016 [42]; Norway	215 dentists; 166 dental hygienists	dentists; dental hygienists in public dental service	public dental service clients—children and adults	X^Professional Type; Patient			
Arheiam et al., 2016 [43]; UK	250	general dental practitioners	children; adults		X^Practice/Prof; Patient		X^Patient
Halawany et al., 2017 [44]; Saudi Arabia	108	pediatric dentists	children; dental caries	X			
Dima et al., 2018 [45]; Taiwan	196	general dentists; pediatric dentists	children; early childhood caries			X^Professional Type	
Mulic et al., 2018 [46]; Iceland	153	dentists	dental erosive wear	X	X		
Kangasmaa et al., 2021 [47]; Finland	814	general dentists; dental specialists	erosive tooth wear	X^Practice/Prof; Professional Type			
Mortensen et al., 2021 [48]; Denmark	419	dentists	erosive tooth wear	X	X		
Dietitians/Nutritionists							
Fuller et al., 2014 [49]; USA	159	WIC program personnel	WIC clients; early childhood caries	X^Practice/Prof			
Gold and Tomar, 2016 [50]; USA	9	WIC nutritionists	WIC clients	X	X	X	
Fernandez et al., 2017 [51]; USA	36	dietitians who completed a pediatric dentistry internship rotation		X^Patient			

Table 3. *Cont.*

Study Authors, Year, and Country	Sample Size *	Professional Type	Population and/or Concern of Focus	General/Unspecific Assessment Practices (e.g., Dietary Analysis)	Use of Specific Assessment Tools, Strategies, or Practices (e.g., Food Records)	Inquiries about Specific Patient Behaviours or Concerns (e.g., Bottle Use, Cariogenic Food Consumption)	Barriers (or Reasons for Lack of Use) Regarding Assessment Practices
CHART REVIEW STUDIES							
Oral Health Professionals							
Sarmadi et al., 2009 [52]; Sweden	432	public dental service (dentists and dental hygienists)	children 6–19 years at high risk of developing dental caries	X[Patient]			
O'Toole et al., 2018 [53]; UK	285	dentists	adults; tooth wear	X[Practice/Prof]			
QUALITATIVE INTERVIEW STUDIES							
Oral Health Professionals							
Threlfall et al., 2007 [54]; UK	93	general dental practitioners	children; dental caries	X[Patient]	X		

* Sample size for survey studies and qualitative interview studies refers to number of professionals included; sample size for chart review studies refers to the number of patients included. WIC: Special Supplemental Nutrition Program for Women, Infants, and Children. (X) = study measure included both assessment and intervention practices combined together (e.g., analyzed diets and gave dietary advice). Patient = examine differences in assessment practices in different types of patients (e.g., children vs. adults, severe dental caries vs. not). Professional Type = examine differences in assessment practices in different types of professionals (e.g., general dentists vs. pediatric dentists, dentists vs. dental hygienists). Practice/Prof = examine differences in assessment practices for different practice characteristics (e.g., public vs. private, rural practice vs. urban practice) and/or health professional characteristics (e.g., demographics, education, attitudes).

General/Unspecific Dietary Assessment Practices

Thirteen articles reported information on general/unspecific dietary assessment practices (e.g., dietary analysis, dietary history, assessment of dietary habits, asking about dietary behaviour, diet history review and analysis) of oral health professionals (cross-sectional survey studies (n = 10) [33,36,38,39,41,42,44,46–48]; chart review studies (n = 2) [52,53], qualitative interview study (n = 1) [54]). Most of the articles reported information regarding these practices in dentists.

Within the cross-sectional survey studies, various self-reported measures were used to capture information on general/unspecific dietary assessment practices. One self-reported measure used in some of these studies was the proportion of respondents who provide this type of service in the population of interest [36,44]. These studies were conducted in pediatric dentists and found that this activity was common in the population of interest (e.g., >90% of pediatric dentists who performed infant oral health evaluations reported this practice [36]; 70.6% of pediatric dentists reported doing a diet history review and analysis regarding dental caries prevention [44]). Several cross-sectional survey studies also reported self-reported information on frequency of providing some type of general/unspecific dietary assessment practice [33,38,39,42,46–48]. Overall, these studies were conducted regarding these practices when assisting patients with specific dental conditions (e.g., root caries [39], erosive tooth wear [38,46–48]) and in children [33,42] and adult [42] patient groups. In articles that focused on specific dental conditions, the percentage of respondents who self-reported always, often, and/or usually providing some type of general/unspecific dietary assessment practice ranged from 45% to 81%, and the percentage of respondents who never or seldom performed this practice ranged from 1% to 25% [38,39,46–48]. In studies focusing on children and/or adults, the percentage of respondents who self-reported never performing this practice ranged from 2% to 6.4% [33,42]. The chart review studies that assessed general/unspecific dietary assessment practices found results that are slightly different compared to results found in the survey studies. These studies, which included one focusing on pediatric patients at high risk for developing dental caries in a public dental service [52] and another focusing on tooth wear in adults in general dental practice [53], found that <25% of patients had this type of assessment documented in their dental records.

The studies of Widström et al. [42] and Kangasmaa et al. [47] were the only studies that compared general/unspecific dietary assessment practices amongst different types of oral health professionals. Widström et al. [42] found in their survey study that dental hygienists were significantly more likely to assess dietary habits in all or most of their patients vs. dentists in both children and adult patients. Kangasmaa et al. [47] found regarding erosive tooth wear that there was no difference in the frequency of assessing a patient's dietary history between general dentists and different types of dental specialists. In addition, four studies [33,41,47,53] examined professional and practice factors that impact the frequency with which dentists provide general/unspecific dietary assessment services for their patients. Overall, these studies found that dentists who were significantly more likely to practice this activity were less experienced (vs. more experienced) [53], work as a community dental officer (vs. general dental practitioner) [33], and have positive attitudes regarding prevention [41].

Three studies examined whether patient-related factors were associated with whether oral health professionals perform general/unspecific dietary assessment activities [42,52,54]. Widström et al. [42] found in their survey study that dentists and dental hygienists were more likely to perform an assessment of dietary habits in children compared to adults (e.g., % of dentists and dental hygienists who perform an assessment of dietary habits in all or most of their child patients: 18.9; % of dentists and dental hygienists who perform an assessment of dietary habits in all or most of their adult patients: 8.3). Threlfall et al. [54] found in their qualitative interview study of general dental practitioners that they were more likely to ask questions about a child's diet if the child had dental caries.

Garton and Ford [39] investigated barriers reported by dentists regarding performing dietary analysis for root caries. They found that 43.3% of respondents reported barriers to providing dietary analysis. Time was the most common barrier (33.9% of respondents); however, other barriers encountered by <10% of respondents included cost, lack of usefulness, lack of authority to order, and dietary analysis not being evidence-based. In addition, these authors found statistically significantly more dentists working in the public sector vs. the private sector reported the barrier of lack of authority to order (public: 8.7% vs. private: 1.7%).

Use of Specific Dietary Assessment Tools

Six studies provide information on self-reported use of specific dietary assessment tools (e.g., diet diary) by oral health professionals (cross-sectional survey studies ($n = 5$) [35,38,43,46,48]; qualitative interview study ($n = 1$) [54]); of note, all of these studies were conducted in dentists. Overall, the survey studies found that less than 50% of dentists self-reported using some type of diet diary with their patients (e.g., 9% of pediatric dentists [35]; 28% of general dental practitioners [43]; 12–31% of dentists when referring to care of patients with erosive tooth wear [38,46,48]). These studies also found that less structured diet assessment approaches (e.g., oral interviews, asking patients to recall usual activities for a specified period) tend to be more commonly used by dentists compared to diet diaries [38,43,46,48].

Arheiam et al. [43] studied the use of diet diaries in UK general dental practitioners, including reasons for using diet diaries, factors that are considered when deciding to use these tools, routines when using diet diaries, and reasons for not using diet diaries. Of note, they found that diet diaries were more commonly used in children vs. adults, and the top reasons for lack of use of diet diaries were inadequate remuneration by the National Health Service (NHS), lack of usefulness, lack of knowledge, and poor compliance. The authors also found statistically significant predictors of diet diary use in a multivariate model were years of service, percentage of NHS patients in practice, and percentage of case-mix children in practice. The authors also reported the median time required to complete a diet diary analysis was 10 min (range: 1–23 min) and that patients were asked to keep a diary for a median of 3 days (range: 1–7 days) [43]. Lastly, a qualitative interview study by Threlfall et al. [54] found that a few general dental practitioners had attempted to use diet sheets in children, but reported little success.

Inquiries about Specific Patient Behaviours or Concerns Related to Diet

In total, four cross-sectional survey studies report information on inquiries by oral health professionals about specific patient behaviours or concerns related to diet [34,37,40,45]; three of these studies were conducted in dentists [34,40,45] and one was conducted in dental hygienists [37]. Three of these studies captured self-reported information on asking about specific behaviours related to dental caries in children (e.g., between-meal exposure to food that causes dental caries, bottle use, juice consumption) [37,40,45], and one study focused on older adults [34].

Overall, the studies that captured information on inquires about specific behaviours in children related to diet and dental caries found that this practice is relatively common [37,40,45]. For example, Clovis et al. [37] found that among dental hygienists who routinely assess their child/youth patients for risk factors related to dental caries (88.7% of respondents), 64.9% self-reported asking about between-meal exposure to cavity-producing foods. In addition, Sim et al. [40] found that the frequency of asking about different feeding practices (including bottle feeding and juice consumption) in infants and toddlers can vary depending on the practice (e.g., 77% of respondents reported asking about bottle contents all of the time vs. 27% of respondents reported asking about age of first juice consumption all of the time). One study captured differences in these types of practices between different types of oral health professionals. Dima et al. [45] found that a significantly higher percentage of pediatric dentists self-report asking about bottle use often or very often compared to general dentists (94.9% vs. 67.2%).

In general dentists, Hawkins and Locker [34] found that asking about different types of behaviours relevant to eating in older adults varied depending on the behaviour (e.g., 55% of respondents usually asked about prevention from eating desired foods because of chewing problems vs. 15% of respondents usually asked about avoiding eating with other people because of chewing problems). These authors [34] also found that numerous practice and dentist demographic characteristics were significantly related to inquiring about various behaviours relevant to eating in older adults in bivariate (and for some variables multivariate) analyses including dentist involvement in taking patient history, self-rated ability to treat older adults who reside in institutional settings, estimated percentage of patients 65+ years of age, continuing education in geriatric dentistry in the last year, time taken to obtain a patient history, dentist age, population size of primary practice location, and dental school experience in geriatric outreach care.

3.1.2. Dietitians and Nutritionists

Three cross-sectional survey studies captured self-reported information about assessment practices of dietitians and/or nutritionists (including WIC personnel) related to nutrition and oral health or oral health only [49–51]; these studies are also described in Table 3. Fuller et al. [49] found that less than 50% of surveyed WIC personnel assessed children for visual evidence of dental caries; they further found that respondents ≥40 years of age were significantly more likely to do this practice compared to respondents 18–39 years of age (53% vs. 28%). Gold and Tomar [50] found in a small study of WIC nutritionists that 33% of respondents frequently asked about women's and caregivers' dental health and no respondents reported frequently examining the teeth of children for dental caries. They also found that 100% of respondents frequently asked about whether the child brought a bottle to bed. In addition, Fernandez et al. [51] found in dietitians who had completed an elective pediatric dentistry rotation during their dietetic internship training that 28% always and 31% never collect information on an adult's oral health history and 24% always and 38% never collect information on a child's oral health history.

3.2. Intervention Practices

3.2.1. Oral Health Professionals

Nutrition intervention practices (e.g., diet counselling, nutrition counselling, dietary advice, dietary instruction, providing information on diet, nutrition advice) in oral health professionals were investigated in $n = 48$ studies (presented in $n = 53$ articles); these studies are described in Table 4. Overall, most articles reported on cross-sectional survey studies ($n = 36$ studies presented in $n = 39$ articles). In addition, there were $n = 8$ chart review studies (one of which had professionals keep detailed documents of encounters over a 2-week period), $n = 1$ observation study that also included a survey and chart review study (presented in $n = 2$ articles), and $n = 3$ qualitative interview/focus group studies (presented in $n = 4$ articles) that were included. In general, most of the studies provided information on general/unspecified nutrition intervention practices (e.g., nutrition counselling, diet advice); however, there were also studies that discussed types of resources/strategies used, information provided to patients, and barriers regarding intervention practices.

Table 4. Intervention practice information reported in the included articles.

Study Authors, Year, and Country	Sample Size *	Professional Type	Population and/or Concern of Focus	General/ Unspecific Intervention Practices (e.g., Nutrition Counselling, Diet Advice)	Types of Resources/ Strategies Used	Information Provided to Patients	Barriers Regarding Intervention Practices	Referrals/ Collaboration between Dentistry and Nutrition/Dietetics
SURVEY STUDIES								
Oral Health Professionals								
Chisick et al., 2000 [55]; USA	606	full-time military or civilian dentists in the Army Dental Care System		X	X	X		X
Anderson et al., 2002 [56]; Wales	568	dentists; dental hygienists; dental therapists				X		
Roshan et al., 2003 [33]; UK	687	general dental practitioners; community dental officers	children	(X)^Practice/Prof				
Dugmore and Rock, 2003 [57]; UK	227	general and community dental practitioners	children; tooth erosion	X^Patient		X^Patient		
Freeman et al., 2005 [58]; Northern Ireland	128 practices	general dental practices	dental caries	X				
Wang, 2005 [59]; Norway	199 (1995); 210 (2004)	dental hygienists from public dental service	children; dental caries	X^Patient				
Huang et al., 2006 [60]; USA	111	orthodontists	children; dental caries	X^Practice/Prof	X	X	X	X
Sajnani-Oommen et al., 2006 [35]; USA	180	pediatric dentists	children	X^Practice/Prof		X		X
Dyer and Robinson, 2006 [61]; UK	166	principal dentists		X			X^Professional Type	
Trueblood et al., 2008 [62]; USA	127	pediatric dentists	children; dental caries	X				
Brickhouse et al., 2008 [63]; USA	~221	general dentists; pediatric dentists	infants	X^Professional Type		X^Professional Type		

Table 4. *Cont.*

Study Authors, Year, and Country	Sample Size *	Professional Type	Population and/or Concern of Focus	General/ Unspecific Intervention Practices (e.g., Nutrition Counselling, Diet Advice)	Types of Resources/ Strategies Used	Information Provided to Patients	Barriers Regarding Intervention Practices	Referrals/ Collaboration between Dentistry and Nutri-tion/Dietetics
				SURVEY STUDIES				
				Oral Health Professionals				
Kelly and Moynihan, 2008 [64]; UK	879	dentists; dental hygienists; other occupations or specialties	periodontal disease	X		X	X	
Csikar et al., 2009 [65]; UK	386	dental practitioners		X[Practice/Prof]				
Satur et al., 2009 [66]; Australia	59	dental therapists		X[Practice/Prof]				
Tseveenjav et al., 2009 [67]; Finland and Norway	682	dental hygienists		X[Practice/Prof]				
Malcheff et al., 2009 [68]; USA	2157	pediatric dentists	infants	X				
Manski and Parker, 2010 [69]; USA	308	dental hygienists	children; early childhood caries	X[Practice/Prof]				
Salama and Kebriaei, 2010 [70]; USA	371	general dentists	infants	X				
Ananaba et al., 2010 [71]; USA	2294	general dentists; pediatric dentists	infants	X[Professional Type; Practice/Prof]				
Cunha-Cruz et al., 2010 [72]; USA	209	dentists	dentin hyper-sensitivity	X				
Bubna et al., 2012 [36]; USA	554	pediatric dentists	infants	(X)				
Lee et al., 2012 [73]; USA	1779	pediatric dentists	children; dental caries	X[Practice/Prof]				
Kakudate et al., 2012 [74]; Yokoyama et al., 2013 [75]; Yokoyama et al., 2013 [76]; Japan	189	dentists		X[Practice/Prof]				
Hussein et al., 2013 [77]; Germany	640	dentists		X[Practice/Prof]				
Sim et al., 2014 [40]; USA	86	pediatric dentists	infants and toddlers; dental caries	X[Practice/Prof]			X	
Gnich et al., 2014 [78]; Scotland	174	dental nurses	children	X[Patient; Practice/Prof]				
Yusuf et al., 2015 [79]; Yusuf et al., 2016 [41]; UK	164	National Health Service general dental practitioners		X[Practice/Prof]				
Arheiam et al., 2016 [43]; UK	250	general dental practitioners		X	X			
Hayes et al., 2016 [80]; Australia	426	dental hygienists; oral health therapists					X	

Table 4. *Cont.*

Study Authors, Year, and Country	Sample Size *	Professional Type	Population and/or Concern of Focus	General/Unspecific Intervention Practices (e.g., Nutrition Counselling, Diet Advice)	Types of Resources/Strategies Used	Information Provided to Patients	Barriers Regarding Intervention Practices	Referrals/Collaboration between Dentistry and Nutrition/Dietetics
SURVEY STUDIES								
Oral Health Professionals								
Baatsch et al., 2017 [81]; Germany	250	dentists						X[Practice/Prof]
Hayes et al., 2017 [82]; Australia	41	dentists; dental hygienists; oral health therapists		X[Professional Type]			X[Professional Type]	
Wright and Casamass-imo, 2017 [83]; USA	1615	pediatric dentists; pediatric dental residents	children; sugar sweetened beverages	X[Practice/Prof]	X	X	X	X
Cole et al., 2018 [84]; USA	919	dental hygienists	children	X[Practice/Prof]	X[Practice/Prof]	X		X[Practice/Prof]
Djokic et al., 2019 [85]; Ireland	467	pediatric dentists; nonpediatric dentists	infants	X[Professional Type]				
Aziz et al., 2020 [86]; New Zealand	325	general dentists		X[Practice/Prof]				
Bakhurji et al., 2021 [87]; Saudi Arabia	335	general dentists; pediatric dentists	infants	X[Professional Type]	X[Professional Type]			
Dietitians/Nutritionists								
Shick et al., 2005 [88]; USA	324	WIC nutritionists	WIC clients					X[Patient; Practice/Prof]
Butani et al., 2006 [89]; USA	126	WIC providers	WIC clients	X[Practice/Prof]				
Fuller et al., 2014 [49]; USA	159	WIC personnel	WIC clients			X[Practice/Prof]		X[Practice/Prof]
Gold and Tomar, 2016 [50]; USA	9	WIC nutritionists	WIC clients			X		X
Fernandez et al., 2017 [51]; USA	36	dietitians who completed a pediatric dentistry internship rotation		X			X	X
CHART REVIEW STUDIES								
Oral Health Professionals								
Kärkkäinen et al., 2001 [90]; Finland	267 in 1992; 590 in 1995	public dental service	children 12 years and 15 years	X[Patient; Practice/Prof]				
Tickle et al., 2003 [91]; UK	677	general dental practices (*n* = 50)	children who regularly attended dental care and have a history of interproximal caries in primary molars	X[Patient]				
Nihtilä and Widström, 2009 [92]; Finland	466	public dental service	children and adolescents	X[Patient]				

Table 4. *Cont.*

Study Authors, Year, and Country	Sample Size *	Professional Type	Population and/or Concern of Focus	General/ Unspecific Intervention Practices (e.g., Nutrition Counselling, Diet Advice)	Types of Resources/ Strategies Used	Information Provided to Patients	Barriers Regarding Intervention Practices	Referrals/ Collaboration between Dentistry and Nutrition/Dietetics
				CHART REVIEW STUDIES				
				Oral Health Professionals				
Wang and Aspelund, 2010 [93]; Norway	576	public dental service (20 clinicians in 16 public dental service clinics)	children and adolescents 3–18 years	X[Patient]				
Sarmadi et al., 2011 [94]; Sweden	432	public dental service (dentists and dental hygienists)	children 6–19 years at high risk of developing dental caries	X[Patient]				
Masoe et al., 2014 [95]; Australia	29,599	public dental service (oral health therapists)	adolescents 12–18 years	X[Patient; Practice/Prof]				
Raindi et al., 2015 [96]; UK		general dental practice	periodontal disease	X				
Skinner et al., 2016 [97]; Australia	~26,000 to ~31,000 per year	public dental service	adolescents 12–17 years	X[Patient]				
				OBSERVATION, CHART REVIEW, AND SURVEY STUDY				
				Oral Health Professionals				
Demko et al., 2008 [98]; Wotman et al., 2010 [99]; USA	3751 patient visits in 120 general dental practices	dentists, dental hygienists		X[Professional Type]				
				QUALITATIVE INTERVIEW AND/OR FOCUS GROUP STUDIES				
				Oral Health Professionals and Dietitians/Nutritionists				
Threlfall et al., 2007 [100]; Threlfall et al., 2007 [54]; UK	93	general dental practitioners	children; dental caries	X[Patient; Practice/Prof]	X	X[Patient]	X	
Cashmore et al., 2011 [101]; Australia	10	dental assistants, dental therapists, pediatric dental specialist, regional co-ordinator of oral health promotion	children waiting for surgery for treatment of severe dental caries				X	
Ong et al., 2015 [102]; Hong Kong	23	dentists, dietitians						X

* Sample size for survey studies and qualitative interview and/or focus group studies refers to number of professionals included; sample size for chart review and observational studies refers to the number of patients included. WIC: Special Supplemental Nutrition Program for Women, Infants, and Children. (X) = study measure included both assessment and intervention practices combined together (e.g., analyzed diets and gave dietary advice). Patient = examine differences in intervention practices in different types of patients (e.g., children vs. adults, severe dental caries vs. not). Professional Type = examine differences in intervention practices in different types of professionals (e.g., general dentists vs. pediatric dentists, dentists vs. dental hygienists). Practice/Prof = examine differences in intervention practices for different practice characteristics (e.g., public vs. private, rural practice vs. urban practice) and/or health professional characteristics (e.g., demographics, education, attitudes).

General/Unspecific Nutrition Intervention Practices

In total, $n = 33$ cross-sectional survey studies presented in $n = 36$ articles, $n = 8$ chart review studies, $n = 1$ observation study presented in $n = 2$ articles, and $n = 1$ qualitative interview study presented in $n = 2$ articles provide information on the delivery of general/unspecific nutrition interventions (e.g., diet counselling, nutrition counselling, dietary advice, dietary instruction, providing information on diet, nutrition advice) by oral health professionals. In general, most of the survey studies that captured self-report information on this topic report on the proportion of oral health professionals providing this service with or without some type of measure of how often they provide this service. Of note, most of these studies reported information on dentists; however, there were eight studies that also captured information on the practices of other oral health professionals (e.g., dental hygienists, dental therapists, dental nurses) [59,64,66,67,69,78,82,84]. Overall, most of these studies find using a variety of different types of measures that many oral health professionals self-report carrying out nutrition interventions at least some of the time. However, within these survey studies, only a few studies captured information on the percentage of patients receiving this care and found it varied from a mean of 21.4% to 63.0% [43,74–76]. In addition, a few survey studies reported that the length of time spent on these activities was brief (approximately five minutes) [35,60].

In contrast to the cross-sectional survey studies which provide self-report data, the chart review studies (one of which includes professionals documenting all preventative activities over a 2-week time frame) and observation studies generally find that this practice is variable and often limited. For example, these studies conducted in children and adolescents have found that nutrition interventions are provided to a range of <10% of children/adolescents to >50% of children/adolescents in both public dental service and other practice settings [91–94,97], that dietary advice represented <10% of clinical activities in public dental service [95], and that the number of diet instruction sessions is low in public dental clinics (e.g., ≤~1 per child/adolescent in the observation periods) [90]. Of note, the study by Sarmadi et al. [94] also found that diet counselling was provided to ~10–20% of children and adolescents whereas diet information was provided to ~40–50% of children and adolescents attending public dental services in Sweden. In addition, Raindi et al. [96] found in a small pilot study that diet advice was not provided for periodontal prevention. As well, an observation study [98,99] conducted in general dental practices in the United States found that overall <~10% of visits had nutrition counselling with the median number of 30 s intervals devoted to nutrition counselling being 0 (range: 0–6 for dentists; 0–23 for dental hygienists). In addition, this study also found that among dentists and dental hygienists who self-reported often/always providing a nutrition discussion using a self-administered survey, only a mean of 3.9%, and 13.7% of the patients of these dentists and dental hygienists, respectively, were observed to actually receive this service. In addition, when this practice occurred, <5% of visit time was spent on this activity.

Very few studies provide information on how general/unspecific nutrition intervention practices of different types of oral health professionals compare to one another [63,71,82,85,87,98,99]. Overall, most of these studies found that pediatric dentists more commonly provided these interventions to infant patients compared to other dentists [63,71,85,87] and that dental hygienists and/or oral health therapists provide these interventions more frequently compared to dentists [82,98,99].

In total, 11 studies [54,57,59,78,90–95,97] examined the provision of general/unspecific nutrition interventions by patient type. Six studies [57,59,90–93] found that the provision of general/unspecific nutrition interventions generally increased as the severity of dental disease (e.g., dental caries, erosion), risk of dental disease, or amount of dental care increased; however, only three studies reported significant results [90,91,93]. Studies also found that in children and adolescent patients, those who are younger (vs. older) [95], those who are less disadvantaged when looking at socioeconomic status (vs. more disadvantaged) [97], and patients/families who the professional felt were more motivated and with whom they had seen success [54] were more likely to receive nutrition interventions from oral health professionals. In addition, one study found that the frequency of delivery of dietary advice by dental nurses was similar for children <2 years of age compared to children >2 years of age [78].

Seventeen survey studies presented in 19 articles investigated various professional and practice factors that impact the provision or the intent to provide general/unspecific nutrition interventions, with some of these studies finding statistically significant results. First, some studies found that oral health professional demographic variables showed some type of statistically significant relationship with the provision of general/unspecific nutrition interventions, including oral health professional age [79]; sex [73,75,79,86]; knowledge, skills, and/or education in this area [78,84]; and ownership of practice [73]. Studies have also found that attitudes, perceived behavioural control, motivation, and/or confidence in this area were statistically significantly associated with providing nutrition interventions [40,41,60,75,78,83]. A study of dental hygienists found that working more hours per week was associated with increased likelihood of providing nutrition counselling [69]. Studies also found that practice characteristics were statistically significantly associated with providing general/unspecific nutrition interventions, including prevention focus/orientation [75,76], practice location (e.g., rural vs. urban) [66], practice constraints [40], practice busyness [75], and practice type and setting (e.g., private vs. public; community dental service vs. general dental practice) [33,65,67,86]. Moreover, a chart review study of public dental services found that rural health districts provided less dietary advice compared to metropolitan health districts [95]. Lastly, Threlfall et al. [54] found in a qualitative study of general dental practitioners regarding care of children with dental caries that practices with a dental hygienist had an increased focus on providing diet advice.

Types of Resources/Strategies Used

Only a few studies [43,54,55,60,83,84] reported on types of specific nutrition education materials, resources, and/or strategies used when oral health professionals provide nutrition interventions. Most of the studies that have investigated this topic have been cross-sectional survey studies that provide self-reported information. Chisick et al. [55] and Huang et al. [60] found that oral presentations/oral discussions and paper fliers/handouts were the most common ways to deliver this information. Huang et al. [60] reported on the frequency of providing nutrition advice to parents compared to children, and they found similar results between the two groups. In addition, Wright and Casamassimo [83] investigated in pediatric dentists and pediatric dental residents the frequency of using different types of intervention strategies to reduce consumption of sugar-sweetened beverages; they found that speaking to parents about observations if the child has high risk of dental caries was the most common strategy, followed by documenting the high risk of dental caries in the patient's chart. Provision of educational materials on sugar-sweetened beverages and offering motivational interviewing or other behaviour modification programs were also relatively common strategies. They further found that less common intervention strategies included providing parents with a self-administered sugar-sweetened beverage screening tool, and following up on interventions. Cole et al. [84] examined the frequency of provision of different types of nutrition interventions by dental hygienists. They found that nutrition counselling was more common than advocacy and collaborative activities (e.g., advocating to school officials to ensure healthy foods are available in school food services). For advocacy and collaborative activities, they also found that those with continuing education on obesity were more likely to do those activities compared to those who had obesity education only within an entry-level dental hygiene program. Arheiam et al. [43] also found that 40% of general dental practitioner respondents referred patients to other oral health professionals (e.g., dental hygienists) for advice on diet for an average of 11% of their patients. Lastly, Threlfall et al. [54] found in a qualitative study of general dental practitioners regarding caring for children with dental caries that oral advice was the most common way to provide dietary information, but providing leaflets was also done. They also found that general dental practices that had a dental hygienist often had preventative activities (e.g., diet advice) delegated to those professionals.

Types of Nutrition Information Provided

Few details on the types of nutrition information provided to patients by oral health professionals were present in the included articles; only 10 survey studies reported this type of finding [35,55–57,60,63,64,83,84,87]. Topics that were captured in the survey studies included nursing caries/baby bottle decay risk [55,63,87]; consumption of sugary foods and drinks (including timing) [35,56,83,84]; consumption of between-meal snacks [84], supplements (including recommending vitamins) [35,64]; and consumption of erosion-causing foods, specifically carbonated soft drinks, fruit juice, acidic drinks, and citrus fruit [57]. In addition, Huang et al. [60] provided information on the proportion of orthodontists who provided patients handouts on foods to avoid (56% of respondents) and foods to encourage (32% of respondents).

Very few studies examined differences between different types of oral health professionals for this type of finding. Brickhouse et al. [63] found that discussing baby bottle decay risk during infant oral health exams was common and similar between pediatric dentists and general dentists (pediatric dentists: 98%; general dentists: 100%). In addition, Bakhurji et al. [87] found that 60% of pediatric dentists and 64% of general dentists provided nutrition counselling and talked about baby bottle decay in infant oral health care. The work by Dugmore and Rock [57] was the only study to examine the proportion of dentists who provided specific dietary messages in different patient populations. They reported the proportions of dentists who provided advice on carbonated soft drinks, fruit juice, acidic drinks, and citrus fruit for patients presenting with tooth erosion into (a) the enamel and (b) the dentine. The percentage of dentists who gave the specific types of advice ranged from 6.6% to 31.7% depending on the food/beverage topic and whether the tooth erosion was into the enamel or dentine.

A qualitative interview study by Threlfall et al. [54,100] provided in-depth information on the content of dietary advice provided by general dental practitioners to children who are dealing with dental caries and their parents. In this study, all general dental practitioners reported providing dietary advice. Dietary advice was primarily centred on decreasing consumption of sugar, and sugar intake frequency was often considered a key message. Sugary beverages were also a common topic for dietary advice. The authors reported that there were variations in dietary advice content and emphasis (e.g., some participants provided advice on extrinsic sugars while others did not; some participants said to limit carbonated drinks due to erosion, and others said to reduce intake of these drinks because of sugar). Some participants also reported that they emphasized oral hygiene instead of diet because they felt it was easier to change, and some participants also reported trying to provide advice that was practical knowing that children like sugary foods and beverages (e.g., providing strategies on how to consume sugar-rich foods to decrease risk of caries). The authors also found that participants tailored the advice to parents based on their perception of the level of ignorance.

Barriers Regarding Intervention Practices

In total, six survey studies [40,60,61,80,82,83] examined the prevalence of barriers associated with the provision of nutrition interventions by oral health professionals using quantitative methods; five studies examined these barriers in dentists [40,60,61,82,83], and three studies examined these barriers in other types of oral health professionals (i.e., dental hygienists, oral health therapists) [61,80,82]. The most common barriers studied were compensation, funding, and/or reimbursement [40,60,61,80,82,83]; time [40,60,61,80,82,83]; lack of professional training, knowledge, and/or skills [40,61,80,82,83]; and patient motivation, compliance, and/or interest (including difficulties in changing behaviour) [40,80,83]. Other barriers examined in two studies included patient knowledge and demographics (e.g., literacy, education level, socioeconomic status) [80,82]; lack of trained staff [40,83]; lack of resources [60,83]; communication, language, and/or cultural barriers [60,82]; lack of likelihood of effectiveness or benefit [61,82]; and fear of judging, alienating, and/or offending patients [61,83]. Of note, time was among the top three most commonly reported barriers in four of those studies [60,61,80,82]. Additionally, lack of patient motivation, compliance, and/or interest (including difficulties in changing behaviour) [40,80,83]; compensation, funding, and/or reimbursement [40,61,82]; and lack of professional training, knowledge, and/or skills [61,80,82] were among the top three most commonly reported barriers in three of those studies.

Dyer and Robinson [61] examined differences in the prevalence of perceived barriers reported by principal dentists to providing advice on diet/calorie intake by dentists and professionals complementary to dentistry (PCDs). The authors found statistically significant differences in the following barriers between the two types of professionals: time (dentists: 30.7%; PCDs: 16.9%) and lack of training/knowledge (dentists: 22.3%; PCDs: 7.8%). The authors found no differences for other investigated barriers (i.e., funding, effectiveness, patient alienation).

Two studies examined the relationship between barriers and implementation of nutrition interventions in pediatric dentists. Sim et al. [40] found that when practitioners were grouped into those who provide dietary recommendations all of the time and those who do not, those who provide dietary recommendations all of the time had a significantly lower proportion of respondents who reported the following barriers: infant/toddler oral health is not a practice focus, recommendations are confusing/ambiguous, deficiency of trained auxiliaries, and time constraints. Wright and Casamassimo [83] found in pediatric dentists and dental residents that there was a significant relationship between provision of interventions regarding sugar-sweetened beverages and several different barriers, including reimbursement, time, lack of knowledge/skills, concern about offending patients, lack of educational materials, and legal concerns.

In addition, three articles captured qualitative data using various methods (e.g., interviews, focus groups, open-ended survey questions) on barriers to providing nutrition interventions from the perspectives of oral health professionals [54,64,101]. Lack of oral health professional confidence and knowledge [64,101], lack of evidence-based guidance [64], funding and/or time [54,64], and lack of patient motivation and knowledge [54] were all identified.

3.2.2. Dietitians and Nutritionists

Four cross-sectional survey studies examined provision of interventions for oral health provided by dietitians or nutritionists (including WIC personnel) [49–51,89]. Importantly, three of these studies were conducted in WIC personnel [49,50,89].

First, Butani et al. [89] assessed how often oral health was discussed by WIC personnel with clients. In total, they found that 37% of respondents discussed oral health issues most of the time or every time and 21% of respondents discussed it none of the time or a little of the time. They also found that 69% of respondents discussed oral health with more than 50% of their clients. Nursing training and oral health training were significant predictors for WIC personnel to discuss oral health with their clients. Fuller et al. [49] found that a significantly higher percentage of WIC personnel from rural districts self-reported advising parents/guardians on fluoride treatments or supplements compared to those from urban districts (rural: 58%; urban: 42%). Tooth brushing counselling provision in WIC clients by WIC personnel was assessed in two studies. Fuller et al. [49] found that more than 50% of surveyed WIC personnel provide tooth brushing counselling and that it was significantly related to practitioner years of experience. In addition, Gold and Tomar [50] found that 67% of WIC nutritionists frequently advise caregivers on the significance of frequent tooth brushing for their child. They also found that 67% of WIC nutritionists frequently advise caregivers on the importance of dental visits and 11% frequently discuss how the women's oral health and the child's oral health are linked. Gold and Tomar [50] also found that 100% of respondents frequently talk about how sugary drinks and snacks have a role in dental caries.

Only one study examined the intervention practices of dietitians outside of a WIC setting related to oral health. Fernandez et al. [51] surveyed dietitians who completed an elective pediatric dentistry rotation during their dietetic internship training. This study found that among participants, 20% always and 20% never include information about oral health as part of diet counselling; 40% always and 17% never consider the impact on oral health when recommending healthy foods; 34% always and 14% never consider the impact on teeth when providing counselling regarding sugary beverages. The authors also found that 17% always and 34% never provide education on oral health.

The study of Fernandez et al. [51] was the only study that provided information on the perceived barriers of dietitians in providing their services to dental patients. They investigated different types of barriers, and their results are as follows: cost/reimbursement of dietitian services (significant barrier: 57% of respondents; possible barrier: 43%), interest of clients in diet and oral health (significant barrier: 29%; possible barrier: 63%; not a barrier: 9%), dentist reluctance to refer their patients to a dietitian (significant barrier: 37%; possible barrier: 51%; not a barrier: 11%), and dietitian confidence in providing counselling and/or information in this area (possible barrier: 62%; not a barrier: 38%).

3.2.3. Collaboration between Dietitians and Oral Health Professionals

Cross-sectional survey studies of oral health professionals investigated collaboration between nutrition/dietetics and dentistry using various outcomes, including referrals to dietitians/nutritionists [35,60,83,84], nutrition referrals [55,60], and/or recommendation of dietetics [81]. Although slightly different outcomes were used, they reported that the majority of oral health professionals never provide referrals to dietitians/nutritionists.

Four survey studies examined referrals to dentists by dietitians, nutritionists and/or WIC personnel [49–51,88]; three of those studies were conducted in WIC personnel [49,50,88]. For example, Gold and Tomar [50] found that 44% of WIC nutritionists frequently referred children or women to dental care. Fuller et al. [49] found that a significantly higher percentage of WIC personnel from urban districts referred clients to a dentist compared to those from rural districts (urban: 54%; rural: 46%). Shick et al. [88] comprehensively studied the dental care referral practices of WIC personnel. The authors found that 95.6% of respondents reported making dental referrals for children 1–5 years, and of those, 52.3% conducted this activity very frequently or frequently; referrals for infants were much less common. These authors also found that statistically significant predictors of referring children aged 1–5 years to dental care included older practitioner age (i.e., ≥40 years vs. younger), higher frequency of seeing dental concerns in patients (vs. lower), higher frequency of parents asking about obtaining dental care for their children (vs. lower), higher confidence in performing oral health risk assessment (vs. lower), higher confidence in making dental referrals (vs. lower), and higher confidence that patients will access dental care if advised (vs. lower). This study also reported that the most often used referral locations were local health departments (60.3% of respondents) and private dental offices (31.7% of respondents). The study of Fernandez et al. [51] was the only survey study that examined referrals to oral health professionals by dietitians outside of a WIC setting. The authors found that 54% of dietitians referred patients to pediatric or general dentists in their practice.

The qualitative study by Ong et al. [102] examined interdisciplinary collaboration between dietitians, dentists, and physicians in Hong Kong in regards to diet. The authors found that barriers included those associated with electronic health records (e.g., not used by all the different professions), limited contact between the professions, lack of financial coverage, and inconsistent diet advice between different professions due to a lack of understanding of the advice given by others and different focuses of treatment administered by the different professions. Ideas presented to facilitate collaboration included more collaboration in undergraduate education, interprofessional education events, and development of guidelines with input from different professions.

4. Discussion

To our knowledge, this is the first scoping review to comprehensively examine the literature on the nutrition care practices of oral health professionals and dietitians/nutritionists to optimize oral health (and specifically conditions that affect the dentition and periodontium). This review provides valuable information on the types of published evidence available in this area and a summary of key findings of these studies. The information gathered through conducting this review helps to provide direction on future strategies needed to move this area of research forward, which is important as oral health issues are prevalent in Canada and worldwide.

Although there appears to be substantial interest in this topic due to the volume of studies published that report information in this area, most articles provide only general and unspecific findings (e.g., capturing how often oral health professionals provide dietary advice) and focus mainly on oral health professionals (and especially dentists). Most of the data are also self-reported, which has limitations. Moreover, more than half of the studies were conducted in two regions (the United States and the United Kingdom), and there was only one study from Canada. In addition, many more studies focus on intervention practices compared to assessment practices despite assessment being an essential component to develop an appropriate intervention plan. Of note, very few studies provided specific details about the nutrition care encounters (e.g., types of dietary assessment tools used, types of information provided to patients, strategies used to provide the information, length of time spent on the encounter, follow-up on encounters). A consideration for future research in this area is that the standardized Nutrition Care Process (NCP) could be used when thinking about how to approach conducting research on this topic. This framework was developed by the Academy of Nutrition and Dietetics (formerly the American Dietetic Association) [103] and distinguishes nutrition care into four components: Nutrition Assessment, Nutrition Diagnosis, Nutrition Intervention, and Nutrition Monitoring and Evaluation. Use of this framework may be useful for structuring future research in this area.

Several studies did not specifically outline the oral health issue and patient population that was being studied; when studies examined nutrition care practices in oral health professionals, it was assumed that they were referring to oral health (and specifically the dentition and periodontium). Although this assumption is likely relatively safe, a limitation of this review is that through the process of conducting this project, we found evidence that oral health professionals may also provide some nutrition care in other areas such as diabetes [104,105] and obesity/weight management [106–109]. We felt that the inclusion of these articles that did not mention the specific oral health condition and patient population was important as they represent an important group of studies in this area.

Another interesting finding from this review was that information on nutrition care practices for oral health (and specifically the dentition and periodontium) was captured using various study designs both in terms of the research methodology (e.g., cross-sectional survey, observation, chart review, qualitative interview) and the overall focus of the articles. In addition, many studies collecting information on nutrition care practices of oral health professionals capture this information as part of a study with a non-nutrition focus such as examining overall practice patterns of oral health professionals (e.g., [66,67]), dental prevention activities (including for dental caries) (e.g., [41,42,55,58,59,77,79]), or infant oral health care (e.g., [36,63,68,70,71,85,87]). However, a few studies focused primarily on diet and oral health (e.g., [35,40,43,75,80,82]). Because diet was often not the focus of the included studies (and instead a subcomponent), one major challenge encountered when conducting this review was that many of the included articles were difficult to locate solely from database searching. As can be seen in Figure 1, many articles were located using other approaches (e.g., citations, hand searching). With diet being such an important component of optimal oral health, researchers conducting work in this area should consider including words related to diet/nutrition in the title, abstract, and keywords of articles to ensure that these studies will be found using database searches. In addition, more studies with a focus on diet and oral health should be conducted to focus on these specific activities, particularly because these activities are complex and multifaceted.

Overall, most of the articles included in this review found that nutrition care is provided by most oral health professionals at least some of the time. Survey studies and studies capturing self-report data found that provision of nutrition care was more common compared to when it was examined in chart review and observation studies. Some studies included as part of this review provide information on both barriers to providing nutrition care by oral health professionals and factors that affect the provision of these types of services, including the professional type, patient type, and various professional and practice factors. Together, this information suggests that many different factors can influence whether professionals provide this type of service and that there are many barriers that they experience when attempting to provide this type of care. This information is helpful for both dietitians and oral health professionals aspiring to provide this care, as well as managers interested in facilitating this process in different types of practice settings. Capturing this type of information in future studies is important to help optimize the provision of these types of services.

Dietitians are a professional group possessing the capability to offer substantial support in this area and have the knowledge, expertise, and time to focus on providing nutrition care to individuals who are in need of improving their diet to optimize oral health. Nutrition care by dietitians may also be a solution to address some of the barriers to performing these types of interventions identified by oral health professionals, including time (as they have more time to devote to nutrition care); lack of patient motivation, compliance, and/or interest (as they are trained to provide nutrition care to address these barriers such as motivational interviewing); and lack of knowledge/confidence among oral health professionals in providing this type of care (as dietitians are specifically trained to provide nutrition care). Despite the skillset of dietitians, this review identified only a handful of studies that captured information on nutrition care for oral health provided by dietitians and collaboration between dietitians and oral health professionals. Importantly, within the studies identifying collaboration between dietitians and dental professionals, findings suggest that this activity is uncommon despite various organizations and peer-review articles highlighting the importance of collaboration between these professionals [8,110,111]. In addition, dietitians have identified barriers in this area, including cost, lack of client interest in this area, dietitian confidence in providing support in this area, and concerns about reluctance of oral health professions to provide referrals to dietitians. Finding new ways to stimulate collaboration between the different professions will likely be very important in this area and overcoming barriers in this area is needed. Increased training on this topic for both professionals and students is important to consider.

There are a few limitations of this review. Although we did our best to locate articles using different strategies and are confident that we were able to locate the vast majority of the research studies in this area that met inclusion criteria, there are likely articles that were missed. Only studies written in English were included; there could have been relevant studies available in other languages that may have been excluded. We also did not assess nutrition care practices regarding oral health by professionals other than oral health professionals and dietitians, and there may be others who also provide these services. In addition, this review did not assess study quality.

5. Conclusions

Many different types of studies have captured information on nutrition care practices related to oral health (and specifically dentition and periodontium) in oral health professionals, and very few are available focusing on dietitians. In addition, there are limited data available on the specific details of the care that is provided. Few studies have captured information on interprofessional collaboration between dietitians and oral health professionals. This review article provides insight into how to move this area of research forward.

Author Contributions: Conceptualization, J.R.L.L.; methodology, J.R.L.L., A.G.T.V., J.R.d.M. and A.C.; formal analysis, J.R.L.L., A.G.T.V., J.R.d.M. and A.C.; investigation, J.R.L.L., A.G.T.V., J.R.d.M. and A.C.; writing—original draft preparation, J.R.L.L.; writing—review and editing, A.G.T.V., J.R.d.M. and A.C.; project administration, J.R.L.L. All authors have read and agreed to the published version of the manuscript.

Funding: J. Rover de Mello was funded by a New Faculty Graduate Student Support Program Scholarship from the University of Saskatchewan, a Saskatchewan Centre for Patient Oriented Research Traineeship, and through a Saskatchewan Health Research Foundation Establishment Grant awarded to JRLL. A. Vanzan was funded by a Saskatchewan Centre for Patient Oriented Research Traineeship. An undergraduate student who assisted with article screening was funded by a Saskatchewan Health Research Foundation Establishment Grant awarded to JRLL.

Acknowledgments: We would like to thank Jenna Thomson for her assistance with screening articles for this review. In addition, we would like to thank Megan Kennedy and Vicky Duncan (health science librarians) for their advice with the literature searches. The funders had no role in scoping review design, data collection and analysis, decision to publish, or manuscript preparation.

Conflicts of Interest: The authors declare no conflict of interest. The funders had no role in the design of the study; in the collection, analyses, or interpretation of data; in the writing of the manuscript; or in the decision to publish the results.

References

1. James, S.L.; Abate, D.; Abate, K.H.; Abay, S.M.; Abbafati, C.; Abbasi, N.; Abbastabar, H.; Abd-Allah, F.; Abdela, J.; Abdelalim, A.; et al. Global, regional, and national incidence, prevalence, and years lived with disability for 354 diseases and injuries for 195 countries and territories, 1990–2017: A systematic analysis for the Global Burden of Disease Study 2017. *Lancet* **2018**, *392*, 1789–1858. [CrossRef]
2. Bernabe, E.; Marcenes, W.; Hernandez, C.R.; Bailey, J.; Abreu, L.G.; Alipour, V.; Amini, S.; Arabloo, J.; Arefi, Z.; Arora, A.; et al. Global, Regional, and National Levels and Trends in Burden of Oral Conditions from 1990 to 2017: A Systematic Analysis for the Global Burden of Disease 2017 Study. *J. Dent. Res.* **2020**, *99*, 362–373. [PubMed]
3. Health Canada. *Report on the Findings of the Oral Health Component of the Canadian Health Measures Survey 2007–2009*; Health Canada: Ottawa, ON, Canada, 2010; ISBN 9781100156606.
4. Schroth, R.J.; Quiñonez, C.; Shwart, L.; Wagar, B. Treating Early Childhood Caries under General Anesthesia: A National Review of Canadian Data. *J. Can. Dent. Assoc.* **2016**, *82*, g20. [PubMed]
5. World Health Organization. Oral Health. 2020. Available online: https://www.who.int/news-room/fact-sheets/detail/oral-health (accessed on 30 September 2021).
6. Jensen, M.E. Diet and dental caries. *Dent. Clin. N. Am.* **1999**, *43*, 615–633.
7. Touger-Decker, R.; van Loveren, C. Sugars and dental caries. *Am. J. Clin. Nutr.* **2003**, *78*, 881S–892S. [CrossRef]
8. Touger-Decker, R.; Mobley, C. Position of the Academy of Nutrition and Dietetics: Oral health and nutrition. *J. Acad. Nutr. Diet.* **2013**, *113*, 693–701. [CrossRef]
9. Moynihan, P.J. Dietary advice in dental practice. *Br. Dent. J.* **2002**, *193*, 563–568. [CrossRef]
10. Salas, M.M.S.; Nascimento, G.G.; Vargas-Ferreira, F.; Tarquinio, S.B.C.; Huysmans, M.C.D.N.J.M.; Demarco, F.F. Diet influenced tooth erosion prevalence in children and adolescents: Results of a meta-analysis and meta-regression. *J. Dent.* **2015**, *43*, 865–875. [CrossRef]
11. Buzalaf, M.A.R.; Magalhães, A.C.; Rios, D. Prevention of erosive tooth wear: Targeting nutritional and patient-related risks factors. *Br. Dent. J.* **2018**, *224*, 371–378. [CrossRef]
12. Palmer, C.A. Important Relationships Between Diet, Nutrition, and Oral Health. *Nutr. Clin. Care* **2001**, *4*, 4–14. [CrossRef]
13. Tinanoff, N.; Palmer, C.A. Dietary determinants of dental caries and dietary recommendations for preschool children. *J. Public Health Dent.* **2000**, *60*, 197–199. [CrossRef]
14. Moynihan, P.; Petersen, P.E. Diet, nutrition and the prevention of dental diseases. *Public Health Nutr.* **2004**, *7*, 201–226. [CrossRef]
15. Scardina, G.A.; Messina, P. Good oral health and diet. *J. Biomed. Biotechnol.* **2012**, *2012*, 720692. [CrossRef]
16. Najeeb, S.; Zafar, M.S.; Khurshid, Z.; Zohaib, S.; Almas, K. The Role of Nutrition in Periodontal Health: An Update. *Nutrients* **2016**, *8*, 530. [CrossRef]
17. Bhattacharya, P.T.; Misra, S.R.; Hussain, M. Nutritional Aspects of Essential Trace Elements in Oral Health and Disease: An Extensive Review. *Scientifica* **2016**, *2016*, 5464373. [CrossRef]
18. Dietitians Association of Australia; Dental Health Services Victoria. Joint Position Statement on Oral Health and Nutrition October 2015. 2015. Available online: https://dietitiansaustralia.org.au/wp-content/uploads/2016/05/DAA-DHSV-Joint-Statement-Oral-Health-and-Nutrition.pdf (accessed on 30 September 2021).
19. NHS Health Scotland. Oral Health and Nutrition Guidance for Professionals June 2012. 2012. Available online: https://www.scottishdental.org/wp-content/uploads/2014/10/OralHealthAndNutritionGuidance.pdf (accessed on 30 September 2021).

20. American Academy of Pediatric Dentistry Clinical Affairs Committee; American Academy of Pediatric Dentistry Council on Clinical Affairs. Policy on Dietary Recommendations for Infants, Children, and Adolescents. *Pediatr. Dent.* **2017**, *39*, 64–66.
21. Jones, A.C.; Kirkpatrick, S.I.; Hammond, D. Beverage consumption and energy intake among Canadians: Analyses of 2004 and 2015 national dietary intake data. *Nutr. J.* **2019**, *18*, 60. [CrossRef]
22. Canadian Dental Association. CDA Position on Early Childhood Caries. 2010. Available online: https://www.cda-adc.ca/en/about/position_statements/ecc/ (accessed on 30 September 2021).
23. Canadian Dental Association. The State of Oral Health in Canada. 2017. Available online: https://www.cda-adc.ca/stateoforalhealth/_files/TheStateofOralHealthinCanada.pdf (accessed on 30 September 2021).
24. Petersen, P.E. Global policy for improvement of oral health in the 21st century–implications to oral health research of World Health Assembly 2007, World Health Organization. *Community Dent. Oral Epidemiol.* **2009**, *37*, 1–8. [CrossRef]
25. Franki, J.; Hayes, M.J.; Taylor, J.A. The provision of dietary advice by dental practitioners: A review of the literature. *Community Dent. Health* **2014**, *31*, 9–14.
26. Arksey, H.; O'Malley, L. Scoping studies: Towards a methodological framework. *Int. J. Soc. Res. Methodol.* **2005**, *8*, 19–32. [CrossRef]
27. Levac, D.; Colquhoun, H.; O'Brien, K.K. Scoping studies: Advancing the methodology. *Implement. Sci.* **2010**, *5*, 69. [CrossRef]
28. FDI. World Dental Federation FDI's Definition of Oral Health. Available online: https://www.fdiworlddental.org/fdis-definition-oral-health (accessed on 12 May 2021).
29. Suga, U.S.G.; Terada, R.S.S.; Ubaldini, A.L.M.; Fujimaki, M.; Pascotto, R.C.; Batilana, A.P.; Pietrobon, R.; Vissoci, J.R.N.; Rodrigues, C.G. Factors that drive dentists towards or away from dental caries preventive measures: Systematic review and metasummary. *PLoS ONE* **2014**, *9*, e107831. [CrossRef]
30. Kay, E.; Vascott, D.; Hocking, A.; Nield, H.; Dorr, C.; Barrett, H. A review of approaches for dental practice teams for promoting oral health. *Community Dent. Oral Epidemiol.* **2016**, *44*, 313–330. [CrossRef]
31. U.S Department of Agriculture Food and Nutrition Service. Special Supplemental Nutrition Program for Women, Infants, and Children (WIC). Available online: https://www.fns.usda.gov/wic (accessed on 30 September 2021).
32. Ouzzani, M.; Hammady, H.; Fedorowicz, Z.; Elmagarmid, A. Rayyan—A web and mobile app for systematic reviews. *Syst. Rev.* **2016**, *5*, 210. [CrossRef]
33. Roshan, D.; Curzon, M.E.J.; Fairpo, C.G. Changes in dentists' attitudes and practice in paediatric dentistry. *Eur. J. Paediatr. Dent.* **2003**, *4*, 21–27.
34. Hawkins, R.J.; Locker, D. Non-clinical information obtained by dentists during initial examinations of older adult patients. *Spec. Care Dent.* **2005**, *25*, 12–18. [CrossRef]
35. Sajnani-Oommen, G.; Perez-Spiess, S.; Julliard, K. Comparison of nutritional counseling between provider types. *Pediatr. Dent.* **2006**, *28*, 369–374.
36. Bubna, S.; Perez-Spiess, S.; Cernigliaro, J.; Julliard, K. Infant oral health care: Beliefs and practices of American Academy of Pediatric Dentistry members. *Pediatr. Dent.* **2012**, *34*, 203–209.
37. Clovis, J.B.; Horowitz, A.M.; Kleinman, D.V.; Wang, M.Q.; Massey, M. Maryland dental hygienists' knowledge, opinions and practices regarding dental caries prevention and early detection. *J. Dent. Hyg.* **2012**, *86*, 292–305.
38. Mulic, A.; Vidnes-Kopperud, S.; Skaare, A.B.; Tveit, A.B.; Young, A. Opinions on Dental Erosive Lesions, Knowledge of Diagnosis, and Treatment Strategies among Norwegian Dentists: A Questionnaire Survey. *Int. J. Dent.* **2012**, *2012*, 716396. [CrossRef]
39. Garton, B.J.; Ford, P.J. Root caries: A survey of Queensland dentists. *Int. J. Dent. Hyg.* **2013**, *11*, 216–225. [CrossRef] [PubMed]
40. Sim, C.J.; Iida, H.; Vann, W.F.J.; Quinonez, R.B.; Steiner, M.J. Dietary recommendations for infants and toddlers among pediatric dentists in North Carolina. *Pediatr. Dent.* **2014**, *36*, 322–328. [PubMed]
41. Yusuf, H.; Kolliakou, A.; Ntouva, A.; Murphy, M.; Newton, T.; Tsakos, G.; Watt, R.G. Predictors of dentists' behaviours in delivering prevention in primary dental care in England: Using the theory of planned behaviour. *BMC Health Serv. Res.* **2016**, *16*, 44. [CrossRef] [PubMed]
42. Widström, E.; Tillberg, A.; Byrkjeflot, L.I.; Skudutyte-Rysstad, R. Chair-side preventive interventions in the Public Dental Service in Norway. *Br. Dent. J.* **2016**, *221*, 179–185. [CrossRef] [PubMed]
43. Arheiam, A.; Brown, S.L.; Burnside, G.; Higham, S.M.; Albadri, S.; Harris, R.V. The use of diet diaries in general dental practice in England. *Community Dent. Health* **2016**, *33*, 267–273.
44. Halawany, H.S.; Salama, F.; Jacob, V.; Abraham, N.B.; Moharib, T.N.; Alazmah, A.S.; Al Harbi, J.A. A survey of pediatric dentists' caries-related treatment decisions and restorative modalities-A web-based survey. *Saudi Dent. J.* **2017**, *29*, 66–73. [CrossRef] [PubMed]
45. Dima, S.; Chang, W.-J.; Chen, J.-W.; Teng, N.-C. Early Childhood Caries-Related Knowledge, Attitude, and Practice: Discordance between Pediatricians and Dentists toward Medical Office-Based Prevention in Taiwan. *Int. J. Environ. Res. Public Health* **2018**, *15*, 1067. [CrossRef]
46. Mulic, A.; Arnadottir, I.B.; Jensdottir, T.; Kopperud, S.E. Opinions and Treatment Decisions for Dental Erosive Wear: A Questionnaire Survey among Icelandic Dentists. *Int. J. Dent.* **2018**, *2018*, 8572371. [CrossRef]
47. Kangasmaa, H.; Tanner, T.; Laitala, M.-L.; Mulic, A.; Kopperud, S.E.; Vähänikkilä, H.; Anttonen, V.; Alaraudanjoki, V. Knowledge on and treatment practices of erosive tooth wear among Finnish dentists. *Acta Odontol. Scand.* **2021**, *79*, 499–505. [CrossRef]

48. Mortensen, D.; Mulic, A.; Pallesen, U.; Twetman, S. Awareness, knowledge and treatment decisions for erosive tooth wear: A case-based questionnaire among Danish dentists. *Clin. Exp. Dent. Res.* **2021**, *7*, 56–62. [CrossRef]
49. Fuller, L.A.; Stull, S.C.; Darby, M.L.; Tolle, S.L. Oral health promotion: Knowledge, confidence, and practices in preventing early-severe childhood caries of Virginia WIC program personnel. *J. Dent. Hyg.* **2014**, *88*, 130–140. [PubMed]
50. Gold, J.T.; Tomar, S. Oral Health Knowledge and Practices of WIC Staff at Florida WIC Program. *J. Community Health* **2016**, *41*, 612–618. [CrossRef] [PubMed]
51. Fernandez, J.B.; Ahearn, K.; Atar, M.; More, F.G.; Sasson, L.; Rosenberg, L.; Godfrey, E.; Sehl, R.; Daronch, M. Interprofessional Educational Experience among Dietitians after a Pediatric Dentistry Clinical Rotation. *Top. Clin. Nutr.* **2017**, *32*, 193–201. [CrossRef]
52. Sarmadi, R.; Gabre, P.; Gahnberg, L. Strategies for caries risk assessment in children and adolescents at public dental clinics in a Swedish county. *Int. J. Paediatr. Dent.* **2009**, *19*, 135–140. [CrossRef]
53. O'Toole, S.; Khan, M.; Patel, A.; Patel, N.J.; Shah, N.; Bartlett, D.; Movahedi, S. Tooth wear risk assessment and care-planning in general dental practice. *Br. Dent. J.* **2018**, *224*, 358–362. [CrossRef]
54. Threlfall, A.G.; Hunt, C.M.; Milsom, K.M.; Tickle, M.; Blinkhorn, A.S. Exploring factors that influence general dental practitioners when providing advice to help prevent caries in children. *Br. Dent. J.* **2007**, *202*, E10; discussion 216–217. [CrossRef]
55. Chisick, M.C.; Richter, P.; Piotrowski, M.J. Dental health promotion and preventive dentistry practices of U.S. Army dentists. *Mil. Med.* **2000**, *165*, 604–606. [CrossRef]
56. Anderson, R.; Treasure, E.T.; Sprod, A.S. Oral health promotion practice: A survey of dental professionals in Wales. *Int. J. Health Promot. Educ.* **2002**, *40*, 9–14. [CrossRef]
57. Dugmore, C.R.; Rock, W.P. Awareness of tooth erosion in 12 year old children and primary care dental practitioners. *Community Dent. Health* **2003**, *20*, 223–227.
58. Freeman, R.; Kerr, G.; Salmon, K.; Speedy, P. Patient-active prevention in primary dental care: A characterisation of general practices in Northern Ireland. *Prim. Dent. Care* **2005**, *12*, 42–46. [CrossRef]
59. Wang, N.J. Caries preventive methods in child dental care reported by dental hygienists, Norway, 1995 and 2004. *Acta Odontol. Scand.* **2005**, *63*, 330–334. [CrossRef]
60. Huang, J.S.; Becerra, K.; Walker, E.; Hovell, M.F. Childhood overweight and orthodontists: Results of a survey. *J. Public Health Dent.* **2006**, *66*, 292–294. [CrossRef]
61. Dyer, T.A.; Robinson, P.G. General health promotion in general dental practice—The involvement of the dental team Part 2: A qualitative and quantitative investigation of the views of practice principals in South Yorkshire. *Br. Dent. J.* **2006**, *201*, 45–51; discussion 31. [CrossRef]
62. Trueblood, R.; Kerins, C.A.; Seale, N.S. Caries risk assessment practices among Texas pediatric dentists. *Pediatr. Dent.* **2008**, *30*, 49–53.
63. Brickhouse, T.H.; Unkel, J.H.; Kancitis, I.; Best, A.M.; Davis, R.D. Infant oral health care: A survey of general dentists, pediatric dentists, and pediatricians in Virginia. *Pediatr. Dent.* **2008**, *30*, 147–153.
64. Kelly, S.A.M.; Moynihan, P.J. Attitudes and practices of dentists with respect to nutrition and periodontal health. *Br. Dent. J.* **2008**, *205*, E9; discussion 196–197. [CrossRef]
65. Csikar, J.; Williams, S.A.; Beal, J. Do smoking cessation activities as part of oral health promotion vary between dental care providers relative to the NHS/private treatment mix offered? A study in West Yorkshire. *Prim. Dent. Care* **2009**, *16*, 45–50. [CrossRef]
66. Satur, J.; Gussy, M.; Marino, R.; Martini, T. Patterns of dental therapists' scope of practice and employment in Victoria, Australia. *J. Dent. Educ.* **2009**, *73*, 416–425. [CrossRef] [PubMed]
67. Tseveenjav, B.; Virtanen, J.I.; Wang, N.J.; Widström, E. Working profiles of dental hygienists in public and private practice in Finland and Norway. *Int. J. Dent. Hyg.* **2009**, *7*, 17–22. [CrossRef] [PubMed]
68. Malcheff, S.; Pink, T.C.; Sohn, W.; Inglehart, M.R.; Briskie, D. Infant oral health examinations: Pediatric dentists' professional behavior and attitudes. *Pediatr. Dent.* **2009**, *31*, 202–209. [CrossRef] [PubMed]
69. Manski, M.C.; Parker, M.E. Early childhood caries: Knowledge, attitudes, and practice behaviors of Maryland dental hygienists. *J. Dent. Hyg.* **2010**, *84*, 190–195.
70. Salama, F.; Kebriaei, A. Oral care for infants: A survey of Nebraska general dentists. *Gen. Dent.* **2010**, *58*, 182–187.
71. Ananaba, N.; Malcheff, S.; Briskie, D.; Inglehart, M.R. Infant oral health examinations: Attitudes and professional behavior of general and pediatric dentists in Michigan and pediatric dentists in the U.S. *J. Mich. Dent. Assoc.* **2010**, *92*, 38–43.
72. Cunha-Cruz, J.; Wataha, J.C.; Zhou, L.; Manning, W.; Trantow, M.; Bettendorf, M.M.; Heaton, L.J.; Berg, J. Treating dentin hypersensitivity: Therapeutic choices made by dentists of the northwest PRECEDENT network. *J. Am. Dent. Assoc.* **2010**, *141*, 1097–1105. [CrossRef]
73. Lee, J.Y.; Caplan, D.J.; Gizlice, Z.; Ammerman, A.; Agans, R.; Curran, A.E. US pediatric dentists' counseling practices in addressing childhood obesity. *Pediatr. Dent.* **2012**, *34*, 245–250.
74. Kakudate, N.; Sumida, F.; Matsumoto, Y.; Manabe, K.; Yokoyama, Y.; Gilbert, G.H.; Gordan, V.V. Restorative treatment thresholds for proximal caries in dental PBRN. *J. Dent. Res.* **2012**, *91*, 1202–1208. [CrossRef]
75. Yokoyama, Y.; Kakudate, N.; Sumida, F.; Matsumoto, Y.; Gilbert, G.H.; Gordan, V.V. Dentists' dietary perception and practice patterns in a dental practice-based research network. *PLoS ONE* **2013**, *8*, e59615. [CrossRef]

76. Yokoyama, Y.; Kakudate, N.; Sumida, F.; Matsumoto, Y.; Gilbert, G.H.; Gordan, V.V. Dentists' practice patterns regarding caries prevention: Results from a dental practice-based research network. *BMJ Open* **2013**, *3*, e003227. [CrossRef]
77. Hussein, R.J.; Schneller, T.; Walter, U. Preventive activity of dentists and its associations with dentist and dental practice characteristics in northern Germany. *J. Public Health* **2013**, *21*, 455–463. [CrossRef]
78. Gnich, W.; Deas, L.; Mackenzie, S.; Burns, J.; Conway, D.I. Extending dental nurses' duties: A national survey investigating skill-mix in Scotland's child oral health improvement programme (Childsmile). *BMC Oral Health* **2014**, *14*, 137. [CrossRef]
79. Yusuf, H.; Tsakos, G.; Ntouva, A.; Murphy, M.; Porter, J.; Newton, T.; Watt, R.G. Differences by age and sex in general dental practitioners' knowledge, attitudes and behaviours in delivering prevention. *Br. Dent. J.* **2015**, *219*, E7. [CrossRef] [PubMed]
80. Hayes, M.J.; Wallace, J.P.; Coxon, A. Attitudes and barriers to providing dietary advice: Perceptions of dental hygienists and oral health therapists. *Int. J. Dent. Hyg.* **2016**, *14*, 255–260. [CrossRef] [PubMed]
81. Baatsch, B.; Zimmer, S.; Rodrigues Recchia, D.; Bussing, A. Complementary and alternative therapies in dentistry and characteristics of dentists who recommend them. *Complement. Ther. Med.* **2017**, *35*, 64–69. [CrossRef] [PubMed]
82. Hayes, M.J.; Cheng, B.; Musolino, R.; Rogers, A.A. Dietary analysis and nutritional counselling for caries prevention in dental practise: A pilot study. *Aust. Dent. J.* **2017**, *62*, 485–492. [CrossRef]
83. Wright, R.; Casamassimo, P.S. Assessing attitudes and actions of pediatric dentists toward childhood obesity and sugar-sweetened beverages. *J. Public Health Dent.* **2017**, *77* (Suppl. S1), S79–S87. [CrossRef]
84. Cole, D.D.M.; Boyd, L.D.; Vineyard, J.; Giblin-Scanlon, L.J. Childhood Obesity: Dental hygienists' beliefs attitudes and barriers to patient education. *J. Dent. Hyg.* **2018**, *92*, 38–49.
85. Djokic, J.; Bowen, A.; Dooa, J.S.; Kahatab, R.; Kumagai, T.; McKee, K.; Tan, C.; FitzGerald, K.; Duane, B.; Sagheri, D. Knowledge, attitudes and behaviour regarding the infant oral health visit: Are dentists in Ireland aware of the recommendation for a first visit to the dentist by age 1 year? *Eur. Arch. Paediatr. Dent.* **2018**, *20*, 65–72. [CrossRef]
86. Aziz, S.A.; Kuan, S.; Jin, E.; Loch, C.; Thomson, W.M. Do as I say and not as I do? New Zealand dentists' oral health practices and advice to patients. *J. R. Soc. N. Z.* **2020**, *50*, 178–188. [CrossRef]
87. Bakhurji, E.A.; Al-Saif, H.M.; Al-Shehri, M.A.; Al-Ghamdi, K.M.; Hassan, M.M. Infant Oral Healthcare and Anticipatory Guidance Practices among Dentists in a Pediatric Care Shortage Area. *Int. J. Dent.* **2021**, *2021*, 6645279. [CrossRef]
88. Shick, E.A.; Lee, J.Y.; Rozier, R.G. Determinants of Dental Referral Practices Among WIC Nutritionists in North Carolina. *J. Public Health Dent.* **2005**, *65*, 196–202. [CrossRef]
89. Butani, Y.; RA, K.; Qian, F.; Lampiris, L. Predictors of oral health counseling by WIC providers. *J. Dent. Child.* **2006**, *73*, 146–151.
90. Kärkkäinen, S.; Seppa, L.; Hausen, H. Dental check-up intervals and caries preventive measures received by adolescents in Finland. *Community Dent. Health* **2001**, *18*, 157–161.
91. Tickle, M.; Milsom, K.M.; King, D.; Blinkhorn, A.S. The influences on preventive care provided to children who frequently attend the UK General Dental Service. *Br. Dent. J.* **2003**, *194*, discussion 318. [CrossRef]
92. Nihtilä, A.; Widström, E. Heavy use of dental services among Finnish children and adolescents. *Eur. J. Paediatr. Dent.* **2009**, *10*, 7–12.
93. Wang, N.J.; Aspelund, G.Ø. Preventive care and recall intervals. Targeting of services in child dental care in Norway. *Community Dent. Health* **2010**, *27*, 5–11.
94. Sarmadi, R.; Gahnberg, L.; Gabre, P. Clinicians' preventive strategies for children and adolescents identified as at high risk of developing caries. *Int. J. Paediatr. Dent.* **2011**, *21*, 167–174. [CrossRef]
95. Masoe, A.V.; Blinkhorn, A.S.; Taylor, J.; Blinkhorn, F.A. Preventive and clinical care provided to adolescents attending public oral health services New South Wales, Australia: A retrospective study. *BMC Oral Health* **2014**, *14*, 142. [CrossRef]
96. Raindi, D.; Thornley, A.; Thornley, P. Explaining diet as a risk factor for periodontal disease in primary dental care. *Br. Dent. J.* **2015**, *219*, 497–500. [CrossRef]
97. Skinner, J.; Byun, R.; Blinkhorn, A. Utilization of public oral health services by New South Wales teenagers, 2004-05 to 2014-15. *Aust. Dent. J.* **2016**, *61*, 514–520. [CrossRef]
98. Demko, C.A.; Victoroff, K.Z.; Wotman, S. Concordance of chart and billing data with direct observation in dental practice. *Community Dent. Oral Epidemiol.* **2008**, *36*, 466–474. [CrossRef]
99. Wotman, S.; Demko, C.A.; Victoroff, K.; Sudano, J.J.; Lalumandier, J.A. A multimethod investigation including direct observation of 3751 patient visits to 120 dental offices. *Clin. Cosmet. Investig. Dent.* **2010**, *2*, 27–39. [CrossRef]
100. Threlfall, A.G.; Milsom, K.M.; Hunt, C.M.; Tickle, M.; Blinkhorn, A.S. Exploring the content of the advice provided by general dental practitioners to help prevent caries in young children. *Br. Dent. J.* **2007**, *202*, E9; discussion 148–149. [CrossRef]
101. Cashmore, A.W.; Noller, J.; Ritchie, J.; Johnson, B.; Blinkhorn, A.S. Reorienting a paediatric oral health service towards prevention: Lessons from a qualitative study of dental professionals. *Heal. Promot. J. Aust.* **2011**, *22*, 17–21. [CrossRef]
102. Ong, H.H.; Wan, C.C.; Gao, X. Interprofessional Collaboration in Addressing Diet as a Common Risk Factor: A Qualitative Study. *J. Res. Interprof. Pract. Educ.* **2015**, *5*. [CrossRef]
103. Lacey, K.; Pritchett, E. Nutrition Care Process and Model: ADA adopts road map to quality care and outcomes management. *J. Am. Diet. Assoc.* **2003**, *103*, 1061–1072. [CrossRef]
104. Boyd, L.D.; Hartman-Cunningham, M.L. Survey of diabetes knowledge and practices of dental hygienists. *J. Dent. Hyg.* **2008**, *82*, 43.

105. Efurd, M.G.; Bray, K.K.; Mitchell, T.V.; Williams, K. Comparing the risk identification and management behaviors between oral health providers for patients with diabetes. *J. Dent. Hyg.* **2012**, *86*, 130–140. [PubMed]
106. Braithwaite, A.S.; Vann, W.F.J.; Switzer, B.R.; Boyd, K.L.; Lee, J.Y. Nutritional counseling practices: How do North Carolina pediatric dentists weigh in? *Pediatr. Dent.* **2008**, *30*, 488–495. [PubMed]
107. Curran, A.E.; Caplan, D.J.; Lee, J.Y.; Paynter, L.; Gizlice, Z.; Champagne, C.; Ammerman, A.S.; Agans, R. Dentists' attitudes about their role in addressing obesity in patients: A national survey. *J. Am. Dent. Assoc.* **2010**, *141*, 1307–1316. [CrossRef] [PubMed]
108. da Gomes, F.J.S.; Paula, A.B.P.; Curran, A.E.; Rodrigues, M.A.; Ferreira, M.M.; Carrilho, E.V.P. Portuguese Dentists' Attitudes Towards Their Role in Addressing Obesity. *Oral Health Prev. Dent.* **2016**, *14*, 13–20.
109. Clark, E.; Tuthill, D.; Hingston, E.J. Paediatric dentists' identification and management of underweight and overweight children. *Br. Dent. J.* **2018**, *225*, 657–661. [CrossRef]
110. Bennett, S. Reducing Dental Disease A Canadian Oral Health Framework. 2013. Available online: https://www.caphd.ca/sites/default/files/FrameworkOctober%202014%20-%20FINAL%20English.pdf (accessed on 30 September 2021).
111. Saskatchewan Prevention Institute. Improving the Oral Health of Pregnant Women and Young Children: Opportunities for Oral Care and Prenatal Care Providers—A Saskatchewan Consensus Document. 2014. Available online: https://skprevention.ca/wp-content/uploads/2016/07/2-804_Improving_Oral_Health_Consensus_Document.pdf?x98285 (accessed on 30 September 2021).

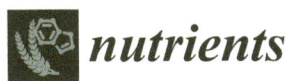

Review

The Association between Malnutrition and Oral Health in Older People: A Systematic Review

Yne Algra [1], Elizabeth Haverkort [1], Wilhelmina Kok [1], Faridi van Etten-Jamaludin [2], Liedeke van Schoot [1], Vanessa Hollaar [3], Elke Naumann [3], Marian de van der Schueren [3,4] and Katarina Jerković-Ćosić [1,*]

1 Research Group Innovations in Preventive Health Care, HU University of Applied Sciences, 3584 Utrecht, The Netherlands; yne.fennema@gmail.com (Y.A.); liesbeth.haverkort@hu.nl (E.H.); seline.kok@hu.nl (W.K.); liedeke.vanschoot@hu.nl (L.v.S.)
2 Research Support, Medical Library AMC, Amsterdam UMC-Location AMC, University of Amsterdam, 1105 Amsterdam, The Netherlands; f.s.vanetten@amsterdamumc.nl
3 Research Group Nutrition, Dietetics and Lifestyle, HAN University of Applied Sciences, 6525 Nijmegen, The Netherlands; vanessa.hollaar@han.nl (V.H.); e.naumann@han.nl (E.N.); Marian.devanderSchueren@han.nl (M.d.v.d.S.)
4 Division of Human Nutrition and Health, Wageningen University and Research, 6708 Wageningen, The Netherlands
* Correspondence: Katarina.Jerkovic@hu.nl

Citation: Algra, Y.; Haverkort, E.; Kok, W.; Etten-Jamaludin, F.v.; Schoot, L.v.; Hollaar, V.; Naumann, E.; Schueren, M.d.v.d.; Jerković-Ćosić, K. The Association between Malnutrition and Oral Health in Older People: A Systematic Review. *Nutrients* 2021, 13, 3584. https://doi.org/10.3390/nu13103584

Academic Editor: Kirstin Vach

Received: 17 August 2021
Accepted: 7 October 2021
Published: 13 October 2021

Publisher's Note: MDPI stays neutral with regard to jurisdictional claims in published maps and institutional affiliations.

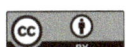
Abstract: The aim of this systematic review was to examine the association between malnutrition and oral health in older people (≥60 years of age). A comprehensive systematic literature search was performed in four databases (PubMed, CINAHL, Dentistry and Oral Sciences Source, and Embase) for literature from January 2000 to May 2020. Both observational and intervention studies were screened for eligibility. Two reviewers independently screened the search results to identify potential eligible studies, and assessed the methodological quality of the full-text studies. A total of 3240 potential studies were identified. After judgement for relevance, 10 studies (cross-sectional ($n = 9$), prospective cohort ($n = 1$)) met the inclusion criteria. Three studies described malnourished participants as having fewer teeth, or functional (tooth) units (FTUs), compared to well-nourished participants. Four studies reported soft tissue problems in malnourished participants, including red tongue with blisters, and dry or cracked lips. Subjective oral health was the topic in six studies, with poorer oral health and negative self-perception of oral health in malnourished elderly participants. There are associations between (at risk of) malnutrition and oral health in older people, categorized in hard and soft tissue conditions of the mouth, and subjective oral health. Future research should be focused on longitudinal cohort studies with proper determination of malnutrition and oral health assessments, in order to evaluate the actual association between malnutrition and oral health in older people.

Keywords: malnutrition; undernutrition; oral health; dental status; older people; elderly people; systematic review

1. Introduction

Aging is a complex phenomenon that, partially due to the occurrence of chronic diseases, can result in frailty, limited mobility, and other aspects of physical and cognitive decline [1–3]. Major concerns for older people are poor general health and poor nutrition [1,3]. In the Netherlands, it is estimated that one in three older people receiving formal home care is malnourished, and nearly 20% of the independently living older people (>85 y) suffer from a poor nutritional status [4]. Prevalence rates of high risk for malnutrition in older people in Europe are 28% (hospital), 17.5% (residential care), and 8.5% (community settings), according to a recent systematic review [5]. Malnutrition risk is associated with older age, presence of disease, and gender [5]. Consequences of malnutrition include reduced immunity, frequent infections, overall physical and psychological decline, and higher mortality [6–8].

Malnutrition can be defined as "a state resulting from lack of intake or uptake of nutrition that leads to altered body composition (decreased fat free mass) and body cell mass leading to diminished physical and mental function and impaired clinical outcome from disease" [9]. Malnutrition is often demonstrated by reductions in body weight and body mass index (BMI), primarily as a result of inadequate nutritional intake of proteins and/or energy from calories [7]. Malnutrition can also be present in persons with normal body weight or overweight, when there is a substantial reduction in fat-free mass (FFM), also called sarcopenia.

In addition to the risk of malnutrition, older people also have an increased risk of developing oral health problems [10]. Worldwide, the burden of oral diseases in older people is growing, as there are high levels of tooth loss, periodontal disease, xerostomia, dental caries, and oral cancer [11]. Several studies have shown an association between malnutrition/poor nutritional status and oral health in older people [10,12–16]. Poor oral health can cause oral pain, chewing problems, periodontal disease, and tooth loss, which have a negative impact on nutritional intake, leading to poor nutritional status and risk of malnutrition. Inadequate intake of micronutrients and macronutrients can, in turn, lead to an increased risk of oral health problems such as gum disease, caries, and hyposalivation [17–19].

The association between nutritional status and oral health in older people seems evident. There is tentative evidence indicating a negative association between malnutrition and oral health, according to several systematic reviews [20–22]. Still, the association seems general, without focusing on detailed information about observed oral health conditions in terms of hard tissues of the mouth (e.g., dental caries, decayed/missing/filled teeth), soft tissues of the mouth (e.g., periodontitis, gingivitis), hyposalivation or xerostomia, and (general) subjective oral health (e.g., oral hygiene, oral-health-related quality of life, autonomy for oral care) in malnourished older people. Prevention of malnutrition and optimizing oral health conditions in older people can result in better overall health, increased self-dependency, and higher quality of life.

The aim of this systematic review was to examine the association between malnutrition and oral health in terms of hard and soft tissue conditions of the mouth, xerostomia and salivary flow, and general (subjective) oral health in older people ($\geq$60 years of age).

2. Materials and Methods

This systematic review was conducted in adherence to the guidelines of the Preferred Reporting Items for Systematic Reviews and Meta-Analyses (PRISMA) statement.

2.1. Search Strategy

Four electronic databases—PubMed, Embase (Ovid), CINAHL (EBSCO), and Dentistry and Oral Sciences Source (DOSS)—were searched for literature from January 2000 to May 2020 with a combination of MeSH terms, terms in titles or abstracts (TIAB), free-text terms, and synonyms. Since approximately 2000, there has been an increase in published literature about malnutrition and oral health in PubMed. Therefore, studies were included from January 2000 to May 2020. In view of the exploratory character of this systematic review, the following MeSH terms were used: oral health, mouth diseases, jaw diseases, tooth diseases, taste disorders, dentition, malnutrition, nutritional status, sarcopenia, aged, and geriatrics. The search strategy of this systematic review is available from the first author (Y.A.) upon request.

Two reviewers (Y.A. and W.K.) independently screened the studies for eligibility. Only when a consensus was not possible was a third reviewer (E.H.) consulted. Reference lists of every selected publication were also screened for eligibility using the same procedure.

2.2. Selection Criteria for Studies

In view of the exploratory character of this systematic review, observational and interventional studies were included. Case reports, expert opinions, conference meetings, animal studies, summaries, papers, overviews, and reviews were excluded. The search was limited to the English and Dutch languages. Articles were eligible for inclusion only if they (1) described malnutrition, (2) described oral health, and (3) described the association between both. The definition and determination of both malnutrition and oral health were defined beforehand in order to assess the eligibility of the studies.

There are several screening and assessment tools for malnutrition. For this systematic review, malnutrition—or risk of malnutrition—had to be determined based on at least one or more anthropometric measures (BMI, weight loss, or fat-free mass), preferably together with the use of a validated nutritional screening or assessment tool for older adults (e.g., Short Nutritional Assessment Questionnaire (SNAQ), Malnutrition Universal Screening Tool (MUST), Subjective Global Assessment (SGA), Mini Nutritional Assessment (MNA), or MNA Short Form (MNA-SF)).

Oral health was defined as the condition of hard and soft tissues of the mouth, hyposalivation, xerostomia, and general (subjective) oral health (oral hygiene, mouth pain, oral-health-related quality of life (OHRQoL)). Hard tissues of the mouth comprises he mineralized tissues: alveolar bone (jaw bone), enamel, root cement, and natural teeth [23]. Soft tissues of the mouth comprise the mouth membranes: gingiva, alveolar mucosa, periodontal ligament, and mucous membranes [23], with common oral diseases including periodontitis, gingivitis, candidiasis, and denture stomatitis [24,25]. Xerostomia is the (subjective) feeling of dry mouth, while hyposalivation refers to an objectively measured lower salivary rate [26].

2.3. Selection Criteria Populaton

The population of interest was older people, of 60 years or older. Studies were excluded if participants (1) had cancer or malignancies, (2) were terminally ill, (3) had dysphagia or chewing problems due to medical conditions such as cerebral vascular accident or musculoskeletal disease, or (4) received (complete) enteral or parenteral tube feeding.

2.4. Methodological Quality Assessment

Methodological quality was assessed independently by two reviewers (Y.A. and W.K.) using the Newcastle–Ottawa Scale (NOS) for non-randomized trials and observational studies [27]. Assessment was based on selection, comparability, and outcome, with a maximum score of 10. Studies with a score of 6 or less were excluded to guarantee the quality of the included studies. A level of evidence was adjudged to each article by two reviewers independently (Y.A. and W.K.). Any disagreement between the two reviewers about assigning a methodological quality score and level of evidence to the articles was resolved through discussion with a third review author (E.H.).

2.5. Data Extraction

Information with regard to study design, population, measures, and outcomes was extracted from the included studies by one reviewer (Y.A.), and reviewed by a second reviewer (W.K.). This information included first author, year, country, number and mean age of participants, setting, measures of malnutrition, and oral health status.

2.6. Clinical and Methodological Heterogeneity

Study results were summarized using descriptive statistics. Meta-analysis was impossible due to clinical and methodological diversity as a result of the broadly formulated research question, the various definitions of malnutrition and oral health in the included studies, and the variability of the participants, measurements, outcomes, and study designs.

3. Results

3.1. Study Selection

The electronic database search resulted in 3240 studies, refined to 1988 potential studies after removing duplicates. Titles and abstracts were screened based on study design, population, reporting on malnutrition and oral health, and outcome measures (malnutrition or oral health). After screening of titles and abstracts, 207 studies remained to be reviewed in their full text, out of which 195 did not meet the selection criteria and were excluded, resulting in a total of 12 potentially eligible studies (Figure 1). An overview of studies (references) excluded, by reason for exclusion, is available upon request from the first author (Y.A.).

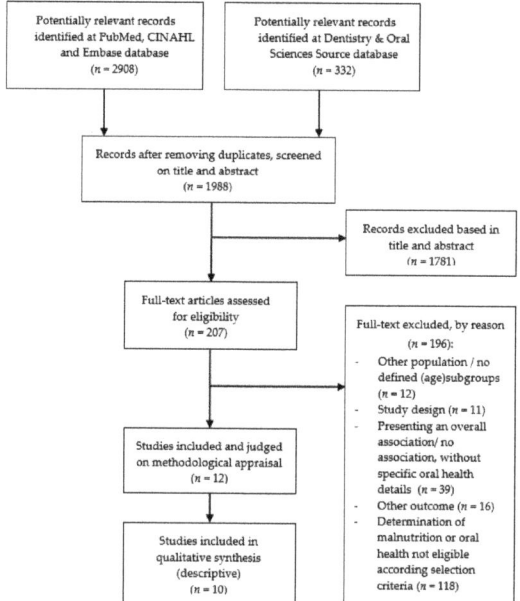

Figure 1. Flow chart of study selection.

3.2. Methodological Quality of the Studies

Eleven studies had a cross-sectional design and one study was a longitudinal cohort study. The methodological quality scores from these studies ranged from 5 to 10. Two studies were excluded due to having an NOS methodological quality score less than 7. Ten studies were included in this systematic review, with a mean quality score of 8.9 ± 0.54 (Supplementary Table S1).

3.3. Study Characteristics

General study characteristics are presented in Table 1. The 10 included studies had a cross-sectional design (n = 9) or longitudinal design (n = 1), with wide variation in outcome variables and statistics (mean and standard deviations, percentages, odds ratio or hazard ratio with 95% confidence interval, p-values). The numbers of participants in the studies ranged from 159 to 3320, with a total number of 9093 participants in this systematic review. In most of the studies, the proportion of women was higher than that of men. Participants were derived from different settings: nursing homes, dental clinics, community -welling older people, or hospital units (acute care units or rehabilitation). The prevalence of malnourished participants in the studies varied from 11.7% to 60%, and the reported range of participants "at risk of malnutrition" was 21–60%.

Table 1. Main study characteristics.

First Author	Publication Year, Country	Number of Participants	Mean Age	Setting	Measurement of Malnutrition	Measurement of Oral Health	Methodological Quality Score
Andersson [28]	2004, Sweden	n = 161 M: 43 F: 118	81.7 (range 65–89)	Three rehabilitation wards at a university hospital	SGA	ROAG	9
El Osta [29]	2013, Lebanon	n = 201 F: 121 M: 80	F: 71.6 ± 6 M: 72.7 ± 7	Older people attending two acute care units	MNA	GOHAI, DMTF/DTF, prosthetic status, posterior dental FUs	9
Huppertz [30]	2017, The Netherlands	n = 3320 M: 1059 F: 2261	84.3 ± 7.4	Nursing homes	BMI in combination with unintentional weight loss	Standardized questionnaire on potential indicators of poor oral health	9
Kiesswetter [31]	2019, The Netherlands	n = 893 M: 418 F: 475	67.6 ± 6.1	Community-dwelling older people	BMI, time-specific weight loss	Self-administered questionnaire (22 items) on four oral health domains	8
Lindmark [32]	2017, Sweden	n = 1156 M: 443 F: 713	82.8 ± 7.9	Nursing homes and hospitals	MNA-SF	ROAG-J	8
Mesas [33]	2010, Sweden	n = 267 M: 107 F: 160	66.5 ± 4.1	Community-dwelling older people	MNA	GOHAI, number of teeth, prosthesis, posterior occlusion, stimulated salivary flow, CPITN	10
Poisson [34]	2014, France	n = 159 M: 51 F: 108	85.3 ± 5.7	Patients hospitalized in acute care units: 78% (n = 124) from home, 22% (n = 35) from nursing homes	Weight loss, BMI, MNA	Oral examination by dentist, DMTF index, gingival inflammation, oral candidiasis, salivary test (insufficiency if salivary flow < 0.1 g/min/weight compress < 0.35 g)	9
Samnieng [35]	2011, Thailand	n = 612 M: 158 F: 454	68.8 ± 5.9	Community-dwelling older people	MNA	Dental status assessed by dentist; DMFT, prostheses, FTUs	9
Soini [36]	2006, Finland	n = 3088 M: 649 F: 2439	NH: 81 LT: 83	Institutionalized older people from NH (n = 2036) and LT (n = 1052)	MNA	Oral status evaluated by trained ward nurses	9
Takahashi [37]	2018, Japan	n = 279 M: 106 F: 173	76 ± 7.5	Older people at a dental clinic	Sarcopenia (GS, HS, MNA-SF, BMI, EAT-10, CC).	Number of teeth, FTUs. Primary outcome: OHIP to evaluate OHRQoL. Secondary outcome: OHAT	9

Level of evidence of all studies level 4. Legend: ±: standard deviation; ADD-GOHAI: Additive Geriatric Oral Health Assessment Instrument; BMI: body mass index; CC: calf circumference; CPITN: periodontal condition; DMTF: decayed/missing/filled teeth; DFT: decayed/filled teeth; EAT-10: 10-item Eating Assessment Tool; F: female; FUs: (posterior dental) functional units; FTUs: functional tooth units; g: gram; GOHAI: Geriatric Oral Health Assessment Tool; GS: gait speed; HS: handgrip strength; LT: long-term care wards; M: male; MNA: Mini Nutritional Assessment; MNS-SF: Mini Nutritional Assessment Short Form; N: number; NH: nursing homes; OHAT: Oral Health Assessment Tool; OHRQoL: oral-health-related quality of life (OHRQoL); OHIP: Oral Health Impact Profile; ROAG: Revised Oral Assessment Guide; ROAG-J: Revised Oral Assessment Guide-Jönköping; SGA: Subjective Global Assessment.

Malnutrition was assessed via the Mini Nutritional Assessment (MNA) ($n = 4$), MNA Short Form (MNA-SF) ($n = 1$), Subjective Global Assessment (SGA) ($n = 1$), body mass index (BMI) in combination with unintentional or time-specific weight loss ($n = 2$), or MNA in combination with BMI and weight loss ($n = 1$). Sarcopenia was assessed by low handgrip strength and/or low gait speed, with CC measurement of <33 (female)/<34 (male) ($n = 1$).

Several measurement instruments were used to assess subjective and objective oral health aspects, or a combination of both. Objective oral health was evaluated by using the Revised Oral Assessment Guide (ROAG) or ROAG-Jönköping (ROAG-J) ($n = 2$), oral examination or evaluation by a professional ($n = 3$), or the Oral Health Assessment Tool (OHAT) ($n = 1$). Additional data on objective oral health were reported with regard to the use of dentures ($n = 4$), decayed/missing/filled teeth (DMFT) or decayed/filled teeth (DFT) ($n = 3$), functional tooth units (FTUs) or functional units (FUs) ($n = 3$), number of teeth ($n = 2$), stimulated salivary flow ($n = 2$), and gingival inflammation ($n = 1$). Subjective oral health was assessed using the Geriatric Oral Health Assessment Instrument (GOHAI) ($n = 2$), self-administered or standardized questionnaires ($n = 2$), and the Oral Health Impact Profile (OHIP) ($n = 1$). Additional data on subjective oral health were reported regarding xerostomia ($n = 2$), chewing problems ($n = 3$), general mouth problems ($n = 2$), pain ($n = 1$), oral candidiasis ($n = 1$), and oral hygiene ($n = 2$).

3.4. Malnutrition and Hard Tissue Conditions of the Mouth

Three studies explored the number of dental functional units (Table 2). The number of functional tooth units (FTUs) was defined as pairs of upper and lower opposing natural teeth and/or artificial teeth on removable or fixed dentures [35,37]. Functional units (FUs) were defined as a pair of posterior antagonist teeth with at least one contact area during chewing [29]. Two studies showed that malnourished older people had significantly less FUs (<4) [29] or FTUs (8.3 ± 1.1) [35] compared to older people without malnutrition. In one study, there were no significant differences in terms of FTUs between older people with and without sarcopenia [37].

Table 2. Outcome measures regarding hard tissue conditions in malnourished older people compared to well-nourished older people.

Item	[Ref]	Prevalence (N(%)), or No. of Teeth/FU		
		MN	At Risk of MN	Well-Nourished
No. of FUs: <4 FUs 5 or 6 FUs 7 or 8 FUs	[29]	n total = 85 n = 52 (61%) ** n = 6 (7.1%) n = 27 (31.8%)	- - -	n total = 116 n = 38 (32.8%) ** n = 24 (20.7%) 54 (46.6%)
No. of decayed teeth	[35]	1.6 ± 0.3 *	1.3 ± 0.1 *	1.1 ± 0.2 *
No. of teeth	[35] [37]	8.7 ± 1.4 * 13.4 ± 9.3	10.1 ± 0.4 * -	13.2 ± 0.7 * 18.9 ± 7.8
No. of FTUs	[35] [37]	8.3 ± 1.1 * 10.0 ± 3.5	8.4 ± 0.3 *	10.3 ± 0.5 * 10.5 ± 2.5
Association ND and edentulism	[33]	Crude OR: 1.44 [a] (95% CI 0.61–3.33) Adjusted OR [b]: 0.65 (95% CI 0.23–1.83)		

Legend: *: $p < 0.05$; **: $p < 0.0001$; ±: standard deviation; [a]: chi-squared test or Fisher's exact test; [b]: logistic regression of the association between each indicator of oral health and nutrition deficit adjusted for gender, age, schooling, economic class, smoking, depression, and medication use; CI: confidence interval; FUs: (posterior dental) functional units; FTUs: functional tooth units; MN: malnourished; ND: nutritional deficit; No.: number.

Two studies explored the associations based on number of teeth (Table 2). Samnieng et al. [35] reported a significantly increased malnutrition risk in older people with fewer teeth, compared to older people with more teeth. A second study demonstrated significantly lower numbers of teeth in older people with sarcopenia, compared to those without sarcopenia [37]. On the other hand, Mesas et al. [33] reported a non-significant association between the oral health indicator "edentulous" and (at risk of) malnutrition. In addition, Andersson et al. [28] found that the mean values for decayed/missing/filled teeth (DMFT) and decayed/filled teeth (DFT) did not differ between malnourished older people and older people with normal nutritional status. Furthermore, the associations between nutritional status and both DMFT and prosthetic status were not significant ($p > 0.05$).

3.5. Malnutrition and Soft Tissue Conditions of the Mouth

Conditions with regard to soft tissues of the mouth related to malnutrition were presented in four studies (Table 3). Malnourished participants had a higher proportion of oral problems in soft tissues. This included, for example, a tongue with no papillae, white coating, blisters, or ulceration. According to the ROAG items, lips were dry or cracked, and gums were edematous or red. Moreover, dry, red tick mucous membranes or ulcerations with bleeding were spotted [28,32]. Poisson et al. [34] reported low salivary flow in malnourished older people. Malnourished older people had the highest proportion of oral problems in soft tissues according to Lindmark et al. [32].

Table 3. Outcome measures regarding soft tissue conditions in malnourished older people compared to well-nourished older people.

Item	[Ref]	Prevalence's		
		MN	At Risk of MN	Well-Nourished
Tongue	[32]	40 (20.3%)	38 (7.4%)	21 (4.7%)
	[28]	43 (49%)	-	-
Mucous membranes	[32]	41 (21.3%)	37 (7.2%)	14 (3.2%)
	[28]	26 (30%)	-	-
Lips	[32]	35 (17.8%)	26 (5.0%)	17 (3.8%)
	[28]	48 (55%)	-	-
Gums	[32]	26 (14.4%)	42 (8.7%)	20 (5.0%)
	[28]	14 (16%)	-	-
Candidiasis	[34]	12 (15.6%) $p < 0.001$	-	-
Association MN and tongue problems	[28]	OR 4.4 (95 % CI 2.0–9.6; $p < 0.0005$)		

Legend: CI: confidence interval; MN: malnourished; OR: odds ratio; *p*: *p*-value

Andersson et al. [28] presented a significant association between malnutrition and tongue problems according to the ROAG. The study of Mesas et al. [33] found a significant association between the nutritional deficit (MNA score < 24 points) and advanced periodontal disease (defined as at least one sextant with pocket depths ≥ 6 mm). The presence of candidiasis in the mouth was associated with malnutrition as estimated by low MNA scores, according to Poisson et al. [34].

3.6. Malnutrition and Hyposalivation or Xerostomia

Conditions with regard to hyposalivation or xerostomia were presented in eight studies (Table 4).

Table 4. Outcome measures regarding hyposalivation and xerostomia in malnourished older people compared to well-nourished older people.

Outcomes	First Author [Ref]
Hyposalivation	
Association nutritional deficit and stimulated salivary flow < 0.7 mL/min: Crude OR 1.96 (95% CI 1.06–3.83) Adjusted OR 2.18 (95% CI 1.06–4.50).	Mesas [33]
Association salivary flow rate < 0.7 (mL/min) and nutritional deficit: Adjusted OR 2.18 (95% CI 1.06–4.50).	Poisson [34]
Xerostomia	
Perception of xerostomia as parameter of explaining MNA variation: OR 3.49 (95% CI 1.657–7.337; *p* = 0.001).	El Osta [29]
Association between xerostomia and incident malnutrition HR 2.63 (95% CI 1.18–6.26).	Kiesswetter [31]

Legend: CI: confidence interval; HR: hazard ratio; MNA: Mini Nutritional Assessment; OR: odds ratio; *p*: *p*-value.

Hyposalivation: Malnourished older people had the highest proportion of oral problems, including low salivary flow [32,34]. In the study of Andersson et al. [28], low salivary flow according to the ROAG was associated with the presence of malnutrition. Stimulated salivary flow rate (hyposalivation) was measured in the study of Mesas et al. [33], and a salivary flow rate < 0.7 (mL/min) was associated with nutritional deficit (MNA score < 24 points).

Xerostomia: Weak and non-significant associations between malnutrition and xerostomia were demonstrated by Huppertz et al. [30]. However, three studies showed significant associations between malnutrition and xerostomia. According to El Osta et al. [29], participants with xerostomia were more likely to be malnourished. Kiesswetter et al. [31] demonstrated associations between xerostomia and incident malnutrition. In addition, xerostomia was more pronounced in people without teeth and with incident malnutrition. In the study of Soini et al. [36], malnutrition increased consistently with the increasing number of oral health problems (including chewing problems, oral pain, and xerostomia).

3.7. Malnutrition and Subjective Oral Health

Eight studies demonstrated associations between malnutrition and other (general) subjective oral health indicators (Table 5). In the study of El Osta et al. [29], discomfort when eating, trouble biting/chewing, and lower mean Additive Geriatric Oral Health Assessment Instrument (ADD-GOHAI) scores were associated with malnutrition (*p* < 0.0001). Of the malnourished participants in the study of Huppertz et al. [30], 58.8% complained of poor oral health and 24.3% complained of general mouth problems (not further specified). According to Soini et al. [36], lower MNA values had a significant relationship with the number of oral health problems, such as chewing problems, swallowing difficulties, and oral pain. Lindmark et al. [32] demonstrated at least one oral health problem in one-third of the older people at risk of malnutrition; problems were seen in lips, mucous membranes, tongues, and saliva (*p* < 0.001). Mesas et al. [33] reported an association between nutritional deficit (MNA score < 24 points) and negative self-perception of oral health. Poisson et al. [34] reported that decreases in autonomy of oral care were independently associated with malnutrition according to the MNA (*p* = 0.004). The study of Takahashi et al. [37] demonstrated sarcopenia to be an independent exploratory factor of OHIP-14 scores. However, Kiesswetter et al. [31] reported that no differences were found between groups with and without malnutrition, with regard to their self-perceived oral health characteristics (relating to teeth, dentures and oral hygiene).

Table 5. Outcome measures regarding subjective oral health.

Outcomes and Prevalence: Subjective Oral Health	First Author [Ref]
Negative self-perception of oral health: Crude OR: 3.95 (95% CI 2.04–7.67) Adjusted OR: 3.41 (95% CI 1.59–7.33)	Mesas [33]
OHRQoL/oral status: Poorer OHRQoL and oral health status (all $p < 0.001$). GOHAI score explains MNA variation: OR: 2.905 (95% CI 1.40–6.00; $p = 0.004$).	Takahashi [37] El Osta [29]
OHRQoL/oral status: Negative correlation between the ROAG-J total score and MNA total score (r = −0.241; $p < 0.001$).	Lindmark [32]
Association between toothache while chewing (adjusted) HR 2.14 (95% CI 1.10–4.19; $p = 0.026$).	Huppertz [30]

Legend: CI: confidence interval; GOHAI: Geriatric Oral Health Assessment Instrument; HR: hazard ratio; MNA: Mini Nutritional Assessment; OHRQoL: oral-health-related quality of life; OR: odds ratio; *p*: *p*-value; ROAG-J: Revised Oral Assessment Guide-Jönköping.

4. Discussion

This systematic review describes the associations between malnutrition and hard and soft tissue conditions of the mouth, hyposalivation, xerostomia, and subjective oral health in older people. Ten cross-sectional studies were included, and demonstrated an association between malnutrition and poor oral health conditions. Five studies indicated an association between number of F(T)Us and number of teeth, while one study described this association for edentulism and malnutrition. Four studies demonstrated associations between different soft tissue conditions of the mouth in malnourished older people. Periodontal disease, candidiasis, red or bleeding gums, blisters, tongue problems, and dry or cracked lips were more frequently present in malnourished older people, compared to older people with normal nutritional status. The association between (stimulated) low salivary flow or xerostomia and malnutrition was demonstrated in four studies. Seven studies reported subjective oral health aspects that were associated with malnutrition, or were more frequently reported by malnourished participants, such as pain (when chewing), autonomy of oral care, and negative self-perception of oral health.

These results confirm the previously demonstrated association between malnutrition, or nutritional status, and oral health problems in older people [11,13–17].

4.1. Measurement and Definition of Malnutrition and Oral Health

In 2018, consensus criteria were published by the Global Leadership Initiative on Malnutrition (GLIM) to define malnutrition in adults. However, there still is variation in the definition of malnutrition. The studies included in this systematic review frequently used nutritional assessment tools, such as the MNA.

Although BMI is often not the most valid method to determine malnutrition, the published literature demonstrates significant associations with oral health problems. Studies reported an association between low BMI and tooth loss, BMI and dry mouth when eating, and association between underweight and dryness, pain, uncomfortable sores, and irritation in the mouth [38–41].

Similarly to malnutrition, oral health is not unambiguously measured. Several measurement instruments were used to assess oral health, based on questionnaires and/or oral clinical assessment performed by a dentist or a nurse. The review of Everaars et al. [42] showed the methodological limitations of the available oral health assessments for non-dental healthcare professionals, and the limited quality of their measurement properties. Furthermore, the difference between hyposalivation and xerostomia should be stressed here. Xerostomia is the (subjective) feeling of dry mouth, and it can also occur while someone has normal salivation [26], while hyposalivation refers to an objectively measured lower salivary rate. As these two terms are sometimes used interchangeably, in some of the included studies it is not clear how the information about xerostomia was collected.

4.2. Methodological Limitations of Included Studies

Firm conclusions based on this systematic review are hampered by the statistical and clinical heterogeneity of the included studies, as well as the cross-sectional design of the included studies. All studies had a cross-sectional design, with low levels of evidence, measurement at one timepoint, and no control group or intervention. The methodological quality of the studies varied from 8 to 10 (mean score of 8.9 ± 0.54), with the lowest scores for complete description regarding methodological processes, non-respondents, comparability of the subjects, controlling for confounding, and statistical tests. Adjustment for confounding was described in a few studies; however, with the use of (partially) self-reported data in cross-sectional studies (subjective oral health, xerostomia, weight loss, or BMI), confounding factors and measurement bias can be a problem.

4.3. Strengths and Limitations

This systematic review was strengthened by the broadly formulated inclusion criteria regarding study designs and types of participants. Moreover, a large number of participants from different settings were included, with ages of 60 years or older. However, only a few studies included community-dwelling older people, which suggests that the studies are not representative of the general older population.

A comprehensive search strategy was conducted in four electronic databases, with search strategy support from two medical librarians. In all of the included studies, malnutrition was the actual outcome, and not a surrogate outcome. Furthermore, the literature was independently evaluated by two reviewers, as was the methodological quality of the potential eligible studies. Older (published before the year 2000) systematic reviews on the topic of malnutrition and oral health were examined to ensure that no relevant literature was excluded beforehand. Finally, we acknowledge the risk of publication bias. The 10 included studies often presented significant associations. However, publication bias is difficult to identify.

4.4. Implications for Practice

In this systematic review, malnourished older people had significantly more impaired soft tissue conditions related to mucous membranes, periodontium, gums, and tongue, such as a tongue with no papillae, white coating, blisters, or ulceration. Oral health appears to be important in nutritional care. Preventive healthcare and multidisciplinary cooperation will be important with regard to the aging population over the next few decades. The knowledge from this systematic review can contribute to the development of screening instruments and guidelines. In addition, it can help healthcare professionals to better identify problems in the field of malnutrition and oral health. Reducing the prevalence or severity of malnutrition and oral health conditions in older people can result in better overall health, increased self-dependency, and higher quality of life.

5. Conclusions

Despite the limitations of this review, there are indications that the presence of malnutrition is related to the state of hard and soft tissues of the mouth, salivary flow, and xerostomia, as well as other subjective oral health aspects. In the end, there is an extensive interrelation between oral health and malnutrition; however, it remains unclear whether this is a two-way association, or whether poor oral health increases the risk of being malnourished, or vice versa: that being malnourished results in poor oral health in older people.

Future research should be focused on longitudinal cohort studies with proper determination of malnutrition and oral health assessments, so as to evaluate the actual association between malnutrition and oral health in older people.

Nutrients **2021**, *13*, 3584

Supplementary Materials: The following are available online at https://www.mdpi.com/article/10.3390/nu13103584/s1, Table S1: Methodological quality assessment of the included studies.

Author Contributions: All authors approved the submitted version, agree to be personally accountable for their contribution to this review, and ensure that questions related to the accuracy or integrity of any part of this work will be appropriately investigated, resolved, and documented. Individual contributions: Y.A. conceptualized the research question, commissioned by E.H. and W.K. Y.A., E.H. and W.K. developed the search strategy with the support of F.v.E.-J. and L.v.S., who helped in designing the search string and carried out the searches of the databases. Y.A. and W.K. screened search results, obtained papers, screened retrieved papers against inclusion criteria, and carried out quality assessment. Y.A. extracted the data from included papers, designed tables and figures, and wrote the review. E.H. commented on drafts of the review. V.H., E.N., M.d.v.d.S. and K.J.-Ć. commented on the final manuscript. K.J.-Ć. supervised the project and was available for advice. All authors have read and agreed to the published version of the manuscript.

Funding: This research as funded by the Taskforce for Applied Research SIA, part of the Dutch Research Council, NOW.

Institutional Review Board Statement: Not applicable.

Informed Consent Statement: Not applicable.

Data Availability Statement: Not applicable—because this is a systematic review, all data are available in the primary studies.

Conflicts of Interest: The authors declare no conflict of interest.

References

1. Suzman, R.; Beard, J. *Global Health and Aging*; WHO: Geneva, Switzerland, 2011; p. 26. Available online: https://www.who.int/ageing/publications/global_health.pdf (accessed on 3 February 2020).
2. LoketGezondleven.nl. Facts and Figures Elderly People in the Netherlands. National Institute for Public Health and the Environment Ministry of Health, Welfare and Sport. Available online: https://www.loketgezondleven.nl/gezonde-gemeente/themadossiers/gezond-en-vitaal-ouder-worden/feiten-en-waarden-ouderen (accessed on 23 November 2019).
3. Guigoz, P.Y.; Vellas, M.B.; Garry, P.P.J. Assessing the Nutritional Status of the Elderly: The Mini Nutritional Assessment as Part of the Geriatric Evaluation. *Nutr. Rev.* **2009**, *54*, S59–S65. [CrossRef]
4. Son, N.; Kavak, B.; Nazan, S.; Buket, K. Evaluation of nutritional status of elderly patients presenting to the Family Health Center. *Pak. J. Med. Sci.* **2018**, *34*, 446–451. [CrossRef]
5. Leij-Halfwerk, S.; Verwijs, M.H.; van Houdt, S.; Borkent, J.W.; Guaitoli, P.R.; Pelgrim, T.; Heymans, M.W.; Power, L.; Visser, M.; Corish, C.A.; et al. Prevalence of protein-energy mal-nutrition risk in European older adults in community, residential and hospital settings, according to 22 malnutrition screening tools validated for use in adults ≥65 years: A systematic review and meta-analysis. *Maturitas* **2019**, *126*, 80–89. [CrossRef]
6. Voedingscentrum. Dutch Nutrition Center. Malnutrition. Available online: https://www.voedingscentrum.nl/encyclopedie/ondervoeding.aspx (accessed on 20 November 2019).
7. Definition and Diagnosis Malnutrition. Available online: https://www.steeringgroepondervoeding.nl/toolkits/wat-is-ondervoeding (accessed on 15 November 2019).
8. Kruizenga, H.; Beijer, S.; Huisman-de Waal, G.; Jonkers-Schuitema, C.; Klos, M.; Remijnse-Meester, W.; Thijs, A.; Witteman, B.; Tieland, M. *Guideline for Malnutrition Recognition, Diagnosis and Treatment of Malnutrition in Adults*; Steering Committee Malnutrition: The Netherlands, 2009; pp. 1–39.
9. Sobotka, L.; Allison, S.P.; Forbes, A.; Meier, R.F.; Schneider, S.M.; Soeters, P.B.; Stanga, Z.; Van Gossum, A. *Basics in Clinical Nutrition*, 4th ed.; Galén: Praha, Czech Republic, 2019.
10. Gil-Montoya, J.; Ponce, G.; Lara, I.S.; Barrios, R.; Llodra, J.; Bravo, M. Association of the oral health impact profile with malnutrition risk in Spanish elders. *Arch. Gerontol. Geriatr.* **2013**, *57*, 398–402. [CrossRef]
11. Petersen, P.; Kandelman, D.; Arpin, S.; Ogawa, H. Global oral health of older people–call for public health action. *Community Dent. Health* **2010**, *27*, 21313969.
12. Wang, T.-F.; Chen, Y.-Y.; Liou, Y.-M.; Chou, C. Investigating tooth loss and associated factors among older Taiwanese adults. *Arch. Gerontol. Geriatr.* **2014**, *58*, 446–453. [CrossRef]
13. Kshetrimayum, N.; Reddy, C.V.K.; Siddhana, S.; Manjunath, M.; Rudraswamy, S.; Sulavai, S. Oral health-related quality of life and nutritional status of institutionalized elderly population aged 60 years and above in Mysore City, India. *Gerodontology* **2013**, *30*, 119–125. [CrossRef] [PubMed]
14. Chen, C.C.-H.; Tang, S.T.; Wang, C.; Huang, G.-H. Trajectory and determinants of nutritional health in older patients during and six-month post-hospitalisation. *J. Clin. Nurs.* **2009**, *18*, 3299–3307. [CrossRef] [PubMed]

15. Boulos, C.; Salameh, P.; Barberger-Gateau, P. Factors associated with poor nutritional status among community dwelling Lebanese elderly subjects living in rural areas: Results of the AMEL study. *J. Nutr. Health Aging* **2014**, *18*, 487–494. [CrossRef] [PubMed]
16. De Marchi, R.J.; Hugo, F.; Hilgert, J.; Padilha, D.M.P. Association between oral health status and nutritional status in south Brazilian independent-living older people. *Nutrients* **2008**, *24*, 546–553. [CrossRef] [PubMed]
17. Gil-Montoya, J.; de Mello, A.L.F.; Barrios, R.; Gonzalez-Moles, M.A.; Bravo, M. Oral health in the elderly patient and its impact on general well-being: A nonsystematic review. *Clin. Interv. Aging* **2015**, *10*, 461–467. [CrossRef]
18. Sheetal, A.; Hiremath, V.K.; Patil, A.G.; Sajjansetty, S.; Kumar, S.R. Malnutrition and its Oral Outcome—A Review. *J. Clin. Diagn. Res.* **2013**, *7*, 178–180. [CrossRef]
19. Morris, A.M.; Engelberg, J.K.; Orozco, M.; Schmitthenner, B. The Link between Malnutrition and Poor Oral Health in Older Adults. 4 June 2019. Available online: https://www.westhealth.org/the-link-between-malnutrition-and-poor-oral-health-in-older-adults/ (accessed on 16 October 2019).
20. Toniazzo, M.P.; Amorim, P.D.S.; Muniz, F.W.M.G.; Weidlich, P. Relationship of nutritional status and oral health in elderly: Systematic review with meta-analysis. *Clin. Nutr.* **2018**, *37*, 824–830. [CrossRef] [PubMed]
21. Kazemi, S.; Savabi, G.; Khazaei, S.; Savabi, O.; Esmaillzadeh, A.; Keshteli, A.H.; Adibi, P. Association between food intake and oral health in elderly: SEPAHAN systematic review no. 8. *Dent. Res. J.* **2011**, *8*, S15–S20.
22. Van Lancker, A.; Verhaeghe, S.; Van Hecke, A.; Vanderwee, K.; Goossens, J.; Beeckman, D. The association between malnutrition and oral health status in elderly in long-term care facilities: A systematic review. *Int. J. Nurs. Stud.* **2012**, *49*, 1568–1581. [CrossRef] [PubMed]
23. Van Steenberghe, D.; Beertsen, W.; van der Velden, U.; Quirynen, M. *Periodontology*, 1st ed.; Bohn Stafleu van Loghum: Houten, The Netherlands, 2015; p. 533.
24. Gonsalves, W.C.; Wrightson, A.S.; Henry, R.G. Common oral conditions in older persons. *Am. Fam. Phys.* **2008**, *78*, 18841733.
25. Professional Association of Nursing Home Doctors and Social Geriatricians. Oral Care Guideline for Care Dependent Clients in Nursing Homes. Available online: http://www.platformouderenzorg.nl/dossiers/richtenmondzorgnvva_web.pdf (accessed on 10 March 2020).
26. Wiener, R.C.; Wu, B.; Crout, R.; Wiener, M.; Plassman, B.; Kao, E.; McNeil, D. Hyposalivation and Xerostomia in Dentate Older Adults. *J. Am. Dent. Assoc.* **2010**, *141*, 279–284. [CrossRef]
27. Wells, G.A.; Shea, B.; O'Connell, D.; Peterson, J.; Welch, V.; Losos, M.; Tugwell, P. The Newcastle-Ottawa Scale for Assessing the Quality of Nonrandomised Studies in Meta-Analyses. 2014. Available online: http://www.ohri.ca/programs/clinical_epidemiology/oxford.asp (accessed on 4 July 2020).
28. Andersson, P.; Hallberg, I.; Lorefält, B.; Unosson, M.; Renvert, S. Oral health problems in elderly rehabilitation patients. *Int. J. Dent. Hyg.* **2004**, *2*, 70–77. [CrossRef] [PubMed]
29. El Osta, N.; Hennequin, M.; Tubert-Jeannin, S.; Naaman, N.B.A.; El Osta, L.; Geahchan, N. The pertinence of oral health indicators in nutritional studies in the elderly. *Clin. Nutr.* **2014**, *33*, 316–321. [CrossRef]
30. Huppertz, V.A.; van der Putten, G.-J.; Halfens, R.J.; Schols, J.M.; de Groot, L. Association between Malnutrition and Oral Health in Dutch Nursing Home Residents: Results of the LPZ Study. *J. Am. Med. Dir. Assoc.* **2017**, *18*, 948–954. [CrossRef]
31. Kiesswetter, E.; Hengeveld, L.M.; Keijser, B.J.; Volkert, D.; Visser, M. Oral health determinants of incident malnutrition in community-dwelling older adults. *J. Dent.* **2019**, *85*, 73–80. [CrossRef]
32. Lindmark, U.; Jansson, H.; Lannering, C.; Johansson, L. Oral health matters for the nutritional status of older persons-A population-based study. *J. Clin. Nurs.* **2017**, *27*, 1143–1152. [CrossRef]
33. Mesas, A.E.; De Andrade, S.; Cabrera, M.A.S.; Bueno, V.L.R.D.C. Salud oral y déficit nutricional en adultos mayores no institucionalizados en Londrina, Paraná, Brasil. *Rev. Bras. Epidemiol.* **2010**, *13*, 434–445. [CrossRef]
34. Poisson, P.; Laffond, T.; Campos, S.; Dupuis, V.; Bourdel-Marchasson, I. Relationships between oral health, dysphagia and undernutrition in hospitalised elderly patients. *Gerodontology* **2016**, *33*, 161–168. [CrossRef]
35. Samnieng, P.; Ueno, M.; Shinada, K.; Zaitsu, T.; Wright, F.A.C.; Kawaguchi, Y. Oral Health Status and Chewing Ability is Related to Mini-Nutritional Assessment Results in an Older Adult Population in Thailand. *J. Nutr. Gerontol. Geriatr.* **2011**, *30*, 291–304. [CrossRef] [PubMed]
36. Soini, H.; Muurinen, S.; Routasalo, P.; Sandelin, E.; Savikko, N.; Suominen, M.; Ainamo, A.; Pitkala, K.H. Oral and nutritional status–Is the MNA a useful tool for dental clinics. *J. Nutr. Health Aging* **2006**, *10*, 500–501.
37. Takahashi, M.; Maeda, K.; Wakabayashi, H. Prevalence of sarcopenia and association with oral health-related quality of life and oral health status in older dental clinic outpatients. *Geriatr. Gerontol. Int.* **2018**, *18*, 915–921. [CrossRef]
38. Jung, S.H.; Ryu, J.I.; Jung, D.B. Association of total tooth loss with socio-behavioural health indicators in Korean elderly. *J. Oral Rehabilitation* **2010**, *38*, 517–524. [CrossRef]
39. Ikebe, K.; Nokubi, T.; Sajima, H.; Kobayashi, S.; Hata, K.; Ono, T.; Ettinger, R.L. Perception of dry mouth in a sample of community-dwelling older adults in Japan. *Speéc. Care Dent.* **2001**, *21*, 52–59. [CrossRef] [PubMed]
40. Makhija, S.K.; Gilbert, G.H.; Litaker, M.S.; Allman, R.M.; Sawyer, P.; Locher, J.L.; Ritchie, C.S. Association Between Aspects of Oral Healthâ€"Related Quality of Life and Body Mass Index in Community-Dwelling Older Adults. *J. Am. Geriatr. Soc.* **2007**, *55*, 1808–1816. [CrossRef]

41. Alam, I.; Bangash, F. Oral health and nutritional status of the free-living elderly in Peshawar, Pakistan. *Saudi Med. J.* **2010**, *31*, 713–715. [PubMed]

42. Everaars, B.; Weening, L.; Jerković-Ćosić, K.; Schoonmade, L.; Bleijenberg, N.; De Wit, N.J.; Van Der Heijden, G.J.M.G. Measurement properties of oral health assessments for non-dental healthcare professionals in older people: A systematic review. *BMC Geriatr.* **2020**, *20*, 4–18. [CrossRef] [PubMed]

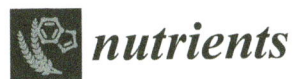

MDPI

Article

Improved Healing after Non-Surgical Periodontal Therapy Is Associated with Higher Protein Intake in Patients Who Are Non-Smokers

David W. Dodington [1], Hannah E. Young [1], Jennifer R. Beaudette [1], Peter C. Fritz [1,2] and Wendy E. Ward [1,*]

1 Department of Kinesiology, Faculty of Applied Health Sciences, Brock University,
St. Catharines, ON L2S 3A1, Canada; david.dodington@mail.utoronto.ca (D.W.D.);
hy19nt@brocku.ca (H.E.Y.); jbeaudette3@gmail.com (J.R.B.); drpeterfritz@me.com (P.C.F.)
2 Periodontal Wellness and Implant Surgery Clinic, Fonthill, ON L0S 1E5, Canada
* Correspondence: wward@brocku.ca

Abstract: The aim of this study was to determine whether a relationship between periodontal healing and protein intake exists in patients undergoing non-surgical treatment for periodontitis. Dietary protein intake was assessed using the 2005 Block food frequency questionnaire in patients with chronic generalized periodontitis undergoing scaling and root planing ($n = 63$ for non-smokers, $n = 22$ for smokers). Protein intake was correlated to post-treatment probing depth using multiple linear regression. Non-smoking patients who consumed ≥ 1 g protein/kg body weight/day had fewer sites with probing depth ≥ 4 mm after scaling and root planing compared to patients with intakes <1 g protein/kg body weight/day (11 ± 2 versus 16 ± 2, $p = 0.05$). This relationship was strengthened after controlling for baseline probing depth, hygienist and time between treatment and follow-up (10 ± 2 versus 16 ± 1, $p = 0.018$) and further strengthened after controlling for potential confounders including age, sex, body mass index, flossing frequency, and bleeding on probing (8 ± 2 versus 18 ± 2, $p < 0.001$). No associations were seen in patients who smoked. Consuming ≥ 1 g protein/kg body weight/day was associated with reductions in periodontal disease burden following scaling and root planing in patients who were non-smokers. Further studies are needed to differentiate between animal and plant proteins.

Keywords: periodontitis; periodontal diseases; scaling and root planning; diet; dietary protein

Citation: Dodington, D.W.; Young, H.E.; Beaudette, J.R.; Fritz, P.C.; Ward, W.E. Improved Healing after Non-Surgical Periodontal Therapy Is Associated with Higher Protein Intake in Patients Who Are Non-Smokers. *Nutrients* **2021**, *13*, 3722. https://doi.org/10.3390/nu13113722

Academic Editors: Kirstin Vach and Johan Peter Woelber

Received: 25 September 2021
Accepted: 19 October 2021
Published: 22 October 2021

Publisher's Note: MDPI stays neutral with regard to jurisdictional claims in published maps and institutional affiliations.

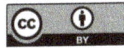

1. Introduction

It is estimated that 70% of Canadians will experience periodontal disease in their lifetime [1]. Globally, the prevalence of periodontal disease is 11.2%, and severe periodontitis is the sixth most prevalent disease worldwide [2,3]. In the United States, the prevalence of periodontitis is 38% for adults over 30 years of age, and it increases to 64% in those over 65 years [4,5]. Periodontal disease has also been associated with numerous chronic illnesses including obesity, diabetes, metabolic syndrome, and rheumatoid arthritis [3,6,7]. While there are many known risk factors for periodontal disease, such as diet and smoking, there is a paucity of data on the roles of these factors in periodontal healing after scaling and root planing (SRP), the first-line non-surgical treatment modality for periodontitis [8]. Healing after SRP is dependent on the resolution of inflammation and reactive oxygen species and can result in reductions in probing depth (PD) and bleeding on probing (BOP) due to the repair and regeneration of damaged tissues [9,10]. SRP followed by routine periodontal maintenance appointments can prevent disease progression and ultimately, tooth loss. Tooth loss can have negative effects on speech, food intake, self-esteem and quality of life, and is independently associated with several chronic systemic inflammatory diseases [7]. Thus, it is important to understand the factors that may support periodontal healing post-SRP.

Nutrients **2021**, 13, 3722

Smoking is a risk factor for numerous chronic diseases through increased inflammation and/or a compromised inflammatory response [11,12] and is a variable of interest due to its known negative effects on periodontal health [13]. Negative associations between smoking and periodontal bone loss, BOP, PD and clinical attachment loss have been found in patients following periodontal treatment [13–15]. While there is evidence to suggest diet is a risk factor for periodontal disease, this evidence is much weaker. Some associations are observed between periodontal health and nutrients with known anti-inflammatory, osteogenic and antioxidant activity [16–21]—these include calcium, vitamin C, flavonoids and omega 3 fatty acids. A previous study by our team reported associations between diet and healing post-SRP and found intakes of fruits and vegetables, β-carotene, vitamin C, α-tocopherol and long chain omega-3 fatty acids (EPA, DHA) to be positively associated with periodontal healing in patients who did not smoke [18]. There was no association between these same components in individuals who currently smoked [18]. It was hypothesized that the lack of an association was due to the negative effect of smoking on the periodontium, though it may also have been due to a small sample size.

With the paucity of data on protein intake and periodontal healing, protein was the primary nutrient of interest in the present study. Periodontal disease is most prevalent in adults over 65 years of age and has been associated with age-related diseases [22,23]. This, along with the fact that protein is the most important macronutrient for supporting immune function and wound healing [24], provided a rationale to determine if there is an association between higher protein intakes and periodontal healing. Of note, several organizations advocate that protein intakes of 1.0 to 1.5 g/kg body weight/day rather than the current recommended dietary allowance (RDA) for protein intake (0.8 g/kg body weight/day) are more appropriate for older adults ($\geq$65 years) to reduce sarcopenia and its resultant loss in quality of life [25–27]. Sarcopenia is defined as a reduction in muscle mass and muscle function that occurs with aging [25,26]. The destruction of alveolar bone tissue is a prominent feature of periodontal disease; sufficient protein intake is associated with higher bone mineral density and slower rates of bone loss, again supporting a potential role of protein in periodontal healing [21,27,28]. Protein also has known anabolic effects on bone and may increase calcium absorption from the gut, leading to increased bone mineralization [28]. Moreover, two recent studies suggest a significant relationship between increased dairy consumption and decreased prevalence of periodontal disease [29,30]. Finally, a study in a rat model of periodontal disease found that consuming a higher level of milk basic protein (MBP) (1% versus 0.2%) supported greater recovery of alveolar bone that was lost as a result of previous ligature placement [31].

Given the widespread interest in higher protein intakes and health and indirect evidence suggesting a potential benefit in periodontal healing, the primary objective of this study was to determine whether the intake of dietary protein ($\geq$1 g/kg body weight/day) was associated with a reduction in periodontal disease burden (i.e., fewer sites with PD $\geq$ 4 mm) following non-surgical treatment of periodontitis.

2. Materials and Methods

2.1. Study Population and Design

The data presented in this study are a retrospective analysis from a patient cohort initially investigated to study the relationship between fruits and vegetables, antioxidants, vitamins and omega-3 fatty acid intake and healing following SRP [18]. The study took place at a specialty periodontal clinic (Fonthill, ON, Canada) between January 2013 and July 2014. All patients undergoing SRP during this time were invited to participate in the study. Patients were excluded from the study analysis if they did not meet the requirements for chronic generalized periodontitis set by the American Academy of Periodontology (PD of $\geq$4 mm in at least 30% of sites) [32]. While a new periodontal classification system was developed in 2017, after this study was conducted, and the term 'chronic periodontitis' is no longer used, reporting the number and proportion of teeth with PD $\geq$ 4 mm remains a clinically meaningful periodontal measure in the new classification system [33]. During the enrolment visit, a comprehensive baseline dental examination including medical/dental history and periodontal charting was completed (see Section 2.2, Periodontal Examination, for more details). Full mouth SRP was then performed by one of four calibrated hygienists using hand and ultrasonic instruments as necessary. Individualized oral hygiene instructions were also provided to all patients. Participants were provided with a food frequency questionnaire (FFQ) to be completed at home and returned at the follow-up appointment. Follow-up occurred between 8 and 16 weeks after SRP and included a complete periodontal examination. The Bioscience Research Ethics Board at Brock University approved the study protocol and all participants provided written informed consent. This trial was registered at clinicaltrials.gov (accessed on 18 October 2021) as NCT02291835.

2.2. Periodontal Examination

Baseline and follow-up periodontal charting included measurement of PD, BOP and plaque index (PI). PD was measured using a periodontal probe as the distance from the gingival margin to the bottom of the periodontal pocket at six sites per tooth (mesiobuccal, buccal, distobuccal, mesiolingual, lingual, and distolingual) on all teeth present, and the number of sites ≥ 4 mm were counted. Teeth to be extracted were not included in the count. BOP and PI were assessed by visual inspection after probing, and PI was measured using the O'Leary Plaque Index [34]. The baseline examinations were all performed by the same periodontist (P.C.F.) and occurred 1 to 19 weeks prior to SRP. Follow-up examinations were performed by one of four hygienists at 8 to 16 weeks post-SRP. Prior to the study, the hygienists were calibrated to apply 25 N of pressure when probing by repeated probing simulations against an electronic scale.

2.3. Diet Assessment

Nutrient intakes were assessed using the 2005 Block FFQ, which has been previously validated against multiple diet records [35] (https://www.nutritionquest.com/assessment/list-of-questionnaires-and-screeners/ (accessed on 21 October 2021)). The FFQ queried 110 food items for frequency (never, a few times a year, once per month, 2–3 times per month, once per week, 2 times per week, 3–4 times per week, 5–6 times per week, every day) and portion size. Portion size pictures were provided to enhance the accuracy of quantification. Nutrient intake estimates were calculated using a database of nutrient values derived from the Canadian Nutrient File. Assessment of reporting accuracy in this cohort has been previously published [18]. Nutrient intakes were energy adjusted and standardized to a 2000 Kcal diet using the residual method [36]. Protein intake was expressed in grams per kilogram of body weight and participants were classified by protein intake level (<1 g/kg body weight/day or ≥ 1 g/kg body weight/day). The 1 g/kg bodyweight/day cut-off was chosen due to evidence suggesting protein intakes ≥ 1 g/kg body weight/day may be more appropriate for older adults (>65 years) [25–27].

2.4. Assessment of Covariates

Self-reported age, sex, health conditions, medication use and smoking status (never, former or current) were recorded from the patient's medical history form. Dental hygiene information was gathered by a hygienist and included brushing and flossing frequency, electronic toothbrush use, frequency of professional dental cleaning and any previous periodontal therapy. Participants also met with a study nurse during their initial visit and had their height and body weight measured (Health-O-Meter Professional) to calculate their BMI. Blood was also drawn at this time for the measurement of serum 25-hydroxyvitamin D, which was analyzed by a third-party provider (Life Labs, Thorold, ON, Canada) using the Liaison chemiluminescence system (DiaSorin Inc., Mississauga, Canada). The laboratory participates in the Vitamin D External Quality Assessment Scheme (DEQAS).

2.5. Statistical Analysis

Patients were stratified by smoking status for two main reasons: i. patients who smoke are known to have compromised healing after SRP [15,37] and ii. no associations between periodontal health and any of the previously analyzed nutrient intakes was previously observed in patients who smoke [18]. Descriptive statistics and nutrient intakes were compared between the protein intake groups using an independent sample t test for continuous variables and chi-square test for categorical variables. When the expected cell count was <5 for categorical variables, Fisher's exact test was used in place of the chi-square test. Due to the small sample size and the violation of the assumption of normality in the group of patients who smoked, a Mann–Whitney U Test was used instead of the independent sample t test. The relationship between protein intake and periodontal healing was assessed by multiple linear regression using PD as a continuous dependent variable. Protein intake was entered into the model as a dichotomous variable (<1 versus $\geq$1 g protein/kg/day), first in an unadjusted model, then in subsequent models with adjustment for covariates. All models were assessed for normality of residuals and multicollinearity. Data were analyzed with SPSS v.20 (IBM, Inc., Armonk, NY, USA), and statistical significance was defined as $p < 0.05$.

3. Results

Main Findings

In total, 129 patients were recruited for the study (Figure 1). Of those, 17 patients were lost to follow-up, 11 did not return within the 16-week follow-up period, and 3 did not complete the food frequency questionnaire and were thus excluded from the analysis. Subsequently, 12 did not meet the criteria for chronic generalized periodontitis and were excluded. One additional patient was excluded as their body weight was not measured, so protein intake per kg of bodyweight could not be calculated. There were no differences in age, sex, BMI, smoking status, baseline clinical outcomes, or serum 25-hydroxyvitamin D concentration between those included and those excluded from the analysis (Table S1).

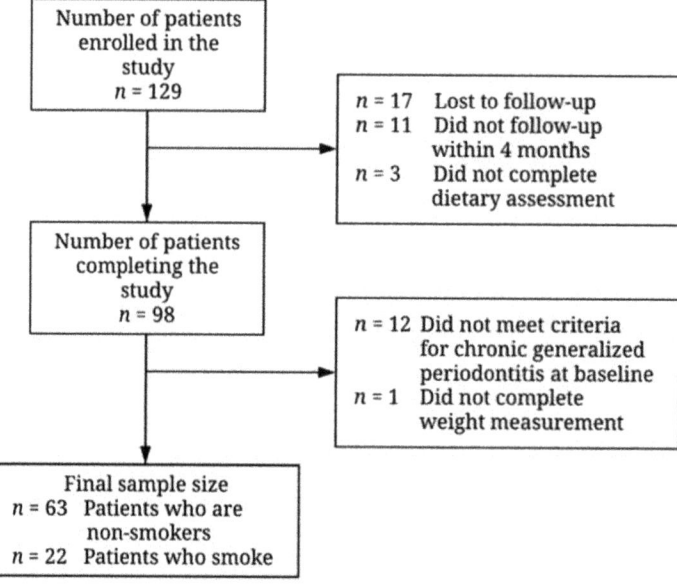

Figure 1. Flowchart illustrating recruitment and final sample size for patients undergoing non-surgical periodontal therapy. Reasons for exclusion of participants are given to the right of the arrows denoting the transitions between stages.

Participant characteristics by level of protein intake and smoking status are shown in Table 1. Regardless of smoking status, participant age and comorbidities did not differ between the two levels of protein intake. For patients who were non-smokers, former smoking status did not differ based on protein intake. For both non-smokers and smokers, the ≥ 1 g/kg body weight/day protein group had significantly more female participants and they had a lower average BMI. In terms of dental hygiene, there were no differences in brushing frequency, electric toothbrush use, professional cleaning frequency and previous periodontal therapy based on protein intake levels in both the smoking and non-smoking groups. Patients who were non-smokers and consumed ≥ 1 g/kg/day of protein reported significantly higher flossing frequencies compared to those who consumed <1 g/kg body weight/day of protein; however, this difference was not observed in patients who smoked.

Table 1. Descriptive statistics and clinical parameters of patients undergoing non-surgical periodontal therapy grouped by protein intake and current smoking status [1].

	Patients Who Did Not Smoke			Patients Who Did Smoke		
	Protein Intake g/kg Body Weight/Day		*p* Value	Protein Intake g/kg Body Weight/Day		*p* Value
	<1	≥1		<1	≥1	
	n = 34	*n* = 29		*n* = 10	*n* = 12	
Patient Characteristics						
Male	25 (73%)	8 (28%)	<0.001	7 (70%)	2 (17%)	**0.027**
Female	9 (27%)	21 (72%)	<0.001	3 (30%)	10 (83%)	**0.027**
Age (years)	57 ± 10	61 ± 13	0.10	54 ± 8	52 ± 7	0.72
BMI (kg/m^2)	31.8 ± 5.0	26.6 ± 3.8	<0.001	31.8 ± 6.1	24.6 ± 4.2	**0.004**
Former smokers	15 (44%)	18 (62%)	0.16	-	-	-
Comorbidities						
Diabetes	4 (12%)	2 (7%)	0.68	1 (10%)	1 (8.3%)	1.00
HTN or CAD	14 (41%)	10 (35%)	0.59	3 (30%)	2 (17%)	0.62
Osteoporosis	1 (3%)	5 (17%)	0.09	0	0	-
# of medications	3 ± 3	3 ± 4	0.75	2 ± 1	1 ± 2	0.25
Dental hygiene						
Brushing (times/day)	2.2. ± 0.6	2.4 ± 1.1	0.37	1.0 ± 0.7	2.3 ± 0.75	0.35
Flossing (times/week)	2.7 ± 4.4	5.3 ± 3.6	**0.016**	2.4 ± 4.7	5.0 ± 6.1	0.069
Electric toothbrush use	11 (32%)	10 (35%)	0.83	3 (27%)	3 (25%)	1.00
Cleanings (months)	5 ± 3	5 ± 3	0.54	5 ± 3	7 ± 6	0.67
Previous therapy	10 (29%)	8 (28%)	0.89	3 (30%)	3 (25%)	1.00
Baseline clinical outcomes						
Number of teeth	25 ± 4	25 ± 4	0.81	25 ± 4	26 ± 2	0.25
PD (# sites ≥ 4 mm)	93 ± 37	93 ± 33	0.96	102 ± 39	107 ± 34	0.77
BOP (# sites)	76 ± 46	77 ± 50	0.92	79 ± 61	73 ± 43	0.77
Plaque index (%)	78 ± 27	67 ± 30	0.19	83 ± 24	57 ± 37	0.080
Follow-up time (days)	74 ± 17	78 ± 15	0.37	79 ± 17	80 ± 16	0.92
Follow-up clinical outcomes						
Number of teeth	24 ± 4	24 ± 5	0.95	24 ± 4	26 ± 3	0.35
PD (# sites ≥ 4 mm)	16 ± 11	11 ± 8	0.05	22 ± 21	20 ± 15	1.00
BOP (# sites)	8 ± 9	3 ± 6	**0.009**	13 ± 18	4 ± 7	0.069
Plaque index (%)	36 ± 19	28 ± 25	0.14	47 ± 26	30 ± 25	0.50

Table 1. *Cont.*

	Patients Who Did Not Smoke			Patients Who Did Smoke		
	Protein Intake g/kg Body Weight/Day		*p* Value	Protein Intake g/kg Body Weight/Day		*p* Value
	<1	≥1		<1	≥1	
	n = 34	*n* = 29		*n* = 10	*n* = 12	
Nutritional intake and status						
Calories (Kcal/day)	1625 ± 586	1583 ± 649	0.79	1828 ± 530	1525 ± 674	0.28
Protein (g/day)	79 ± 10	88 ± 9	<0.001	69 ± 13	84 ± 13	0.025
Carbohydrate (g/day)	244 ± 34	230 ± 37	0.14	231 ± 51	227 ± 33	0.72
Fats (g/day)	76 ± 12	78 ±13	0.43	77 ± 12	80 ±18	1.00
EPA + DHA (mg/day)	320 ± 463	380 ± 365	0.58	99 ± 61	253 ± 163	0.021
Vitamin C (mg/day)	130 ± 51	129 ± 37	0.90	105 ± 61	137 ± 73	0.25
25-OH-D (nmol/L)	59 ± 21	70 ± 25	0.074	44 ± 12	57 ± 21	0.159

[1] All values are means ± SDs for continuous variables and counts (%) for categorical variables. Non-standard abbreviations: HTN, hypertension; CAD, coronary artery disease; PD, probing depth; BOP, bleeding on probing; EPA, eicosapentaenoic acid; DHA, docosahexaenoic acid; 25-OH-D, 25-hydroxyvitamin D.

Importantly, there were no differences in periodontal outcomes between protein intake groups at baseline, including the number of teeth, PD, BOP and PI, as well as the time between treatment and follow-up regardless of smoking status. By design, protein intakes differed between groups. Other nutritional intakes, including total energy, total carbohydrate, total fat, omega-3 fatty acid, vitamin C intakes and serum 25-hydroxyvitamin D were not significantly different between the two levels of dietary protein intake in those who did not smoke. In patients who smoked, only omega-3 fatty acid intake was significantly higher in those with protein intakes ≥1 g/kg body weight/day.

In the unadjusted regression analysis, non-smoking patients who consumed ≥1 g/kg body weight/day of protein had fewer sites with PD ≥ 4 mm at the time of follow-up compared to those who consumed <1 g/kg/day of protein. This difference was borderline significant (11 ± 2 versus 16 ± 2, *p* = 0.05) (Model 1, Table 2 and Figure 2a). To improve the fit of the model, additional study design factors were considered in the regression model. This included the patient's baseline PD, the hygienist performing their treatment and the time between treatment and follow-up.

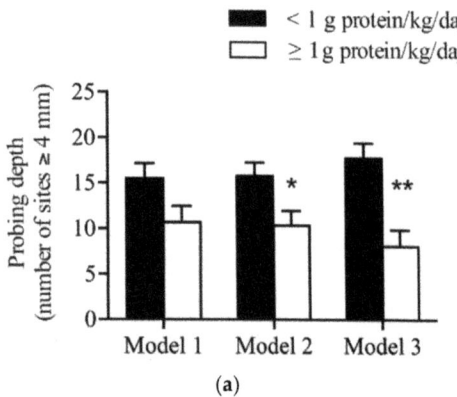

(a)

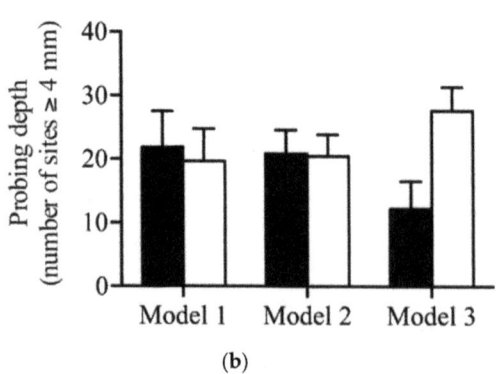

(b)

Figure 2. Comparison of dietary protein levels with probing depth after non-surgical periodontal therapy in patients who (a) did not smoke and (b) did smoke. Model 1 is unadjusted. Model 2 adjusted for baseline probing depth, hygienist and time between treatment and follow-up. Model 3 adjusted for variables in Model 2 plus age, sex, BMI, flossing frequency and bleeding on probing. Data presented are estimated marginal means ± SEM. * Indicates a significant difference between groups (*p* < 0.05), ** indicates a significant difference between the two levels of protein intake (*p* < 0.01).

Table 2. Multiple linear regression of probing depth sites > 4 mm in patients after non-surgical periodontal therapy who did not smoke [1].

	Model 1		Model 2		Model 3	
	B (95% CI)	p	B (95% CI)	p	B (95% CI)	p
Protein intake						
<1 g/kg body weight/day	Reference		Reference		Reference	
≥1 g/kg body weight/day	−4.8 (−9.6, 0.0)	0.050	−5.4 (−9.9, −1.0)	**0.018**	−9.7 (−15.5, −3.9)	**0.001**
Hygienist						
Hygienist 1			Reference		Reference	
Hygienist 2			−7.3 (−12.8, −1.8)	**0.011**	−7.2 (−12.4, −1.9)	**0.009**
Hygienist 3			−4.8 (−10.7, 1.0)	0.11	−6.1 (−11.9, −0.4)	**0.037**
Hygienist 4			−4.2 (−0.1, 0.2)	0.23	−6.3 (−13.7, 1.0)	0.09
Baseline PD (# ≥ 4 mm)			0.1 (0.01, 0.2)	**<0.001**	0.2 (0.1, 0.2)	**<0.001**
Follow-up time (days)			0.0 (−0.1, 0.2)	0.54	0.0 (−0.1, 0.2)	0.54
Sex						
Male					Reference	
Female					4.1 (−0.8, 9.0)	0.10
Age (years)					0.2 (0.0, 0.4)	**0.041**
BMI (kg/m²)					−0.5 (−1.0, 0.0)	**0.038**
Flossing (times/week)					0.0 (−0.5, 0.6)	0.89
BOP (# sites)					0.3 (0.0, 0.6)	0.09

[1] Regression of probing depth (number of sites ≥ 4 mm) using low (<1 g/kg/day) and high (≥1 g/kg/day) protein intake as a categorical variable. Unstandardized regression coefficients (B) and 95% confidence intervals (CI) are shown. Non-standard abbreviations: BOP, bleeding on probing; PD, probing depth.

In this second model, patients who consumed ≥1 g/kg/day of protein had significantly fewer numbers of sites with PD ≥ 4 mm compared to patients who consumed <1 g/kg body weight/day (10 ± 2 versus 16 ± 1, $p = 0.018$) (Model 2, Table 2 and Figure 2a). Lastly, to control for potential confounders and to better understand the association between protein intake and PD, the confounders identified in Table 1 were added to the model: sex, BMI, flossing frequency, as well as age and BOP at follow-up as an objective measure of oral hygiene.

In the fully adjusted model, there continued to be a significant association between the consumption of ≥1 g/kg body weight/day of protein and a reduction in the number of sites with PD ≥ 4 mm compared to patients who consumed <1 g/kg body weight/day (8 ± 2 versus 18 ± 2, $p < 0.001$) (Model 3, Table 2 and Figure 2a). In patients who smoked, no significant differences in the number of sites with probing depths ≥ 4 mm were observed based on protein intake in any of the models (Table 3 and Figure 2b).

Table 3. Multiple linear regression of probing depth sites ≥ 4 mm after non-surgical periodontal therapy in patients who smoked [1].

	Model 1		Model 2		Model 3	
	B (95% CI)	p	B (95% CI)	p	B (95% CI)	p
Protein intake						
<1 g/kg body weight/day	Reference		Reference		Reference	
≥1 g/kg body weight/day	−2.2 (−18.3, 13.8)	0.77	−0.4 (11.9, 11.1)	0.95	16.3 (−1.4, 34.0)	0.066

Table 3. *Cont.*

	Model 1		Model 2		Model 3	
	B (95% CI)	*p*	*B* (95% CI)	*p*	*B* (95% CI)	*p*
Hygienist						
Hygienist 1			Reference		Reference	
Hygienist 2			−18.2 (−32.7, −3.8)	**0.017**	−25.0 (−44.7, −5.2)	**0.016**
Hygienist 3			−7.0 (−28.4, 14.4)	0.49	−9.8 (−35.3, 15.7)	0.45
Hygienist 4			−20.7 (−46.1, 4.8)	0.10	−26.2 (−55.2, 2.8)	**0.033**
Baseline PD (# ≥ 4 mm)			0.2 (0.0, 0.4)	**0.025**	0.1 (−0.2, 0.3)	0.38
Follow-up time (days)			0.3 (−0.1, 0.6)	0.17	0.0 (−0.5, 0.5)	0.98
Sex						
Male					Reference	
Female					−9.6 (−27.1, 7.9)	0.30
Age (years)					0.2 (−0.6, 0.9)	0.60
BMI (kg/m^2)					0.3 (−1.0, 1.6)	0.66
Flossing (times/week)					−0.3 (−1.3, 0.7)	0.47
BOP (# sites)					0.8 (0.1, 1.4)	**0.017**

[1] Regression of probing depth (number of sites ≥ 4 mm) using low (<1 g/kg/day) and high (≥1 g/kg/day) protein intake as a categorical variable. Unstandardized regression coefficients (*B*) and 95% confidence intervals (CI) are shown. Non-standard abbreviations: BOP, bleeding on probing; PD, probing depth.

4. Discussion

A key finding from this study is the association between higher consumption of dietary protein (≥1 g/kg body weight/day) and a greater reduction in the number of sites with a PD ≥ 4 mm in patients who were non-smokers after SRP. Moreover, this relationship was strengthened by controlling for baseline PD, hygienist and time between treatment and follow-up. It was even further strengthened after accounting for additional confounding factors such as age, sex, BMI, flossing frequency and BOP. While there is little literature available on the relationship between dietary protein and periodontal disease in non-smokers, that which is available supports the current findings. For example, feeding milk basic protein, containing whey protein and other potential bioactives, improved healing in a rat model of periodontal disease [31]. Periodontal disease was induced in rats by placing a ligature on the second maxillary molar for 20 days. The ligature was then removed, and varying levels of milk basic protein were added into the control diet at a level of 0.2% or 1.0% MBP while keeping the total level of protein similar among diets. The rats fed the diet containing a higher level of MPB (1.0%) had greater alveolar bone regeneration following 90 days compared to rats fed the control diet or the diet containing 0.2% MBP.

Additional evidence supporting a relationship between dietary protein and periodontal disease comes from data from the fifth and sixth Korean National Health and Nutrition Examination Survey (*n* = 9798), which found that consuming ≥ 7 servings of dairy products per week was associated with a 24% lower prevalence of periodontal disease after controlling for confounding factors including calcium intake, BMI and smoking status [29]. Given that dairy foods tend to be high in protein, the authors hypothesized that whey proteins may prevent alveolar bone loss and attenuate periodontal disease. Similar findings were reported in a cohort study using Danish Health Examination Survey data (*n* = 3287) which found adults consuming ≥ 9.6 g of whey/day and/or ≥32 g casein/day had a lower likelihood of severe periodontal disease as defined by the American Academy of Periodontology [30,38].

A similar relationship between protein intake and the number of sites with PD ≥ 4 mm was not observed in patients who smoked. This may be a result of smoking having negative effects on oral health and healing—this was previously shown for other nutrients [18]. Smoking is one of the largest risk factors for periodontal disease and is thought to impact periodontal health through various mechanisms, including decreased vascular flow, decreased lymphocyte proliferation, and impairing neutrophil function, thus compromising wound healing [11,13,15,39]. However, it is important to note that there were relatively few patients who smoked within the study and as such, this specific analysis was underpowered but helps inform the design of future studies. Based on the results of this study, a retrospective power calculation was performed. Detecting a difference in the PD depth of 2.2 sites with a standard deviation of 18.0, ($\alpha = 0.05$, $\beta = 0.80$) would require a sample size of $n = 1050$ per group, assuming a relationship exists in smokers. Given the small difference in PD seen in smokers, it is likely that either no relationship exists or that the effect size is too small to be clinically meaningful.

It is possible that protein has both direct and indirect effects on periodontal health. One possible explanation of the observed relationship between probing depth and protein intake could be due to its direct effects on wound repair. For example, studies have found that protein malnutrition leads to delayed wound healing [40]. Moreover, in a randomized clinical trial of elderly home-nursed patients, consuming a nutrient- and protein-dense supplement resulted in improved wound healing [41]. The level and quality of protein intake are known to affect collagen deposition and other factors that result in delayed wound healing [39–42]. However, no studies have specifically studied protein intake and oral healing. Additionally, given that periodontal disease can result in a loss of bone and teeth, the osteogenic effects of protein are hypothesized to contribute to long-term periodontal health; however, these effects might not be expected to contribute directly to changes in probing depth during the 8 to 16 week follow-up. Studies of protein intake and bone health indicate that there is little benefit of increasing protein intake beyond levels of 0.8–1.3 g/kg body weight/day in healthy adults—and no detrimental effects of such higher protein intakes to bone mineral density or fracture risk provided calcium intake is at the recommended level [28]. However, levels of protein intake below 0.8 g/kg body weight/day could potentially have negative implications for bone health and periodontal disease.

Strengths and Limitations

One of the strengths of this study was that there were no significant differences in baseline periodontal outcomes between protein intake groups. Given that baseline PD was associated with periodontal outcomes 8 to 16 weeks post-SRP in our original study [18], this reduces the likelihood that baseline periodontal health served as a confounding factor in this study. Additionally, there were no differences in participant age, former smoking status, comorbidities, brushing frequency, electric toothbrush use, professional cleaning frequency and previous periodontal therapy between protein intake groups regardless of smoking status. The study also included approximately equal proportions of male and female participants.

Some of the limitations are the use of FFQ to measure dietary intake, multiple hygienists performing periodontal examinations, variation in the length of time before SRP and follow-up time after SRP, and potential confounding variables such as dental hygiene practices. Due to the tendency of FFQs to overestimate food intakes [43], caution should be used when interpreting intake levels derived from this study and comparisons to the RDA. Additionally, the FFQ used was unable to differentiate between dairy, animal, and plant proteins. Thus, we are unable to draw specific conclusions based on protein type. The effects of multiple examiners were minimized by calibrating hygienists and performing statistical control for this variable. The variation in the length of time prior to and after SRP reflect the real-life situation of clinical practice, in which patients need to find time in busy schedules for these appointments. Baseline examinations occurred 1 to 19 weeks prior to SRP, and follow-up time ranged from 8 to 16 weeks, which was the standard of care at the time of the study. In patients who were non-smokers, flossing frequency was significantly higher in the group who consumed ≥ 1 g protein/kg body weight/day. While this may serve as a confounding factor, it is unlikely to have a large effect, given that all other oral hygiene variables showed no significant difference between groups, which suggests overall that patients had relatively similar oral hygiene behaviors. Additionally, including flossing frequency as a covariate in statistical models had minimal effect on the strength of the associations observed. The small sample size for the group of patients who were smokers is a limitation, though it was also encouraging that there were far fewer participants who smoked given the known detriment that smoking has on overall health.

5. Conclusions

This study shows a positive association between protein intakes ≥ 1 g/kg body weight/day and better periodontal healing following SRP in patients who do not smoke, but not in patients who smoke. Albeit there were few patients who were current smokers, so this association requires verification. Future dietary intervention studies during the post-SRP healing phase are warranted in order to determine the potential benefits of protein intake as an adjunct to SRP. Additionally, long-term studies should be carried out to measure the relationship between dietary protein intake, tooth loss and alveolar bone loss, as these measures may be better indicators of the long-term benefit of higher protein intakes for periodontal health.

Supplementary Materials: The following are available online at https://www.mdpi.com/article/10.3390/nu13113722/s1, Table S1: descriptive statistics and clinical parameters of excluded participants.

Author Contributions: Conceptualization, D.W.D., P.C.F. and W.E.W.; methodology, D.W.D.; formal analysis, D.W.D., H.E.Y. and J.R.B.; investigation, D.W.D.; resources, P.C.F. and W.E.W.; data curation, D.W.D., H.E.Y. and J.R.B.; writing—original draft preparation, D.W.D. and W.E.W.; writing—review and editing, H.E.Y., J.R.B., D.W.D., W.E.W. and P.C.F.; visualization, D.W.D. and H.E.Y.; supervision, P.C.F. and W.E.W.; project administration, D.W.D., P.C.F. and W.E.W. All authors have read and agreed to the published version of the manuscript.

Funding: Funding was provided by start-up funding to W.E.W. from Brock University. D.W.D. held a Frederick Banting and Charles Best Canada Graduate Scholarship. W.E.W. holds a Canada Research Chair in Bone and Muscle Development. H.E.Y. held an Ontario Graduate Scholarship.

Institutional Review Board Statement: The study was conducted according to the guidelines of the Declaration of Helsinki and approved by the Bioscience Research Ethics Board of Brock University (12-068-WARD, November 2012).

Informed Consent Statement: Informed consent was obtained from all subjects involved in the study.

Data Availability Statement: The data presented in this study are available upon request from the corresponding authors. The data are not publicly available due to ethics restrictions.

Acknowledgments: The authors are grateful to the clinical team at PCF's Periodontal Wellness and Implant Surgery Clinic, who assisted with patient recruitment, the measurement of clinical outcomes, and the collection of samples.

Conflicts of Interest: The authors declare no conflict of interest. The funders had no role in the design of the study; in the collection, analyses, or interpretation of data; in the writing of the manuscript, or in the decision to publish the results.

References

1. Canadian Dental Association. Available online: https://www.cda-adc.ca/en/oral_health/faqs/gum_diseases_faqs.asp (accessed on 3 April 2020).
2. GBD 2016 Disease and Injury Incidence and Prevalence Collaborators. Global, regional, and national incidence, prevalence, and years lived with disability for 328 diseases and injuries for 195 countries, 1990–2016: A systematic analysis for the Global Burden of Disease Study 2016. *Lancet* **2017**, *390*, 1211–1259. [CrossRef]
3. Tonetti, M.S.; Jepsen, S.; Jin, L.; Otomo-Corgel, J. Impact of the global burden of periodontal diseases on health, nutrition and wellbeing of mankind: A call for global action. *J. Clin. Periodontol.* **2017**, *44*, 456–462. [CrossRef] [PubMed]
4. Eke, P.I.; Dye, B.A.; Wei, L.; Thornton-Evans, G.O.; Genco, R.J. Prevalence of periodontitis in adults in the United States: 2009 and 2010. *J. Dent. Res.* **2012**, *91*, 914–920. [CrossRef]
5. Billings, M.; Holtfreter, B.; Papapanou, P.N.; Mitnik, G.L.; Kocher, T.; Dye, B.A. Age-dependent distribution of periodontitis in two countries: Findings from NHANES 2009 to 2014 and SHIP-TREND 2008 to 2012. *J. Clin. Periodontol.* **2018**, *45*, S130–S148. [CrossRef]

6. Chapple, I.L.C.; Bouchard, P.; Cagetti, M.G.; Campus, G.; Carra, M.C.; Cocco, F.; Nibali, L.; Hujoel, P.; Laine, M.L.; Lingstrom, P.; et al. Interaction of lifestyle, behaviour or systemic diseases with dental caries and periodontal diseases: Consensus report of group 2 of the joint EFP/ORCA workshop on the boundaries between caries and periodontal diseases. *J. Clin. Periodontol.* **2017**, *44*, S39–S51. [CrossRef] [PubMed]

7. Chapple, I.L.C.; van der Weijden, F.; Doerfer, C.; Herrera, D.; Shapira, L.; Polak, D.; Madianos, P.; Louropoulou, A.; Machtei, E.; Donos, N.; et al. Primary prevention of periodontitis: Managing gingivitis. *J. Clin. Periodontol.* **2015**, *42*, 71–76. [CrossRef] [PubMed]

8. Sanz, M.; Herrera, D.; Kebschull, M.; Chapple, I.; Jepsen, S.; Beglundh, T.; Sculean, A.; Tonetti, M.S.; EFP Workshop Participants and Methodological Consultants. Treatment of Stage I–III Periodontitis—The EFP S3 Level Clinical Practice Guideline. *J. Clin. Periodontol.* **2020**, *47* (Suppl. 22), 4–60. [CrossRef] [PubMed]

9. Damgaard, C.; Kantarci, A.; Holmstrup, P.; Hasturk, H.; Nielsen, C.H.; van Dyke, T.E. Porphyromonas Gingivalis-induced production of reactive oxygen species, tumor necrosis factor-α, interleukin-6, CXCL8 and CCL2 by neutrophils from localized aggressive periodontitis and healthy donors: Modulating actions of red blood cells and resolvin E1. *J. Periodontal. Res.* **2017**, *52*, 246–254. [CrossRef] [PubMed]

10. Reis, C.; da Costa, A.V.; Guimarães, J.T.; Tuna, D.; Braga, A.C.; Pacheco, J.J.; Arosa, F.A.; Salazar, F.; Cardoso, E.M. Clinical improvement following therapy for periodontitis: Association with a decrease in IL-1 and IL-6. *Exp. Ther. Med.* **2014**, *8*, 323–327. [CrossRef] [PubMed]

11. Rom, O.; Avezov, K.; Aizenbud, D.; Reznick, A.Z. Cigarette smoking and inflammation revisited. *Respir. Physiol. Neurobiol.* **2013**, *187*, 5–10. [CrossRef]

12. Barbieri, S.S.; Zacchi, E.; Amadio, P.; Gianellini, S.; Mussoni, L.; Weksler, B.B.; Tremoli, E. Cytokines present in smokers' serum interact with smoke components to enhance endothelial dysfunction. *Cardiovasc. Res.* **2011**, *90*, 475–483. [CrossRef] [PubMed]

13. Naji, A.; Edman, K.; Holmlund, A. Influence of smoking on periodontal healing one year after active treatment. *J. Clin. Periodontol.* **2020**, *47*, 343–350. [CrossRef] [PubMed]

14. Boström, L.; Linder, L.E.; Bergström, J. Influence of smoking on the outcome of periodontal surgery: A 5-year follow-up. *J. Clin. Periodontol.* **1998**, *25*, 194–201. [CrossRef]

15. Heasman, L.; Stacey, F.; Preshaw, P.M.; McCracken, G.I.; Hepburn, S.; Heasman, P.A. The effect of smoking on periodontal treatment response: A review of clinical evidence. *J. Clin. Periodontol.* **2006**, *33*, 241–253. [CrossRef] [PubMed]

16. Lau, B.Y.; Johnston, B.D.; Fritz, P.C.; Ward, W.E. Dietary strategies to optimize wound healing after periodontal and dental implant surgery: An evidence-based review. *Open Dent. J.* **2013**, *7*, 36–46. [CrossRef] [PubMed]

17. Iwasaki, M.; Manz, M.C.; Taylor, G.W.; Yoshihara, A.; Miyazaki, H. Relations of serum ascorbic acid and α-tocopherol to periodontal disease. *J. Dent. Res.* **2012**, *91*, 167–172. [CrossRef] [PubMed]

18. Dodington, D.W.; Fritz, P.C.; Sullivan, P.J.; Ward, W.E. Higher intakes of fruits and vegetables, β-Carotene, Vitamin C, α-Tocopherol, EPA, and DHA are positively associated with periodontal healing after nonsurgical periodontal therapy in nonsmokers but not in smokers. *J. Nutr.* **2015**, *145*, 2512–2519. [CrossRef]

19. Abou Sulaiman, A.E.; Shehadeh, R.M.H. Assessment of total antioxidant capacity and the use of vitamin C in the treatment of non-smokers with chronic periodontitis. *J. Periodontol.* **2010**, *81*, 1547–1554. [CrossRef] [PubMed]

20. Martinon, P.; Fraticelli, L.; Giboreau, A.; Dussart, C.; Bourgeois, D.; Carrouel, F. Nutrition as a key modifiable factor for periodontitis and main chronic diseases. *J. Clin. Med.* **2021**, *10*, 197. [CrossRef] [PubMed]

21. O'Connor, J.L.P.; Milledge, K.L.; O'Leary, F.; Cumming, R.; Eberhard, J.; Hirani, V. Poor dietary intake of nutrients and food groups are associated with increased risk of periodontal disease among community-dwelling older adults: A systematic literature review. *Nutr. Rev.* **2020**, *78*, 175–188. [CrossRef]

22. Baima, G.; Romandini, M.; Citterio, F.; Romano, F.; Aimetti, M. Periodontitis and Accelerated Biological Aging: A Geroscience Approach. *J. Dent. Res.* **2021**. Advance online publication. [CrossRef] [PubMed]

23. Clark, D.; Kotronia, E.; Ramsay, S.E. Frailty, aging, and periodontal disease: Basic biologic considerations. *Periodontol. 2000* **2021**, *87*, 143–156. [CrossRef] [PubMed]

24. McClave, S.A.; Martindale, R.G.; Vanek, V.W.; McCarthy, M.; Roberts, P.; Taylor, B.; Ochoa, J.B.; Napolitano, L.; Cresci, G. Guidelines for the provision and assessment of nutrition support therapy in the adult critically ill patient. *J. Parenter. Enter. Nutr.* **2009**, *33*, 277–316. [CrossRef] [PubMed]

25. Phillips, S.M. Determining the protein needs of "older" persons one meal at a time. *Am. J. Clin. Nutr.* **2017**, *105*, 291–292. [CrossRef] [PubMed]

26. Baum, J.I.; Kim, I.Y.; Wolfe, R.R. Protein Consumption and the elderly: What is the optimal level of intake? *Nutrients* **2016**, *8*, 359. [CrossRef] [PubMed]

27. Bauer, J.; Biolo, G.; Cederholm, T.; Cesari, M.; Cruz-Jentoft, A.J.; Morley, J.E.; Phillips, S.; Sieber, C.; Stehle, P.; Teta, D.; et al. Evidence-based recommendations for optimal dietary protein intake in older people: A position paper from the Prot-Age study group. *J. Am. Med. Dir. Assoc.* **2013**, *14*, 542–559. [CrossRef] [PubMed]

28. Darling, A.L.; Manders, R.J.F.; Sahni, S.; Zhu, K.; Hewitt, C.E.; Prince, R.L.; Millward, D.J.; Lanham-New, S.A. Dietary protein and bone health across the life-course: An updated systematic review and meta-analysis over 40 years. *Osteoporos. Int.* **2019**, *30*, 741–761. [CrossRef] [PubMed]

29. Lee, K.; Kim, J. Dairy food consumption is inversely associated with the prevalence of periodontal disease in Korean adults. *Nutrients* **2019**, *11*, 1035. [CrossRef] [PubMed]

30. Adegboye, A.R.A.; Boucher, B.J.; Kongstad, J.; Fiehn, N.E.; Christensen, L.B.; Heitmann, B.L. Calcium, Vitamin D, casein and whey protein intakes and periodontitis among Danish adults. *Public Health Nutr.* **2016**, *19*, 503–510. [CrossRef] [PubMed]

31. Seto, H.; Toba, Y.; Takada, Y.; Kawakami, H.; Ohba, H.; Hama, H.; Horibe, M.; Nagata, T. Milk basic protein increases alveolar bone formation in rat experimental periodontitis. *J. Periodontal. Res.* **2007**, *42*, 85–89. [CrossRef] [PubMed]

32. Wiebe, C.; Putnins, E. The Periodontal Disease Classification System of the American Academy of Periodontology—An Update. *J. Can. Dent. Assoc.* **2000**, *66*, 594–597. [PubMed]

33. Papapanou, P.N.; Sanz, M.; Buduneli, N.; Dietrich, T.; Feres, M.; Fine, D.H.; Flemmig, T.F.; Garcia, R.; Giannobile, W.V.; Graziani, F.; et al. Periodontitis: Consensus report of workgroup 2 of the 2017 World Workshop on the Classification of Periodontal and Peri-Implant Diseases. *J. Periodontol.* **2018**, *89*, S173–S182. [CrossRef] [PubMed]

34. O'Leary, T.J.; Drake, R.B.; Naylor, J.E. The plaque control record. *J. Periodontol.* **1972**, *43*, 38. [CrossRef] [PubMed]

35. Block, G.; Woods, M.; Potosky, A.; Clifford, C. Validation of a self-administered diet history questionnaire using multiple diet records. *J. Clin. Epidemiol.* **1990**, *43*, 1327–1335. [CrossRef]

36. Willett, W.C.; Howe, R. Adjustment for total energy intake in epidemiologic studies. *Am. J. Clin. Nutr.* **1997**, *65*, 1220S–1228S. [CrossRef]

37. Patel, R.A.; Wilson, R.F.; Palmer, R.M. The effect of smoking on periodontal bone regeneration: A systematic review and meta-analysis. *J. Periodontol.* **2012**, *83*, 143–155. [CrossRef] [PubMed]

38. Page, R.C.; Eke, P.I. Case definitions for use in population-based surveillance of periodontitis. *J. Periodontol.* **2007**, *78*, 1387–1399. [CrossRef] [PubMed]

39. Tomar, S.L.; Asma, S. Smoking-attributable periodontitis in the United States: Findings from NHANES III. *J. Periodontol.* **2000**, *71*, 743–751. [CrossRef]

40. Yamane, T.; Konno, R.; Iwatsuki, K.; Oishi, Y. Negative Effects of a Low-Quality Protein Diet on Wound Healing via Modulation of the MMP2 activity in rats. *Amino Acids* **2020**, *52*, 505–510. [CrossRef] [PubMed]

41. Collins, C.E.; Kershaw, J.; Brockington, S. Effect of nutritional supplements on wound healing in home-nursed elderly: A randomized trial. *Nutrition* **2005**, *21*, 147–155. [CrossRef] [PubMed]

42. Wolfe, R.R.; Miller, S.L.; Miller, K.B. Optimal protein intake in the elderly. *Clin. Nutr.* **2008**, *27*, 675–684. [CrossRef] [PubMed]

43. Shu, X.O.; Yang, G.; Jin, F.; Liu, D.; Kushi, L.; Wen, W.; Gao, Y.T.; Zheng, W. Validity and reproducibility of the food frequency questionnaire used in the Shanghai Women's Health Study. *Euro. J. Clin. Nutr.* **2004**, *58*, 17–23. [CrossRef]

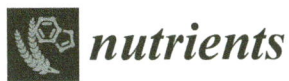

Article

Antimicrobial Effects of *Inula viscosa* Extract on the In Situ Initial Oral Biofilm

Hannah Kurz [1], Lamprini Karygianni [2], Aikaterini Argyropoulou [3], Elmar Hellwig [1], Alexios Leandros Skaltsounis [3], Annette Wittmer [4], Kirstin Vach [5] and Ali Al-Ahmad [1,*]

1   Department of Operative Dentistry and Periodontology, Faculty of Medicine and Medical Center, University of Freiburg, 79085 Freiburg, Germany; hannahkurz@gmx.net (H.K.); elmar.hellwig@uniklinik-freiburg.de (E.H.)
2   Clinic of Conservative and Preventive Dentistry, Center of Dental Medicine, University of Zurich, 8006 Zurich, Switzerland; Lamprini.Karygianni@zzm.uzh.ch
3   Department of Pharmacognosy and Natural Products Chemistry, Faculty of Pharmacy, National and Kapodistrian University of Athens, 157 72 Athens, Greece; katarg@pharm.uoa.gr (A.A.); skaltsounis@pharm.uoa.gr (A.L.S.)
4   Institute of Medical Microbiology and Hygiene, Faculty of Medicine, University of Freiburg, 79085 Freiburg, Germany; annette.wittmer@uniklinik-freiburg.de
5   Institute for Medical Biometry and Statistics, Faculty of Medicine and Medical Center, University of Freiburg, 79085 Freiburg, Germany; kv@imbi.uni-freiburg.de
*   Correspondence: ali.al-ahmad@uniklinik-freiburg.de; Tel.: +49-761-27048940

Citation: Kurz, H.; Karygianni, L.; Argyropoulou, A.; Hellwig, E.; Skaltsounis, A.L.; Wittmer, A.; Vach, K.; Al-Ahmad, A. Antimicrobial Effects of *Inula viscosa* Extract on the In Situ Initial Oral Biofilm. *Nutrients* 2021, *13*, 4029. https://doi.org/10.3390/nu13114029

Academic Editors: LaVerne L. Brown and Maria Luz Fernandez

Received: 8 September 2021
Accepted: 8 November 2021
Published: 11 November 2021

Publisher's Note: MDPI stays neutral with regard to jurisdictional claims in published maps and institutional affiliations.

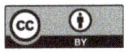
Abstract: Given the undesirable side effects of commercially used mouth rinses that include chemically synthesized antimicrobial compounds such as chlorhexidine, it is essential to discover novel antimicrobial substances based on plant extracts. The aim of this study was to examine the antimicrobial effect of *Inula viscosa* extract on the initial microbial adhesion in the oral cavity. Individual test splints were manufactured for the participants, on which disinfected bovine enamel samples were attached. After the initial microbial adhesion, the biofilm-covered oral samples were removed and treated with different concentrations (10, 20, and 30 mg/mL) of an *I. viscosa* extract for 10 min. Positive and negative controls were also sampled. Regarding the microbiological parameters, the colony-forming units (CFU) and vitality testing (live/dead staining) were examined in combination with fluorescence microscopy. An *I. viscosa* extract with a concentration of 30 mg/mL killed the bacteria of the initial adhesion at a rate of 99.99% ($\log_{10}$ CFU value of 1.837 ± 1.54). Compared to the negative control, no killing effects were determined after treatment with *I. viscosa* extract at concentrations of 10 mg/mL ($\log_{10}$ CFU value 3.776 ± 0.831; median 3.776) and 20 mg/mL ($\log_{10}$ CFU value 3.725 ± 0.300; median 3.711). The live/dead staining revealed a significant reduction ($p < 0.0001$) of vital adherent bacteria after treatment with 10 mg/mL of *I. viscosa* extract. After treatment with an *I. viscosa* extract with a concentration of 30 mg/mL, no vital bacteria could be detected. For the first time, significant antimicrobial effects on the initial microbial adhesion in in situ oral biofilms were reported for an *I. viscosa* extract.

Keywords: *Inula viscosa*; initial adhesion; colony-forming units (CFU); live/dead staining; fluorescence microscopy

1. Introduction

Biofilms consist of microbial cells that are irreversibly attached to a surface or interface and embedded in a matrix of extracellular polymeric substances that are produced by the microorganisms themselves [1]. Furthermore, the microorganisms within a biofilm have altered growth characteristics and gene expression patterns as compared to their planktonic counterparts [1]. The oral cavity is an ideal niche for biofilm formation, which commences with the development of the acquired salivary pellicle (conditioning layer) on which the early colonizers, including oral streptococci, *Actinomyces* spp., and *Veillonella* spp., adhere in an initial phase [2]. After this initial phase, the different microbial species produce a diverse extracellular matrix and multiply to form a thick mature oral biofilm [3,4]. The oral biofilm consists of a plethora of different microbial species, including bacterial species of the genera *Streptococcus, Actinomyces, Fusobacterium, Rothia, Veillonella, Prevotella, Tannerella*, and *Porphyromonas, Neisseria,* and *Gemella* [5–8]. In addition to bacteria, fungi such as members of the Candida, protozoa, and Archaea species have been detected in oral biofilm [8]. As biofilms cause serious infections in different fields of medicine, novel and alternative methods such as the use of natural products are required to prevent biofilm formation [9]. The oral biofilm consists of more than 700 different bacterial species [10,11]. Biofilms are up to 1000 times more resistant to antibiotics compared to equivalent planktonic microorganisms that remain unbound in free suspension [12]. Alterations in the microbial composition in the oral cavity can lead to an increased risk of tooth decay, periodontitis, and periimplantitis [13]. Alternative disinfection methods based on plant extracts recently started receiving increased attention as potential substitutes for known antibacterial agents. Substantial efforts have been made to identify alternative substances to substitute commonly used mouth rinses such as chlorhexidine (CHX) [14]. Although CHX is still regarded as the gold standard in the prevention of plaque formation and the treatment of gingivitis, it causes diverse side effects including CHX-resistance in oral bacteria [15] and reversible taste disorders [16]. Additionally, CHX use results in undesirable effects such as a discoloration of the tongue, composite fillings, and teeth [17,18]. Moreover, due to the increasing number of antibiotic-resistant microorganisms, plant extracts are gaining importance as potent alternatives to circumvent resistance and remove biofilms [19]. Such plant extracts could feature similar antimicrobial and anti-inflammatory behavior to existing treatments but deliver remedial effects more gently, thereby reducing side effects [20]. In 2014, the World Health Organization (WHO) published recommendations in which they emphasized the importance of traditional and alternative phytomedicine for the well-being of mankind and presented a large number of proposals to establish more plant-based medicine and drugs [21]. Since nature yields a large, complex, and mostly unexplored reservoir of phytotherapeutic agents that provide alternatives to common pharmaceuticals for oral antibiosis, it is of crucial importance to find effective antimicrobial mouth rinses based on natural substances [14]. Phytotherapy is used in modern dentistry, mainly for the anti-inflammatory, antibiotic, analgesic, or sedative effects of herbal remedies or as a component of root canal irrigations [22].

To date, several studies have been conducted to examine the effects of natural extracts on different bacterial species in vitro, ex vivo, and in situ [9]. It could be shown that especially *Vitis vinifera, Pinus* spp., *Coffea canephora, Clonorchis sinensis, Vaccinium macrocarpon, Psidium cattleianum,* and Manuka honey have a significant antimicrobial effect on oral biofilms. The antibacterial, antiviral, and antifungal effects of the tested *Inula viscosa* extract have been confirmed in several studies [23–25]. Especially with regard to oral pathogens, the effectiveness of the ethyl acetate extract and the methanol extract of *I. viscosa* against both Gram-negative (*Porphyromonas gingivalis, Prevotella intermedia, Fusobacterium nucleatum*) and Gram-positive (*Staphylococcus aureus, Streptococcus mutans, Streptococcus sobrinus, Streptococcus oralis*) species, and also against the fungus *Candida albicans* in concentrations between 0.15 and 5.00 mg/mL, was shown [14].

The *I. viscosa* plant (*Dittricha viscosa*) belongs to the Asteraceae family and mainly grows in the Mediterranean area [26]. *I. viscosa* shrubs can be found in southern Europe, Turkey, and the Middle East. Due to its adaptive behavior, *I. viscosa* also grows as a neophyte in Great Britain, Belgium, and North America [27]. *I. viscosa* is a stem hemicryptophyte or nanophanerophyte that reaches heights of 40 to 130 cm. The leaves are 6 to 12 mm wide, slim to lancet-like, sticky, and have an unpleasant smell [28]. In a previous study, the effect of *I. viscosa* on selected oral bacterial species was tested in vitro and yielded minimum inhibitory concentrations (MIC) ranging from 0.07 mg/mL (*P. gingivalis*) up to 2.50 mg/mL (*S. sobrinus*), and showed the elimination of obligate anaerobes such as *P. gingivalis* at a minimal bactericidal concentration (MBC) of 0.15 mg/mL [14]. To date, there are no clinical data on the antimicrobial impact of *I. viscosa* on in situ initial oral biofilms. *I. viscosa* has been used for a long time as a herb in folk medicine to treat skin inflammations and diseases such as scabies [29,30]. Different health benefits were reported for the use of *I. viscosa* extract, including its anticancer, antioxidant, antifungal, antibacterial, and hypoglycemic effects [31]. Phytochemical analysis of *I. viscosa* revealed the presence of compounds that have the potential to be used as food additives such as flavonoids, triterpenoids, and sesquiterpenoids [31,32]. Additionally, the application of *I. viscosa* tea yielded a significant reduction of adherent bacteria of the initial in vivo oral biofilm without any negative impact on the acid protective properties of the salivary pellicle [27]. Subsequently, the aforementioned reports on *I. viscosa* show the great potential for this species to be used in maintaining oral health, especially due to the direct contact of its different ingredients with the oral mucosa. Therefore, the antimicrobial effect of *I. viscosa* on the initial adhesion of in situ oral biofilms was investigated in the present study to acquire new knowledge in dental phytotherapy. The aim of the present study was to evaluate if there are any antimicrobial effects of *I. viscosa* extract on the initial oral biofilm and hence to clarify if there is a potential for using this extract for the treatment of dental diseases caused by the oral biofilm.

2. Materials and Methods

All reagents used in the study are depicted in Table S1 (Supplementary Material).

2.1. Selection of Study Participants and Test Specimens

Six healthy volunteers participated in this study and wore appliances that included bovine enamel samples to acquire in situ initial oral biofilm samples. The volunteers were between 23 and 50 years old and had neutral saliva (pH 6.6–7.4) with an average salivary flow rate of 1.49 mL/min. None of the volunteers suffered from carious lesions, insufficient restorations, or periodontal diseases at the time of wearing the specimen. A stable hold of the support rails and sufficient space for the enamel platelets was ensured. The prerequisites for participation in the study included: (i) no use of antibiotics and mouthwashes in the three months prior to wearing the appliance, (ii) no pregnancy or breastfeeding, (iii) no systemic diseases, and in addition, (iv) no oral hygiene was to be carried out in the two hours prior to wearing the appliance, (v) the consumption of food, liquids, alcohol, and nicotine was not permitted while wearing the appliances, and finally, (vi) the subjects had not participated in any other clinical examination up to 30 days before the commencement of the study. The use of chewing gum was also not permitted while the splint was worn. All participants were non-smokers. Since all volunteers remained in the Department for Operative Dentistry and Periodontology while wearing the splint systems, all prerequisites for the sample collection were ensured. The test persons provided written consent prior to participation and the study was approved by the Ethics Committee of the University of Freiburg (no. 91/31).

Bovine front teeth were extracted from caries- and bovine spongiform encephalopathy (BSE)-free cattle. The test specimens were manufactured as described earlier in detail [33] so that the resulting enamel platelets had a constant thickness of 1.5 mm, which corresponded to a total surface area of 19.63 mm^2. The enamel side of the cylinder was ground and polished flat on a hand sanding pad with sandpaper in ascending order of grain size (220–4000 grit), so that no irregularities or facets could be seen under a light microscope (Wild M3Z; Leica GmbH, Wetzlar, Germany) prior to being cleansed.

The disinfection of the bovine enamel platelets took place in different solutions in an ultrasonic bath. First, the produced platelets were exposed to a 3% sodium hypochlorite (NaOCl) solution and ultrasound in plastic cups for three minutes to remove the superficial smear layer. After air drying, the next step was the disinfection with 70% ethanol in an ultrasonic bath for a further three minutes. Finally, the platelets were treated twice for 10 min each in double-distilled water in an ultrasonic bath. Following the disinfection protocol, the enamel samples were stored in distilled water (H_2O) for at least 24 h in order to ensure the formation of a hydration layer [34].

Individual upper-jaw acrylic splints were fabricated for each study participant. The plastic splints were disinfected with 70% ethanol before insertion. The enamel platelets were fixed in the depressions with adhesive wax (Supradent; Oppermann-Schwedler, Bonn, Germany) immediately prior to the start of the timed period, whereby the enamel surface was not covered by adhesive wax and remained untouched. The surfaces of the enamel platelets were at a distance of approximately 1 mm from the buccal surfaces of the posterior teeth. In this position, normal saliva flow and protection against manipulation from the tongue or cheek could be ensured (Figure 1).

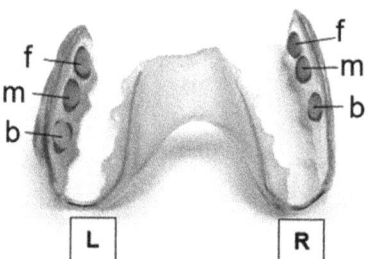

Figure 1. Individual upper-jaw acrylic appliance with the enamel slabs placed in different locations on each side in front (f), in the middle (m), or at the back (b). The samples were positioned on the right (R) and left (L) in the splint. The exposed surfaces were attached to the splint with adhesive wax.

2.2. Extract Preparation

The *I. viscosa* extract was prepared using pressure liquid extraction. A Dionex 300 system (ASE, accelerated solvent extraction) with 100 mL stainless-steel vessels was used. In the following, 20 g of ground *I. viscosa* aerial parts was introduced into the cells. Extraction was carried out under the following conditions: 70 °C, 120 bar, 1 min preheating time, 5 min heating time, two extraction cycles of 5 min each, 100% flush volume, and 120 s cleaning. The final ethyl acetate extract was then produced using a rotary evaporator until it was dried at 40 °C under reduced pressure. The yield was 2.08 g of ethyl acetate extract [19].

2.3. Protocol for Treatment of the Initial Adhesion

Each specimen covered with initial biofilm was assigned a later treatment, with the controls on each side (negative control: 0.9% NaCl, positive control: 0.2% chlorhexidine (CHX), toxicity control: 10% dimethyl sulfoxide (DMSO)), and on the opposite side, the treatments with the extract to be tested. Each volunteer carried an individual upper-jaw acrylic appliance to which six specimens were fixed for two hours. This procedure was performed twice for each subject. After the initial adhesion had been obtained in situ, the appliances were removed from the oral cavity. Sterile tweezers were used to detach the adhesive wax from the samples, which were then rinsed off with sterile 0.9% NaCl for 30 s. The following solutions were prepared in 6 wells in a 24-well plate (μ-Slide 8 Well; Ibidi GmbH, Munich, Germany): 0.9% NaCl, 0.2% CHX, 10% DMSO. The extract to be tested was vortexed in 300 μL of DMSO until it was completely dissolved. This was followed by dilution with phosphate-buffered saline (PBS) so that the corresponding concentrations of the natural substances to be tested were reached. The adherent bacteria on the enamel platelets were treated in the solutions for 10 min.

2.4. Determination of Colony-Forming Units (CFU)

For the quantification of viable bacterial counts, the specimens with the adherent bacteria were transferred to Eppendorf tubes after the 10 min treatments with the *I. viscosa* extract. Each Eppendorf tube contained 500 μL of 0.9% NaCl solution. To desorb the microorganisms, the samples were placed in an ultrasonic bath (Sonorex Digital 10p; Bandelin, Berlin, Germany) for 1 min. The Eppendorf tubes were then carefully vortexed, and the specimens were removed with sterilized dental tweezers. A dilution series was prepared to obtain countable single bacterial colonies. This was carried out by diluting them to 1:5, 1:50, and 1:500 with 0.9% NaCl solution. After further vortexing, 100 μL of the solutions that remained was removed from each tube with a pipette and plated on agar plates. Yeast-cysteine blood agar (HCB) plates were used to cultivate anaerobic bacteria at 7 °C, and Columbia blood agar (CBA) plates were used to enable the growth of aerobic and facultative anaerobic bacteria at 5–10% CO_2 and 37 °C. The CBA plates were incubated for 5 days, whereas the HCB plates were incubated for 10 days using GasPaks (GENbox® Anaer GasPaks; bioMérieux, Marcy l'Etoile, France). At the end of the incubation period, the CFUs were counted for each plate and a CFU mean value was calculated from the identical dilutions and incubation conditions. The number determined was based on the intraorally exposed surface of the samples of 0.196 cm^2 ($\pi \times 2.5^2$ cm^2), taking the respective dilution into account, to calculate the number of CFU per cm^2.

2.5. Live/Dead Staining and Fluorescence Microscopy

For the live/dead staining and fluorescence microscopy (FM) assay, the fluorescent SYTO 9 stain and propidium iodide (PI) (Live/Dead BacLight bacterial viability kit; Life Technologies GmbH, Darmstadt, Germany) were used. The two dyes, SYTO 9 and propidium iodide (PI), were mixed 1:1 and added to the samples [35]. The green fluorescent nucleic acid SYTO 9 penetrates living and dead bacterial cells. When SYTO 9 binds to nucleic acids, the fluorescence signal is amplified, in contrast to unbound SYTO 9. In order to be able to differentiate dead cells, the second dye (PI) is required [36]. This dye only penetrates cells whose membrane is damaged, and there binds to nucleic acids, which appear red under a fluorescence microscope. Components A (SYTO 9, 1.67 mM) and B (PI, 1.67 mM) were mixed 1:1. This mixture was then diluted with 0.9% NaCl solution to achieve a final concentration of 0.1 pM. The enamel samples were subsequently stained in the solution with the intraorally exposed side facing upward at room temperature and in a dark room for 10 min. Any residues were then washed off by swirling the platelets several times in 0.9% saline solution. Afterwards, the specimens were placed with the plaque side down on a drop of 0.9% NaCl solution in an 8-chamber cover disk (μ-Slide 8 Well; ibidi, Munich, Germany) and were analyzed using FM with a 63× oil immersion objective (ApoTome.2, Zeiss, Oberkochen, Germany). For quantification, 10 representative locations on the enamel sample surface were selected, which resulted in 60 images to be evaluated per test person. The respective living or dead bacteria on these were then determined using the image analysis program ZEN 2 pro (Zeiss, Oberkochen, Germany). The data obtained were used to calculate the coverage rates from living and dead bacteria [37]. Representative images were acquired for demonstration of the results.

2.6. Statistical Analysis

For the descriptive analysis of the data, the mean values and standard deviations were calculated and a graphic representation with boxplots was carried out. Diagrams of the viable bacterial counts on the $\log_{10}$ scale per cm^2 ($\log_{10}/cm^2$) were graphically displayed. Linear mixed models with the patient as the random effect were used to analyze treatment differences in bacterial counts, and the Bonferroni method was used to correct for multiple testing. All calculations were carried out with STATA (StataCorp LT, College Station, TX, USA, version 14.1) and the level of significance was $p < 0.05$.

3. Results

3.1. I. viscosa Extract Significantly Decreased the Viable Counts of Oral Microorganisms during Initial Adhesion

Figure 2A,B show the high eradication rates of initially adherent oral aerobic (Figure 2A) and anaerobic (Figure 2B) microorganisms after the treatment with *I. viscosa* extract at a concentration of 30 mg/mL, plus the untreated negative (NaCl) and positive (CHX) controls. The *I. viscosa* extract induced a substantial reduction of more than 99.99% in the viable bacterial count after two hours of initial microbial adhesion in situ. When using *I. viscosa* at a concentration of 30 mg/mL, a $\log_{10}$ CFU value of 1.837 ± 1.54 (median 1.754) was found. Thus, there was a highly significant reduction ($p < 0.0001$) in CFU compared with the negative control and with the enamel platelets treated with DMSO. With regard to the adherent aerobic oral microorganisms (Figure 2A), the untreated control showed a $\log_{10}$ CFU value of 3.299 ± 1.045 (median 3.772). The positive control showed a significant reduction in viable bacteria of more than 99.99% ($\log_{10}$ CFU value of 0 ± 0) after 10 min of treatment with 0.2% CHX. The treatment with DMSO (10%) did not result in any significant change of viable bacterial count compared to the negative control ($\log_{10}$ CFU value 3.796 ± 0.6412; median 3.946). No killing effects were determined after treatment with *I. viscosa* at concentrations of 10 mg/mL ($\log_{10}$ CFU value 3.776 ± 0.8306; median 3.776) and 20 mg/mL ($\log_{10}$ CFU value 3.725 ± 0.2999; median 3.711). Figure 2B shows the $\log_{10}$ counts of adherent anaerobic bacteria on the enamel samples after 10 min of treatment with NaCl, CHX, DMSO, and *I. viscosa* extract (10, 20, and 30 mg/mL). The negative control had a CFU value of $3.226 \pm 1.17 \log_{10}$ (median 3.662). Here, a significant reduction ($p < 0.0001$) of adherent microorganisms during treatment with the positive control ($\log_{10}$ CFU value 0.0383 ± 0.1382; median 0) was also demonstrated.

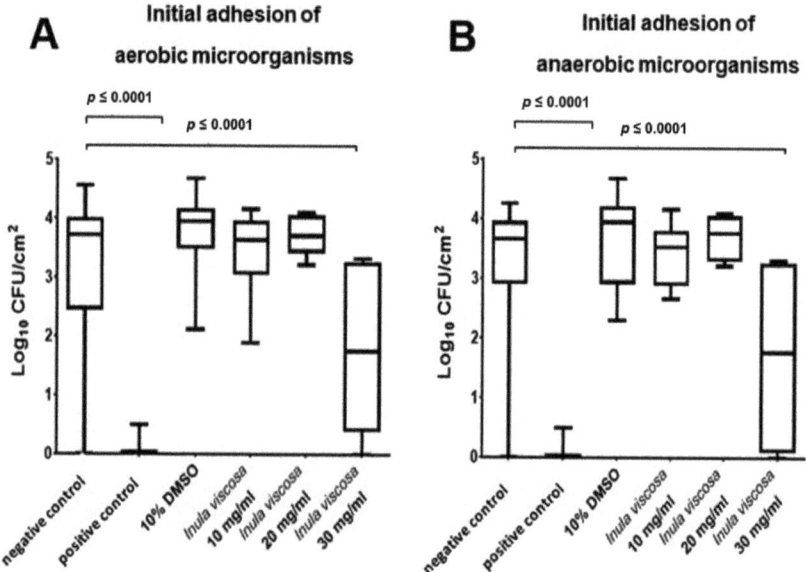

Figure 2. The graphs show the number of CFUs that demonstrate the antimicrobial effect of the tested substances on aerobic (**A**) and anaerobic (**B**) bacteria after an oral exposure time of two hours. An untreated negative control (NaCl 0.9%), a positive control (CHX 0.2%), and a control with DMSO (10%) were also used, as was the natural *I. viscosa* extract (10, 20, and 30 mg/mL) with a 10 min exposure time. The CFU values were shown on a $\log_{10}$ scale per cm^2 ($\log_{10}/\text{cm}^2$). The box shows the area in which the middle 50% of the data lies. The line dividing the box shows the median. The *p*-values of the significantly different data are marked on the graphs.

The toxicity control with DMSO ($\log_{10}$ CFU value 3.7 ± 0.8072; median 3.944) showed no significant change ($p \geq 0.05$) compared to the negative control. Treatment with *I. viscosa* extract at concentrations of 10 mg/mL ($\log_{10}$ CFU value 3.425 ± 0.534; median 3.532) and 20 mg/mL ($\log_{10}$ CFU value 3.706 ± 0.4028; median 3.758) did not yield a significant reduction. However, the anaerobic CFUs decreased significantly ($p < 0.0001$) after treatment with 30 mg/mL of *I. viscosa* extract in comparison to the treatments with NaCl and DMSO. The result was a $\log_{10}$ CFU value of 1.71 ± 1.774 (median 1.768).

3.2. Live/Dead Assays Revealed High Bactericidal Activity for I. viscosa Extract against Oral Initial Adhesion

The quantitative results of the remaining vital bacteria detected by the live/dead assay during initial adhesion two hours after treatment with *I. viscosa* extract in two concentrations (10 and 30 mg/mL) are depicted in Figure 3 in the form of boxplots. In the negative control (Figure 3), 68.93% of the bacteria adhering to the enamel were vital ($\pm$26.89, median 75.0). In the positive control (treatment with 0.2% CHX), the coverage rate of vital bacteria was significantly reduced ($p < 0.0001$) to 16.59% ($\pm$29.05 median 15.8). The toxicity control showed 69.99% vital adherent microorganisms ($\pm$21.3, median 77.52). After treatment with *I. viscosa* extract at a concentration of 10 mg/mL, there was a significant reduction ($p < 0.0001$) compared to the negative and toxicity control, with only 20.87% of the bacteria being vital ($\pm$22.86, median 27.4). In an *I. viscosa* extract concentration of 30 mg/mL, no vital microorganisms could be detected.

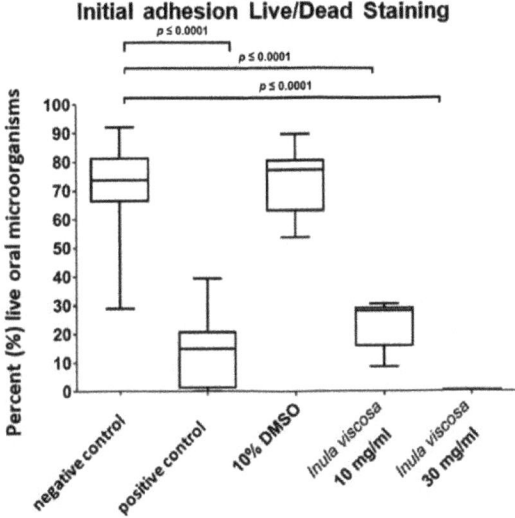

Figure 3. The boxplots represent the percentage of vital oral microorganisms that were evaluated by live/dead staining under the fluorescence microscope (FM). A negative control (NaCl 0.9%), a positive control (CHX 0.2%), a toxicity control (DMSO 10%), and the initial biofilm treated with *I. viscosa* extract at different concentrations (10 and 30 mg/mL) were evaluated. The line dividing the box shows the median. The *p*-values of the significantly different data are marked on the graphs.

Figure 4 shows representative FM images of live/dead-stained initial oral biofilms two hours after the treatment with different concentrations of the *I. viscosa* extract. In the untreated control (Figure 4A) and the control treated with DMSO (Figure 4C), a dense accumulation of viable (green) bacteria was detected on the specimens. Very few cells were avital (red). Most microorganisms exhibited diverse arrangements of single cocci, mono- or multi-stratified chains, and three-dimensional bacterial aggregates varying in size. In contrast to the negative controls, the structure of initial oral biofilms treated with CHX (Figure 4B) and *I. viscosa* extract (Figure 4D,E) was markedly different. In fact, most of the initially adhered bacteria were avital (red), which aligns with the results shown in Figure 3.

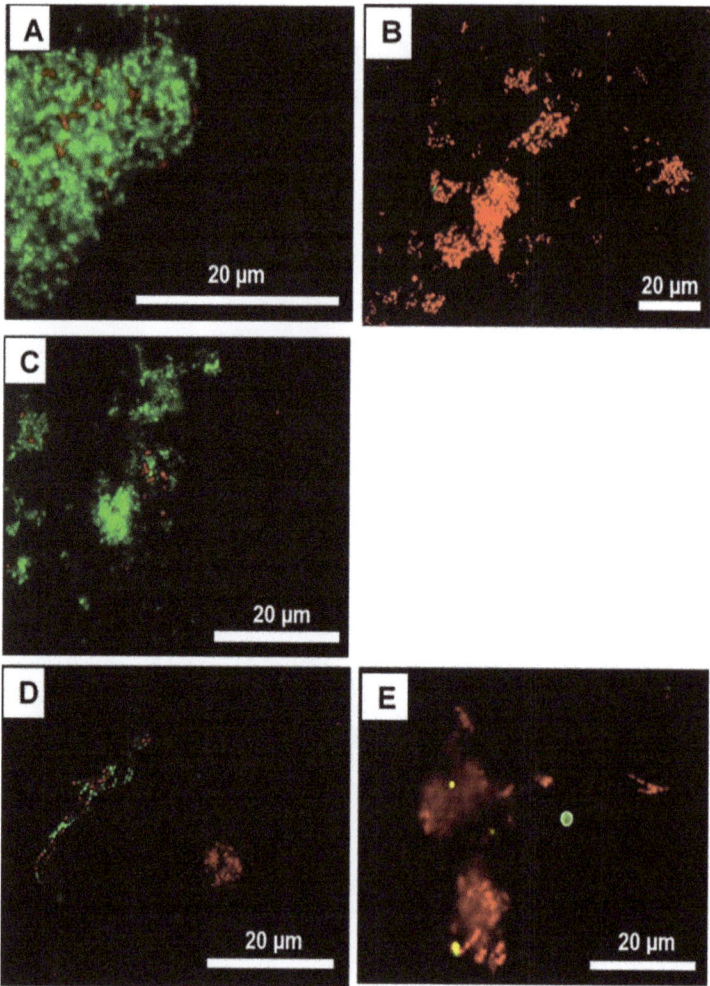

Figure 4. Fluorescence microscopy (FM) images after live/dead staining with BacLight®. The vital bacteria fluoresce in green, the avital in red. The effects on the initial adhesion (2 h) after 10 min of 0.9% NaCl treatment (negative control) (**A**), 0.2% CHX treatment (positive control) (**B**), 10% DMSO treatment (toxicity control) (**C**), as well as after treatment with *I. viscosa* extract in two concentrations: 10 mg/mL (**D**) and 30 mg/mL (**E**), are shown.

4. Discussion

For the first time, the present study established *I. viscosa* extract as a potent agent with an antimicrobial effect on initial oral biofilms in situ.

Enamel samples from BSE-negative cattle were used, as constant quality is assumed for bovine front teeth [38,39]. In addition, bovine enamel is very similar to human enamel in terms of its physico-chemical structure, mineral composition, density, and structure [40,41]. Bovine enamel is also the most similar to human enamel when comparing the enamel of sheep, cattle, and pigs [42]. After successful production, the enamel platelets were treated with various reagents (sodium hypochlorite, ethanol, double-distilled water) in an ultrasonic bath in order to rid the enamel samples of bacteria [43]. The enamel samples were stored in distilled water until they were used, so that a hydration layer could be formed on the clean enamel surface. This is a prerequisite for the in situ pellicle formation without the effect of surface-active substances [44]. The approach used in the present work to obtain an initial biofilm by means of bovine enamel platelets attached to a plastic splint has frequently been used and is described in previous clinical studies [45,46]. The CFU method was used to determine the total adherent number of bacteria on the enamel slabs. Individual or aggregated bacterial cells from a single colony were cultivated. The CFU quantification showed high standard deviations, which can be attributed to the fact that active bacterial communities are heterogeneous, dynamic systems that are influenced by multiple internal and external factors, and in which death and growth processes constantly occur in the framework of homeostasis [47]. Individual differences in the microbial counts among the samples can also lead to high standard deviations. Furthermore, extremely high CFU numbers can lead to errors in quantification, due to overlay or accumulation [48]. The large dispersion could be explained by the fact that biofilm formation is also a dynamic process and includes various cell–cell communications, such as quorum sensing and horizontal gene transfer. The complexity of a structured microbial biofilm affords microorganisms a high resistance against diverse antimicrobials and distinct physical and chemical properties, which enhance the biofilm resilience [3]. The use of a live/dead viability assay not only supplemented the CFU quantification but also enabled visualization of the *I. viscosa*-treated initial oral biofilms. Vital staining with the BacLight® kit using the dyes SYTO 9 and propidium iodide (PI) is a reliable method to differentiate vital from non-vital microorganisms [49]. The examination took place under a fluorescence microscope (FM). In comparison to conventional methods such as light microscopy, FM achieves high optical resolutions. FM is ideal for examining cell physiology, as it is specified for proteins, lipids, or ions in cells [50]. When counting under the FM, 10 different representative grid fields were selected for each melt platelet. Different bacterial agglomerates could be recorded and counted. This confirmed a high intra- and inter-individual variability in the distribution of live/dead bacteria within the biofilm as well as the resulting coverage rates, as already shown in earlier studies [49,51]. The determined coverage rates are therefore just an approximation and only serve as a basic assessment of the relationship between vital and non-vital microorganisms. A major limitation of FM was the fact that natural extracts, namely *I. viscosa*, showed a high level of self-fluorescence. Thus, some areas on the enamel slabs could not be evaluated because of the high levels of self-fluorescence of the extract. However, there were still enough spots to allow for a proper quantification. The total number of vital microorganisms declined significantly after the treatment with *I. viscosa* extract. In the present work, the differences between the vital staining and the CFU can be attributed to the fact that bacterial aggregates are shaken up by the ultrasonic bath and thus falsify the result, as without treatment they might only have formed a single CFU [52].

In a previous report, Karygianni et al. tested the effect of both the ethyl acetate extract and the methanol extract of *I. viscosa* on certain planktonic oral bacterial species [14]. The microbial species were *S. mutans*, *S. sobrinus*, *S. oralis*, *Enterococcus faecalis*, *C. albicans*, *Escherichia coli*, *S. aureus*, *P. gingivalis*, *P. intermedia*, *F. nucleatum*, and *Parvimonas micra*. This study revealed that the minimum inhibitory concentration (MIC) of *P. gingivalis* was 0.07 mg/mL, and *S. sobrinus*, *E. faecalis*, and *E. coli* showed an MIC of up to 2.50 mg/mL. At a minimum bactericidal concentration (MBC) of 0.15 mg/mL, obligate anaerobes such as *P. gingivalis* could be eliminated, whereas *E. faecalis* was more resistant. Taking the above results into account, one could have expected a significant reduction of the initial adherent bacteria at a concentration of 10 mg/mL. However, the concentration had to be increased up to 30 mg/mL to observe a significant effect on the number of CFUs. Our previously reported results on the effects of *I. viscosa* extract on diverse planktonic bacteria provide a strong indication of possible bacteriostatic effects on the initial oral adhesion. The antibacterial effect can mainly be attributed to the polyphenols and the essential oils contained in *I. viscosa*. These oils are flavonoids/aglycones, genkwanin, naringenin, quercetin, camphor, luteolin, and apigenin, whose antimicrobial effects have been proven [53–55]. Particularly apigenin, luteolin, and naringenin show high antibacterial effectiveness against oral streptococci, which make up the largest portion of oral microflora [56–58]. Regarding the antimicrobial effects of the ingredient apigenin, it was shown that it inhibits glycosyltransferases [57], resulting in the production of fewer glucans required for the synthesis of extracellular polymeric substances (EPS), a compound crucial for biofilm formation and microbial resistance [59]. Quercetin has been shown to be able to damage the cell walls of *Bacillus cereus* and *C. albicans* [25]. Furthermore, polyphenols also have an antimicrobial effect on the growth of biofilms by denaturing or obscuring functional groups of the receptor proteins and thus reducing the interaction between different bacterial species. Therefore, a negative effect on biofilm formation could also be achieved with *Cistus* tea, which is rich in polyphenols [60]. Hertel et al. investigated the effect of *I. viscosa* tea on initial oral biofilm formation [27]. The test subjects carried splints with bovine enamel slabs similar to the ones used in the present study and rinsed for 10 min with *I. viscosa* tea, and afterwards the splints remained intraorally for eight hours. It could be shown that the percentage of viable adherent bacteria was affected by the tea. After rinsing with *I. viscosa* tea, the proportion of dead bacteria increased (38% viable: 62% dead). In the present study, the inhibitory effect was even stronger, as *I. viscosa* extract at a concentration of 10 mg/mL led to 21% viable and 79% dead bacteria, whereas 30 mg/mL yielded even better results (0% viable: 100% dead). This discrepancy in outcomes could be attributed to the fact that the boiled *I. viscosa* tea reduced the concentration of the actual effective ingredients to a concentration lower than 10 or 30 mg/mL. The difference between the two studies was that Hertel et al. [27] examined bacterial growth after rinsing with *I. viscosa*, whereas the current study investigated how the extract affected the microbiological composition after bacterial colonization. Our data do not support that an *I. viscosa* extract (10 or 20 mg/mL) can replace common mouthwash solutions such as CHX (0.2%) since the effect is inferior to that produced by 0.2% CHX, which almost always resulted in no viable bacterial species. However, *I. viscosa* extract at a concentration of 30 mg/mL is certainly a bacteriostatic alternative, as the CFU could be significantly reduced at this concentration. A comprehensive testing of a dilution series that includes both lower concentrations and concentrations higher than 30 mg/mL is necessary to identify the optimal inhibitory concentration of the extract and to evaluate a possible higher eradication effect on the initial and mature oral biofilm. Moreover, the reported adverse effects of frequent use of CHX solution in the oral cavity should be taken into consideration in the comparison to mouthwashes based on natural products [17,18]. Even if it seems generally accepted that natural products are safe and devoid of side effects, natural products can also have toxic properties, react with other drugs, and cause severe side effects [61]. They can also cause allergies, for example contact dermatitis after the use of *Magnolia officinalis* and *Allium sativum* [62]. *Verbena officinalis* can also cause gastrointestinal dysfunction and heartburn [63,64]. Therefore, interactions with other drugs should always be monitored and adequately tested. The identification of single active components of the tested extract and an analysis of their antimicrobial activity should also be conducted in future studies since the concentration of such ingredients can depend on the geographical location the plant was harvested in. Additionally, there are some indications in the literature that *I. viscosa* extract inhibits cancer cells at concentrations of 150 or 300 mg/kg in mice experiments [65]. Hence, the toxicity of the *I. viscosa* extract used towards human oral mucosal cells should be examined in future studies. In a comprehensive phythochemical analysis, Mahmoudi et al. [66] reported that *I. viscosa* leaves are rich in the unsaturated essential fatty acids (UFAs) α-linolenic (C18:3) and linoleic (C18:2) acid. The authors recommended the use of *I. viscosa* as a safe source of such essential UFAs and hence as a beneficial supplement to the human diet. Furthermore, in the total leaf lipid fraction of *I. viscosa*, the authors found a ω-3/ω-6 ratio of 4.42, which is similar to the intake values (5) recommended by nutritionists. Additionally, a high total phenol content (TPH) and total flavonoid content (TFC) were determined in *I. viscosa* leaves [66]. Considering the reduction of both azino-bis(ethylbenzothiazoline 6-sulfonic acid) and 2, 2-diphenyl-1-picrylhydrazyl, the high antioxidant effect of these contents that was shown by the authors again indicates a possible use of certain compounds from the *I. viscosa* extract as a food supplement [66]. In general, the phenolic compounds identified in *I. viscosa* comprised caffeic acid-O-hexoside, p-coumaric acid, chlorogenic acid, 1,3-O-dicaffeoylquinic acid, taxifolin hexoside, hydroxybenzoic acid hexoside, isorhamnetin-O-hexoside, 3,4-dicaffeoylquinic acid, 3,5-dicaffeoylquinic acid, 4,5-dicaffeoylquinic acid, coumaroyl caffeoylquinic acid, dimers of caffeic acid-O-hexoside, luteolin, isorhamnetin-3-O-(6-O-feruloyl)-glucoside, isorhamnetin, acetyl taxifolin, and an unknown dihydroflavonol [66]. Many of these compounds contribute to the antioxidant and antifungal activity reported for *I. viscosa* extract [29]. Considering the aforementioned detailed composition of *I. viscosa* leaves, *I. viscosa* could be used as a source of bioactive components such as phenolic compounds and volatile oils. Additionally, its antioxidant, antibacterial, and antifungal properties indicate its potential use for the development of natural preservatives with applications in agro-food.

5. Conclusions

In conclusion, the growing relevance and importance of phytotherapy for providing novel treatments in the field of dental research can be clearly shown. Many natural extracts have the potential to feature extensive medicinal efficacy and could therefore supplement, or even completely replace, chemically produced drugs in the long term. However, further clinical studies must be carried out to be able to comprehensively demonstrate the interactions of the natural extracts within the human body and with other pharmaceuticals. Additionally, clinical studies are required to evaluate such a mouthwash product and to compare it with standard mouth rinses based on CHX or cetylpyridinium chloride (CPC). On the other hand, the properties of the natural extracts such as their consistency, solubility, and interactions with surfaces must be investigated in order to be able to guarantee a user-friendly, durable, and stable application as a common mouthwash solution. The antioxidant, antibacterial, and antifungal activities of *I. viscosa* extract indicate its potential use for the development of natural preservatives with applications in agro-food.

Supplementary Materials: The following are available online at https://www.mdpi.com/article/10.3390/nu13114029/s1, Table S1: Overview of the reagents used, including their brands and the countries where they were purchased.

Author Contributions: H.K.: drafted and critically revised the manuscript, methodology, data analysis, and interpretation; A.A.: methodology; L.K., E.H., A.L.S. and A.A.-A.: conception and design of the study, supervision, and critically revised the manuscript; A.W.: methodology; K.V.: statistical analysis of the data. All authors have read and agreed to the published version of the manuscript.

Funding: This study was supported in part by the German Research Foundation (DFG; Grant AL 1179/4-1).

Institutional Review Board Statement: The study was conducted according to the guidelines of the declaration of Helsinki, and approved by the Ethics Committee of the University of Freiburg (No. 91/31). All experiments and data collections were performed in accordance with relevant guidelines and regulations.

Informed Consent Statement: Written informed consent was obtained from all participants involved in the study.

Data Availability Statement: The data are available upon request from the authors.

Acknowledgments: Bettina Spitzmüller is acknowledged for skillful technical laboratory assistance during the live/dead assay.

Conflicts of Interest: The authors declare no conflict of interest. The funders had no role in the design of the study; in the collection, analyses, or interpretation of data; in the writing of the manuscript, or in the decision to publish the results.

References

1. Donlan, R.M.; Costerton, J.W. Biofilms: Survival mechanisms of clinically relevant microorganisms. *Clin. Microbiol. Rev.* **2002**, *15*, 167–193. [CrossRef]
2. Hannig, C.; Hannig, M. The oral cavity—A key system to understand substratum-dependent bioadhesion on solid surfaces in man. *Clin. Oral Investig.* **2009**, *13*, 123–139. [CrossRef] [PubMed]
3. Kolenbrander, P.E.; Palmer, R.J.; Periasamy, S.; Jakubovics, N.S. Oral multispecies biofilm development and the key role of cell-cell distance. *Nat. Rev. Microbiol.* **2010**, *8*, 471–480. [CrossRef] [PubMed]
4. Cugini, C.; Shanmugam, M.; Landge, N.; Ramasubbu, N. The Role of Exopolysaccharides in Oral Biofilms. *J. Dent. Res.* **2019**, *98*, 739–745. [CrossRef] [PubMed]
5. Dewhirst, F.E.; Chen, T.; Izard, J.; Paster, B.J.; Tanner, A.C.R.; Yu, W.-H.; Lakshmanan, A.; Wade, W.G. The human oral microbiome. *J. Bacteriol.* **2010**, *192*, 5002–5017. [CrossRef] [PubMed]
6. Griffen, A.L.; Beall, C.J.; Campbell, J.H.; Firestone, N.D.; Kumar, P.S.; Yang, Z.K.; Podar, M.; Leys, E.J. Distinct and complex bacterial profiles in human periodontitis and health revealed by 16S pyrosequencing. *ISME J.* **2012**, *6*, 1176–1185. [CrossRef] [PubMed]
7. Mark Welch, J.L.; Rossetti, B.J.; Rieken, C.W.; Dewhirst, F.E.; Borisy, G.G. Biogeography of a human oral microbiome at the micron scale. *Proc. Natl. Acad. Sci. USA* **2016**, *113*, E791–E800. [CrossRef] [PubMed]
8. Marsh, P.D.; Zaura, E. Dental biofilm: Ecological interactions in health and disease. *J. Clin. Periodontol.* **2017**, *44* (Suppl. 18), S12–S22. [CrossRef]
9. Karygianni, L.; Al-Ahmad, A.; Argyropoulou, A.; Hellwig, E.; Anderson, A.C.; Skaltsounis, A.L. Natural Antimicrobials and Oral Microorganisms: A Systematic Review on Herbal Interventions for the Eradication of Multispecies Oral Biofilms. *Front. Microbiol.* **2015**, *6*, 1529. [CrossRef]
10. Whittaker, C.J.; Klier, C.M.; Kolenbrander, P.E. Mechanisms of adhesion by oral bacteria. *Annu. Rev. Microbiol.* **1996**, *50*, 513–552. [CrossRef]
11. Saini, R.; Saini, S.; Sharma, S. Biofilm: A dental microbial infection. *J. Nat. Sci. Biol. Med.* **2011**, *2*, 71–75. [CrossRef] [PubMed]
12. Davies, D. Understanding biofilm resistance to antibacterial agents. *Nat. Rev. Drug Discov.* **2003**, *2*, 114–122. [CrossRef] [PubMed]
13. Åberg, C.H.; Kelk, P.; Johansson, A. Aggregatibacter actinomycetemcomitans: Virulence of its leukotoxin and association with aggressive periodontitis. *Virulence* **2015**, *6*, 188–195. [CrossRef] [PubMed]
14. Karygianni, L.; Cecere, M.; Skaltsounis, A.L.; Argyropoulou, A.; Hellwig, E.; Aligiannis, N.; Wittmer, A.; Al-Ahmad, A. High-level antimicrobial efficacy of representative Mediterranean natural plant extracts against oral microorganisms. *Biomed. Res. Int.* **2014**, *2014*, 839019. [CrossRef] [PubMed]
15. Kampf, G. Acquired resistance to chlorhexidine—Is it time to establish an 'antiseptic stewardship' initiative? *J. Hosp. Infect.* **2016**, *94*, 213–227. [CrossRef] [PubMed]
16. Gent, J.F.; Frank, M.E.; Hettinger, T.P. Taste confusions following chlorhexidine treatment. *Chem. Senses* **2002**, *27*, 73–80. [CrossRef]
17. Eley, B.M. Antibacterial agents in the control of supragingival plaque—A review. *Br. Dent. J.* **1999**, *186*, 286–296. [CrossRef]
18. Cieplik, F.; Jakubovics, N.S.; Buchalla, W.; Maisch, T.; Hellwig, E.; Al-Ahmad, A. Resistance Toward Chlorhexidine in Oral Bacteria—Is There Cause for Concern? *Front. Microbiol.* **2019**, *10*, 587. [CrossRef]
19. Karygianni, L.; Ruf, S.; Follo, M.; Hellwig, E.; Bucher, M.; Anderson, A.C.; Vach, K.; Al-Ahmad, A. Novel Broad-Spectrum Antimicrobial Photoinactivation of In Situ Oral Biofilms by Visible Light plus Water-Filtered Infrared A. *Appl. Environ. Microbiol.* **2014**, *80*, 7324–7336. [CrossRef]
20. Cai, H.; Chen, J.; Panagodage Perera, N.K.; Liang, X. Effects of Herbal Mouthwashes on Plaque and Inflammation Control for Patients with Gingivitis: A Systematic Review and Meta-Analysis of Randomised Controlled Trials. *Evid. Based Complement. Alternat. Med.* **2020**, *2020*, 2829854. [CrossRef]
21. World Health Organization. *WHO Traditional Medicine Strategy 2014–2023*; WHO: Geneva, Switzerland, 2013.
22. Groppo, F.C.; Bergamaschi, C.d.C.; Cogo, K.; Franz-Montan, M.; Motta, R.H.L.; de Andrade, E.D. Use of phytotherapy in dentistry. *Phytother. Res.* **2008**, *22*, 993–998. [CrossRef]
23. Maoz, M.; Neeman, I. Effect of *Inula viscosa* extract on chitin synthesis in dermatophytes and *Candida albicans*. *J. Ethnopharmacol.* **2000**, *71*, 479–482. [CrossRef]
24. Gökbulut, A.; Ozhan, O.; Satilmiş, B.; Batçioğlu, K.; Günal, S.; Sarer, E. Antioxidant and antimicrobial activities, and phenolic compounds of selected Inula species from Turkey. *Nat. Prod. Commun.* **2013**, *8*, 475–478. [CrossRef] [PubMed]
25. Talib, W.H.; Zarga, M.H.A.; Mahasneh, A.M. Antiproliferative, antimicrobial and apoptosis inducing effects of compounds isolated from Inula viscosa. *Molecules* **2012**, *17*, 3291–3303. [CrossRef] [PubMed]
26. Omezzine, F. In vitro assessment of Inula spp. organic extracts for their antifungal activity against some pathogenic and antagonistic fungi. *Afr. J. Microbiol. Res.* **2011**, *5*, 3527–3531. [CrossRef]
27. Hertel, S.; Graffy, L.; Pötschke, S.; Basche, S.; Al-Ahmad, A.; Hoth-Hannig, W.; Hannig, M.; Hannig, C. Effect of Inula viscosa on the pellicle's protective properties and initial bioadhesion in-situ. *Arch. Oral Biol.* **2016**, *71*, 87–96. [CrossRef]
28. Jahn, R.; Schönfelder, P. *Exkursionsflora für Kreta*; Ulmer: Stuttgart, Germany, 1995; ISBN 3800134780.
29. Danino, O.; Gottlieb, H.E.; Grossman, S.; Bergman, M. Antioxidant activity of 1,3-dicaffeoylquinic acid isolated from Inula viscosa. *Food Res. Int.* **2009**, *42*, 1273–1280. [CrossRef]

30. Hernández, V.; Recio, M.C.; Máñez, S.; Giner, R.M.; Ríos, J.-L. Effects of naturally occurring dihydroflavonols from Inula viscosa on inflammation and enzymes involved in the arachidonic acid metabolism. *Life Sci.* **2007**, *81*, 480–488. [CrossRef]
31. Andolfi, A.; Zermane, N.; Cimmino, A.; Avolio, F.; Boari, A.; Vurro, M.; Evidente, A. Inuloxins A-D, phytotoxic bi-and tri-cyclic sesquiterpene lactones produced by Inula viscosa: Potential for broomrapes and field dodder management. *Phytochemistry* **2013**, *86*, 112–120. [CrossRef]
32. Máñez, S.; Hernández, V.; Giner, R.-M.; Ríos, J.-L.; Recio, M.D.C. Inhibition of pro-inflammatory enzymes by inuviscolide, a sesquiterpene lactone from Inula viscosa. *Fitoterapia* **2007**, *78*, 329–331. [CrossRef]
33. Karygianni, L.; Follo, M.; Hellwig, E.; Burghardt, D.; Wolkewitz, M.; Anderson, A.; Al-Ahmad, A. Microscope-based imaging platform for large-scale analysis of oral biofilms. *Appl. Environ. Microbiol.* **2012**, *78*, 8703–8711. [CrossRef]
34. Jung, D.J.; Al-Ahmad, A.; Follo, M.; Spitzmüller, B.; Hoth-Hannig, W.; Hannig, M.; Hannig, C. Visualization of initial bacterial colonization on dentine and enamel in situ. *J. Microbiol. Methods* **2010**, *81*, 166–174. [CrossRef]
35. Hannig, C.; Follo, M.; Hellwig, E.; Al-Ahmad, A. Visualization of adherent micro-organisms using different techniques. *J. Med. Microbiol.* **2010**, *59*, 1–7. [CrossRef]
36. Stiefel, P.; Schmidt-Emrich, S.; Maniura-Weber, K.; Ren, Q. Critical aspects of using bacterial cell viability assays with the fluorophores SYTO9 and propidium iodide. *BMC Microbiol.* **2015**, *15*, 36. [CrossRef] [PubMed]
37. Hannig, C.; Basche, S.; Burghardt, T.; Al-Ahmad, A.; Hannig, M. Influence of a mouthwash containing hydroxyapatite microclusters on bacterial adherence in situ. *Clin. Oral Investig.* **2013**, *17*, 805–814. [CrossRef] [PubMed]
38. Al-Ahmad, A.; Müller, N.; Wiedmann-Al-Ahmad, M.; Sava, I.; Hübner, J.; Follo, M.; Schirrmeister, J.; Hellwig, E. Endodontic and salivary isolates of Enterococcus faecalis integrate into biofilm from human salivary bacteria cultivated in vitro. *J. Endod.* **2009**, *35*, 986–991. [CrossRef]
39. Al-Ahmad, A.; Follo, M.; Selzer, A.-C.; Hellwig, E.; Hannig, M.; Hannig, C. Bacterial colonization of enamel in situ investigated using fluorescence in situ hybridization. *J. Med. Microbiol.* **2009**, *58*, 1359–1366. [CrossRef] [PubMed]
40. Davidson, C.L.; Boom, G.; Arends, J. Calcium distribution in human and bovine surface enamel. *Caries Res.* **1973**, *7*, 349–359. [CrossRef]
41. Nakamichi, I.; Iwaku, M.; Fusayama, T. Bovine teeth as possible substitutes in the adhesion test. *J. Dent. Res.* **1983**, *62*, 1076–1081. [CrossRef]
42. Teruel, J.d.D.; Alcolea, A.; Hernández, A.; Ruiz, A.J.O. Comparison of chemical composition of enamel and dentine in human, bovine, porcine and ovine teeth. *Arch. Oral Biol.* **2015**, *60*, 768–775. [CrossRef]
43. Hannig, C.; Hannig, M.; Rehmer, O.; Braun, G.; Hellwig, E.; Al-Ahmad, A. Fluorescence microscopic visualization and quantification of initial bacterial colonization on enamel in situ. *Arch. Oral Biol.* **2007**, *52*, 1048–1056. [CrossRef]
44. Hannig, M.; Joiner, A. The structure, function and properties of the acquired pellicle. *Monogr. Oral Sci.* **2006**, *19*, 29–64. [CrossRef] [PubMed]
45. Al-Ahmad, A.; Wiedmann-Al-Ahmad, M.; Fackler, A.; Follo, M.; Hellwig, E.; Bächle, M.; Hannig, C.; Han, J.-S.; Wolkewitz, M.; Kohal, R. In vivo study of the initial bacterial adhesion on different implant materials. *Arch. Oral Biol.* **2013**, *58*, 1139–1147. [CrossRef] [PubMed]
46. Hannig, C.; Spitzmüller, B.; Lux, H.C.; Altenburger, M.; Al-Ahmad, A.; Hannig, M. Efficacy of enzymatic toothpastes for immobilisation of protective enzymes in the in situ pellicle. *Arch. Oral Biol.* **2010**, *55*, 463–469. [CrossRef] [PubMed]
47. Sutherland, I. The biofilm matrix—An immobilized but dynamic microbial environment. *Trends Microbiol.* **2001**, *9*, 222–227. [CrossRef]
48. Amann, R.I.; Ludwig, W.; Schleifer, K.H. Phylogenetic identification and in situ detection of individual microbial cells without cultivation. *Microbiol. Rev.* **1995**, *59*, 143–169. [CrossRef]
49. Tawakoli, P.N.; Al-Ahmad, A.; Hoth-Hannig, W.; Hannig, M.; Hannig, C. Comparison of different live/dead stainings for detection and quantification of adherent microorganisms in the initial oral biofilm. *Clin. Oral Investig.* **2013**, *17*, 841–850. [CrossRef] [PubMed]
50. Giepmans, B.N.G.; Adams, S.R.; Ellisman, M.H.; Tsien, R.Y. The fluorescent toolbox for assessing protein location and function. *Science* **2006**, *312*, 217–224. [CrossRef] [PubMed]
51. Hannig, C.; Attin, T.; Hannig, M.; Henze, E.; Brinkmann, K.; Zech, R. Immobilisation and activity of human alpha-amylase in the acquired enamel pellicle. *Arch. Oral Biol.* **2004**, *49*, 469–475. [CrossRef]
52. Al-Ahmad, A.; Wiedmann-Al-Ahmad, M.; Auschill, T.M.; Follo, M.; Braun, G.; Hellwig, E.; Arweiler, N.B. Effects of commonly used food preservatives on biofilm formation of Streptococcus mutans in vitro. *Arch. Oral Biol.* **2008**, *53*, 765–772. [CrossRef]
53. Grande, M.; Piera, F.; Cuenca, A.; Torres, P.; Bellido, I.S. Flavonoids from *Inula viscosa*. *Planta Med.* **1985**, *51*, 414–419. [CrossRef] [PubMed]
54. Wollenweber, E.; Mayer, K.; Roitman, J.N. Exudate flavonoids of *Inula viscosa*. *Phytochemistry* **1991**, *30*, 2445–2446. [CrossRef]
55. Cushnie, T.P.T.; Lamb, A.J. Antimicrobial activity of flavonoids. *Int. J. Antimicrob. Agents* **2005**, *26*, 343–356. [CrossRef] [PubMed]
56. Osawa, K.; Yasuda, H.; Maruyama, T.; Morita, H.; Takeya, K.; Itokawa, H. Isoflavanones from the heartwood of *Swartzia polyphylla* and their antibacterial activity against cariogenic bacteria. *Chem. Pharm. Bull.* **1992**, *40*, 2970–2974. [CrossRef]
57. Koo, H.; Schobel, B.; Scott-Anne, K.; Watson, G.; Bowen, W.H.; Cury, J.A.; Rosalen, P.L.; Park, Y.K. Apigenin and tt-farnesol with fluoride effects on S. mutans biofilms and dental caries. *J. Dent. Res.* **2005**, *84*, 1016–1020. [CrossRef]
58. Petti, S.; Scully, C. Polyphenols, oral health and disease: A review. *J. Dent.* **2009**, *37*, 413–423. [CrossRef]

59. Fulaz, S.; Vitale, S.; Quinn, L.; Casey, E. Nanoparticle-Biofilm Interactions: The Role of the EPS Matrix. *Trends Microbiol.* **2019**, *27*, 915–926. [CrossRef]
60. Hannig, C.; Spitzmüller, B.; Al-Ahmad, A.; Hannig, M. Effects of Cistus-tea on bacterial colonization and enzyme activities of the in situ pellicle. *J. Dent.* **2008**, *36*, 540–545. [CrossRef]
61. Little, J.W. Complementary and alternative medicine: Impact on dentistry. *Oral Surg. Oral Med. Oral Pathol. Oral Radiol. Endod.* **2004**, *98*, 137–145. [CrossRef]
62. West, I.; Maibach, H.I. Contact urticaria syndrome from multiple cosmetic components. *Contact Dermat.* **1995**, *32*, 121. [CrossRef]
63. Hadley, S.; Petry, J.J. Valerian. *Am. Fam. Phys.* **2003**, *67*, 1755–1758. [PubMed]
64. Huntley, A.L.; Thompson Coon, J.; Ernst, E. The safety of herbal medicinal products derived from Echinacea species: A systematic review. *Drug Saf.* **2005**, *28*, 387–400. [CrossRef] [PubMed]
65. Bar-Shalom, R.; Bergman, M.; Grossman, S.; Azzam, N.; Sharvit, L.; Fares, F. Inula Viscosa Extract Inhibits Growth of Colorectal Cancer Cells in vitro and in vivo Through Induction of Apoptosis. *Front. Oncol.* **2019**, *9*, 227. [CrossRef]
66. Mahmoudi, H.; Hosni, K.; Zaouali, W.; Amri, I.; Zargouni, H.; Hamida, N.B.; Kaddour, R.; Hamrouni, L.; Nasri, M.B.; Ouerghi, Z. Comprehensive Phytochemical Analysis, Antioxidant and Antifungal Activities of Inula viscosa Aiton Leaves. *J. Food Saf.* **2016**, *36*, 77–88. [CrossRef]

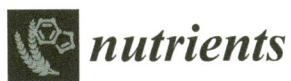

nutrients

MDPI

Article

Association between Dietary Pattern and Periodontitis—A Cross-Sectional Study

Ersin Altun [1,†], Carolin Walther [1,*,†], Katrin Borof [1], Elina Petersen [2,3], Berit Lieske [1], Dimitros Kasapoudis [1], Navid Jalilvand [1], Thomas Beikler [1], Bettina Jagemann [4], Birgit-Christiane Zyriax [4,‡] and Ghazal Aarabi [1,‡]

[1]   Department of Periodontics, Preventive and Restorative Dentistry, University Medical Centre Hamburg-Eppendorf, 20246 Hamburg, Germany; ersin.altun@live.de (E.A.); k.borof@uke.de (K.B.); b.lieske@uke.de (B.L.); d.kasapoudis@outlook.com (D.K.); n.jalilvand@uke.de (N.J.); t.beikler@uke.de (T.B.); g.aarabi@uke.de (G.A.)

[2]   Department of Cardiology, University Heart and Vascular Center, 20246 Hamburg, Germany; e.petersen@uke.de

[3]   Population Health Research Department, University Heart and Vascular Center, 20246 Hamburg, Germany

[4]   Midwifery Science—Health Services Research and Prevention, Institute for Health Services Research in Dermatology and Nursing (IVDP), University Medical Center Hamburg-Eppendorf (UKE), 20246 Hamburg, Germany; b.jagemann@uke.de (B.J.); b.zyriax@uke.de (B.-C.Z.)

*   Correspondence: c.walther@uke.de; Tel.: +49-40-7410-52284

†   These authors contributed equally to this work.

‡   These authors contributed equally to this work.

Citation: Altun, E.; Walther, C.; Borof, K.; Petersen, E.; Lieske, B.; Kasapoudis, D.; Jalilvand, N.; Beikler, T.; Jagemann, B.; Zyriax, B.-C.; et al. Association between Dietary Pattern and Periodontitis—A Cross-Sectional Study. *Nutrients* **2021**, *13*, 4167. https://doi.org/10.3390/nu13114167

Academic Editors: Kirstin Vach and Johan Peter Woelber

Received: 27 October 2021
Accepted: 19 November 2021
Published: 21 November 2021

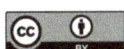
Abstract: The aim of the study was to investigate the relationship between specific known dietary patterns and the prevalence of periodontal disease in a northern population-based cohort study. We evaluated data from 6209 participants of the Hamburg City Health Study (HCHS). The HCHS is a prospective cohort study and is registered at ClinicalTrial.gov (NCT03934957). Dietary intake was assessed with the food frequency questionnaire (FFQ2). Periodontal examination included probing depth, gingival recession, plaque index, and bleeding on probing. Descriptive analyses were stratified by periodontitis severity. Ordinal logistic regression models were used to determine the association. Ordinal regression analyses revealed a significant association between higher adherence to the DASH diet/Mediterranean diet and lower odds to be affected by periodontal diseases in an unadjusted model (OR: 0.92; 95% CI: 0.87, 0.97; $p < 0.001$/OR: 0.93; 95% CI: 0.91, 0.96; $p < 0.001$) and an adjusted model (age, sex, diabetes) (OR: 0.94; 95% CI: 0.89, 1.00; $p < 0.0365$/OR: 0.97; 95% CI: 0.94, 1.00; $p < 0.0359$). The current cross-sectional study identified a significant association between higher adherence to the DASH and Mediterranean diets and lower odds to be affected by periodontal diseases (irrespective of disease severity). Future randomized controlled trials are needed to evaluate to which extent macro- and micronutrition can affect periodontitis initiation/progression.

Keywords: dietary patterns; nutrition; oral health; periodontal disease; clinical attachment loss; DMFT

1. Introduction

According to the Fifth German Oral Health Survey, periodontitis affects up to 11.5 million people in Germany [1] and is one of the main reasons for tooth loss [2]. A primary risk factor for periodontitis is the accumulation of intraoral dysbiotic microflora at the tooth surface [3]. The host immune system responds to the bacterial colonization via destruction/degradation of the periodontal ligament and the surrounding bone structure [4]. Additionally, the host immune system is modulated by genetic, environmental, and behavioral factors [5].

It has been demonstrated that the reduction of oxidative stress in combination with an increased intake of antioxidants through diet has beneficial effects on gingival and periodontal inflammation due to the modulation of host immune responses [6,7]. A clinical controlled trial with 15 participants demonstrated that fewer carbohydrates, more omega-3 fatty acids, and more vitamins C and D, antioxidants, and fiber in the diet significantly reduce periodontal inflammatory parameters [8]. Higher levels of fiber and lower levels of fat in the diet improve markers of periodontitis in high-risk subjects [9].

The Dietary Approach to Stop Hypertension (DASH) and the Mediterranean diet consider these aspects. The Mediterranean diet refers to a traditional diet rich in plant-based foods, fish, and olive oil from the Mediterranean region. It is based on a low consumption of red meat and processed foods [10]. A high consumption of polyphenols through olive oil can increase the health benefits of the Mediterranean diet [11,12]. The DASH diet aims to control the blood pressure with a plant-based diet [13]. A Key aspect of this diet is a high intake of plant-based foods, low-fat dairy products, fish, and whole grains. Sodium, red meat, and processed foods should be reduced [14].

In 2013, those dietary approaches were initially recommended to prevent heart disease and stroke [15], as it was already well known that dietary habits influence the onset/progression of, e.g., coronary heart disease (CHD) and type 2 diabetes [16]. Unsaturated fatty acids, particularly polyunsaturated fatty acids (PUFA), and/or high-quality carbohydrates from whole grains, have been associated with a lower risk of CHD. In fact, high adherence to the Mediterranean diet or the DASH diet seems to have preventive effects against stroke and CHD [17,18].

Only a few studies investigated the effect of distinct dietary patterns on oral inflammation in large epidemiological settings [19–22] and, to the best of our knowledge, only one study specifically considered the DASH or the Mediterranean diet [23].

Consequently, the aim of the current cross-sectional study was to investigate the relationship between specific known dietary patterns (DASH and Mediterranean Diet) and the prevalence of periodontal disease in a northern population-based cohort study.

2. Materials and Methods

2.1. Subjects, Study Design, and Setting

In total, 6209 participants of the Hamburg City Health Study (HCHS) fitted the required inclusion criteria and were selected for analysis. The HCHS is a prospective cohort study conducted at the University Medical Center Hamburg-Eppendorf, with the aim to gain substantial knowledge on major chronic disease initiation and development [24]. Prior general and oral examination, all participants answered a questionnaire regarding their environmental conditions and lifestyle (e.g., physical condition and activity, dietary habits). The HCHS has been registered at ClinicalTrial.gov (NCT03934957). The Landesärztekammer Hamburg (State of Hamburg Chamber of Medical Practitioners, PV5131) approved the study protocol, and all participants signed an informed consent. The manuscript was written according to the STROBE Guidelines [25].

2.2. Sample Size Calculation

The periodontal cohort consisted of 1453 participants with none/mild periodontitis and 1176 participants with severe periodontitis. For the estimation of detectable effects due to healthy dietary patterns, we compared a change in the dietary score corresponding to the interquartile range [22], i.e., the half of the participants with "worse" dietary scores to the half with the "best" dietary scores. With a binomial response (mild/none vs. severe) and a significance level of 5%, we found that the study detected an effect of OR = 1.25 with 80% power. This effect is considered realistic and clinically relevant.

2.3. Assessment of Dietary Patterns

Initially developed for the European Prospective Investigation into Cancer and Nutrition (EPIC) study, the corresponding validated questionnaires were used to collect information on dietary intake [26]. The current version of the food frequency questionnaire (FFQ2) records the portion size and frequency of 102 food items eaten within the previous year [27]. Subsequently, energy intake, relevant food groups, and nutrients were assessed.

2.4. DASH Adherence Score

The scoring scheme adapted from Folsom et al. was used to determine adherence to the DASH diet [28]. Ten equally weighted food items (frequency consumption of fruits, dairy, grains, vegetables, nuts/seeds/legumes, meat/poultry/fish, and sweets obtained from raw data) and average daily nutrients intake (e.g., saturated fat, fat, sodium) were included. The DASH adherence score could be assessed for 9020 participants. For each dietary component, a score of 0–1 was given and summed across the 10 items [29] (Table 1; score of 10 = full adherence, score of 0 = nonadherence). A score from 0 to 3.5 was classified as low adherence, from 4 to 6.5 as medium adherence, and from 7 to 10 as high adherence.

Table 1. Scoring criteria for DASH Dietary Adherence according to Epstein et al. [29].

Score Items	DASH-Component	Scoring
	Total Grain	
1	≥7 servings/day	1
	5–6 servings/day	0.5
	<5 servings/day	0
	Vegetables	
2	≥4 servings/day	1
	2–3 servings/day	0.5
	<2 servings/day	0
	Fruits	
3	≥4 servings/day	1
	2–3 servings/day	0.5
	<2 servings/day	0
	Total dairy	
4	≥2 servings/day	1
	1 servings/day	0.5
	<1 serving/day	0
	Meat, poultry, and fish	
5	≤2 servings/day	1
	3 servings/day	0.5
	≥4 serving/day	0
	Nuts, seeds, and legumes	
6	≥4 servings/day	1
	2–3 servings/day	0.5
	<2 servings/day	0
	% kcal from fat	
7	≤27%	1
	≥28 ≤ 29%	0.5
	≥30%	0
	% kcal from saturated fat	
8	≤6%	1
	≤7 ≥8%	0.5
	≥9%	0
	Sweets	
9	≤5 servings/week	1
	6–7 servings/week	0.5
	≥8 serving/week	0

Table 1. *Cont.*

Score Items	DASH-Component	Scoring
	Sodium	
10	≤2.400 mg/day	1
	2.400–3.000 mg/day	0.5
	>3.000 mg/day	0

2.5. Mediterranean Adherence Score (MEDAS)

The validated German translation of the original MEDAS was used to determine adherence to the Mediterranean diet [30]. Twelve questions on food items (consumption of food groups and frequency by using raw data, mean daily intake of animal fat and vegetable oil) and additional 2 questions on characteristic food habits of the Mediterranean diet were included (Table 2). The MEDAS score could be assessed for 9020 participants and ranged from 0 to 14 points, with items scoring either 0 (condition not met) or 1 (adherent). A score from 0 to 4 was classified as low adherence, from 5 to 9 as medium adherence, and from 10 to 14 as high adherence.

Table 2. Scoring criteria for Mediterranean Dietary score according to Hebestreit et al. [30].

Score Items	MEDAS Question	Data Recorded by FFQ 1 Point Given, If . . .
1	Do you use olive oil as the principal source of fat for cooking?	use of olive oil for the preparation of at least 2 of the following groceries: salad, vegetable, meat/fish
2	How much olive oil do you consume per day (including that used in frying, salads, meals eaten away from home, etc.)?	based on FFQ calculation, if >48 g vegetable oil per day
3	How many servings of vegetables do you consume per day?	based on FFQ calculation, if ≥2 portions of vegetables per day (including raw and cooked vegetables, salad, olives, mushrooms, except potatoes and legumes)
4	How many pieces of fruit (including fresh-squeezed juice) do you consume per day?	based on FFQ calculation, if ≥3 portions of fruit (including fruit, mixed fruit, fruit salad, mixed stewed fruit, and fruit juices, excluding sweetened beverages)
5	How many servings of red meat, hamburger, or sausages do you consume per day?	based on FFQ calculation, if <100 g red meat (e.g., beef, veal, pork, lamb) and processed meat products
6	How many servings (12 g) of butter, margarine, or cream do you consume per day?	based on FFQ calculation, if <1 portion butter, margarine, and cream and other animal fat
7	How many carbonated and/or sugar-sweetened beverages do you consume per day?	based on FFQ calculation, sugar-sweetened beverages <1 portion per day (including lemonade and colas)
8	Do you drink wine? How much do you consume per week?	based on FFQ calculation, if ≥7 portions wine (red and white wine)
9	How many servings of pulses do you consume per week?	≥3 portions pulses (e.g., beans, lentils, peas, chickpeas)
10	How many servings of fish/seafood do you consume per week?	based on FFQ calculation, if ≥3 portions fish, fish products, and seafood per week

Table 2. *Cont.*

Score Items	MEDAS Question	Data Recorded by FFQ 1 Point Given, If ...
11	How many times do you consume commercial (not homemade) pastry such as cookies or cake per week?	based on FFQ calculation, if <3 portions cakes, chocolate, cookies, sweets with and without chocolate per week
12	How many times do you consume nuts per week?	based on FFQ calculation, if ≥3 portions nuts per week
13	Do you prefer to eat chicken, turkey, or rabbit instead of beef, pork, hamburgers, or sausages?	Based on FFQ calculation, if g white meat (e.g., chicken, hen, and other poultry) > g red meat (e.g., beef, veal, pork, lamb, and processed meat products)
14	How many times per week do you consume boiled vegetables, pasta, rice, or other dishes with a sauce of tomato, garlic, onion, or leeks sautéed in olive oil?	> 1–2 times/week tomato sauce

2.6. Assessment of Dental Variables

The 6209 participants received a full dental examination (excluding wisdom teeth). Study nurses were trained and regularly calibrated. Calibration took place every two months and was performed by a trained dentist. Prior to oral examination, all participants were asked to undergo a necessary endocarditis prophylaxis. Oral examination included: probing depth (mm), gingival recession (mm), bleeding on probing (BOP) (6 sites per tooth; PCP-12 probe), and determination of the plaque index (4 sites per tooth). Subsequently, two secondary variables were calculated, i.e., DMFT (decayed, missing, filled teeth) and CAL (clinical attachment loss). All participants were then categorized in one out of three severity levels of periodontitis [31]: (1) no periodontitis/mild periodontitis, (2) moderate periodontitis, and (3) severe periodontitis.

2.7. Assessment of Additional Variables

For all participants, the following information was retrieved from the HCHS Database: gender, age (years), education (according to ISCED [32]), cardiovascular risk factors, i.e., BMI (in kg/m^2), smoking (ever/non-smoking), diabetes (positive self-declaration and/or taking medication of the A10 group (insulin and analogues), and/or fasting glucose >126 mg/dL, not fasting glucose >200 mg/dL), and hypertension. High-sensitivity interleukin 6 (IL-6) and C-reactive protein (CRP) were assessed via established ELISA. Nutrition was reported as gram/day and included fiber, protein, fat, carbohydrates, and alcohol. Participants were asked about their physical activity level and hours of sport/week.

2.8. Statistical Analysis

Descriptive analyses were stratified by periodontitis severity (and by gender in supplementary Tables S1–S3). Continuous variables are displayed as median and interquartile range [median (IQR)]. Consequently, categorical variables are displayed as absolute numbers and percentages [n (%)]. Differences within groups were tested using the Chi-squared test for categorical variables and the Kruskal–Wallis test for continuous variables. Dietary patterns were categorized into terciles, resulting in three groups: "Low", "Medium", and "High". Ordinal logistic regression models were applied to determine the association between periodontitis (dependent variable) and dietary patterns (independent variable). Simplified logistic regression model is presented in supplementary material (supplementary Tables S4 and S5). Dietary patters were categorized using a numerical range. All statistical analyses were performed in R Studio Version 4.0.3 (Free Software Foundation's GNU project) with standard 0.05 statistical significance.

3. Results

3.1. Descriptive Statistics Stratified According to Periodontitis Severity

Data from 6209 participants with fully completed periodontal examination were included. Participants with severe periodontitis were more likely men (60.9 vs. 39,6%), of higher age (66 vs. 59 years), with less frequent higher education (39.8 vs. 47.6 %) when compared to participants with none/mild periodontitis. Participants with severe periodontitis presented higher BMI values (26.4 vs. 25.5 kg/m^2), were current smokers (25.1 vs. 16.2%), had more often diabetes (11.3 vs. 6.2 %), suffered from hypertension (72.5 vs. 54.8%), and differed in their CRP values (0.10 vs. 0.13 mg/l). Participants with severe periodontitis consumed (g/day) more proteins (72.64 vs. 69.20), more fat (91.41 vs. 86.81), more carbohydrates (198.21 vs. 195.19), and more alcohol (10.44 vs. 9.33) when compared to participants with none/mild periodontitis. Participants with severe periodontitis presented higher BOP Indices (21.05 vs. 2.08) and plaque indices (22.00 vs. 0.00) (Table 3).

Table 3. Baseline characteristics.

	None/Mild Periodontitis	Moderate Periodontitis	Severe Periodontitis	p-Value for Trend
n (%), median; IQR, * mean/SD	1453	3580	1176	
DEMOGRAPHICS				
Female sex	878 (60.4)	1814 (50.7)	460 (39.1)	<0.001
Age	59.00; 52.00, 66.00	63.00; 55.00, 69.00	66.00; 59.00, 71.00	<0.001
Education				0.001
Low	37 (2.7)	112 (3.4)	44 (4.1)	
Medium	678 (49.7)	1701 (51.0)	609 (56.2)	
High	650 (47.6)	1521 (45.6)	431 (39.8)	
CARDIOVASCULAR RISK				
BMI	25.56; 23.01, 28.67	26.02; 23.55, 29.01	26.44; 24.11, 29.65	<0.001
Smoking	235 (16.2)	608 (17.1)	293 (25.1)	<0.001
Diabetes	85 (6.2)	242 (7.4)	122 (11.3)	<0.001
Hypertension	768 (54.8)	2266 (66.3)	810 (72.5)	<0.001
LABORATORIES				
IL6	1.45; 1.01, 2.04	1.55; 1.15, 2.16	1.77; 1.33, 2.63	<0.001
CRP	0.10; 0.06, 0.23	0.11; 0.06, 0.25	0.13; 0.07, 0.30	<0.001
NUTRITION				
Total energy (kcal/day)	1989; 1569, 2543	2048; 1629, 2594	2069; 1639, 2602	0.057
Fibre (g/day)	18.88; 14.91, 24.29	18.94; 14.98, 24.07	18.23; 14.46, 23.41	0.023
Protein (g/day)	69.20; 54.97, 87.42	71.35; 56.41, 90.35	72.64; 57.27, 91.34	0.003
Fat (g/day)	86.81; 68.39, 113.25	90.04; 70.98, 114.56	91.41; 70.64, 115.76	0.023
Carbohydrates (g/day)	195.19; 153.19, 254.80	198.36; 153.70, 255.73	198.21; 150.12, 248.81	0.554
Alcohol (g/day)	9.33; 2.69, 21.52	9.38; 2.70, 22.94	10.44; 2.78, 26.41	0.140
Saccharides	89.21; 68.76, 116.66	89.81; 68.06, 119.89	87.83; 66.93, 114.71	0.187
DASH diet *	4.55/1.06	4.51/1.08	4.39/1.07	0.001
Mediterranean Diet *	4.77/1.92	4.58/1.88	4.38/1.87	<0.001
PHYSICAL ACTIVITY				
Physical activity	983 (75.5)	2286 (72.4)	657 (64.7)	<0.001
Sport (h/week)	2.00; [0.38, 4.00]	2.00; 0.00, 4.00	2.00; 0.00, 3.50	<0.001
DENTAL VARIABLES				
DMFT index	17.00; 14.00, 21.00	19.00; 16.00, 23.00	21.00; 17.00, 24.25	<0.001
BOP index	2.08; 0.00, 7.14	8.33; 2.17, 19.23	21.05; 9.26, 41.67	<0.001
Plaque index	0.00; 0.00, 10.71	8.93; 0.00, 27.78	22.00; 5.77, 54.76	<0.001

Abbreviations: BMI = Body Mass Index, BOP Index = Bleeding on Probing Index, DMFT Index = Decayed, Missing, Filled, Teeth Index, CRP = High-sensitivity C-reactive protein, IL6 = Interleukin 6, PA = periodontitis, * values for adherence score are displayed as Mean and Standard deviation.

Participants with low adherence to the DASH diet presented higher BOP Indices (8.70 vs. 7.14) and higher plaque indices (10.71 vs. 6.25) and were more affected by severe periodontitis (21.3 vs. 13.3%) when compared to participants with high adherence (Table 4).

Table 4. Baseline dental characteristics stratified according to adherence to the DASH diet.

	DASH Score			
	Low	**Medium**	**High**	***p*-Value**
n *	2259	6718	43	
DMFT index	20.00; 16.00, 24.00	19.00; 16.00, 23.00	19.00; 14.00, 22.00	<0.001
BOP index	8.70; 2.00, 22.00	7.50; 1.92, 19.44	7.14; 2.07, 14.98	0.081
Plaque index	10.71; 0.00, 35.36	7.41; 0.00, 26.92	6.25; 0.00, 29.63	<0.001
Periodontitis				0.046
None/mild	304 (22.2)	1014 (23.9)	9 (30.0)	
Moderate	775 (56.5)	2472 (58.3)	17 (56.7)	
Severe	292 (21.3)	755 (17.8)	4 (13.3)	

Abbreviations: BOP Index = Bleeding on Probing Index, DMFT Index = Decayed, Missing, Filled, Teeth Index, *n* * = Adherence score could be assessed for 9020 participants–not all columns sum up to 100%, because of missing values for different variables.

We could detect a similar trend in participants with low adherence to the Mediterranean diet, with higher plaque index (10.42 vs. 3.57) and, overall, more cases with severe periodontitis (20.4 vs. 18.8%) when compared with participants with high adherence to the diet (Table 5).

Table 5. Baseline dental characteristics stratified according to adherence to the Mediterranean diet.

	Mediterranean Score			
	Low	**Medium**	**High**	***p*-Value**
n *	4589	4380	51	
DMFT index	20.00; 16.00, 23.00	19.00; 15.00, 23.00	21.00; 15.00, 25.00	<0.001
BOP index	8.93; 2.00, 22.36	7.14; 1.85, 18.18	9.99; 1.34, 25.45	<0.001
Plaque index	10.42; 0.00, 33.33	6.82; 0.00, 25.00	3.57; 0.00, 23.30	<0.001
Periodontitis				0.010
None/mild	644 (22.5)	676 (24.6)	7 (21.9)	
Moderate	1633 (57.1)	1612 (58.6)	19 (59.4)	
Severe	584 (20.4)	461 (16.8)	6 (18.8)	

Abbreviations: BOP Index = Bleeding on Probing Index, DMFT Index = Decayed, Missing, Filled, Teeth Index, *n* * = Adherence score could be assessed for 9020 participants–not al columns sum up to 100%, because of missing values for different variables.

3.2. Regression Analyses

Ordinal regression analyses revealed significant association between higher adherence to the DASH diet and lower odds to present periodontitis in an unadjusted model (OR: 0.92; 95% CI: 0.87, 0.97; $p < 0.001$), adjusted model 1 (age, sex, diabetes) (OR: 0.94; 95% CI: 0.89, 1.00; $p < 0.0365$), and adjusted model 2 (age, sex, and physical activity) (OR: 0.95; 95% CI: 0.89, 1.00; $p < 0.0507$) (Table 6).

We detected a similar trend for the Mediterranean diet with significant association between higher adherence to the diet and lower odds to present periodontitis in an unadjusted model (OR: 0.93; 95% CI: 0.91, 0.96; $p < 0.001$), adjusted model 1 (age, sex, diabetes) (OR: 0.97; 95% CI: 0.94, 1.00; $p < 0.0359$), and adjusted model 2 (age, sex, and physical activity) (OR: 0.97; 95% CI: 0.94, 1.00; $p < 0.0515$) (Table 7).

Table 6. Ordinal logistic regression: outcome periodontitis, exposure DASH diet.

Variable	Units	Odds Ratio	95% CI	*p*-Value
DASH diet		0.92	0.87; 0.97	<0.001
DASH diet		0.94	0.88; 0.99	0.0122
Age		1.05	1.05; 1.06	<0.001
Sex	Male	Ref		
	Female	0.64	0.53; 0.75	<0.001
DASH diet		0.94	0.89; 1.00	0.0365
Age		1.05	1.04; 1.06	<0.001
Sex	Male	Ref		
	Female	0.65	0.53; 0.76	<0.001
Diabetes	No	Ref		
	Yes	1.13	0.92; 1.34	0.2494
DASH diet		0.95	0.89; 1.00	0.0507
Age		1.05	1.04; 1.06	<0.001
Sex	Male	Ref		
	Female	0.64	0.53; 0.76	<0.001
Physical activity	No	Ref		
	Yes	0.81	0.69; 0.94	<0.001

Abbreviations: DASH = Dietary Approach to Stop Hypertension, CI = confidence interval. Unadjusted and stepwise adjusted for age, sex, diabetes, and physical activity.

Table 7. Ordinal logistic regression: outcome periodontitis, exposure Mediterranean Diet.

Variable	Units	Odds Ratio	95% CI	*p*-Value
Mediterranean Diet		0.93	0.91; 0.96	<0.001
Mediterranean Diet		0.96	0.94; 0.99	0.0157
Age		1.05	1.04; 1.06	<0.001
Sex	Male	Ref		
	Female	0.64	0.53; 0.75	<0.001
Mediterranean Diet		0.97	0.94; 1.00	0.0359
Age		1.05	1.04; 1.06	<0.001
Sex	Male	Ref		
	Female	0.65	0.53; 0.76	<0.001
Diabetes	No	Ref		
	Yes	1.13	0.93; 1.34	0.2368
Mediterranean Diet		0.97	0.94; 1.00	0.0515
Age		1.05	1.04; 1.06	<0.001
Sex	Male	Ref		
	Female	0.64	0.53; 0.76	<0.001
Physical activity	No	Ref		
	Yes	0.81	0.69; 0.93	<0.001

Abbreviations: CI = confidence interval. Unadjusted and stepwise adjusted for age, sex, diabetes, and physical activity.

4. Discussion

In this cross-sectional study, dental and nutritional parameters were collected from 6209 individuals. Older men with higher cardiovascular burden appeared to be more affected by the severe form of periodontitis. Participants with poor adherence to the DASH diet and Mediterranean diet more often presented insufficient oral hygiene (higher BOP and plaque index) when compared to participants with high adherence to these diets. This trend was also perceptible in regression analyses: a higher adherence to the DASH diet as well as to the Mediterranean diet was significantly associated with lower odds to present periodontitis.

A recently published cross-sectional study included rather young (mean age = 20.2 years) and healthy Moroccan individuals, with only 71 (6.6%) participants presenting periodontitis [23]. Logistic regression revealed no significant association between adherence to the

Mediterranean diet and periodontitis, though the lack of a significant association might be because of (1) the small number of diseased participants and (2) the fact that the study population only consisted of undergraduate university students, who probably present overall better health and oral health literacy.

Nielsen et al. analyzed data of 6052 adults participating in the National Health and Nutrition Examination Survey (NHANES 2011–2012) to investigate dietary fiber intake and periodontal disease prevalence [22]. The periodontal cohort was quite comparable to our cohort, with approximately 50% of female participants over 50 years of age and a majority of non-Hispanic white, who never smoked and graduated from college. Although the authors chose not to include the DASH diet or the Mediterranean diet specifically, they included fiber consumption, whole-grain consumption, and fruit and vegetable consumption. The authors reported a significant association between a low fiber consumption and moderate to severe periodontitis (referenced as mild–no periodontitis) compared with the association of periodontitis with a high fiber intake (OR: 1.30; 95% CI: 1.00, 1.69).

The current case–control study design cannot address causality. Thus, the impact of the participants' adherence to a diet can directly affect periodontitis via quite complex biological mechanisms (reviewed in detail [33]). In brief, carbohydrates can alter the microbial diversity and directly affect periodontal ligament cells. Saturated fatty acids are suspected to increase oxidative stress and thereby promote periodontal damage.

However, participants' adherence to a diet can also just act as confounding mediating factor. For example, behavioral patterns modify the association between dietary patterns and periodontitis. In fact, (1) women of all ages, unfortunately, are more often concerned about weight control and dieting, eating especially lower fat and lower sugar foods, as well as increasing the intake of fruits and vegetables [34], (2) men present lower health literacy, meaning lower understanding and application of health information for healthcare and disease prevention [35]. Consequently, it is possible that the significant association between lower adherence to dietary approaches and severe periodontitis is solely because of the accumulation of poor (oral) healthcare choices.

Moreover, the DASH and Mediterranean diets were selected as examples of healthy plant-based diets recommended by international (AHA) and European guidelines (EAS). However, the two scores were not specifically developed for the HCHS study population. Therefore, the two dietary patterns may not fully reflect the specific dietary behaviors of the target population, although we observed a clear trend across all groups."

5. Limitation

The population of the HCHS cohort is middle-aged white Caucasian, and our findings cannot be generalized to other ethnicities or to a much younger population. For periodontal classification, we used the reported gold standard: the AAP/CDC case definition for epidemiologic surveillance [31]. However, during the 2017 World Workshop on the Classification of Periodontal and Peri-Implant Diseases and Conditions, a new classification, "Staging and Grading", was introduced [36]. Yet, this classification is not routinely used for epidemiological approaches. Thus, we set higher priority for the comparability of our study results. Lastly, the sample size of participants with severe periodontitis and high adherence to the DASH diet and the Mediterranean diet was small (<1%), which can be improved by, for example, purposeful over-sampling.

6. Conclusions

The current cross-sectional study identified a significant association between higher adherence to the DASH and Mediterranean diets and lower odds to be affected by periodontal diseases. Future randomized controlled trials are needed to evaluate to which extent macro- and micronutrition can affect periodontitis initiation/progression.

Supplementary Materials: The following are available online at https://www.mdpi.com/article/ 10.3390/nu13114167/s1, Table S1: Baseline characteristics, Table S2: Baseline dental characteristics stratified according to DASH Diet, Table S3: Baseline dental characteristics stratified according to Mediterranean Diet, Table S4: Logistic regression: outcome binary variable periodontitis (no vs. severe periodontitis), exposure DASH Diet, Table S5: Logistic regression: outcome binary variable periodontitis (no vs. severe periodontitis), exposure Mediterranean Diet.

Author Contributions: Conceptualization, E.A., D.K., N.J., G.A., B.-C.Z.; methodology, E.A., C.W., G.A., B.-C.Z.; software K.B., E.P.; validation E.A., C.W., G.A., B.-C.Z., T.B.; formal analysis K.B., E.P., E.A., C.W.; investigation E.A., C.W.; resources G.A., B.-C.Z., T.B.; data curation K.B., E.P.; writing— original draft preparation E.A., C.W.; writing—review and editing G.A., B.-C.Z., B.L., B.J., T.B.; visualization C.W., K.B.; supervision G.A., B.-C.Z.; project administration G.A., B.-C.Z. All authors have read and agreed to the published version of the manuscript.

Funding: This research received no external funding.

Institutional Review Board Statement: The study was conducted according to the guidelines of the Declaration of Helsinki and approved by the Institutional Review Board (or Ethics Committee) of The Landesärztekammer Hamburg (State of Hamburg Chamber of Medical Practitioners, PV5131). The HCHS has been registered at ClinicalTrial.gov (NCT03934957).

Informed Consent Statement: Informed consent was obtained from all subjects involved in the study.

Conflicts of Interest: The authors declare no conflict of interest.

References

1. Jordan, A.R.; Micheelis, W. (Eds.) *Fünfte Deutsche Mundgesundheitsstudie (DMS V)*; Deutscher Zahnärzte Verlag DÄV: Köln, Germany, 2016; p. 617.
2. Kassebaum, N.J.; Smith, A.G.C.; Bernabe, E.; Fleming, T.D.; Reynolds, A.E.; Vos, T.; Murray, C.J.L.; Marcenes, W.; GBD 2015 Oral Health Collaborators. Global, Regional, and National Prevalence, Incidence, and Disability-Adjusted Life Years for Oral Conditions for 195 Countries, 1990-2015: A Systematic Analysis for the Global Burden of Diseases, Injuries, and Risk Factors. *J. Dent. Res.* **2017**, *96*, 380–387. [CrossRef] [PubMed]
3. Axelsson, P.; Albandar, J.M.; Rams, T.E. Prevention and control of periodontal diseases in developing and industrialized nations. *Periodontol 2000* **2002**, *29*, 235–246. [CrossRef] [PubMed]
4. Kinane, D.F.; Stathopoulou, P.G.; Papapanou, P.N. Periodontal diseases. *Nat. Rev. Dis. Prim.* **2017**, *3*, 17038. [CrossRef]
5. Benakanakere, M.; Abdolhosseini, M.; Hosur, K.; Finoti, L.S.; Kinane, D.F. TLR2 promoter hypermethylation creates innate immune dysbiosis. *J. Dent. Res.* **2015**, *94*, 183–191. [CrossRef] [PubMed]
6. Chapple, I.L. Potential mechanisms underpinning the nutritional modulation of periodontal inflammation. *J. Am. Dent. Assoc.* **2009**, *140*, 178–184. [CrossRef] [PubMed]
7. Mazur, M.; Ndokaj, A.; Jedlinski, M.; Ardan, R.; Bietolini, S.; Ottolenghi, L. Impact of Green Tea (Camellia Sinensis) on periodontitis and caries. Systematic review and meta-analysis. *Jpn. Dent. Sci. Rev.* **2021**, *57*, 1–11. [CrossRef]
8. Woelber, J.P.; Bremer, K.; Vach, K.; Konig, D.; Hellwig, E.; Ratka-Kruger, P.; Al-Ahmad, A.; Tennert, C. An oral health optimized diet can reduce gingival and periodontal inflammation in humans - a randomized controlled pilot study. *BMC Oral Health* **2016**, *17*, 28. [CrossRef]
9. Kondo, K.; Ishikado, A.; Morino, K.; Nishio, Y.; Ugi, S.; Kajiwara, S.; Kurihara, M.; Iwakawa, H.; Nakao, K.; Uesaki, S.; et al. A high-fiber, low-fat diet improves periodontal disease markers in high-risk subjects: A pilot study. *Nutr. Res.* **2014**, *34*, 491–498. [CrossRef]
10. Trichopoulou, A.; Costacou, T.; Bamia, C.; Trichopoulos, D. Adherence to a Mediterranean diet and survival in a Greek population. *N. Engl. J. Med.* **2003**, *348*, 2599–2608. [CrossRef]
11. Covas, M.I.; Nyyssönen, K.; Poulsen, H.E.; Kaikkonen, J.; Zunft, H.J.; Kiesewetter, H.; Gaddi, A.; de la Torre, R.; Mursu, J.; Bäumler, H.; et al. The effect of polyphenols in olive oil on heart disease risk factors: A randomized trial. *Ann. Intern. Med.* **2006**, *145*, 333–341. [CrossRef]
12. Bunte, K.; Hensel, A.; Beikler, T. Polyphenols in the prevention and treatment of periodontal disease: A systematic review of in vivo, ex vivo and in vitro studies. *Fitoterapia* **2019**, *132*, 30–39. [CrossRef] [PubMed]
13. Moore, T.J.; Conlin, P.R.; Ard, J.; Svetkey, L.P. DASH (Dietary Approaches to Stop Hypertension) diet is effective treatment for stage 1 isolated systolic hypertension. *Hypertension* **2001**, *38*, 155–158. [CrossRef] [PubMed]
14. Vollmer, W.M.; Sacks, F.M.; Ard, J.; Appel, L.J.; Bray, G.A.; Simons-Morton, D.G.; Conlin, P.R.; Svetkey, L.P.; Erlinger, T.P.; Moore, T.J.; et al. Effects of diet and sodium intake on blood pressure: Subgroup analysis of the DASH-sodium trial. *Ann. Intern. Med.* **2001**, *135*, 1019–1028. [CrossRef] [PubMed]

15. Mancia, G.; Fagard, R.; Narkiewicz, K.; Redon, J.; Zanchetti, A.; Böhm, M.; Christiaens, T.; Cifkova, R.; De Backer, G.; Dominiczak, A.; et al. 2013 ESH/ESC guidelines for the management of arterial hypertension: The Task Force for the Management of Arterial Hypertension of the European Society of Hypertension (ESH) and of the European Society of Cardiology (ESC). *Eur. Heart J.* **2013**, *34*, 2159–2219. [CrossRef]

16. Micha, R.; Shulkin, M.L.; Penalvo, J.L.; Khatibzadeh, S.; Singh, G.M.; Rao, M.; Fahimi, S.; Powles, J.; Mozaffarian, D. Etiologic effects and optimal intakes of foods and nutrients for risk of cardiovascular diseases and diabetes: Systematic reviews and meta-analyses from the Nutrition and Chronic Diseases Expert Group (NutriCoDE). *PLoS ONE* **2017**, *12*, e0175149. [CrossRef]

17. Chen, G.C.; Neelakantan, N.; Martin-Calvo, N.; Koh, W.P.; Yuan, J.M.; Bonaccio, M.; Iacoviello, L.; Martinez-Gonzalez, M.A.; Qin, L.Q.; van Dam, R.M. Adherence to the Mediterranean diet and risk of stroke and stroke subtypes. *Eur. J. Epidemiol.* **2019**, *34*, 337–349. [CrossRef]

18. Yang, Z.Q.; Yang, Z.; Duan, M.L. Dietary approach to stop hypertension diet and risk of coronary artery disease: A meta-analysis of prospective cohort studies. *Int. J. Food Sci. Nutr.* **2019**, *70*, 668–674. [CrossRef]

19. Zong, G.; Holtfreter, B.; Scott, A.E.; Völzke, H.; Petersmann, A.; Dietrich, T.; Newson, R.S.; Kocher, T. Serum vitamin B12 is inversely associated with periodontal progression and risk of tooth loss: A prospective cohort study. *J. Clin. Periodontol.* **2016**, *43*, 2–9. [CrossRef] [PubMed]

20. Lula, E.C.; Ribeiro, C.C.; Hugo, F.N.; Alves, C.M.; Silva, A.A. Added sugars and periodontal disease in young adults: An analysis of NHANES III data. *Am. J. Clin. Nutr.* **2014**, *100*, 1182–1187. [CrossRef]

21. Wright, D.M.; McKenna, G.; Nugent, A.; Winning, L.; Linden, G.J.; Woodside, J.V. Association between diet and periodontitis: A cross-sectional study of 10,000 NHANES participants. *Am. J. Clin. Nutr.* **2020**, *112*, 1485–1491. [CrossRef] [PubMed]

22. Nielsen, S.J.; Trak-Fellermeier, M.A.; Joshipura, K.; Dye, B.A. Dietary Fiber Intake Is Inversely Associated with Periodontal Disease among US Adults. *J. Nutr.* **2016**, *146*, 2530–2536. [CrossRef] [PubMed]

23. Iwasaki, M.; Ennibi, O.K.; Bouziane, A.; Erraji, S.; Lakhdar, L.; Rhissassi, M.; Ansai, T.; Yoshida, A.; Miyazaki, H. Association between periodontitis and the Mediterranean diet in young Moroccan individuals. *J. Periodontal Res.* **2021**, *56*, 408–414. [CrossRef] [PubMed]

24. Jagodzinski, A.; Johansen, C.; Koch-Gromus, U.; Aarabi, G.; Adam, G.; Anders, S.; Augustin, M.; der Kellen, R.B.; Beikler, T.; Behrendt, C.A.; et al. Rationale and Design of the Hamburg City Health Study. *Eur. J. Epidemiol.* **2020**, *35*, 169–181. [CrossRef] [PubMed]

25. von Elm, E.; Altman, D.G.; Egger, M.; Pocock, S.J.; Gøtzsche, P.C.; Vandenbroucke, J.P. Strengthening the reporting of observational studies in epidemiology (STROBE) statement: Guidelines for reporting observational studies. *BMJ* **2007**, *335*. [CrossRef] [PubMed]

26. Riboli, E.; Hunt, K.J.; Slimani, N.; Ferrari, P.; Norat, T.; Fahey, M.; Charrondière, U.R.; Hémon, B.; Casagrande, C.; Vignat, J.; et al. European Prospective Investigation into Cancer and Nutrition (EPIC): Study populations and data collection. *Public Health Nutr.* **2002**, *5*, 1113–1124. [CrossRef]

27. Nöthlings, U.; Hoffmann, K.; Bergmann, M.M.; Boeing, H. Fitting portion sizes in a self-administered food frequency questionnaire. *J. Nutr.* **2007**, *137*, 2781–2786. [CrossRef]

28. Folsom, A.R.; Parker, E.D.; Harnack, L.J. Degree of concordance with DASH diet guidelines and incidence of hypertension and fatal cardiovascular disease. *Am. J. Hypertens.* **2007**, *20*, 225–232. [CrossRef] [PubMed]

29. Epstein, D.E.; Sherwood, A.; Smith, P.J.; Craighead, L.; Caccia, C.; Lin, P.H.; Babyak, M.A.; Johnson, J.J.; Hinderliter, A.; Blumenthal, J.A. Determinants and consequences of adherence to the dietary approaches to stop hypertension diet in African-American and white adults with high blood pressure: Results from the ENCORE trial. *J. Acad. Nutr. Diet.* **2012**, *112*, 1763–1773. [CrossRef]

30. Hebestreit, K.; Yahiaoui-Doktor, M.; Engel, C.; Vetter, W.; Siniatchkin, M.; Erickson, N.; Halle, M.; Kiechle, M.; Bischoff, S.C. Validation of the German version of the Mediterranean Diet Adherence Screener (MEDAS) questionnaire. *BMC Cancer* **2017**, *17*, 341. [CrossRef]

31. Eke, P.I.; Page, R.C.; Wei, L.; Thornton-Evans, G.; Genco, R.J. Update of the case definitions for population-based surveillance of periodontitis. *J. Periodontol.* **2012**, *83*, 1449–1454. [CrossRef]

32. Organisation for Economic Co-Operation and Development. *Classifying Educational Programmes: Manual for ISCED-97 Implementation in OECD Countries*; Organisation for Economic Co-Operation and Development: Paris, France, 1999.

33. Martinon, P.; Fraticelli, L.; Giboreau, A.; Dussart, C.; Bourgeois, D.; Carrouel, F. Nutrition as a Key Modifiable Factor for Periodontitis and Main Chronic Diseases. *J. Clin. Med.* **2021**, *10*, 197. [CrossRef] [PubMed]

34. Wardle, J.; Haase, A.M.; Steptoe, A.; Nillapun, M.; Jonwutiwes, K.; Bellisle, F. Gender differences in food choice: The contribution of health beliefs and dieting. *Ann. Behav. Med.* **2004**, *27*, 107–116. [CrossRef] [PubMed]

35. Sørensen, K.; Pelikan, J.M.; Röthlin, F.; Ganahl, K.; Slonska, Z.; Doyle, G.; Fullam, J.; Kondilis, B.; Agrafiotis, D.; Uiters, E.; et al. Health literacy in Europe: Comparative results of the European health literacy survey (HLS-EU). *Eur. J. Public Health* **2015**, *25*, 1053–1058. [CrossRef]

36. Tonetti, M.S.; Greenwell, H.; Kornman, K.S. Staging and grading of periodontitis: Framework and proposal of a new classification and case definition. *J. Clin. Periodontol.* **2018**, *45*, S149–S161. [CrossRef] [PubMed]

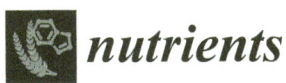

Article

Effects of a Non-Energy-Restricted Ketogenic Diet on Clinical Oral Parameters. An Exploratory Pilot Trial

Johan Peter Woelber [1,*,†] , Christian Tennert [2,†] , Simon Fabian Ernst [1], Kirstin Vach [3] , Petra Ratka-Krüger [1], Hartmut Bertz [4] and Paul Urbain [4]

1 Department of Operative Dentistry and Periodontology, Faculty of Medicine, University of Freiburg, Hugstetter Str. 55, 79106 Freiburg, Germany; si.-fa._ernst@web.de (S.F.E.); petra.ratka-krueger@uniklinik-freiburg.de (P.R.-K.)

2 Department of Restorative, Preventive and Pediatric Dentistry, University of Berne, Freiburgstrasse 7, 3010 Bern, Switzerland; christian.tennert@zmk.unibe.ch

3 Institute of Medical Biometry and Statistics, Faculty of Medicine, University of Freiburg, Zinkmattenstr. 6A, 79108 Freiburg, Germany; kv@imbi.uni-freiburg.de

4 Department of Medicine I, Medical Center-University of Freiburg, Faculty of Medicine, University of Freiburg, Hugstetter Str. 55, 79106 Freiburg, Germany; hartmut.bertz@uniklinik-freiburg.de (H.B.); paul.urbain@uniklinik-freiburg.de (P.U.)

* Correspondence: johan.woelber@uniklinik-freiburg.de

† These authors contributed equally to this work.

Abstract: Ketogenic diets (KDs) may be a helpful complement in the prevention of and therapy for several diseases. Apart from their non-cariogenic properties, it is still unclear how KDs affect oral parameters. The aim of this study was to investigate the influence of a KD on clinical periodontal parameters. Twenty generally healthy volunteers with an average age of 36.6 years underwent a KD for 6 weeks. Their compliance was monitored by measuring their urinary ketones daily and by keeping 7-day food records. Clinical oral parameters included plaque (PI), gingival inflammation (GI), a complete periodontal status (probing depths, bleeding on probing), and general physical and serologic parameters at baseline and after 6 weeks. The results showed a trend towards lower plaque values, but with no significant changes from baseline to the end of the study with regard to the clinical periodontal parameters. However, their body weight and BMI measurements showed a significant decrease. The regression analyses showed that the fat mass and the BMI were significantly positively correlated to periodontal inflammation, while HDL, fiber, and protein intake were negatively correlated to periodontal inflammation. The KD change did not lead to clinical changes in periodontal parameters in healthy participants under continued oral hygiene, but it did lead to a significant weight loss.

Keywords: ketogenic diet; periodontal inflammation; gingivitis; oral health

Citation: Woelber, J.P.; Tennert, C.; Ernst, S.F.; Vach, K.; Ratka-Krüger, P.; Bertz, H.; Urbain, P. Effects of a Non-Energy-Restricted Ketogenic Diet on Clinical Oral Parameters. An Exploratory Pilot Trial. *Nutrients* **2021**, *13*, 4229. https://doi.org/10.3390/nu13124229

Academic Editor: Anna Tagliabue

Received: 19 October 2021
Accepted: 23 November 2021
Published: 25 November 2021

Publisher's Note: MDPI stays neutral with regard to jurisdictional claims in published maps and institutional affiliations.

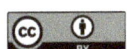
1. Introduction

Ketogenic diets (KDs) are characterized by a very low-carbohydrate intake (<10% energy) which induces a state of physiological ketosis with increased use of ketone bodies as an energy source [1]. KDs are used and investigated as potential dietary supports or as therapy for a wide range of diseases, such as intractable childhood epilepsy [2], type 2 diabetes, polycystic ovary syndrome, neurodegenerative diseases [3], and cancer [4,5]. Furthermore, the KD is a popular approach for achieving weight loss [3,6]. While its safety and efficacy were investigated with regard to various anthropomorphic outcomes (body weight, body mass index (BMI), waist circumference, etc.), serological outcomes (cholesterol, markers of blood sugar and insulin resistance, etc.), and body functions (blood pressure, peak oxygen uptake (VO2peak) and peak power, handgrip strength, etc.) [7–9], there is a lack of data with regard to clinical oral parameters. This seems surprising since caries are a process that is fundamentally dependent on digested fermentable carbohydrates [10]. Furthermore, there is growing evidence that avoiding sugar and processed carbohydrates in a diet can significantly reduce gingival inflammation, which is a prerequisite for periodontitis, even without changes in plaque values [11–14]. There are two basic mechanisms assumed about how processed carbohydrates can lead to an alteration of gingival inflammation by a local and a systemic pro-inflammatory effect. Kashket et al. were able to show that the supragingival plaque can metabolize processed carbohydrates to short-chain fatty acids, which, in turn, promote an inflammatory reaction of the gingiva [15]. The systemic effect is assumed to be mediated by high blood sugar peaks with an associated increase in oxidative stress and the formation of advanced glycation end products [10,16]. However, there is also evidence that carbohydrate consumption significantly alters the plaque formation on both teeth and dental implants [17,18], which also has an impact on gingival inflammation [19]. Since caries and periodontitis are the most common diseases in mankind [20], there is a fundamental need for research in therapeutics.

On the other side, there are aspects of KDs which may have a negative impact on periodontal parameters, such as a possible higher intake of saturated fatty acids or an increase in LDL values [16,21]. Furthermore, to the best of the author's knowledge, it is not described if a drop in serum pH values might have a negative impact on the oral system [22].

Thus, the aim of the current study was to exploratively evaluate the effect of a six-week ketogenic diet on clinical periodontal parameter participants within a larger main study about KDs. Due to the lack of studies regarding KDs and oral parameters, this study focused on generally healthy participants with continued oral hygiene as a first step.

2. Materials and Methods

2.1. Ethics and Trial Registration

The study was a part of a larger study titled "Impact of a 6-week non-energy-restricted ketogenic diet on physical fitness, body composition and biochemical parameters in healthy adults" [8]. The aim of the main study was to evaluate a six-week KD on endurance and physical performance in young healthy adults because prior studies to this time were only available for athletes. The results showed that KDs had no relevant impact on physical fitness that would impair daily activities or aerobic training [8]. The study protocol was approved by the Ethics Commission of the Albert-Ludwigs-University of Freiburg, Germany (494/14). All subjects signed a written consent form. The study was registered in an international trial register (German Clinical Trial Register number DRKS00009605).

2.2. Study Design and Recruitment

This study was designed as an interventional uncontrolled clinical trial. The participants were recruited from employees of the University Medical Center Freiburg via advertising from February to June 2016 at the Department of Medicine I. Besides their participation in the main study, participants were asked to take part in the oral examination conducted at the Department of Operative Dentistry and Periodontology, Faculty of Medicine, University of Freiburg, Germany.

2.3. Participants

All participants needed to meet the following inclusion criteria:

- Adults in good general health with a BMI in the range of 19–30 kg/m^2;
- Age $\geq$ 18 years.

The exclusion criteria were as follows:

- low-carbohydrate nutrition already prior to the study;
- Impaired liver and renal function, kidney stones;
- Pregnancy or lactation period;
- Diabetes mellitus and any fatty acid-metabolism disorders;
- Smoking.

2.4. Intervention

The experimental intervention consisted of a KD without caloric restriction over a period of 6 weeks in accordance with a modified Atkins diet [23]. Prior to the study period, the participants were instructed by a dietitian. The participants were provided with handouts describing the main aspects of a KD and given a list of suitable foods with a very low carbohydrate content. They were advised to eat ad libitum but to limit their carbohydrate intake to a maximum of 20–40 g/day to derive at least 75%, 15–20%, and 5–10% of total energy from fats, protein, and carbohydrates, respectively. The participants were allowed to vary the food according to their preferences within the framework of the KD. In addition, they were instructed to make the change gradually, step by step, during the first week in order to avoid unwanted side effects (such as constipation) [8]. A detailed description of the foods recommended to avoid and to eat can be found in the supplementary material of Cervenka et al. [24]. Their compliance was monitored by taking daily measurements of urinary ketones using self-testing strips (Ketostix, Bayer Vital GmbH, Leverkusen, Germany) and two semi-quantitative 7-day food records before and during the last week of the intervention. The participants were instructed to measure ketonuria in the morning time since a pre-study with 12 participants measuring both ketonuria and ß-hydroxybutyrate (BHB) in the serum showed that this was the most reliable time for testing [25]. The measurements in the evening and night time showed much higher values for ketonuria compared to serum BHB.

The participants were instructed to accurately record the amounts and types of food and beverages using a digital portable scale (KS 22, Beurer GmbH, Ulm, Germany). The nutrient analysis of the 7-day food records was performed with nutritional database software (Prodi 6.5 basis, Nutri-Science GmbH, Stuttgart, Germany). All participants were advised not to alter their physical activities during the study period. Physical activity was assessed using a validated questionnaire [26].

2.5. General and Clinical Oral Measurements

As part of the main study, the fat mass (FM), the body weight, the BMI, and the serological measurements were assessed. The FM was determined via air displacement plethysmography (ADP) using a calibrated BodPod device (Cosmed USA Inc., Concord, CA, USA). The serological measurements included the C-reactive protein (CRP), the blood glucose concentration, insulin, cholesterol, triglycerides (TG), the high-density lipoprotein (HDL), the low-density lipoprotein (LDL), and the insulin-like growth factor (IGF-1).

The clinical oral measurements were assessed by a dentist (SE) and included plaque, gingival inflammation, and a periodontal status including pocket probing depths (PPD), bleeding on probing (BOP), gingival recessions, and the clinical attachment loss (CAL). Based on PPDs and BOP, the periodontal inflamed surface area (PISA) was calculated [27]. Furthermore, participants were interviewed with regard to their oral hygiene behavior, including oral hygiene products and the frequency of use. Plaque was measured with the plaque index (PI) described by Silness and Löe [28] using a dental probe (Emil Huber GmbH, Karlsruhe, Germany). Gingival inflammation (GI) was measured according to Löe and Silness [28]. Periodontal measurements were performed with a pressure-sensitive periodontal probe DB764R (Aesculap AG, Tuttlingen, Germany). In order to assess the intra-rater reliability regarding the PPDs, half of the participants were measured twice in the first quadrant after the assessment of the periodontal status.

2.6. Statistical Analysis

The sample size calculation was carried out within the main study for the primary outcome peak oxygen uptake (VO2peak) [8]. Accordingly, the current study had no predefined primary and secondary outcomes but followed an explorative approach. The median, mean, standard deviation, minimum and maximum were calculated for a descriptive description of the data. A graphical representation was made by boxplots. By means of t-tests for paired samples, a before–after comparison was performed. A linear regression model was fitted per time point for an investigation of the influence of different influencing variables on the clinical parameters. It was also used to examine the changes in the clinical parameters. Due to the explorative character of this study, no correction for multiple testing was carried out. All data were analyzed using STATA 14.1 (StataCorp LP, Lakeway Drive College Station, TX, USA). $p < 0.05$ was considered as statistically significant.

3. Results

Twenty participants were recruited and completed the investigation, without any dropouts. The group consisted of 16 women and 4 men with a mean age of 36.6 years varying from 25 to 57 years. With regard to oral hygiene procedures, all participants brushed their teeth between 1 and 3 times daily and used additional oral hygiene products in varying frequencies (Table 1).

Table 1. Oral hygiene behavior of the experimental group.

Oral Hygiene Behavior	Mean Frequency (Per Day)	Standard Deviation	Minimum–Maximum
Tooth brushing	1.95	0.39	1–3
Interdental cleaning	0.49	0.55	0–2
Use of mouth rinse	0.41	0.68	0–2

3.1. Intragroup Differences

The factors PI, GI, BOP, PPD, CAL, and PISA did not change significantly from baseline to the end. With regard to PI, there was a trend toward lower scores at the final examination ($p = 0.096$; Table 2). The repeated measurements of the first quadrant showed high intra-rater reliability with an intraclass-correlation (ICC) of 0.98.

Table 2. Intragroup differences for clinical periodontal parameters from baseline to the final examination.

Oral Parameter	Time	Mean (Standard Deviation)	(95%Conf. Interval)	Intra-p-Value (Baseline vs. End)
PI	Baseline	0.49 (0.33)	0.34–0.65	
	End	0.42 (0.27)	0.29–0.55	0.0969
GI	Baseline	0.68 (0.28)	0.55–0.82	
	End	0.62 (0.23)	0.51–0.73	0.1814
BOP	Baseline	0.29 (0.09)	0.24–0.33	
	End	0.27 (0.11)	0.22–0.32	0.2601
PPD	Baseline	2.25 (0.22)	2.15–2.36	
	End	2.19 (0.17)	2.11–2.27	0.2743
CAL	Baseline	2.59 (0.41)	2.40–2.78	
	End	2.60 (0.40)	2.41–2.79	0.8156
PISA	Baseline	370.1 (141.5)	303.9–436.4	
	End	341.3 (149.0)	271.5–411.1	0.2545

PI = plaque index; GI = gingival index; BOP = bleeding on probing; PPD = pocket probing depth; CAL = clinical attachment level; PISA = periodontal inflamed surface area. With regard to the anthropomorphic data and physical activity, body weight and BMI showed a significant decrease from baseline to the end (Table 3). Regarding the fat mass, there was a trend towards lower values at the final examination.

Table 3. Intragroup differences for anthropomorphic parameters and physical activity from baseline to the final examination.

Parameter	Time	Mean (Standard Deviation)	(95% Conf. Interval)	Intra-p-Value (Baseline vs. End)
Body weight (kg)	Baseline	69.20 (10.65)	64.21–74.17	
	End	67.34 (9.26)	63.01–71.67	0.0003 **
BMI (kg/m^2)	Baseline	23.60 (3.25)	22.08–25.13	
	End	22.97 (2.77)	21.67–24.26	0.0002 **
Fat mass (kg)	Baseline	22.75 (9.32)	18.39–27.11	
	End	21.99 (8.33)	18.09–25.89	0.0675
Physical activity (MET-hours/week)	Baseline	39.31 (19.51)	30.17–48.44	
	End	43.29 (24.47)	31.83–54.74	0.1600

MET = metabolic equivalent of task., ** $p < 0.01$.

The serological parameters, glucose, and IGF-1 showed a significant decrease from baseline to the end (Table 4). The LDL value showed a significant increase from baseline to the end, while the HDL did not change from baseline to the end. Changes in nutrient intake from baseline to the final examination are presented in Table 5.

Table 4. Intragroup differences for serological parameters from baseline to the final examination.

Serological Parameter	Time	Mean (Standard Deviation)	(95% Conf. Interval)	Intra-*p*-Value (Baseline vs. End)
CRP (mg/L)	Baseline	1.75 (2.31)	0.67–2.83	0.2127
	End	3.05 (5.00)	0.71–5.39	
Glucose (mg/dL)	Baseline	90.55 (6.66)	87.43–93.67	0.0436 *
	End	87.75 (5.56)	85.15–90.35	
IGF-1 (ng/mL)	Baseline	197.15 (86.10)	156.85–237.45	0.0055 **
	End	154.50 (66.83)	123.22–185.78	
Insulin (pmol/L)	Baseline	53.00 (27.77)	40.00–66.00	0.2259
	End	45.50 (20.12)	36.08–54.92	
HDL (mg/dL)	Baseline	75.65 15.11)	68.58–82.72	0.6235
	End	76.65 (16.65)	68.86–84.44	
LDL (mg/dL)	Baseline	107.80 (38.00)	90.01–125.59	0.0495 *
	End	118.40 (37.51)	100.85–135.95	
Total cholesterol (mg/dL)	Baseline	187.70 (40.59)	168.70–206.70	0.3283
	End	193.05 (37.02)	175.72–210.38	
Triglycerides (mg/dL)	Baseline	76.70 (45.96)	55.19–98.21	0.3505
	End	68.10 (29.52)	54.29–81.91	

CRP = C-reactive Protein, IGF-1 = insulin-like growth factor 1, HDL = high-density lipoprotein, LDL = low-density lipoprotein. * $p < 0.05$, ** $p < 0.01$.

Table 5. Intragroup differences for nutrient intake from baseline to the final examination.

Nutritional Parameter	Time	Mean (Standard Deviation)	(95% Conf. Interval)	Intra-*p*-Value (Baseline vs. End)
Kcal	Baseline	2245.03 (371.00)	2071.40–2418.66	0.7576
	End	2209.53 (561.18)	1956.89–2472.17	
Proteins (g)	Baseline	77.68 (13.15)	71.52–83.83	<0.0001 **
	End	104.54 (20.77)	94.82–114.26	
Fat (g)	Baseline	96.39 (28.23)	83.18–109.61	<0.0001 **
	End	173.38 (56.20)	147.08–199.68	
Carbohydrates (g)	Baseline	230.93 (46.43)	209.20–252.66	<0.0001 **
	End	42.10 (13.18)	35.93–48.27	
Fibre (g)	Baseline	23.72 (6.02)	20.91–26.54	0.9497
	End	23.62 (7.07)	20.31–26.92	
Cholesterol (mg)	Baseline	318.69 (132.90)	256.49–380.89	<0.0001 **
	End	457.04 (120.86)	400.47–513.60	
Saturated fats (g)	Baseline	41.18 (12.11)	35.51–46.85	<0.0001 **
	End	67.30 (25.10)	55.55–79.04	
Monounsaturated fats (g)	Baseline	31.84 (11.12)	26.63–37.04	<0.0001 **
	End	63.01 (22.47)	52.49–73.52	
Polyunsaturated fats (g)	Baseline	13.38 (5.72)	10.71–16.06	<0.0001 **
	End	24.20 (8.69)	20.14–28.27	
Linolenic acid (n-3) (g)	Baseline	1.91 (1.56)	1.18–2.64	0.0036 **
	End	3.71 (2.78)	2.41–5.01	
Linoleic acid (n-6) (g)	Baseline	10.90 (4.44)	8.82–12.98	<0.0001 **
	End	17.44 (7.34)	14.00–20.88	
Eicosapentaenoic acids (EPA) (g)	Baseline	0.05 (0.08)	0.01–0.08	0.0055 **
	End	0.17 (0.15)	0.10–0.24	
Docosahexaenoic acids (DHA) (g)	Baseline	0.13 (0.15)	0.06–0.20	0.0204 *
	End	0.29 (0.24)	0.18–0.40	

* $p < 0.05$, ** $p < 0.01$.

3.2. Regression Analysis

Regarding the age, gender, and oral hygiene behavior parameters (interdental cleaning and use of oral mouthwashes), there were no significant associations to clinical parameters neither at baseline nor in the end. The results of the regression analysis with regard to anthropomorphic parameters, physical activity, serological parameters, and dietary parameters are shown in Table 6. With regard to the clinical inflammatory parameter (GI, BOP), there were significant pro-inflammatory associations to the BMI and fat mass and significantly anti-inflammatory associations to the HDL, fiber, and protein intake. With regard to plaque, there were also significantly positive associations to the BMI and fat mass and significantly negative associations to the MET, HDL, Kcal, and fat and protein intake.

Table 6. Regression coefficients of the linear regression of different parameters on clinical oral parameters at baseline (T1) and at the end of the study period (T2).

	Clinical Oral Parameter									
	PI		GI		PPD		BOP		PISA	
Parameter	T1	T2	T1	T2	T1	T2	T1	T2	T1	T2
BMI	0.053 *	0.064 *	0.052 *	0.032	0.005	0.033 *	0.014 *	0.011	22.323 *	21.807
MET	−0.010 **	−0.006 *	−0.005	−0.004	−0.004	−0.002	−0.001	−0.001	−2.282	−2.472
Fat mass	0.012	0.019 *	0.013	0.006	0.001	0.010 *	0.005 *	0.005	6.902 *	8.312 *
Glucose	−0.014	−0.001	−0.007	−0.008	−0.009	0.001	0.004	0.002	4.451	4.909
CRP	0.009	0.015	0.034	0.014	−0.008	−0.001	0.013	0.002	16.121	2.636
HDL	−0.009	−0.007 *	−0.007	−0.007 *	−0.001	−0.004	−0.001	−0.002	−1.056	−2.867
LDL	0.004	0.003	0.002	0.001	0.001	0.001	0.001	−0.001	1.378	−0.841
Kcal	0.001	−0.001 *	0.001	−0.001	−0.001	−0.001 *	−0.001	−0.001	−0.106	−0.113
CHOs	−0.001	0.001	−0.001	0.001	−0.001	0.001	−0.001	0.001	−1.393 *	1.399
Fat	0.001	−0.003 *	0.001	−0.001	−0.001	−0.002 *	−0.001	−0.001	−0.409	−1.062
Proteins	0.001	−0.007 *	0.005	−0.003	−0.005	−0.005 **	0.001	−0.003 *	−0.081	−3.860 *
Fibre	−0.020	−0.016	−0.014	−0.018 *	−0.005	−0.002	−0.003	−0.005	−7.768	−6.899
EPA	−0.741	0.366	0.237	0.660	0.577	−0.187	0.253	0.102	652.12	91.365
DHA	−0.523	0.247	0.006	0.383	0.224	−0.107	0.138	0.077	358.164	88.329

PI = plaque index; GI = gingival index; PPD = pocket probing depth; BOP = bleeding on probing; PISA = periodontal inflamed surface area; CRP = C-reactive Protein; HDL = high-density lipoprotein, LDL = low-density lipoprotein; BMI = body mass index; MET = metabolic equivalent of task; CHOs = carbohydrates; EPA = Eicosapentaenoic acids; DHA = Docosahexaenoic acids; * $p < 0.05$, ** $p < 0.01$.

4. Discussion

4.1. Changes in Clinical Oral Parameters

The aim of the present study was to exploratively investigate the effects of a very low-carb, ketogenic diet on clinical oral parameters along with serological, anthropomorphic, and nutritional parameters in an uncontrolled clinical trial. The results showed that after six weeks of intervention, there were no significant changes in the clinical oral parameters, except a trend towards lower plaque values. Accordingly, the ketogenic diet did not lead to a worsening nor an increase in periodontal health. This result must be discussed with regard to various factors. First, it must be mentioned that the investigated population consisted of healthy, relatively young volunteers with adequate oral hygiene and low baseline plaque and gingivitis values. The mean GI value of 0.68 represented a value between 0 (=no gingivitis) to 1 (=mild gingivitis), with no participants showing severe gingivitis [28]. Compared to an epidemiological study by Li et al. showing a mean GI-value of 1.06 in a population of 1000 US participants with a comparable mean age of 37.9 years, the investigated population showed less gingivitis. This might be due to continued oral hygiene measures since oral hygiene is very effective in gingivitis reduction [21]. This is in accordance with the presented low mean PI of 0.49, which is in a comparable low range of young, healthy adults evaluated in a German population [29]. With regard to the found trend towards lower plaque values at the end of the study, an additional post hoc power analysis showed that with 20 patients, a difference in PI of 0.2 could have been detected with 80% power and an alpha of 5%.

Against the background of the rather low GI and PI values, the current study setting was both limited to allow a further deterioration due to the high efforts in oral hygiene as well as to show further positive effects on GI since the baseline values were in a low range already. This might be very different to an obese, periodontitis- or gingivitis-affected population. Considering this together, further investigations of ketogenic diets on participants with higher plaque values would be interesting. Baumgartner et al. showed that even under the total absence of oral hygiene for four weeks, participants did experience a stable low level of gingivitis (G = ~0.4) and even a significant decrease in BOP (Δ−12.2%) during a sugar-free stone-age-adapted diet [14]. This is in accordance with a meta-analysis of Hujoel showing a profound gingivitis-decreasing effect when reducing the dietary sugar [11] and previous investigations of our own working group looking at low-carb diets and related gingival effects [12,13]. These studies indicate that the classically assumed correlation between plaque and gingival inflammation might only apply to pro-inflammatory Western diet conditions with high consumption of processed carbohydrates, sugar, saturated fats and animal proteins.

With regard to the study duration and the anticipated quick response of the gingival tissues based on previous findings (within even 4 weeks of intervention), the current study duration of 6 weeks would have been able to show clinical changes [12–14].

Additionally, from a cariogenic point of view, it would be interesting to study the effects of ketogenic diets on the oral microbiome since there is a tremendous lack of interventional studies on sugar-free (or even very low-carb diets) and caries development and/or progression. Behind the background of current theories on caries etiology, the almost total absence of fermentable carbohydrates would not allow any cariogenic shifts in the oral microbiome or demineralization of dental hard tissues [10]. To the best knowledge of the authors, there are only two interventional studies looking at the effects of a sugar-free diet on oral microbiota [30,31]. Both studies showed a significant reduction of the cariogenic strain *Streptococcus mutans* due to the omitted sugar. Translating these results into the practical applications of a ketogenic diet, patients might also benefit from caries protection. This is highly relevant for cancer patients since they are often compromised with xerostomia due to radiation or immunotherapy [32].

4.2. Changes in Non-Oral Parameters

With regard to the anthropomorphic parameters, there was a significant decrease in body weight and BMI. This result is in line with several investigations showing a weight-reducing effect of ketogenic diets [3,6], which is hypothesized to be due to higher rates of resting energy expenditure, lower levels of insulin, and higher satiety [33,34]. Compared to the general German population, this mean weight loss of about 1.9 kg happened in participants with a normal BMI, whereas more than half of the age-matched general population suffers from overweight or obesity [35].

Even if the long-term suitability of ketonic diets has to be questioned, periodontitis patients who are overweight might benefit from the recommendation to at least reduce the intake of processed carbohydrates since being overweight is also a dominant risk factor for periodontal inflammation [36]. Interestingly, in this study, BMI also showed several significant correlations to oral inflammatory parameters such as GI, BOP, and PISA. However, the current ketogenic diet intervention was also accompanied by an increase in serological LDL and total cholesterol levels and an increased intake of saturated fats and dietary cholesterol. This has to be discussed critically since these parameters are not only associated with higher periodontal inflammation but also with general diseases, such as cardiovascular diseases [37,38], and the increase in LDL cholesterol seems to be common in ketogenic diets [9,33]. However, compared to a general Western population, the observed LDL values were still in a low range [38].

With regard to the possible anti-inflammatory properties of omega-3 fatty acids on periodontal inflammation [39], the study could not show any associations. This could be due to the generally low clinical effect previously discussed or to the simultaneous increase in omega-3 and omega-6 fatty acids, whose balance is shown to be an important factor for the clinical effects of omega-3 fatty acids [40]. This factor could be improved in future studies to recommend the intake of mainly plant-derived fats and proteins instead of animal products, which—also within a low-carb diet—would be beneficial to overall health [41]. The recommendations of the current intervention included both animal- and plant-based products and foods. This further differentiation between the sources of macronutrients would also be very important with regard to the effects on the gut microbiome due to the marked difference between the included pre- and probiotics [42].

4.3. Limitations

The study was clearly limited by a low number of participants and a missing control group, which could verify the association of the observed effects to the intervention. However, with regards to the clinical oral effects, it would be unlikely to observe different outcomes under continued oral hygiene measures. Another aspect is that the intervention and control groups can hardly be blinded, which, however, also applies to other dietary studies. On the other side, the intake of non-blinded foods is the condition of real life.

The anthropomorphic effects were all in line with already described effects in the literature. With regard to the serum values, an additional continuous measurement of serum ketosis would be recommended in future studies to ensure the state of ketosis. This should also include pH measurements of the serum and the saliva.

Furthermore, an investigation of the oral microbiome would have allowed a further interpretation of caries- and periodontitis-associated microbiota. This should be included in further studies. Due to the unequal distribution of women and men, future studies might also stratify with regard to gender.

5. Conclusions

The ketogenic dietary change did not lead to clinical changes in periodontal parameters in healthy participants under continued oral hygiene, but it did lead to significant weight loss.

Author Contributions: Conceptualization, J.P.W., C.T., H.B., P.U., and P.R.-K.; methodology, J.P.W., C.T., and K.V.; formal analysis, K.V.; investigation, S.F.E.; resources, P.R.-K.; data curation, S.F.E.; writing—original draft preparation, J.P.W.; writing—review and editing, J.P.W., C.T., H.B., P.R.-K., K.V., and P.U.; visualization, J.P.W.; supervision, J.P.W. and C.T.; project administration, J.P.W.; funding acquisition, P.U., H.B., P.R.-K., and J.P.W. All authors have read and agreed to the published version of the manuscript.

Funding: The study was funded by the German Research Foundation (BE 5760/1-1) and with institutional funds. The article processing charge was funded by the Baden-Wuerttemberg Ministry of Science, Research and Art and the University of Freiburg in the funding programme Open Access Publishing.

Institutional Review Board Statement: The study was conducted according to the guidelines of the Declaration of Helsinki, and approved by the Ethics Committee of the University of Freiburg, Germany (494/14; date of approval: 2016-01-08). The study was registered in an international trial register (German Clinical Trial Register number DRKS00009605).

Informed Consent Statement: Informed consent was obtained from all subjects involved in the study.

Data Availability Statement: The datasets used and/or analyzed during the current study are available from the corresponding author on reasonable request.

Acknowledgments: The authors want to thank Lena Strom and Heidi Mirandola for their support.

Conflicts of Interest: The authors declare no conflict of interest. The funders had no role in the design of the study; in the collection, analyses, or interpretation of data; in the writing of the manuscript; or in the decision to publish the results.

References

1. Veech, R.L. The Therapeutic Implications of Ketone Bodies: The Effects of Ketone Bodies in Pathological Conditions: Ketosis, Ketogenic Diet, Redox States, Insulin Resistance, and Mitochondrial Metabolism. *Prostaglandins Leukot. Essent. Fatty Acids* **2004**, *70*, 309–319. [CrossRef]
2. Freeman, J.M.; Kossoff, E.H.; Hartman, A.L. The Ketogenic Diet: One Decade Later. *Pediatrics* **2007**, *119*, 535–543. [CrossRef]
3. Krieger, J.W.; Sitren, H.S.; Daniels, M.J.; Langkamp-Henken, B. Effects of Variation in Protein and Carbohydrate Intake on Body Mass and Composition during Energy Restriction: A Meta-Regression 1. *Am. J. Clin. Nutr.* **2006**, *83*, 260–274. [CrossRef] [PubMed]
4. Zorn, S.; Ehret, J.; Schäuble, R.; Rautenberg, B.; Ihorst, G.; Bertz, H.; Urbain, P.; Raynor, A. Impact of Modified Short-Term Fasting and Its Combination with a Fasting Supportive Diet during Chemotherapy on the Incidence and Severity of Chemotherapy-Induced Toxicities in Cancer Patients—A Controlled Cross-over Pilot Study. *BMC Cancer* **2020**, *20*, 578. [CrossRef]
5. Fine, E.J.; Segal-Isaacson, C.J.; Feinman, R.D.; Herszkopf, S.; Romano, M.C.; Tomuta, N.; Bontempo, A.F.; Negassa, A.; Sparano, J.A. Targeting Insulin Inhibition as a Metabolic Therapy in Advanced Cancer: A Pilot Safety and Feasibility Dietary Trial in 10 Patients. *Nutr. Burbank Los Angel. Cty. Calif* **2012**, *28*, 1028–1035. [CrossRef]
6. Coleman, J.L.; Carrigan, C.T.; Margolis, L.M. Body Composition Changes in Physically Active Individuals Consuming Ketogenic Diets: A Systematic Review. *J. Int. Soc. Sports Nutr.* **2021**, *18*, 41. [CrossRef] [PubMed]
7. Tragni, E.; Vigna, L.; Ruscica, M.; Macchi, C.; Casula, M.; Santelia, A.; Catapano, A.L.; Magni, P. Reduction of Cardio-Metabolic Risk and Body Weight through a Multiphasic Very-Low Calorie Ketogenic Diet Program in Women with Overweight/Obesity: A Study in a Real-World Setting. *Nutrients* **2021**, *13*, 1804. [CrossRef] [PubMed]
8. Urbain, P.; Strom, L.; Morawski, L.; Wehrle, A.; Deibert, P.; Bertz, H. Impact of a 6-Week Non-Energy-Restricted Ketogenic Diet on Physical Fitness, Body Composition and Biochemical Parameters in Healthy Adults. *Nutr. Metab.* **2017**, *14*, 17. [CrossRef]
9. Burén, J.; Ericsson, M.; Damasceno, N.R.T.; Sjödin, A. A Ketogenic Low-Carbohydrate High-Fat Diet Increases LDL Cholesterol in Healthy, Young, Normal-Weight Women: A Randomized Controlled Feeding Trial. *Nutrients* **2021**, *13*, 814. [CrossRef]
10. Nyvad, B.; Takahashi, N. Integrated Hypothesis of Dental Caries and Periodontal Diseases. *J. Oral Microbiol.* **2020**, *12*, 1710953. [CrossRef] [PubMed]
11. Hujoel, P. Dietary Carbohydrates and Dental-Systemic Diseases. *J. Dent. Res.* **2009**, *88*, 490–502. [CrossRef] [PubMed]
12. Woelber, J.P.; Bremer, K.; Vach, K.; König, D.; Hellwig, E.; Ratka-Krüger, P.; Al-Ahmad, A.; Tennert, C. An Oral Health Optimized Diet Can Reduce Gingival and Periodontal Inflammation in Humans—A Randomized Controlled Pilot Study. *BMC Oral Health* **2016**, *17*, 28. [CrossRef] [PubMed]
13. Woelber, J.P.; Gärtner, M.; Breuninger, L.; Anderson, A.; König, D.; Hellwig, E.; Al-Ahmad, A.; Vach, K.; Dötsch, A.; Ratka-Krüger, P.; et al. The Influence of an Anti-Inflammatory Diet on Gingivitis. A Randomized Controlled Trial. *J. Clin. Periodontol.* **2019**, *46*, 481–490. [CrossRef]
14. Baumgartner, S.; Imfeld, T.; Schicht, O.; Rath, C.; Persson, R.E.; Persson, G.R. The Impact of the Stone Age Diet on Gingival Conditions in the Absence of Oral Hygiene. *J. Periodontol.* **2009**, *80*, 759–768. [CrossRef] [PubMed]
15. Kashket, S.; Van Houte, J.; Lopez, L.R.; Stocks, S. Lack of Correlation between Food Retention on the Human Dentition and Consumer Perception of Food Stickiness. *J. Dent. Res.* **1991**, *70*, 1314–1319. [CrossRef] [PubMed]
16. Woelber, J.P.; Tennert, C. Chapter 13: Diet and Periodontal Diseases. *Monogr. Oral Sci.* **2020**, *28*, 125–133. [CrossRef]
17. Harjola, U.; Liesmaa, H. Effects of Polyol and Sucrose Candies on Plaque, Gingivitis and Lactobacillus Index Scores. Observations on Helsinki School Children. *Acta Odontol. Scand.* **1978**, *36*, 237–242. [CrossRef]
18. Vilarrasa, J.; Peña, M.; Gumbau, L.; Monje, A.; Nart, J. Exploring the Relationship among Dental Caries, Nutritional Habits and Peri-Implantitis. *J. Periodontol.* **2021**, *92*, 1306–1316. [CrossRef]
19. Löe, H.; Theilade, E.; Jensen, S.B. Experimental Gingivitis in Man. *J. Periodontol.* **1965**, *36*, 177–187. [CrossRef]
20. Kassebaum, N.J.; Smith, A.G.C.; Bernabé, E.; Fleming, T.D.; Reynolds, A.E.; Vos, T.; Murray, C.J.L.; Marcenes, W.; GBD 2015 Oral Health Collaborators; Abyu, G.Y.; et al. Global, Regional, and National Prevalence, Incidence, and Disability-Adjusted Life Years for Oral Conditions for 195 Countries, 1990–2015: A Systematic Analysis for the Global Burden of Diseases, Injuries, and Risk Factors. *J. Dent. Res.* **2017**, *96*, 380–387. [CrossRef]
21. O'Neill, B.; Raggi, P. The Ketogenic Diet: Pros and Cons. *Atherosclerosis* **2020**, *292*, 119–126. [CrossRef]
22. Yancy, W.S.; Olsen, M.K.; Dudley, T.; Westman, E.C. Acid-Base Analysis of Individuals Following Two Weight Loss Diets. *Eur. J. Clin. Nutr.* **2007**, *61*, 1416–1422. [CrossRef] [PubMed]
23. Kossoff, E.H.; McGrogan, J.R.; Bluml, R.M.; Pillas, D.J.; Rubenstein, J.E.; Vining, E.P. A Modified Atkins Diet Is Effective for the Treatment of Intractable Pediatric Epilepsy. *Epilepsia* **2006**, *47*, 421–424. [CrossRef] [PubMed]
24. Cervenka, M.C.; Terao, N.N.; Bosarge, J.L.; Henry, B.J.; Klees, A.A.; Morrison, P.F.; Kossoff, E.H. E-Mail Management of the Modified Atkins Diet for Adults with Epilepsy Is Feasible and Effective. *Epilepsia* **2012**, *53*, 728–732. [CrossRef] [PubMed]
25. Urbain, P.; Bertz, H. Monitoring for Compliance with a Ketogenic Diet: What Is the Best Time of Day to Test for Urinary Ketosis? *Nutr. Metab.* **2016**, *13*, 77. [CrossRef]

26. Frey, I.; Berg, A.; Grathwohl, D.; Keul, J. Freiburg Questionnaire of physical activity–development, evaluation and application. *Soz. Praventivmed.* **1999**, *44*, 55–64. [CrossRef]
27. Nesse, W.; Abbas, F.; van der Ploeg, I.; Spijkervet, F.K.L.; Dijkstra, P.U.; Vissink, A. Periodontal Inflamed Surface Area: Quantifying Inflammatory Burden. *J. Clin. Periodontol.* **2008**, *35*, 668–673. [CrossRef]
28. Loe, H.; Silness, J. Periodontal disease in pregnancy. i. prevalence and severity. *Acta Odontol. Scand.* **1963**, *21*, 533–551. [CrossRef]
29. Jockel-Schneider, Y.; Schlagenhauf, U.; Petsos, H.; Rüttermann, S.; Schmidt, J.; Ziebolz, D.; Wehner, C.; Laky, M.; Rott, T.; Noack, M.; et al. Impact of 0.1% Octenidine Mouthwash on Plaque Re-Growth in Healthy Adults: A Multi-Center Phase 3 Randomized Clinical Trial. *Clin. Oral Investig.* **2021**, *25*, 4681–4689. [CrossRef]
30. Kristoffersson, K.; Birkhed, D. Effects of Partial Sugar Restriction for 6 Weeks on Numbers of Streptococcus Mutans in Saliva and Interdental Plaque in Man. *Caries Res.* **1987**, *21*, 79–86. [CrossRef] [PubMed]
31. Wennerholm, K.; Birkhed, D.; Emilson, C.G. Effects of Sugar Restriction on Streptococcus Mutans and Streptococcus Sobrinus in Saliva and Dental Plaque. *Caries Res.* **1995**, *29*, 54–61. [CrossRef]
32. Bustillos, H.; Indorf, A.; Alwan, L.; Thompson, J.; Jung, L. Xerostomia: An immunotherapy-related adverse effect in cancer patients. *Support Care Cancer* **2021**. Epub ahead of print. [CrossRef] [PubMed]
33. Bueno, N.B.; de Melo, I.S.V.; de Oliveira, S.L.; da Rocha Ataide, T. Very-Low-Carbohydrate Ketogenic Diet v. Low-Fat Diet for Long-Term Weight Loss: A Meta-Analysis of Randomised Controlled Trials. *Br. J. Nutr.* **2013**, *110*, 1178–1187. [CrossRef]
34. Westman, E.C.; Feinman, R.D.; Mavropoulos, J.C.; Vernon, M.C.; Volek, J.S.; Wortman, J.A.; Yancy, W.S.; Phinney, S.D. Low-Carbohydrate Nutrition and Metabolism. *Am. J. Clin. Nutr.* **2007**, *86*, 276–284. [CrossRef] [PubMed]
35. *14. DGE Ernährungsbericht*; Deutsche Gesellschaft für Ernährung: Bonn, Germany, 2020.
36. Martinez-Herrera, M.; Silvestre-Rangil, J.; Silvestre, F.-J. Association between Obesity and Periodontal Disease. A Systematic Review of Epidemiological Studies and Controlled Clinical Trials. *Med. Oral Patol. Oral Cir. Bucal* **2017**, *22*, e708–e715. [CrossRef]
37. Nepomuceno, R.; Pigossi, S.C.; Finoti, L.S.; Orrico, S.R.P.; Cirelli, J.A.; Barros, S.P.; Offenbacher, S.; Scarel-Caminaga, R.M. Serum Lipid Levels in Patients with Periodontal Disease: A Meta-Analysis and Meta-Regression. *J. Clin. Periodontol.* **2017**, *44*, 1192–1207. [CrossRef] [PubMed]
38. Fernández-Friera, L.; Fuster, V.; López-Melgar, B.; Oliva, B.; García-Ruiz, J.M.; Mendiguren, J.; Bueno, H.; Pocock, S.; Ibáñez, B.; Fernández-Ortiz, A.; et al. Normal LDL-Cholesterol Levels Are Associated With Subclinical Atherosclerosis in the Absence of Risk Factors. *J. Am. Coll. Cardiol.* **2017**, *70*, 2979–2991. [CrossRef] [PubMed]
39. Kruse, A.B.; Kowalski, C.D.; Leuthold, S.; Vach, K.; Ratka-Krüger, P.; Woelber, J.P. What Is the Impact of the Adjunctive Use of Omega-3 Fatty Acids in the Treatment of Periodontitis? A Systematic Review and Meta-Analysis. *Lipids Health Dis.* **2020**, *19*, 100. [CrossRef]
40. Simopoulos, A.P. An Increase in the Omega-6/Omega-3 Fatty Acid Ratio Increases the Risk for Obesity. *Nutrients* **2016**, *8*, 128. [CrossRef]
41. Fung, T.T.; van Dam, R.M.; Hankinson, S.E.; Stampfer, M.; Willett, W.C.; Hu, F.B. Low-Carbohydrate Diets and All-Cause and Cause-Specific Mortality: Two Cohort Studies. *Ann. Intern. Med.* **2010**, *153*, 289–298. [CrossRef]
42. Gentile, C.L.; Weir, T.L. The Gut Microbiota at the Intersection of Diet and Human Health. *Science* **2018**, *362*, 776–780. [CrossRef] [PubMed]

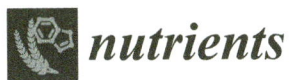

nutrients

MDPI

Article

Radiographic Bone Loss and Its Relation to Patient-Specific Risk Factors, LDL Cholesterol, and Vitamin D: A Cross-Sectional Study

Teresa Thim [1,2], Konstantin Johannes Scholz [1], Karl-Anton Hiller [1], Wolfgang Buchalla [1], Christian Kirschneck [3], Jonathan Fleiner [4], Johan Peter Woelber [5,†] and Fabian Cieplik [1,*,†]

1   Department of Conservative Dentistry and Periodontology, University Hospital Regensburg, 93053 Regensburg, Germany; teresa.thim@web.de (T.T.); konstantin.scholz@ukr.de (K.J.S.); karl-anton.hiller@ukr.de (K.-A.H.); wolfgang.buchalla@ukr.de (W.B.)
2   Private Practice, 63110 Rodgau, Germany
3   Department of Orthodontics, University Hospital Regensburg, 93053 Regensburg, Germany; christian.kirschneck@ukr.de
4   Center of Dental Implantology, Periodontology and 3D-Imaging, 78462 Konstanz, Germany; fleiner@stricker-fleiner.de
5   Department of Operative Dentistry and Periodontology, Faculty of Medicine, University of Freiburg, 79085 Freiburg, Germany; johan.woelber@uniklinik-freiburg.de
*   Correspondence: fabian.cieplik@ukr.de
†   These authors contributed equally to this work.

Citation: Thim, T.; Scholz, K.J.; Hiller, K.-A.; Buchalla, W.; Kirschneck, C.; Fleiner, J.; Woelber, J.P.; Cieplik, F. Radiographic Bone Loss and Its Relation to Patient-Specific Risk Factors, LDL Cholesterol, and Vitamin D: A Cross-Sectional Study. *Nutrients* **2022**, *14*, 864. https://doi.org/10.3390/nu14040864

Academic Editor: Maria Luz Fernandez

Received: 14 January 2022
Accepted: 16 February 2022
Published: 18 February 2022

Publisher's Note: MDPI stays neutral with regard to jurisdictional claims in published maps and institutional affiliations.

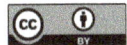
Abstract: The influence of patient-specific factors such as medical conditions, low-density lipoprotein cholesterol (LDL-C) or levels of 25-hydroxyvitamin D (25OHD) on periodontal diseases is frequently discussed in the literature. Therefore, the aim of this retrospective cross-sectional study was to evaluate potential associations between radiographic bone loss (RBL) and patient-specific risk factors, particularly LDL-C and 25OHD levels. Patients from a dental practice, who received full-mouth cone beam CTs (CBCTs) and blood-sampling in the course of implant treatment planning, were included in this study. RBL was determined at six sites per tooth from CBCT data. LDL-C and 25OHD levels were measured from venous blood samples. Other patient-specific risk factors were assessed based on anamnesis and dental charts. Statistical analysis was performed applying non-parametric procedures (Mann–Whitney U tests, error rates method). Data from 163 patients could be included in the analysis. RBL was significantly higher in male patients, older age groups, smokers, patients with high DMFT (decayed/missing/filled teeth) score, lower number of teeth, and high LDL-C levels ($\geq$160 mg/dL). Furthermore, patients with high 25OHD levels ($\geq$40 ng/mL) exhibited significantly less RBL. In summary, RBL was found to be associated with known patient-specific markers, particularly with age and high LDL-C levels.

Keywords: periodontal; bone loss; LDL; vitamin D; CBCT; radiographic bone loss

1. Introduction

Periodontal diseases are among the most prevalent non-communicable diseases in mankind with 1.1 billion prevalent cases of severe periodontitis worldwide according to the Global Burden of Disease 2019 study [1,2]. In Germany, 51.6% of younger adults (35–44 years) and 64.6% of younger seniors (65–74 years) are affected by moderate to severe periodontal disease, as reported in the 5th German Oral Health study (DMS V) [3].

The pathogenesis of periodontal diseases is associated with the presence of subgingival biofilms and considered to be based on a host-mediated dysbiosis of the oral microbiota due to an exaggerated response of the host immune system resulting in a loss of periodontal supporting tissues [4–6]. General medical conditions such as diabetes mellitus or habits like smoking are associated with periodontal disease [7,8]. Recently, also metabolic disorders as well as systemic inflammation were discussed in literature as a risk of causing or accelerating periodontal bone loss [9].

One of these recently discussed conditions is hypercholesterolemia, and in particular high levels of low-density lipoprotein cholesterol (LDL-C) [10]. Hypercholesterolemia is a common phenomenon, and epidemiological data show that increased LDL-C levels ($\geq$130 mg/dL) were prevalent in 29.4% of American adults [11]. High serum levels of LDL-C are often accompanied with a diet high in saturated or trans fats and sugar, physical inactivity, smoking, obesity, type 2 diabetes mellitus, and high blood pressure [12,13]. High LDL-C levels are also a main risk factor for atherosclerotic cardiovascular diseases [14], which represented the leading cause of death among US-Americans in 2017 [11].

Another condition, which was lately brought into focus in context with periodontitis and radiographic bone loss, is vitamin D deficiency [15,16]. Serum levels of 25-hydroxy vitamin D (25OHD), which is an intermediate product in vitamin D metabolism, lower than 20 ng/mL are defined as deficiency [17]. 25OHD deficiency is a widespread condition around the world, especially in northern regions [18], since vitamin D is mostly synthetized in the skin if exposed to sunlight, while just a little part is supplied by nutrition, e.g., by consumption of oily fish [17]. There are several health benefits known which are associated with sufficient 25OHD levels as vitamin D is important for an adequate bone mineralization and for various functions of the immune system [19,20] as well as there is a reduced risk for cardiovascular diseases [21] or cancer [22].

There are some investigations about increased LDL-C and decreased 25OHD levels within periodontitis-patients compared to healthy controls [16,23–28]. However, to the best of the authors' knowledge, there is no study investigating on a "healthy" cross-section of daily dental patients and evaluating potential risk factors for periodontal bone loss using a highly validated method such as cone beam CTs.

Against this background, the aim of this retrospective cross-sectional study was to investigate associations between radiographic bone loss (RBL) and patient-specific general health parameters, particularly levels of LDL-C and 25OHD, in a cohort of patients treated in a private dental practice. The null-hypothesis tested was that levels of LDL-C or 25OHD, respectively, were not associated with RBL.

2. Materials and Methods

2.1. Study Design

The present study was designed as a retrospective cross-sectional study. The objective was to evaluate RBL according to patient-specific parameters including sex, age, smoking history, DMFT (decayed/missing/filled teeth) score, number of teeth, LDL-C, and 25OHD levels. Data were collected from a cohort of patients who received treatment planning for dental implants in a private practice.

The study design was approved by the internal review board of the University of Regensburg, Germany (reference: 21-2431-104; issued on 23 June 2021) in accordance with the 1964 Helsinki Declaration and its later amendments and comparable ethical standards. The study was registered at the German Clinical Trials Register (ref: DRKS00025827).

2.2. Patient Population

All patients from the patient pool of a private practice in Rodgau (Hessen, Germany), who had received a cone beam CT (CBCT) as well as analysis of LDL-C and 25OHD levels in the course of treatment planning for dental implants between February 2017 and October 2020 were screened for inclusion in this study. Patients were excluded if they had less than 16 teeth [29] or in case of insufficient CBCT quality. No other exclusion criteria were applied.

2.3. Medical and Dental History

A detailed anamnesis of the medical history and intake of medications was obtained from the dental charts and anamnesis forms, and if necessary, complemented by telephone interviews. Smoking history was recorded as pack-years (PY), which were calculated by multiplying the number of packs of cigarettes smoked per day by the number of years the person has smoked [30]. Additionally, the intake of statins or vitamin D supplementation was checked. Dental charts were checked for numbers of teeth and teeth were charted as decayed, missing, or filled (DMFT index) according to the clinical oral examination prior to the implant treatment planning, which was double-checked with the CBCT radiographs.

2.4. Radiographic Examination

All CBCTs were conducted with the medical indication of treatment planning for dental implants as full-mouth CBCTs (Orthophos XG 3D, Dentsply-Sirona, Bensheim, Germany). The field of view was set to 8 × 8 cm, voxel size was 160 μm, scan time was 5.1 s, the voltage was 85 kV, and the current was 7 mA.

For evaluation of the radiographic bone loss (RBL), the software package CoPeri-odontiX 9.9 (Dental Wings, Chemnitz, Germany) was used [31]. For each patient, all teeth except the third molars were measured. RBL was defined as distance between alveolar crest (AC) and cemento-enamel junction (CEJ) or restoration margin (RM) in cases of teeth with restorations (e.g., crowns) on six sites per tooth (mesio-buccal, buccal, disto-buccal, mesio-oral, oral, disto-oral). For measurement of RBL, every single tooth was manually positioned three-dimensionally according to its longitudinal axis and its CEJ or RM. After adjusting, CEJ or RM and AC had to be marked on six aspects of the tooth so that RBL could be calculated by the program. Figure 1 shows the workflow for determining RBL in the program package.

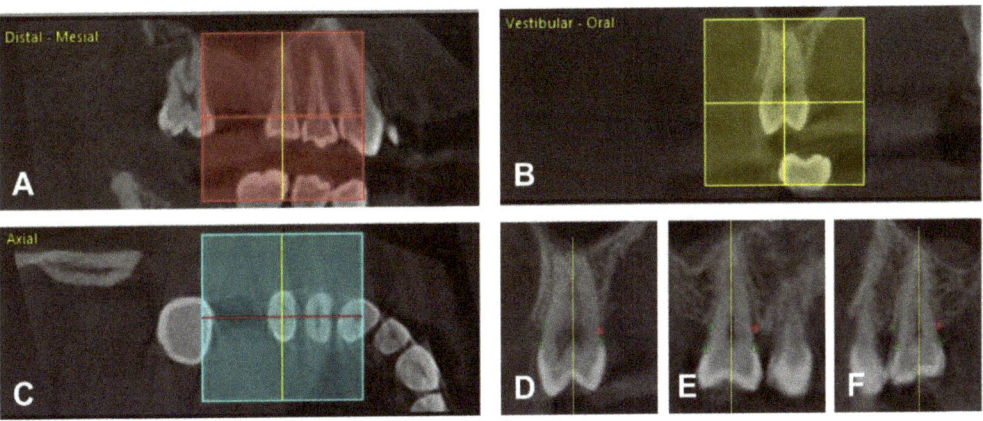

Figure 1. (**A–C**) Tooth selection and positioning. Tooth 15 in a distal-mesial (**A**), vestibular-oral (**B**), and axial (**C**) plane. The crosshair is positioned according to the longitudinal axis and CEJ or RM (**A,B**) and parallel to the cross-axis of the tooth (**C**). Every single tooth was selected and adjusted manually. (**D–F**) Setting the reference points. The yellow line marks the longitudinal axis of tooth 15. It is presented in three different cross-sections, oral/vestibular (**D**), vestibular-distal/oral-mesial (**E**), and vestibular-mesial/oral-distal (**F**). Twelve reference points per tooth (as depicted in green and red color) were set on the CEJ or RM and AC for each side. The red dot marks the AC oral (**D**), oral-mesial (**E**), and oral-distal (**F**). The software measures RBL by calculating the distance between the dots.

All CBCTs were examined by one examiner (TT), who had been extensively trained by an expert (JF). For validation of the accuracy of the RBL measurements, ten randomly chosen CBCTs were re-evaluated and differences between the first and second measurement were assessed for intra-examiner agreement.

2.5. LDL-C and 25OHD Levels

All evaluations of serum LDL-C and 25OHD were conducted in the course of treatment planning for dental implants. Two venous blood samples (2 mL each) were taken in a fasting state by a trained examiner from the basilic vein. The samples were sent to a specialized and accredited laboratory (Institut für medizinische Diagnostik, Berlin, Germany) for evaluation of serum levels of LDL-C and 25OHD. LDL-C levels were determined by enzymatic tests and the physical unit was mg/dL. For evaluation of 25OHD, electrochemiluminescence immunoassay (ECLIA) was conducted and 25OHD levels were measured in ng/mL. All LDL-C and 25OHD data were retrieved retrospectively from the dental charts.

2.6. Data Analysis

The maximum of the six RBL values per tooth was determined as the descriptive value for each tooth. The median of these maxima over all existing teeth of a patient except third molars was used as the RBL value of a patient for analysis. From all patients, medians including first and third quartiles from RBL values were calculated.

Patients were categorized, as follows: Three age groups were formed ($\leq$44 years; 45–59 years; $\geq$60 years). Smoking history was differentiated in "non-smokers", "smokers with $\leq$15 PY", and "smokers with $\geq$16 PY". For DMFT score and number of teeth, the patients were divided in four groups ($\leq$11; 12–18; 19–23; $\geq$24) or two groups ($\leq$24; $\geq$25), respectively. LDL-C levels were subdivided as "optimal" LDL-C ($\leq$99 mg/dL), "near optimal" LDL-C (100–129 mg/dL), "borderline high" LDL-C (130–159 mg/dL) and "high" LDL-C ($\geq$160 mg/dL) according to the U.S. National Cholesterol Education Program [32]. 25OHD levels were categorized as "deficiency" ($\leq$19 ng/mL), "insufficiency" (20–29 ng/mL), "sufficiency" (30–39 ng/mL), and "optimal" ($\geq$40 ng/mL) [17,19].

For analysis of RBL categorized to the different LDL-C groups, patients reporting intake of statins were excluded (n = 5). Accordingly, patients who reported supplementing vitamin D were excluded for RBL analyses categorized to the different 25OHD groups (n = 46).

Differences among experimental groups for matching parameters were evaluated statistically using non-parametric Mann-Whitney U tests on a significance level of α = 0.05. For evaluation of a general influence of a given parameter on all groups, the level of significance was adjusted to $\alpha^*(k) = 1 - (1 - \alpha)^{1/k}$ (k = number of pairwise tests) according to the error rates method, yielding an $\alpha^*(3)$ = 0.01695423 and an $\alpha^*(6)$ = 0.00851244 for three or six pairwise tests (i.e., three or four categorized groups), respectively [33]. All statistical analyses were performed using SPSS for Windows, version 26 (SPSS Inc., Chicago, IL, USA).

RBL, age, and LDL-C or 25OHD levels, respectively, were put into a three-dimensional curve-fitting model and depicted accordingly. TableCurve 3D automated surface fitting analysis software (SYSTAT Software Inc., Systat Software Inc, San Jose, CA, USA; version 4.0) was used to find equations to describe the three-dimensional empirical data.

3. Results

3.1. Patient Population

CBCTs, LDL-C, and 25OHD levels were available from 178 patients. Twelve patients with less than 16 teeth were excluded. Three patients were excluded because quality of CBCT was too poor for further analysis (extensive artifacts due to metal-based restorations). A total of 163 patients could be included in this study.

The patient cohort comprised 100 females (61.3%) and 63 males (38.7%), the median (first; third quartile) age was 53 (44; 62) years and 80.4% were non-smokers. All patients exhibited in median (first; third quartile) 25 (22; 27) teeth, a DMFT score of 19 (14; 22), LDL-C level of 127 (107; 156) mg/dL, and 25OHD level of 29 (20; 43) ng/mL (Table 1). Median (first; third quartile) period of time between the CBCT and taking of the blood samples was 15 (1; 50) days. Figure 2 shows the flow of patients through the stages of this study.

Table 1. Patient characteristics (DMFT score, number of teeth, LDL-C, 25OHD). Depiction of medians (first; third quartiles) and statistically significant differences from pairwise comparisons (Mann–Whitney U tests; $\alpha = 0.05$).

	All Patients	$\leq$44 Years	45–59 Years	$\geq$ 60 Years	$\leq$44 vs. 45–59	$\leq$44 vs. $\geq$60	45–59 vs. $\geq$60
DMFT score §	19 (14; 22)	14.5 (11; 19)	18 (14; 20)	21 (18.3; 23)	0.025	0.000	0.000
Number of teeth §	25 (22; 27)	27 (24.8; 28)	25 (22.5; 27)	23 (19.3; 25)	0.005	0.000	0.002
LDL-C § [mg/dL]	127 (107; 156)	109.5 (91.3; 127.5)	132 (113; 151.5)	146.5 (118.3; 174.3)	0.000	0.000	0.028
25OHD [ng/mL]	29 (20; 42)	27.5 (19.8; 40)	30 (19.5; 47)	30 (20.5; 39)	–	–	–

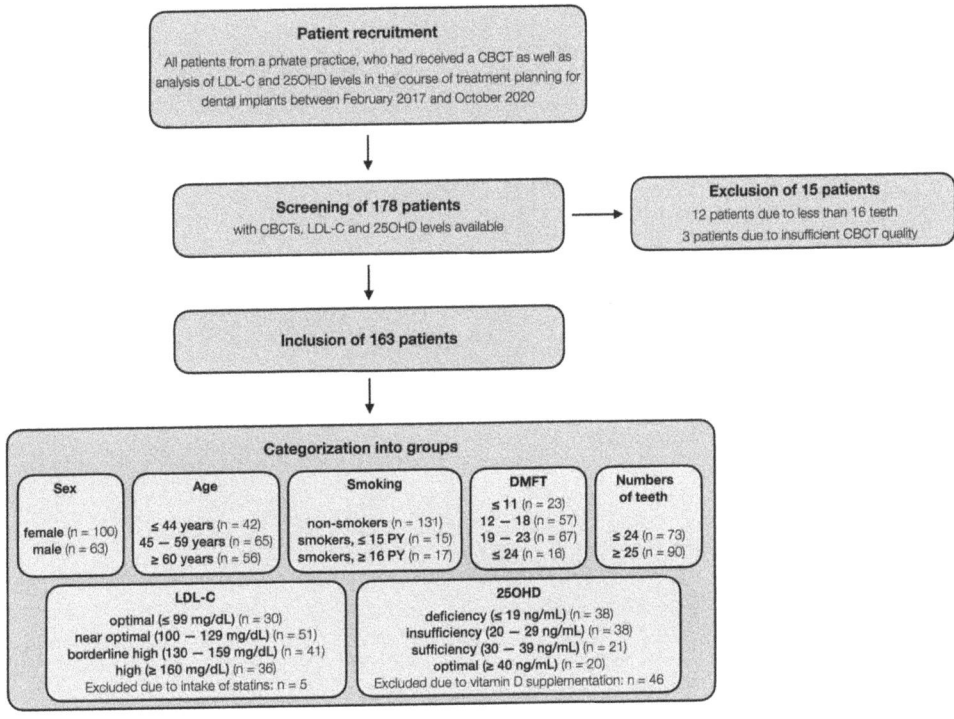

Figure 2. The chart depicts the flow of patients through the stages of this study.

For evaluation of the general influence of age on a given parameter, α was adjusted according to the error rates method to $\alpha^*(3) = 0.01695243$. *p*-value: pairwise significant difference ($p \leq 0.05$); —: no pairwise significant difference; § significant influence of age groups on the respective parameter according to the error rates method.

Table 1 shows DMFT score, number of teeth, LDL-C and 25OHD categorized according to the distinct age groups. According to the error rates method, all age groups showed statistically significant differences with regard to DMFT score, number of teeth, and LDL-C. DMFT score and LDL-C were significantly higher, and number of teeth was significantly lower in older age groups as compared to younger age groups. For 25OHD, there were no statistically significant differences among the age groups.

3.2. RBL

The RBL validation measurements revealed a median (first; third quartile) difference between the first and second measurements of −0.1 (−0.3; 0.1) mm, thus showing sufficient intra-examiner accuracy. Median (first; third quartile) RBL was 3.6 (3.2; 4.2) mm for all patients (Figure 3A). Females had significantly smaller median RBL (3.5 mm) than males (3.8 mm; *p* = 0.026; Figure 3A).

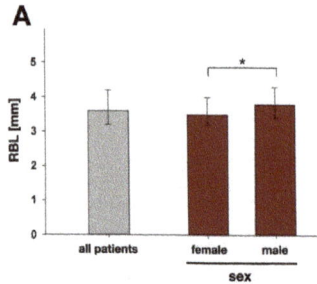 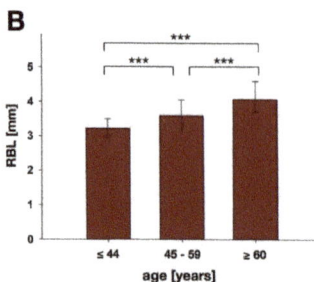 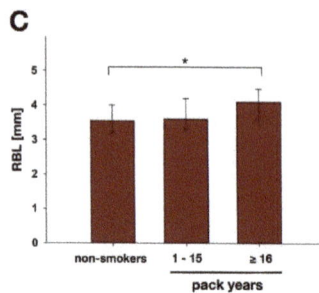

Figure 3. Results of RBL analysis for (**A**) all patients (*n* = 163) and divided into male (*n* = 63) and female (*n* = 100) and according to (**B**) the different age-groups (≤44 y, *n*= 42; 45–59 y, *n* = 65; ≥60 y, *n* = 56) and (**C**) smoking groups (non-smokers, *n* = 131; 1–15 py, *n* = 15; ≥16 py, *n* = 17). Results are depicted as medians, first and third quartiles and asterisks depict statistically significant differences between the groups. * marks significant differences with *p* ≤ 0.05; *** marks significant differences with *p* ≤ 0.001.

Patients ≤ 44 years showed significantly smaller median RBL (3.2 mm) than patients between 45 and 59 years (3.6 mm) and patients ≥ 60 years (4.1 mm). The differences in RBL were statistically significant between all age groups (*p* = 0.000 in all cases; Figure 3B) and accordingly, there was a general influence of the parameter age on RBL according to the error rates method.

Smokers reporting a smoking history of ≥16 PY had significantly higher median RBL values (4.1 mm) than non-smokers (3.6 mm; *p* = 0.029; Figure 3C). There were no significant differences between the two smoking groups or between the non-smokers and the smoking group with 1–15 PY.

DMFT score analysis showed that RBL increased with DMFT (Figure 4A). Patients with DMFT score ≤ 11 showed significantly smaller median RBL (3.5 mm) as compared to patients with DMFT score between 19 and 23 (3.8 mm; *p* = 0.036) and patients with DMFT score ≥ 24 (4.0 mm; *p* = 0.019). Likewise, patients with DMFT score between 12 and 18 showed significantly smaller median RBL (3.5 mm) than those with DMFT score ≥ 24 (*p* = 0.020). It was also found that patients with 24 teeth and less had significantly higher median RBL (3.9 mm) than the ones with ≥25 teeth (3.5 mm; *p* = 0.000), as shown in Figure 4B.

Figure 5 shows RBL according to LDL-C (Figure 5A) and 25OHD groups (Figure 5B). Patients with high LDL-C (≥160 mg/dL) showed significantly higher median RBL (3.9 mm) than those with optimal (≤99 mg/dL; 3.4 mm; *p* = 0.000), near optimal (100–129 mg/dL; 3.5 mm; *p* = 0.009) and borderline high LDL-C (130–159 mg/dL; 3.7 mm; *p* = 0.033). Accordingly, the error rates method revealed a general influence of the parameter LDL-C on RBL. Patients with optimal 25OHD (≥40 ng/mL) showed significantly lower median RBL (3.4 mm) than those with deficient (≤19 ng/mL; 3.6 mm; *p* = 0.029) and sufficient 25OHD (30–39 ng/mL; 3.8 mm; *p* = 0.031). No general influence of the parameter 25OHD on RBL was detected by the error rates method.

RBL, age, and LDL-C or 25OHD levels, respectively, were put into a three-dimensional curve-fitting model and depicted accordingly. When depicting age and LDL-C, Figure 6A shows an irreducible influence of both parameters on RBL. When depicting age and 25OHD, Figure 6B shows that RBL is mainly influenced by age but not by 25OHD levels.

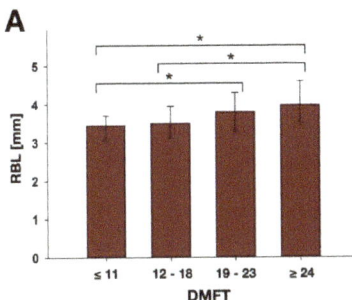

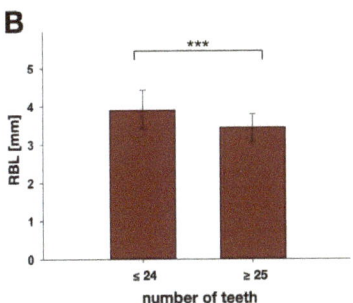

Figure 4. Results of RBL analysis according to (**A**) the different DMFT score groups ($\leq$11, $n = 23$; 12–18, $n = 57$; 19–23, $n = 67$; $\geq$24, $n = 16$) and (**B**) number of teeth ($\leq$24, $n = 73$; $\geq$25, $n = 90$). Results are depicted as medians, first and third quartiles and asterisks depict statistically significant differences between the groups. * marks significant differences with $p \leq 0.05$; *** marks significant differences with $p \leq 0.001$.

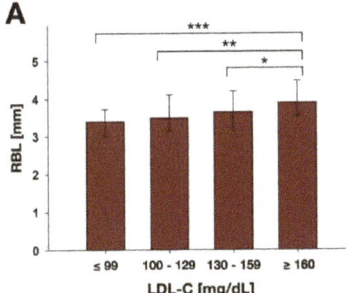

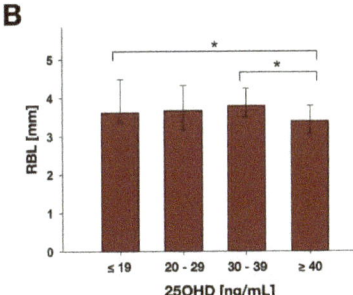

Figure 5. Results of RBL analysis according to the different (**A**) LDL-C groups ($\leq$99, $n = 30$; 100–129, $n = 51$; 130–159, $n = 41$; $\geq$160, $n = 36$) and (**B**) 25OHD groups ($\leq$19, $n = 38$; 20–29, $n = 38$; 30–39, $n = 21$; $\geq$40, $n = 20$). Results are depicted as medians, first and third quartiles and asterisks depict statistically significant differences between the groups. * marks significant differences with $p \leq 0.05$; ** marks significant differences with $p \leq 0.01$; *** marks significant differences with $p \leq 0.001$.

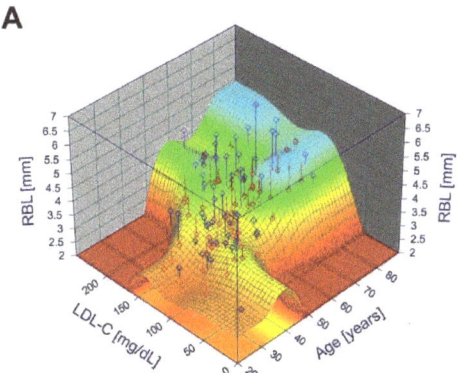

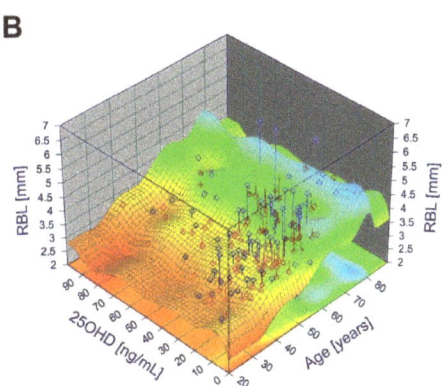

Figure 6. Influence of age and LDL-C or 25OHD levels, respectively, on RBL as fitted three-dimensional curves. (**A**) Influence of age and LDL-C level on RBL as fitted three-dimensional curve (Cosine Series Bivariate Order 5; $r^2 = 0.44$). (**B**) Influence of age and 25OHD level on RBL as fitted three-dimensional curve (Fourier Series Simple Order 2×4; $r^2 = 0.37$).

4. Discussion

The aim of the present study was to investigate potential associations between RBL and patient-specific parameters like sex, age, smoking history, DMFT score, number of teeth, LDL-C, and 25OHD in a cohort of patients, who received treatment planning for dental implants. Focusing on RBL as reference value allowed evaluation of the accumulated history of periodontal destruction and reflected a longer period of time, regardless of the current state of clinical periodontal health.

The data of our study showed that there were significantly higher RBLs in males and in the older age groups, which is in line with other studies. Helmi et al. also evaluated radiographic alveolar bone loss in a cohort-study and revealed significant higher RBLs in men and older age groups [34]. Eke et al. found a higher prevalence of periodontal disease in men as well as an increasing prevalence of periodontitis in the older age groups [35]. Aging is accompanied with modifications of the host immune response, which leads to greater susceptibility to infections and autoimmunity [36]. The higher RBL in males may be explained since men may be less attentive to their (oral) health and consequently may exhibit worse oral hygiene levels, leading to higher RBLs [37]. Furthermore, the immune response is different in men and women, whereby men show higher levels of pro-inflammatory cytokines during infections [37,38].

Furthermore, RBL was also found to be significantly higher in smokers with ≥ 16 PY compared to non-smokers. A similar outcome could be found in other studies, which had measured radiographic alveolar bone loss [34,39]. Smoking is known as a risk factor for onset and progression of periodontitis [40,41] and has also been included as grade modifier in the 2018 classification of periodontal diseases [42]. Smoking is known to impair the host response to the dental plaque biofilm and to be linked to increased levels of potentially destructive inflammatory cytokines and enzymes [43]. Furthermore, smoking diminishes the reparative capacity of periodontal cells, including fibroblasts, osteoblasts and cementoblasts, thus potentially resulting in a higher RBL in smokers [43].

The patient cohort investigated in the present study exhibited a median DMFT score of 19 with a median number of 25 teeth per patient, which clearly outnumbers the results reported in the fifth German Oral Health study for the respective age groups (mean DMFT score of 11.2 or 17.7 for age groups 35–44 or 65–74, respectively) [3]. The reason might be the fact that the investigated cohort were seeking for treatment with dental implants. The older age groups showed significantly higher DMFT score, significantly lower number of teeth, and significantly higher RBL than patients from the other groups. To the best of the authors' knowledge, there has been no other study investigating RBL and DMFT score or numbers of teeth. Levin et al. evaluated the DMFT score and number of missing teeth in periodontitis patients compared to healthy controls [44]. They did not find statistically significant differences regarding DMFT scores but did find a significantly higher number of missing teeth in periodontitis patients. Strauss et al. and Mattila et al. investigated the co-occurrence of periodontitis and caries and found significantly higher numbers of decayed teeth in patients with periodontitis [45,46]. Tooth loss represents the end stage of oral diseases such as periodontitis or caries, thus representing an objective marker for the accumulated inflammatory burden of oral disease. Therefore, there may be common risk factors for caries, periodontitis, and tooth loss such as nutrition, limitations in oral hygiene, and not seeking dental treatment [45].

Pre-conditions such as high LDL-C levels or insufficient levels of 25OHD may be linked to higher RBL [10,15]. Median LDL-C was 127 mg/dL in the patient cohort. According to Virani et al. mean LDL-C among American adults was 112.1 mg/dL and prevalence of LDL-C levels ≥ 130 mg/dL was 29.4% [11]. In our study, 47.9% were found to have LDL-C levels ≥ 130 mg/dL. Thus, the investigated patient cohort had slightly higher values of LDL-C than the average population. As found by Waskiewicz et al., patients suffering from tooth loss and thus seeking for treatment with dental implants might have higher LDL-C values [47]. Significantly higher LDL-C levels were found in the older patient groups which is in line with the literature [48,49], and may be due to an age-associated loss of hepatic

LDL receptors, higher body-mass index, larger waist circumference and lower sex hormone levels [49].

LDL-C was found to have a significant influence on RBL according to the error rates method and the high LDL-C group ($\geq$160 mg/dL) exhibited significantly higher RBL than all other groups in pairwise comparisons. Due to the general influence of age groups on LDL-C as well as RBL according to the error rates method, it cannot be clarified entirely from the data of this study which of both parameters had the bigger influence on RBL (see Figure 6A). However, there are a few more studies, which reported significant associations between high LDL-C and periodontitis when investigating clinical parameters [23–26]. Furthermore, a meta-analysis and meta-regression concluded that periodontitis patients had significantly higher levels of LDL-C [10]. Conversely, Monteiro et al. and Saxlin et al. did not find any significant differences between periodontitis patients and healthy control patients regarding levels of LDL-C [50,51]. Potential associations between LDL-C and periodontal status can be discussed in two ways. The presence of a periodontal infection negatively affects serum lipid levels by an altered immune cell function which leads to a dysregulation of the lipid metabolism [23,52]. On the other hand, high LDL-C levels lead to an increase in periodontal destruction because of an activation of osteoclasts and inhibition of osteoblasts [53] and by the release of pro-inflammatory cytokines [8,54]. Furthermore, higher LDL-C values can be interpreted as a marker of disease-promoting lifestyles, which primarily lead to a higher periodontal inflammation [12,55]. There are also common gen polymorphisms, which are risk factors for both diseases, periodontal disease and hyperlipidemia [56].

The median 25OHD level was 29 ng/mL in the present study, and 23.9% of all patients showed vitamin D deficiency ($\leq$19 ng/mL). Another German investigation found median 25OHD of 44.9 mmol/L, which correspond to 18 ng/mL, and 57.3% of 3,917 subjects were found to be deficient of 25OHD [57]. We found no notable difference regarding 25OHD levels between the different age groups, which is in line with the literature [58,59].

RBL was found to be significantly higher in patients with "deficient" 25OHD levels found as compared to patients with "optimal" ($\geq$40 ng/mL) 25OHD levels. These results are in line with a recently published systematic review and meta-analysis concluding that periodontitis is associated with lower 25OHD levels [15]. This concurs with the known bone-protective effect of higher 25OHD levels, which have been shown to decrease the ratio of RANKL to OPG expression by periodontal ligament fibroblasts controlling osteoclastogenesis [60]. Ketharanathan et al. focused on radiographic bone loss in their cohort study to investigate the impact of 25OHD levels in periodontitis patients. They found that patients with periodontal disease comprised higher radiographic alveolar bone loss (as measured on bitewing radiographs) and lower 25OHD which corresponds to our findings [16]. In another study, clinical attachment loss was evaluated and compared to 25OHD levels [58]. There was significantly less attachment loss in patients with high 25OHD levels, but only in the older age group ($\geq$60 years) [58], which matches with the results from the present study, where age definitely had a higher influence on RBL than 25OHD levels, as depicted in Figure 6B. Similar results have also been shown by other studies [27,28]. Noteworthy, Perić et al. found a tendency for better healing outcomes following non-surgical periodontal therapy in patients who took vitamin D as a supplement than in patients without vitamin D supplementation [61]. There are two potential ways that vitamin D may affect the periodontal status. First, there are effects on bone mineral density especially in the elderly [62], and second, vitamin D may reduce gingival inflammation through anti-inflammatory effects on the general host immune response [15,63,64]. In addition, low salivary levels of 25OHD were found to be associated with higher levels of inflammatory biomarkers in periodontitis patients [65]. Furthermore, there is evidence that vitamin D supplementation reduces systemic inflammation and levels of pro-inflammatory salivary cytokines [66,67] and gingival bleeding [64], whereas vitamin D deficiency is supposed to be a risk factor for periodontal treatment failure [68]. It is also suggested that genetic variants of the vitamin D receptor are a biomarker for periodontitis [69].

Nutrients **2022**, *14*, 864

As a potential limitation of the present study, it must be emphasized that RBL shows a history of periodontal destruction and aging, but gives no information on the current state of clinical periodontal health. Although aging is also strongly associated with RBL (as shown in Figure 6) [70], periodontal disease is considered to be the major cause for alveolar bone loss [71]. Accordingly, other studies showed that there is a reliable relationship between clinical and radiographic bone loss [72–74]. Clinical bone loss precedes radiographic findings six to eight months [75]. In addition, a high accuracy of CBCTs in periodontal diagnosis, especially in visualizing periodontal intra-bony and furcation defects, has been shown [76,77].

While DMFT score, number of teeth, and smoking history also reflect a longer period of time, measurement of LDL-C and 25OHD levels just reflects a current snapshot. Nevertheless, it may be assumed that the determined LDL-C and 25OHD levels are a marker for individual lifestyle and health constitution of the patients and are stable for longer periods of time, particularly due to exclusion of patients receiving "treatment" in the form of statins or vitamin D supplementation.

Although diabetes mellitus and rheumatoid arthritis are known to be associated with periodontal disease [78,79], no sub-analysis regarding those parameters was possible in the present cohort of patients since there were only two diabetes mellitus and four rheumatoid arthritis patients. The small number may be explained by the fact that only patients were included who were treated with dental implants, where diabetes and rheumatoid arthritis are known to be relative contraindications for treatment with dental implants [80,81].

5. Conclusions

The present study detected significant associations between RBL and patient-specific parameters like sex, smoking history, DMFT score, number of teeth, 25OHD levels, and particularly age and LDL-C. While RBL gives no information on the current state of clinical periodontal health, but reflects the cumulated burden of periodontal destruction, the outcomes of this study support similar findings of previous studies investigating clinical periodontal parameters. Future studies using RBL measurements should also include clinical periodontal parameters as well as further investigations of the association between lifestyle- and nutrition-linked conditions such as LDL-C and 25OHD levels and periodontal bone loss.

Author Contributions: Conceptualization, F.C., J.P.W., T.T., K.J.S., J.F.; methodology, T.T., F.C., J.P.W., J.F., K.J.S.; software, J.F., T.T.; validation, K.-A.H., C.K., J.F., W.B.; formal analysis, K.-A.H., T.T., K.J.S., F.C., J.P.W.; investigation, T.T., K.-A.H.; data curation, K.-A.H.; writing—original draft preparation, T.T.; writing—review and editing, F.C., J.P.W., K.J.S., K.-A.H., W.B., C.K., J.F.; visualization, T.T., F.C., K.-A.H.; supervision, F.C., J.P.W. All authors have read and agreed to the published version of the manuscript.

Funding: This research received no external funding and was solely based on institutional funding.

Institutional Review Board Statement: The study was conducted in accordance with the guidelines of the Declaration of Helsinki, and approved by the Institutional Review Board of the University of Regensburg (reference: 21-2431-104; issued on 23 June 2021).

Informed Consent Statement: Patient consent was not applicable for this type of retrospective study.

Data Availability Statement: All data supporting the reported results are available upon request from the corresponding author.

Acknowledgments: Dental Wings (Chemnitz, Germany) is gratefully acknowledged for providing the software package CoPeriodontiX 9.9.

Conflicts of Interest: The authors declare no conflict of interest.

References

1. Chen, M.X.; Zhong, Y.J.; Dong, Q.Q.; Wong, H.M.; Wen, Y.F. Global, regional, and national burden of severe periodontitis, 1990–2019: An analysis of the Global Burden of Disease Study 2019. *J. Clin. Periodontol.* **2021**, *48*, 1165–1188. [CrossRef] [PubMed]

2. James, S.L.; Abate, D.; Abate, K.H.; Abay, S.M.; Abbafati, C.; Abbasi, N.; Abbastabar, H.; Abd-Allah, F.; Abdela, J.; Abdelalim, A.; et al. Global, regional, and national incidence, prevalence, and years lived with disability for 354 diseases and injuries for 195 countries and territories, 1990–2017: A systematic analysis for the Global Burden of Disease Study 2017. *Lancet* **2018**, *392*, 1789–1858. [CrossRef]

3. Jordan, R.A.; Bodechtel, C.; Hertrampf, K.; Hoffmann, T.; Kocher, T.; Nitschke, I.; Schiffner, U.; Stark, H.; Zimmer, S.; Micheelis, W. The Fifth German Oral Health Study (Fünfte Deutsche Mundgesundheitsstudie, DMS V)—Rationale, design, and methods. *BMC Oral Health* **2014**, *14*, 161. [CrossRef]

4. Bartold, P.M.; van Dyke, T.E. Periodontitis: A host-mediated disruption of microbial homeostasis. Unlearning learned concepts. *Periodontology 2000* **2013**, *62*, 203–217. [CrossRef]

5. Hajishengallis, G.; Korostoff, J.M. Revisiting the Page & Schroeder model: The good, the bad and the unknowns in the periodontal host response 40 years later. *Periodontology 2000* **2017**, *75*, 116–151. [CrossRef] [PubMed]

6. Jakubovics, N.S.; Goodman, S.D.; Mashburn-Warren, L.; Stafford, G.P.; Cieplik, F. The dental plaque biofilm matrix. *Periodontology 2000* **2021**, *86*, 32–56. [CrossRef] [PubMed]

7. Grossi, S.G.; Zambon, J.J.; Ho, A.W.; Koch, G.; Dunford, R.G.; Machtei, E.E.; Norderyd, O.M.; Genco, R.J. Assessment of risk for periodontal disease. I. Risk indicators for attachment loss. *J. Periodontol.* **1994**, *65*, 260–267. [CrossRef] [PubMed]

8. Loos, B.G.; van Dyke, T.E. The role of inflammation and genetics in periodontal disease. *Periodontology 2000* **2020**, *83*, 26–39. [CrossRef]

9. Jain, P.; Hassan, N.; Khatoon, K.; Mirza, M.A.; Naseef, P.P.; Kuruniyan, M.S.; Iqbal, Z. Periodontitis and Systemic Disorder—An Overview of Relation and Novel Treatment Modalities. *Pharmaceutics* **2021**, *13*, 1175. [CrossRef]

10. Nepomuceno, R.; Pigossi, S.C.; Finoti, L.S.; Orrico, S.R.P.; Cirelli, J.A.; Barros, S.P.; Offenbacher, S.; Scarel-Caminaga, R.M. Serum lipid levels in patients with periodontal disease: A meta-analysis and meta-regression. *J. Clin. Periodontol.* **2017**, *44*, 1192–1207. [CrossRef]

11. Virani, S.S.; Alonso, A.; Benjamin, E.J.; Bittencourt, M.S.; Callaway, C.W.; Carson, A.P.; Chamberlain, A.M.; Chang, A.R.; Cheng, S.; Delling, F.N.; et al. Heart Disease and Stroke Statistics—2020 Update: A Report from the American Heart Association. *Circulation* **2020**, *141*, e139–e596. [CrossRef] [PubMed]

12. Karr, S. Epidemiology and management of hyperlipidemia. *Am. J. Manag. Care* **2017**, *23*, S139–S148. [PubMed]

13. Stanhope, K.L.; Schwarz, J.M.; Keim, N.L.; Griffen, S.C.; Bremer, A.A.; Graham, J.L.; Hatcher, B.; Cox, C.L.; Dyachenko, A.; Zhang, W.; et al. Consuming fructose-sweetened, not glucose-sweetened, beverages increases visceral adiposity and lipids and decreases insulin sensitivity in overweight/obese humans. *J. Clin. Investig.* **2009**, *119*, 1322–1334. [CrossRef] [PubMed]

14. Ference, B.A.; Ginsberg, H.N.; Graham, I.; Ray, K.K.; Packard, C.J.; Bruckert, E.; Hegele, R.A.; Krauss, R.M.; Raal, F.J.; Schunkert, H.; et al. Low-density lipoproteins cause atherosclerotic cardiovascular disease. 1. Evidence from genetic, epidemiologic, and clinical studies. A consensus statement from the European Atherosclerosis Society Consensus Panel. *Eur. Heart J.* **2017**, *38*, 2459–2472. [CrossRef] [PubMed]

15. Machado, V.; Lobo, S.; Proença, L.; Mendes, J.J.; Botelho, J. Vitamin D and Periodontitis: A Systematic Review and Meta-Analysis. *Nutrients* **2020**, *12*, 2177. [CrossRef] [PubMed]

16. Ketharanathan, V.; Torgersen, G.R.; Petrovski, B.É.; Preus, H.R. Radiographic alveolar bone level and levels of serum 25-OH-Vitamin D3 in ethnic Norwegian and Tamil periodontitis patients and their periodontally healthy controls. *BMC Oral Health* **2019**, *19*, 83. [CrossRef] [PubMed]

17. Holick, M.F.; Chen, T.C. Vitamin D deficiency: A worldwide problem with health consequences. *Am. J. Clin. Nutr.* **2008**, *87*, 1080S–1086S. [CrossRef]

18. Amrein, K.; Scherkl, M.; Hoffmann, M.; Neuwersch-Sommeregger, S.; Köstenberger, M.; Tmava Berisha, A.; Martucci, G.; Pilz, S.; Malle, O. Vitamin D deficiency 2.0: An update on the current status worldwide. *Eur. J. Clin. Nutr.* **2020**, *74*, 1498–1513. [CrossRef] [PubMed]

19. Charoenngam, N.; Holick, M.F. Immunologic Effects of Vitamin D on Human Health and Disease. *Nutrients* **2020**, *12*, 2097. [CrossRef]

20. Prietl, B.; Treiber, G.; Pieber, T.R.; Amrein, K. Vitamin D and immune function. *Nutrients* **2013**, *5*, 2502–2521. [CrossRef] [PubMed]

21. Zhang, R.; Li, B.; Gao, X.; Tian, R.; Pan, Y.; Jiang, Y.; Gu, H.; Wang, Y.; Wang, Y.; Liu, G. Serum 25-hydroxyvitamin D and the risk of cardiovascular disease: Dose-response meta-analysis of prospective studies. *Am. J. Clin. Nutr.* **2017**, *105*, 810–819. [CrossRef] [PubMed]

22. Yin, L.; Ordóñez-Mena, J.M.; Chen, T.; Schöttker, B.; Arndt, V.; Brenner, H. Circulating 25-hydroxyvitamin D serum concentration and total cancer incidence and mortality: A systematic review and meta-analysis. *Prev. Med.* **2013**, *57*, 753–764. [CrossRef] [PubMed]

23. Awartani, F.; Atassi, F. Evaluation of periodontal status in subjects with hyperlipidemia. *J. Contemp. Dent. Pract.* **2010**, *11*, 33–40. [CrossRef]

24. Shivakumar, T.; Patil, V.A.; Desai, M.H. Periodontal status in subjects with hyperlipidemia and determination of association between hyperlipidemia and periodontal health: A clinicobiochemical study. *J. Contemp. Dent. Pract.* **2013**, *14*, 785–789. [CrossRef] [PubMed]

25. Fentoğlu, Ö.; Oz, G.; Taşdelen, P.; Uskun, E.; Aykaç, Y.; Bozkurt, F.Y. Periodontal status in subjects with hyperlipidemia. *J. Periodontol.* **2009**, *80*, 267–273. [CrossRef] [PubMed]

26. Lee, S.; Im, A.; Burm, E.; Ha, M. Association between periodontitis and blood lipid levels in a Korean population. *J. Periodontol.* **2018**, *89*, 28–35. [CrossRef] [PubMed]
27. Anbarcioglu, E.; Kirtiloglu, T.; Öztürk, A.; Kolbakir, F.; Acıkgöz, G.; Colak, R. Vitamin D deficiency in patients with aggressive periodontitis. *Oral Dis.* **2019**, *25*, 242–249. [CrossRef]
28. Kim, H.; Shin, M.H.; Yoon, S.J.; Kweon, S.S.; Lee, Y.H.; Choi, C.K.; Kim, O.; Kim, Y.J.; Chung, H.; Kim, O.S. Low serum 25-hydroxyvitamin D levels, tooth loss, and the prevalence of severe periodontitis in Koreans aged 50 years and older. *J. Periodontal Implant Sci.* **2020**, *50*, 368–378. [CrossRef] [PubMed]
29. Ebersole, J.L.; Lambert, J.; Bush, H.; Huja, P.E.; Basu, A. Serum Nutrient Levels and Aging Effects on Periodontitis. *Nutrients* **2018**, *10*, 1986. [CrossRef]
30. Lebowitz, M.D.; Burrows, B. Quantitative relationships between cigarette smoking and chronic productive cough. *Int. J. Epidemiol.* **1977**, *6*, 107–113. [CrossRef]
31. Fleiner, J.; Hannig, C.; Schulze, D.; Stricker, A.; Jacobs, R. Digital method for quantification of circumferential periodontal bone level using cone beam CT. *Clin. Oral Investig.* **2013**, *17*, 389–396. [CrossRef]
32. National Cholesterol Education Program. Expert Panel on Detection, Evaluation, and Treatment of High Blood Cholesterol in Adults (Adult Treatment Panel III). Third Report of the National Cholesterol Education Program (NCEP) Expert Panel on Detection, Evaluation, and Treatment of High Blood Cholesterol in Adults (Adult Treatment Panel III) Final Report. *Circulation* **2002**, *106*, 3143–3421.
33. Miller, R.G., Jr. *Simultaneous Statistical Inference*, 2nd ed.; Springer: New York, NY, USA, 1981; ISBN 9781461381228.
34. Helmi, M.F.; Huang, H.; Goodson, J.M.; Hasturk, H.; Tavares, M.; Natto, Z.S. Prevalence of periodontitis and alveolar bone loss in a patient population at Harvard School of Dental Medicine. *BMC Oral Health* **2019**, *19*, 254. [CrossRef]
35. Eke, P.I.; Dye, B.A.; Wei, L.; Slade, G.D.; Thornton-Evans, G.O.; Borgnakke, W.S.; Taylor, G.W.; Page, R.C.; Beck, J.D.; Genco, R.J. Update on Prevalence of Periodontitis in Adults in the United States: NHANES 2009 to 2012. *J. Periodontol.* **2015**, *86*, 611–622. [CrossRef]
36. Ebersole, J.L.; Graves, C.L.; Gonzalez, O.A.; Dawson, D.; Morford, L.A.; Huja, P.E.; Hartsfield, J.K.; Huja, S.S.; Pandruvada, S.; Wallet, S.M. Aging, inflammation, immunity and periodontal disease. *Periodontology 2000* **2016**, *72*, 54–75. [CrossRef] [PubMed]
37. Lipsky, M.S.; Su, S.; Crespo, C.J.; Hung, M. Men and Oral Health: A Review of Sex and Gender Differences. *Am. J. Mens. Health* **2021**, *15*, 15579883211016361. [CrossRef]
38. Shiau, H.J.; Reynolds, M.A. Sex differences in destructive periodontal disease: Exploring the biologic basis. *J. Periodontol.* **2010**, *81*, 1505–1517. [CrossRef]
39. Rosa, G.M.; Lucas, G.Q.; Lucas, O.N. Cigarette smoking and alveolar bone in young adults: A study using digitized radiographs. *J. Periodontol.* **2008**, *79*, 232–244. [CrossRef]
40. Knight, E.T.; Liu, J.; Seymour, G.J.; Faggion, C.M.; Cullinan, M.P. Risk factors that may modify the innate and adaptive immune responses in periodontal diseases. *Periodontology 2000* **2016**, *71*, 22–51. [CrossRef]
41. Ryder, M.I.; Couch, E.T.; Chaffee, B.W. Personalized periodontal treatment for the tobacco- and alcohol-using patient. *Periodontology 2000* **2018**, *78*, 30–46. [CrossRef]
42. Papapanou, P.N.; Sanz, M.; Buduneli, N.; Dietrich, T.; Feres, M.; Fine, D.H.; Flemmig, T.F.; Garcia, R.; Giannobile, W.V.; Graziani, F.; et al. Periodontitis: Consensus report of workgroup 2 of the 2017 World Workshop on the Classification of Periodontal and Peri-Implant Diseases and Conditions. *J. Clin. Periodontol.* **2018**, *45* (Suppl. S20), S162–S170. [CrossRef] [PubMed]
43. Chaffee, B.W.; Couch, E.T.; Vora, M.V.; Holliday, R.S. Oral and periodontal implications of tobacco and nicotine products. *Periodontology 2000* **2021**, *87*, 241–253. [CrossRef] [PubMed]
44. Levin, L.; Zini, A.; Levine, J.; Weiss, M.; Lev, R.; Chebath Taub, D.; Hai, A.; Almoznino, G. Demographic profile, Oral Health Impact Profile and Dental Anxiety Scale in patients with chronic periodontitis: A case-control study. *Int. Dent. J.* **2018**, *68*, 269–278. [CrossRef]
45. Strauss, F.-J.; Espinoza, I.; Stähli, A.; Baeza, M.; Cortés, R.; Morales, A.; Gamonal, J. Dental caries is associated with severe periodontitis in Chilean adults: A cross-sectional study. *BMC Oral Health* **2019**, *19*, 278. [CrossRef] [PubMed]
46. Mattila, P.T.; Niskanen, M.C.; Vehkalahti, M.M.; Nordblad, A.; Knuuttila, M.L.E. Prevalence and simultaneous occurrence of periodontitis and dental caries. *J. Clin. Periodontol.* **2010**, *37*, 962–967. [CrossRef]
47. Waskiewicz, K.; Oth, O.; Kochan, N.; Evrard, L. Des facteurs de risque généralement négligés en chirurgie orale et en implantologie: Le taux élevé de LDL-cholestérol et le taux insuffisant de la vitamine D. *Rev. Med. Brux.* **2018**, *39*, 70–77. [CrossRef] [PubMed]
48. Wang, M.; Hou, X.; Hu, W.; Chen, L.; Chen, S. Serum lipid and lipoprotein levels of middle-aged and elderly Chinese men and women in Shandong Province. *Lipids Health Dis.* **2019**, *18*, 58. [CrossRef]
49. Rosada, A.; Kassner, U.; Weidemann, F.; König, M.; Buchmann, N.; Steinhagen-Thiessen, E.; Spira, D. Hyperlipidemias in elderly patients: Results from the Berlin Aging Study II (BASEII), a cross-sectional study. *Lipids Health Dis.* **2020**, *19*, 92. [CrossRef]
50. Monteiro, A.M.; Jardini, M.A.N.; Alves, S.; Giampaoli, V.; Aubin, E.C.Q.; Figueiredo Neto, A.M.; Gidlund, M. Cardiovascular disease parameters in periodontitis. *J. Periodontol.* **2009**, *80*, 378–388. [CrossRef]
51. Saxlin, T.; Suominen-Taipale, L.; Kattainen, A.; Marniemi, J.; Knuuttila, M.; Ylöstalo, P. Association between serum lipid levels and periodontal infection. *J. Clin. Periodontol.* **2008**, *35*, 1040–1047. [CrossRef]
52. Iacopino, A.M.; Cutler, C.W. Pathophysiological relationships between periodontitis and systemic disease: Recent concepts involving serum lipids. *J. Periodontol.* **2000**, *71*, 1375–1384. [CrossRef]

53. Choukroun, J.; Khoury, G.; Khoury, F.; Russe, P.; Testori, T.; Komiyama, Y.; Sammartino, G.; Palacci, P.; Tunali, M.; Choukroun, E. Two neglected biologic risk factors in bone grafting and implantology: High low-density lipoprotein cholesterol and low serum vitamin D. *J. Oral Implantol.* **2014**, *40*, 110–114. [CrossRef] [PubMed]

54. Noack, B.; Jachmann, I.; Roscher, S.; Sieber, L.; Kopprasch, S.; Lück, C.; Hanefeld, M.; Hoffmann, T. Metabolic diseases and their possible link to risk indicators of periodontitis. *J. Periodontol.* **2000**, *71*, 898–903. [CrossRef] [PubMed]

55. Woelber, J.P.; Tennert, C. Chapter 13: Diet and Periodontal Diseases. *Monogr. Oral Sci.* **2020**, *28*, 125–133. [CrossRef] [PubMed]

56. Wang, X.; Li, W.; Song, W.; Xu, L.; Zhang, L.; Feng, X.; Lu, R.; Meng, H. Association of CYP1A1 rs1048943 variant with aggressive periodontitis and its interaction with hyperlipidemia on the periodontal status. *J. Periodontal. Res.* **2019**, *54*, 546–554. [CrossRef] [PubMed]

57. Linseisen, J.; Bechthold, A.; Bischoff-Ferrari, H.A.; Hintzpeter, B.; Leschik-Bonnet, E.; Reichrath, J.; Stehle, P.; Volkert, D.; Wolfram, G.; Zittermann, A. Vitamin D und Prävention Ausgewählter Chronischer Krankheiten—Stellungnahme. Available online: https://www.dge.de/wissenschaft/weitere-publikationen/stellungnahmen/?L=0 (accessed on 13 January 2022).

58. Dietrich, T.; Joshipura, K.J.; Dawson-Hughes, B.; Bischoff-Ferrari, H.A. Association between serum concentrations of 25-hydroxyvitamin D3 and periodontal disease in the US population. *Am. J. Clin. Nutr.* **2004**, *80*, 108–113. [CrossRef] [PubMed]

59. Bettencourt, A.; Boleixa, D.; Reis, J.; Oliveira, J.C.; Mendonça, D.; Costa, P.P.; Da Silva, B.M.; Marinho, A.; Da Silva, A.M. Serum 25-hydroxyvitamin D levels in a healthy population from the North of Portugal. *J. Steroid Biochem. Mol. Biol.* **2018**, *175*, 97–101. [CrossRef]

60. Küchler, E.C.; Schröder, A.; Teodoro, V.B.; Nazet, U.; Scariot, R.; Spanier, G.; Proff, P.; Kirschneck, C. The role of 25-hydroxyvitamin-D3 and vitamin D receptor gene in human periodontal ligament fibroblasts as response to orthodontic compressive strain: An in vitro study. *BMC Oral Health* **2021**, *21*, 386. [CrossRef] [PubMed]

61. Perić, M.; Maiter, D.; Cavalier, E.; Lasserre, J.F.; Toma, S. The Effects of 6-Month Vitamin D Supplementation during the Non-Surgical Treatment of Periodontitis in Vitamin-D-Deficient Patients: A Randomized Double-Blind Placebo-Controlled Study. *Nutrients* **2020**, *12*, 2940. [CrossRef] [PubMed]

62. Dawson-Hughes, B.; Harris, S.S.; Krall, E.A.; Dallal, G.E. Effect of calcium and vitamin D supplementation on bone density in men and women 65 years of age or older. *N. Engl. J. Med.* **1997**, *337*, 670–676. [CrossRef] [PubMed]

63. Botelho, J.; Machado, V.; Proença, L.; Delgado, A.S.; Mendes, J.J. Vitamin D Deficiency and Oral Health: A Comprehensive Review. *Nutrients* **2020**, *12*, 1471. [CrossRef]

64. Dietrich, T.; Nunn, M.; Dawson-Hughes, B.; Bischoff-Ferrari, H.A. Association between serum concentrations of 25-hydroxyvitamin D and gingival inflammation. *Am. J. Clin. Nutr.* **2005**, *82*, 575–580. [CrossRef] [PubMed]

65. Costantini, E.; Sinjari, B.; Piscopo, F.; Porreca, A.; Reale, M.; Caputi, S.; Murmura, G. Evaluation of Salivary Cytokines and Vitamin D Levels in Periodontopathic Patients. *Int. J. Mol. Sci.* **2020**, *21*, 2669. [CrossRef] [PubMed]

66. Garcia, M.N.; Hildebolt, C.F.; Miley, D.D.; Dixon, D.A.; Couture, R.A.; Spearie, C.L.A.; Langenwalter, E.M.; Shannon, W.D.; Deych, E.; Mueller, C.; et al. One-year effects of vitamin D and calcium supplementation on chronic periodontitis. *J. Periodontol.* **2011**, *82*, 25–32. [CrossRef] [PubMed]

67. Meghil, M.M.; Hutchens, L.; Raed, A.; Multani, N.A.; Rajendran, M.; Zhu, H.; Looney, S.; Elashiry, M.; Arce, R.M.; Peacock, M.E.; et al. The influence of vitamin D supplementation on local and systemic inflammatory markers in periodontitis patients: A pilot study. *Oral Dis.* **2019**, *25*, 1403–1413. [CrossRef] [PubMed]

68. Bashutski, J.D.; Eber, R.M.; Kinney, J.S.; Benavides, E.; Maitra, S.; Braun, T.M.; Giannobile, W.V.; McCauley, L.K. The impact of vitamin D status on periodontal surgery outcomes. *J. Dent. Res.* **2011**, *90*, 1007–1012. [CrossRef]

69. Yu, X.; Zong, X.; Pan, Y. Associations between vitamin D receptor genetic variants and periodontitis: A meta-analysis. *Acta Odontol. Scand.* **2019**, *77*, 484–494. [CrossRef]

70. Streckfus, C.F.; Parsell, D.E.; Streckfus, J.E.; Pennington, W.; Johnson, R.B. Relationship between oral alveolar bone loss and aging among African-American and Caucasian individuals. *Gerontology* **1999**, *45*, 110–114. [CrossRef]

71. Jeffcoat, M.K. Bone loss in the oral cavity. *J. Bone Miner. Res.* **1993**, *8* (Suppl. S2), S467–S473. [CrossRef]

72. Machtei, E.E.; Hausmann, E.; Grossi, S.G.; Dunford, R.; Genco, R.J. The relationship between radiographic and clinical changes in the periodontium. *J. Periodontal. Res.* **1997**, *32*, 661–666. [CrossRef] [PubMed]

73. Farook, F.F.; Alodwene, H.; Alharbi, R.; Alyami, M.; Alshahrani, A.; Almohammadi, D.; Alnasyan, B.; Aboelmaaty, W. Reliability assessment between clinical attachment loss and alveolar bone level in dental radiographs. *Clin. Exp. Dent. Res.* **2020**, *6*, 596–601. [CrossRef] [PubMed]

74. Jeffcoat, M.K. Radiographic Methods for the Detection of Progressive Alveolar Bone Loss. *J. Periodontol.* **1992**, *63* (Suppl. S4), 367–372. [CrossRef] [PubMed]

75. Goodson, J.M.; Haffajee, A.D.; Socransky, S.S. The relationship between attachment level loss and alveolar bone loss. *J. Clin. Periodontol.* **1984**, *11*, 348–359. [CrossRef] [PubMed]

76. Walter, C.; Schmidt, J.C.; Dula, K.; Sculean, A. Cone beam computed tomography (CBCT) for diagnosis and treatment planning in periodontology: A systematic review. *Quintessence Int.* **2016**, *47*, 25–37. [CrossRef] [PubMed]

77. Woelber, J.P.; Fleiner, J.; Rau, J.; Ratka-Krüger, P.; Hannig, C. Accuracy and Usefulness of CBCT in Periodontology: A Systematic Review of the Literature. *Int. J. Periodontics Restor. Dent.* **2018**, *38*, 289–297. [CrossRef] [PubMed]

78. Ceccarelli, F.; Saccucci, M.; Di Carlo, G.; Lucchetti, R.; Pilloni, A.; Pranno, N.; Luzzi, V.; Valesini, G.; Polimeni, A. Periodontitis and Rheumatoid Arthritis: The Same Inflammatory Mediators? *Mediat. Inflamm.* **2019**, *2019*, 6034546. [CrossRef]

79. Polak, D.; Shapira, L. An update on the evidence for pathogenic mechanisms that may link periodontitis and diabetes. *J. Clin. Periodontol.* **2018**, *45*, 150–166. [CrossRef]

80. Aghaloo, T.; Pi-Anfruns, J.; Moshaverinia, A.; Sim, D.; Grogan, T.; Hadaya, D. The Effects of Systemic Diseases and Medications on Implant Osseointegration: A Systematic Review. *Int. J. Oral Maxillofac. Implants* **2019**, *34*, s35–s49. [CrossRef] [PubMed]

81. Naujokat, H.; Kunzendorf, B.; Wiltfang, J. Dental implants and diabetes mellitus-a systematic review. *Int. J. Implant Dent.* **2016**, *2*, 5. [CrossRef] [PubMed]

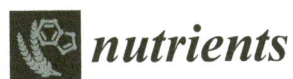

Review

Sarcopenic Dysphagia, Malnutrition, and Oral Frailty in Elderly: A Comprehensive Review

Alessandro de Sire [1,*], Martina Ferrillo [2,*], Lorenzo Lippi [3], Francesco Agostini [4], Roberto de Sire [5], Paola Emilia Ferrara [6], Giuseppe Raguso [7], Sergio Riso [8], Andrea Roccuzzo [9,10], Gianpaolo Ronconi [6], Marco Invernizzi [3,11] and Mario Migliario [12]

1   Department of Medical and Surgical Sciences, University of Catanzaro "Magna Graecia", 88100 Catanzaro, Italy
2   Department of Health Sciences, University of Catanzaro "Magna Graecia", 88100 Catanzaro, Italy
3   Department of Health Sciences, University of Eastern Piedmont "A. Avogadro", 28100 Novara, Italy; lorenzolippi.mt@gmail.com (L.L.); marco.invernizzi@med.uniupo.it (M.I.)
4   Department of Anatomical and Histological Sciences, Legal Medicine and Orthopedics, Sapienza University, 00185 Rome, Italy; francescoagostini.ff@gmail.com
5   Department of Clinical Medicine and Surgery, University Federico II of Naples, 80126 Naples, Italy; roberto.desire@libero.it
6   University Polyclinic Foundation Agostino Gemelli IRCSS, Catholic University of Sacred Heart, 00168 Rome, Italy; paolaemilia.ferrara@policlinicogemelli.it (P.E.F.); gianpaolo.ronconi@policlinicogemelli.it (G.R.)
7   Department of Otolaryngology-Head and Neck Surgery, University of Verona, 37129 Verona, Italy; ragusogiu@gmail.com
8   Dietetic and Clinical Nutrition Unit, Maggiore della Carità Hospital, 28100 Novara, Italy; sergio.riso@maggioreosp.novara.it
9   Department of Periodontology, School of Dental Medicine, University of Bern, Freiburgstrasse 7, 3010 Bern, Switzerland; andrea.roccuzzo@zmk.unibe.ch
10 Department of Oral and Maxillofacial Surgery, Copenhagen University Hospital (Rigshospitalet), 2100 Copenhagen, Denmark
11 Translational Medicine, Dipartimento Attività Integrate Ricerca e Innovazione (DAIRI), Azienda Ospedaliera SS. Antonio e Biagio e Cesare Arrigo, 15121 Alessandria, Italy
12 Dental Clinic, Department of Translational Medicine, University of Eastern Piedmont, 28100 Novara, Italy; mario.migliario@med.uniupo.it
*   Correspondence: alessandro.desire@unicz.it (A.d.S.); martinaferrillo@hotmail.it (M.F.)

Citation: de Sire, A.; Ferrillo, M.; Lippi, L.; Agostini, F.; de Sire, R.; Ferrara, P.E.; Raguso, G.; Riso, S.; Roccuzzo, A.; Ronconi, G.; et al. Sarcopenic Dysphagia, Malnutrition, and Oral Frailty in Elderly: A Comprehensive Review. Nutrients 2022, 14, 982. https://doi.org/10.3390/nu14050982

Academic Editors: Kirstin Vach and Johan Peter Woelber

Received: 11 February 2022
Accepted: 24 February 2022
Published: 25 February 2022

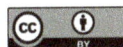
Abstract: Frailty is a highly prevalent condition in the elderly that has been increasingly considered as a crucial public health issue, due to the strict correlation with a higher risk of fragility fractures, hospitalization, and mortality. Among the age-related diseases, sarcopenia and dysphagia are two common pathological conditions in frail older people and could coexist leading to dehydration and malnutrition in these subjects. "Sarcopenic dysphagia" is a complex condition characterized by deglutition impairment due to the loss of mass and strength of swallowing muscles and might be also related to poor oral health status. Moreover, the aging process is strictly related to poor oral health status due to direct impairment of the immune system and wound healing and physical and cognitive impairment might indirectly influence older people's ability to carry out adequate oral hygiene. Therefore, poor oral health might affect nutrient intake, leading to malnutrition and, consequently, to frailty. In this scenario, sarcopenia, dysphagia, and oral health are closely linked sharing common pathophysiological pathways, disabling sequelae, and frailty. Thus, the aim of the present comprehensive review is to describe the correlation among sarcopenic dysphagia, malnutrition, and oral frailty, characterizing their phenotypically overlapping features, to propose a comprehensive and effective management of elderly frail subjects.

Keywords: sarcopenic dysphagia; sarcopenia; dysphagia; malnutrition; oral health; osteoporosis; elderly

1. Introduction

In the last decades, worldwide life expectancy has increased and the proportion of older adults relative to other age groups has continued to grow resulting in ageing of the society, especially in the developed countries [1–3]. Life courses of health and functional status in older people are related to their genetics and environmental backgrounds, as well as other physical and psychological factors [4]. Indeed, a common feature in elderly subjects is the progressive decline in several physiological functions, which might lead to an increased risk of sarcopenia, dysphagia, osteoporosis, and frailty [5–8].

In this context, frailty is a complex and multifaceted public health issue highly prevalent in older adults leading to increased direct and direct sanitary costs and is strictly correlated with a higher risk of falling, fragility fractures and consequent disability, hospitalization, and mortality [5,9–11]. A consistent percentage of frail subjects might present with sarcopenia, a clinical condition, characterized by a reduction in muscle mass, muscle strength, and physical performance [12]. Sarcopenia typically occurs during the fifth decade of life affecting from 9.9 to 40.4% of older people [13] and inducing a muscle mass and strength decline, with a consequent need of a prompt diagnosis and a rehabilitative intervention [6,14,15]. Moreover, it has been recently shown that sarcopenia could be considered as an independent risk factor for dysphagia, reducing the strength of swallowing muscles [5,16,17]. Dysphagia is a dysfunction of the digestive system, characterized by an impairment in chewing and swallowing, with absence or prolonged transit of food or liquids in the upper digestive tract [18]. The oropharyngeal swallowing process involves a coordinated set of neuromuscular actions allowing the transit of the bolus from the oral cavity to the upper esophageal sphincter and is commonly described in three different phases: oral, pharyngeal, and esophageal [19]. Hence, oropharyngeal dysphagia could result in an ineffective deglutition, leading to dehydration and malnutrition with a consequent increased risk of muscle mass loss [20]. In this scenario, sarcopenia and dysphagia share several risk factors and their pathological coexistence has captured the interest of the scientific community in the last few years. Moreover, both conditions could be considered both risk and predictive factors at the same time [17]. Thus, the concept of "sarcopenic dysphagia", a pathological condition caused by a loss of mass and strength of swallowing-related muscles, has been recently proposed and, in light of its detrimental effects on health-related quality of life (HRQoL) and disability requires a multidisciplinary approach and effective management in elderly subjects [21–23].

As previously described, dysphagia might lead to malnutrition through several pathological mechanisms [24,25] with consequent increased risk of developing sarcopenia [26]. At the same time, malnutrition can be caused by a variety of factors including difficulty eating, reduced mobility, psychological stress, and poor access to healthcare, oral health care, and social services [27]. Individuals with impaired masticatory ability usually avoid foods that are difficult to chew, including raw vegetables or fruits. Indeed, an insufficient intake of fibers, linoleic acid, potassium, calcium, magnesium, zinc, selenium, vitamins D, E and K, folate, biotin, and molybdenum have been observed in older adults with dysphagia with reported chewing and swallowing impairments [24,28]. Among all these pathophysiological mechanisms underpinning malnutrition, poor oral hygiene could play a key role in the development of this condition, increasing the risk of progressive periodontal disease and dental decay, as shown in other chronic conditions [29–32]. Indeed, oropharyngeal functional decline culminates in a loss of independence in self-care abilities, including less attention for oral care [33] and activities of daily living (ADL), such as brushing teeth or dentures or periodic visits to the dentist [34]. Moreover, oral cancer, dry mouth (xerostomia), and pathological denture-related conditions (including oral candidiasis and denture stomatitis) [3,35] are more frequent in the elderly [36], resulting in variable degrees of oral disability. Lastly, a reduction in appetite might occur because of decrease in smell and taste senses, leading to a loss of pleasure in eating, which is another well-known risk factor for malnutrition [37,38]. In conclusion, poor oral health might affect nutrient intake, leading to malnutrition and, consequently, to frailty.

In this scenario, age-related conditions are a growing issue and need comprehensive and multidisciplinary interventions for a prompt and effective management. sarcopenia, dysphagia, sarcopenic dysphagia, and oral health seem to be closely linked and share common pathophysiological pathways, overlapping features and disabling sequelae all leading to frailty (see Figure 1).

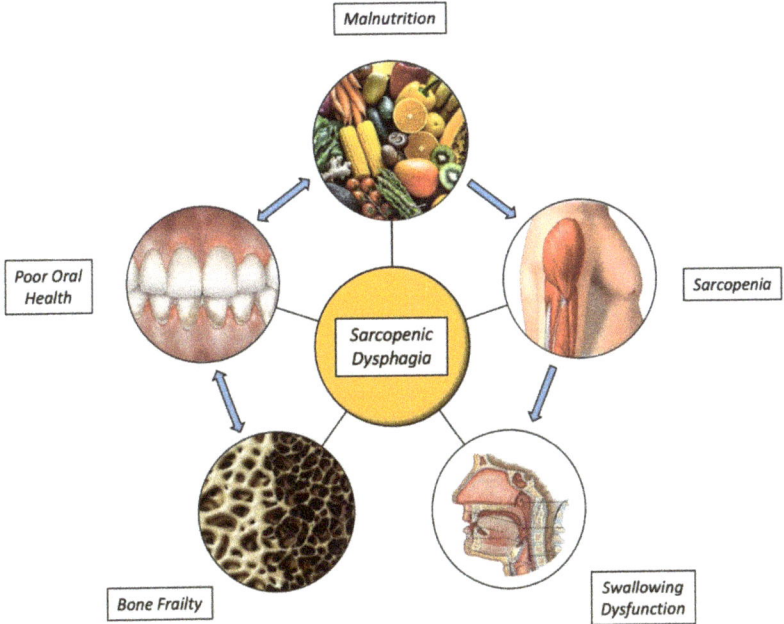

Figure 1. Overview of the vicious circle among malnutrition, sarcopenia, swallowing dysfunction, bone frailty, and poor oral health in older subjects.

However, at present, few reports in the literature focused on these specific issues, their impact on disability and the pathophysiological synergies of these different conditions of older adults.

Therefore, by this comprehensive review we sought to describe the state-of-art about the overlapping features of sarcopenia, sarcopenic dysphagia, malnutrition, and oral frailty in the elderly and their correlation to define the correct framework for an optimal management of these complex pathological conditions.

2. Malnutrition and Aging: A Close but Unclear Link in the Elderly

An adequate nutritional status and physical activity are cornerstones to preserve functioning, wellbeing, and HRQoL in older people, according to the Healthy Aging policy framework of the World Health Organization [39]. However, nutritional disorders are a critical burden in the elderly, affecting physical function and global health with detrimental consequences in well-being and sanitary costs [40].

According to the European Society for Clinical Nutrition and Metabolism (ESPEN), diagnostic criteria for malnutrition are defined by a body mass index (BMI) of <18.5 kg/m^2 or by meeting two of these three criteria: unintentional weight loss of more than 10% (or more than 5% over the last three months), BMI lower 22 kg/m^2 (or lower than 20 kg/m^2 in persons over 70 years old), or a low fat-free mass index (FFMI) score (FFMI < 15 in women and FFMI < 17 kg/m^2 in men) [41].

In recent years, malnutrition prevalence is increasing worldwide due to the aging of the population and the increasing prevalence of age-related pathological conditions [42]. To date, a recent meta-analysis including over 110,000 older persons underlined that malnutrition rate might range between 6% (95% CI, 4.6–7.5) and 29.4% (95% CI, 21.7–36.9) based on the health care setting [43]. In more detail, rehabilitation and subacute care settings were associated with a higher prevalence of malnutrition [43]. In accordance, Wojzischke et al. [44] reported similar results, while approximately 47% (40–54) of geriatric rehabilitation patients were at risk of malnutrition.

Albeit several pathophysiological mechanisms underpinning the strict association between malnutrition and aging have been hypothesized [45], the gap of knowledge remains still consistent. Physical function impairment, social and environmental conditions, acute and chronic diseases, and pharmacological treatments have been identified as independent risk factors potentially responsible to generate malnutrition in the elderly [45]. Moreover, as previously suggested, malnutrition in the elderly might be related to dental problems or to dysphagia due to a reduced performance in swallowing functions that might affect oral intake [46,47]. Therefore, patients who could not achieve full oral intake with support or supplemental strategies might undergo a catabolic state with detrimental consequences in several body tissues tropism and systemic inflammation [48].

The relationship between oral health and nutrition is multidirectional: on the one hand, oral health problems (e.g., tooth loss, toothache) could be contributing factors to malnutrition, through the reduction of chewing skills (e.g., edentulism, dry mouth) [49,50]. In this context, Joshipura et al. showed that edentulous people consumed fewer vegetables, less fiber and carotene and more cholesterol, saturated fat, and calories than did participants with 25 or more teeth [51]; on the other hand, poor dietary intake increased the risk of periodontal disease. Indeed, inverse associations were found between fatty acids, vitamin C, vitamin E, beta-carotene, fiber, calcium, dairy, fruits, and vegetables and risk of periodontal disease [52,53]. Moreover, a strict relationship between the development of periodontal disease and the diet-borne systemic inflammation was supposed [53]. Indeed, nutrients consumption of dairy, fruits and vegetables, fiber, calcium, antioxidants, and fatty acids might regulate the immune-mediated inflammatory responses, starting and propagating pro-inflammatory mechanisms, which are basis of periodontal disease development [54].

Therefore, an early identification of malnutrition is mandatory to optimize the complex management of elderly patients and to prevent the negative clinical consequences of malnutrition. Several screening and grading tools have been proposed to better characterize malnutrition, including Mini Nutritional Assessment (MNA) [55], Malnutrition Screening Tool [56,57], Seniors in the Community: Risk Evaluation for Eating and Nutrition (SCREEN II) [58], Malnutrition Universal Screening Tool [32,59], Simplified Nutrition Assessment Questionnaire (SNAQ) [60], and Nutritional Risk Screening (NRS) [61]. Despite nutritional screening should be routinely performed in the hospital setting, there is still a lack of consensus on the optimal tool to be used in clinical practice to promote the early identification of this condition and an effective and tailored treatment.

To date, it has been widely recognized that malnutrition is related to poor health outcomes due to its clinical consequences in both acute and chronic diseases [62,63]. Moreover, malnutrition is currently considered as one of the main modifiable prognostic factors for worsening outcomes and mortality in elderly patients [64,65]. Lastly, a nutritional deficiency of micronutrients (vitamin D [66,67], vitamin C [66], vitamin B12 and folate [67,68], vitamins A and E [69], vitamin B6 [70], selenium, zinc, magnesium [71], and copper [72]) has been reported to have a potential role in the immune regulation in the elderly. In this scenario, malnutrition is considered as a risk factor for osteoporosis, sarcopenia, and frailty [73,74]. To date, several studies [74–76] highlighted a correlation between protein intake and calcium-phosphate or bone metabolism reporting that deficient protein supply might affect calcium homeostasis. Moreover, protein deficiency might downregulate insulin-like growth factor-I (IGF-I) production which plays a key anabolic role in skeletal muscle, cartilage, and bone [77].

Concurrently, malnutrition consequences might reflect on musculoskeletal system with crucial implications on functional performances and HRQoL of frail elderly patients [78]. Thus, the role of nutritional interventions in the elderly has been widely investigated with increasing evidence supporting the positive role of oral supplementation to optimize the rehabilitative path of frail patients [79].

However, it should be noted that tailored treatment should be proposed in patients affected by concurrent conditions. In particular, it should be noted that dysphagia, malnutrition, and oral frailty frequently coexistent in the elderly [80]. Therefore, nutritional intervention should take into account individual swallowing capacities [81]. Moreover, due to the detrimental effects of malnutrition in musculoskeletal system, sarcopenia and frailty syndrome should be screened in patients with malnutrition due to the high prevalence of these concurrent age-related conditions and the needing for enhancing synergism among therapeutic interventions [82].

Taken together, the evidence reported put in light the needing for early screening for malnutrition in the elderly to minimize malnutrition complications and set-up multidisciplinary strategies to treat this complex and disabling condition and prevent its health-related consequences.

3. Dysphagia in Older Subjects

Swallowing problems have been considered as a growing health concern for the elderly, being a major cause of malnutrition, dehydration, aspiration pneumonia or even death due to asphyxiation [83]. Prevalence ranges from 16% in people aged 70–79 years to 33% in subjects aged more than 80 years [20], reaching 60% in geriatric populations residing in community dwelling settings and nursing homes [84].

Dysphagia is defined as a difficulty in eating and swallowing, characterized by impaired or prolonged transit of food or liquids from the oral cavity to the esophagus [18]. The swallowing process could be divided into four distinct phases: oral preparatory, oral transport, pharyngeal, and esophageal phase. An impairment in any of these phases may lead to dysphagia [85]. The swallowing function may be altered, in every single phase, by the age-related reduction of tissue elasticity, cervical spine changes, oropharyngeal disorders, decrease of oral moisture, and sensory impairments, such as reduction of smell and taste [19]. The coexistence of sarcopenia and dysphagia has recently attracted a considerable amount of interest in the scientific literature, considering that older people with dysphagia might present a loss of muscle mass and strength in both generalized skeletal muscles and swallowing-related muscles [22]. Indeed, this age-related loss of muscle mass might be manifested as a decrease in the thickness of tongue, geniohyoid muscle [86], pharyngeal wall [87], and a reduction of tongue pressure [88] and weaker pharyngeal contractility [89].

Dysphagia management requires a multidisciplinary approach focusing at first on early diagnosis to prevent potential complications [90]. Hence, dysphagia screening can be performed using validated questionnaires designed to rapidly detect signs and symptoms of swallowing impairment, such as the 10-Item Eating Assessment Tool (EAT-10) [91,92]. This tool is composed of 10 items, each one describing a specific risk condition to be scored from 0 (absence of problem) to 4 (severe problem), and a total score of 3 or higher suggests an abnormal swallowing function. This screening tool reported a high specificity (96.8% if $\geq$3 and 98.4% if $\geq$4) for detecting dysphagia in the elderly as shown in a study performed on 534 older people referred to a Rehabilitation Unit after total hip or knee arthroplasty [5]. Another screening test commonly used in the clinical practice is the modified water swallowing test (MWST), which shows a sensitivity and a specificity of 70% and 88%, respectively, for detecting aspiration [93,94]. Similarly, a wide variability of screening tools showed excellent sensitivity and specificity in the assessment of patients with dysphagia, including volume–viscosity swallow test, pharyngo-esophageal manometry, voluntary cough airflow, maximum tongue pressure, surface electromyography, real-time magnetic resonance imaging [95]. These tests might be associated with each other in order to improve specificity and sensibility for a more precise dysphagia assessment [93–95].

Moreover, several rating scales are used to assess the oral intake level of patients, which correlates with deglutition ability, such as the Functional Oral Intake Scale (FOIS), Food Intake Level Scale (FILS), neuromuscular disease swallowing status scale, and Sydney Swallow Questionnaire [96,97].

However, despite these tools being the first-line use in common clinical practice, the instrumental evaluation is mandatory to confirm the diagnosis of dysphagia [20]. The video-fluoroscopic swallowing study (VFSS), also known as modified barium study, is the only diagnostic tool that assesses all four phases of swallowing. It could detect oral and pharyngeal motility problems, ascertain presence of aspiration or penetration, assess the swallow speed and evaluate postural changes and their effect on aspiration/penetration [20]. A video-fluoroscopic study performed on 731 patients complaining of swallowing symptoms showed prolonged oral transit time and aspiration after swallowing in elderly dysphagic patients. Similarly, a study performed on 132 patients with swallowing difficulties using fluoroscopic imaging showed that male sarcopenic patients had lower laryngeal upward movements during swallowing and wider pharyngeal areas compared to healthy controls [88].

Another instrumental technique for dysphagia assessment is the flexible endoscopic evaluation of swallowing (FEES) that allows a direct visualization of the laryngopharynx, whereas patients are asked to eat different consistencies of food with food coloring [98]. It is a very useful tool to assess the presence of penetration or aspiration residue in the valleculate and pyriform sinuses, despite it is limited in exploring the oral and esophageal phases of deglutition. Giraldo-Cadavid et al. showed that aspiration detected by FEES and an age > 65 years were two independent predictors of mortality in 148 patients with oropharyngeal dysphagia [98].

In conclusion, dysphagia is a common and disabling issue in the elderly and need to be managed through a complex multidisciplinary approach, starting from early diagnosis and involving several health professionals such as geriatric, otorhinolaryngoiatric, physical and rehabilitation physicians, nutritionists, dentists, and speech-language pathologists in order to plan the most effective treatment.

4. Oral Frailty: A Detrimental Issue

The oral cavity is the first part of the digestive tract and is involved in several functions including biting the food, chewing, adding saliva for bolus formation and transporting it into the stomach [99]. Poor oral health seems to be strictly related to aging and could be considered as an indicator of frailty [100,101]. It has been shown that poor oral health is associated with poor diet quantity and quality in older adults [102], leading to a consequent reduction of fruits, vegetables, and fibers intake leading to an increased risk of malnutrition [103]. Moreover, the number of teeth is significantly associated with the number of food items that older persons able to eat [103]. Indeed, tooth loss could influence the selection of food of reduced consistency and consequent loss of pleasure in eating [25], explaining the relationship between tooth loss and poor nutritional status in the elderly [104].

In this scenario, Hussein et al. [105] in 2021 performed a systematic review with meta-analysis showing that edentulous patients had a 9.5% higher risk of malnutrition than healthy subjects, evidencing a lack of specific nutrients, that could lead to several disorders. The authors reported that older adults with chewing impairment had twice the risk of malnutrition and those with no daily teeth or denture cleaning had a 52.6% higher risk of malnutrition compared to control subjects. Iwasaki and colleagues [106] investigated the nutritional status among 1054 community-dwelling older adults, reporting that oral frailty is defined as the number of remaining teeth, masticatory performance, articulatory oral motor skill, low tongue pressure and eating and swallowing impairment was present in 20.4% of the patients assessed. Study participants with oral frailty showed a higher odd of more severe malnutrition, evaluated using the Mini-Nutritional Assessment—Short

Form and serum levels of albumin. Furthermore, it should be highlighted that a poor oral health status (in particular edentulism) increased the difficulty in eating hard foods, with a consumption of mashed food and decreasing eating pleasure, leading to a higher risk of malnutrition [107].

Another age-related condition that could affect oral health in the elderly is oral dryness, with a negative impact on oral health status and HRQoL [108–110]. Xerostomia is considered as the subjective sensation of oral dryness, ranging from 17% to 40% among community-dwelling elderly and from 20% to 72% in institutionalized older people [111]. The prevalence of dry mouth increases with increasing numbers of medications used [109,112], especially if used in combination [113]. More than 400 medications could cause xerostomia, including antidepressants, proton pump inhibitors, antihypertensives, antipsychotics, diuretics, and antineoplastics. Xerostomia could also be caused by autoimmune conditions, as the Sjögren's Syndrome [114], radiation therapy for cancers of the head and neck [115], dehydration [116] and infection as hepatitis C virus (HCV) [117]. Moreover, saliva plays a key role in neutralizing potentially damaging food acids and enhancing the ability to taste food and speech facilitation [118]. It contains several enzymes, which start the digestion process, and antibacterial, antifungal, and antiviral agents, which are extremely helpful to prevent oral infections [119]. Older people often present with a reduced salivary flow, with negative consequences for oral health, including dysgeusia, halitosis, burning mouth, oral pain, difficulty in chewing and swallowing, speech impairment, and an increased risk of fungal infections, demineralization/caries, and periodontitis [120–124].

Periodontal disease is a chronic inflammatory pathological condition affecting the tooth-supporting soft and hard tissues, which left untreated leads to tooth mobility and tooth loss [56,125]. The constant deposit of bacterial biofilm on the teeth triggers a chronic inflammatory condition ranging from a reversible low-level (gingivitis) to irreversible higher level of inflammation (periodontitis) and tooth mobility/loss [126]. In this context, microbial products and inflammatory mediators might enter the systemic circulation and reach distant organs, supporting the genesis of systemic pathologies [127–130]. Nutrition is a critical determinant of immune responses [131] because nutrients derived from food sources show a strong interaction with the immune system cells [132] and nutritional deficiency might impair the immune response and predispose the individual to infection [133,134]. In more detail, a low intake of vitamin A, E, C, B6, and B12, pantothenic acid, riboflavin, and folate act on DNA and RNA synthesis, cellular metabolism, and antioxidant activity and a low intake of these micronutrients might affect the host defenses [135,136]. The result is a state of chronic inflammation that might induce an intrinsic production of glucocorticoids and proinflammatory cytokines with consequent body weight loss and skeletal muscle depletion [137,138] Moreover, the high levels of pro-inflammatory cytokines (i.e., interleukin-6 and TNF-α) have been associated with reduced muscle mass and muscle strength [139,140]. Hence, poor oral health conditions characterized by high values of plaque and bleeding on probing scores might be strictly related to dysphagia, sarcopenia, and malnutrition, sharing some pathophysiological mechanisms and phenotypic manifestations with these pathological conditions.

Oral health status is also considered to be a factor associated with sarcopenia [141] and dysphagia [142], and improvement of the oral status and function might be important to conduct dysphagia rehabilitation. Poor oral health status may induce difficulties in chewing and swallowing in older people, as well as malnutrition and consequent sarcopenia. Authors showed a strong relationship between dysphagia and low salivary flow [143], which could induce both a dry feeling in the mouth and a defect in lubrication and the cohesion of the bolus [143,144]. Dysphagia associated with salivary hypofunction can cause a loss of appetite and a restricted choice of dietary intake [143].

Moreover, much attention has been focused on the relationship between oral health and sarcopenia and it was assumed that impaired oral health leads to sarcopenia. In this context, some reports have shown relationships between oral health and handgrip strength, walking speed, and skeletal muscle mass which are measurements used in the diagnosis of sarcopenia [145–147].

Moreover, given the recent evidence underlining a strict muscle–skeletal crosstalk, intriguing implications have been suggested in the relationship between oral health and bone frailty [148,149].

Therefore, in conclusion, impaired oral health can lead to malnutrition and sarcopenia, which can, in turn, cause dysphagia, resulting in a negative cycle that worsens the patient's general condition.

5. Sarcopenic Dysphagia: An Old and New Concept

The term "sarcopenic dysphagia" has been used for the first time in 2012 by Kuroda and Kuroda [21] to define a swallowing impairment due to both systemic and swallowing muscles sarcopenia [22]. To date, this topic has been rising a growing interest in the scientific field with four academic societies that recently published a position paper to better characterize the definition and diagnosis of sarcopenic dysphagia [150]. In this scenario, a progressive decline in skeletal muscle mass in the elderly is widely documented in literature [151–155]. However, this phenomenon might be extremely burdensome in frail patients and might affect even swallowing muscle, including the tongue, geniohyoid muscle, and pharyngeal muscles with negative consequences in terms of swallowing function and consequent increased risk of dysphagia [87,156–158].

Therefore, sarcopenic dysphagia is characterized by specific differences from presbyphagia in elderly. In more detail, although presbyphagia is associated with age-related decline of swallowing mechanisms, sarcopenic dysphagia might be related to a further decline in swallowing muscle strength due to an impairment of whole-body skeletal muscle strength associated with a reduction in swallowing function [22]. The negative bond of events characterizing the evolution from presbyphagia to sarcopenic dysphagia has been not fully understood; however, it has been proposed that energy intake reduction and acute diseases might severely affect the risk for sarcopenic dysphagia in elderly [17,159].

In this context, Ogawa et al. [160] identified the cross-sectional area of the tongue muscle as the most specific factor to assess sarcopenic dysphagia. Moreover, togue muscle area of brightness assessed with ultrasound technique seem to be an independent risk factor for sarcopenic dysphagia [160]. On the other hand, Maeda et al. [17] reported that skeletal muscle index, Barthel Index and BMI were significantly related to sarcopenic dysphagia, supporting the growing evidence on the similar pathophysiological mechanisms underpinning these conditions, with a detrimental synergism in terms of frailty in older people [161,162]. Furthermore, the strict association between sarcopenia and dysphagia has been underlined by the recent systematic review by Zhao et al. [163], that reported a significant association between sarcopenia and dysphagia independently by the diagnostic criteria [163].

However, sarcopenic dysphagia is not simply identified by a concomitant diagnosis of sarcopenia and dysphagia, but it has been characterized by specific diagnostic criteria recently assessed by Mori et al. [164]. The authors emphasized the need for a precise tool to identify sarcopenic dysphagia, aiming at developing specific strategies to counteract this progressive and disabling condition. The authors proposed a diagnostic algorithm consisting of five different items including dysphagia diagnosis, sarcopenia diagnosis, imaging test consistent with loss of swallowing-muscles mass, no other possible cause of dysphagia, or if any, not considered the main cause [164]. Based on these criteria, the authors identified three potential diagnostic categories: probable sarcopenia dysphagia, possible sarcopenic dysphagia, and no sarcopenic dysphagia [164].

However, it has been demonstrated that in stroke patients older than 65 years old, the swallowing muscle mass might be decreased even without a direct neurological deficit, mainly due to the high risk for malnutrition and oral intake reduction [48,165]. In particular, it has been reported that despite stroke-related dysphagia might be associated with common neurological symptoms including dysarthria, aphasia, apraxia, and facial palsy, concurrent or overlapping sarcopenic dysphagia might be related to pre-injury comorbidity, acute illness, immobilization, and inadequate energy intake that might affect post-stroke patients with a major latency of onset but better reversibility with a specific therapeutic intervention [165].

On the other hand, sarcopenic dysphagia has been also reported after severe COVID-19 infection in non-intubated elderly patients [166], leading to an intriguing interest on the screening strategies and therapeutic rehabilitation approach in COVID-19 survivors [167,168].

To date, several barriers have been identified in routine clinical screening of sarcopenia, including the lack of confidence in health care workers in the screening tools, the underestimation of the disease, the lack of specific services to manage sarcopenic patients, or limitations to access these specific services [169–171]. As a result, sarcopenic dysphagia screening has not been fully introduced in routine clinical practice, albeit recent studies [172–175] have emphasized the need for a specific therapeutic intervention including rehabilitation in this condition.

Taken together, these findings underlined that sarcopenic dysphagia is a common and disabling condition in elderly patients. Specific diagnostic criteria have been proposed for the early identification of this condition, and ultrasound imaging might be a useful tool to assess swallowing muscle mass and muscle quality [160].

In this scenario, clinicians should consider the strict associations among sarcopenia, dysphagia, and malnutrition in the therapeutic path of sarcopenic dysphagic patients in order to optimize the comprehensive management of elderly patients.

Moreover, precise identification of these concurrent conditions might have a key role in the optimal treatment strategy prescription directly targeting functional impairment related to these conditions and etiological causes at the basis of the onset of the disease.

Figure 2 describes the overlapping features among different age-related conditions, underlining the key role of sarcopenic dysphagia.

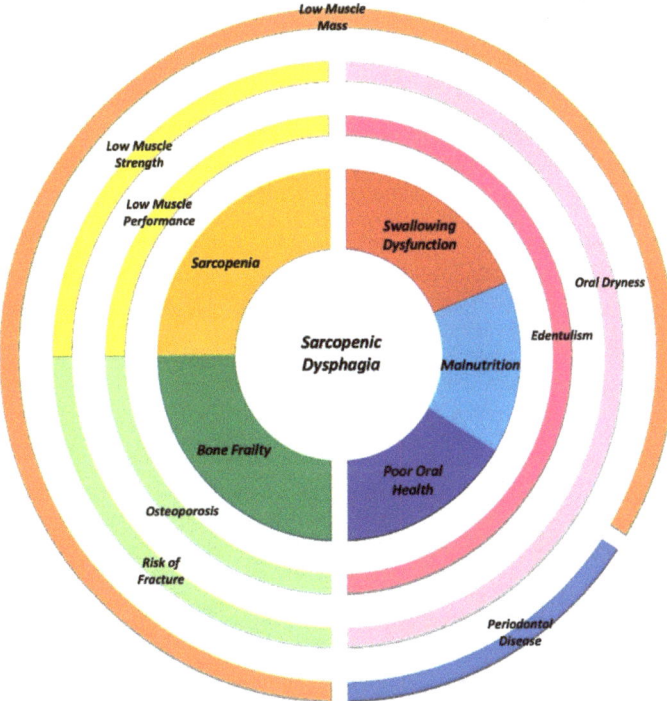

Figure 2. Sarcopenic dysphagia: overlapping features among different age-related conditions.

Lastly, a routine clinical screening to assess sarcopenic dysphagia should be introduced in the clinical practice to support an early rehabilitative treatment and improve functional outcomes in sarcopenic elderly patients, potentially preventing malnutrition and frailty along with their burdensome consequences.

6. Nutritional Supplementation to Counteract Sarcopenic Dysphagia

Nutritional interventions are a cornerstone of the integrated therapeutic path aimed at counteracting sarcopenia and malnutrition in the elderly [176,177]. In more detail, the ESPEN [176] recently recommended an energy intake of 30 kcal/kg of body weight/day and a protein intake of at least 1.0 g/kg body weight/day in the elderly. However, the protein intake may reach 1.2–1.5 g/kg body weight/day in acute or chronic illness [176]. In sarcopenic patients, it has been shown that 1.2 g/ideal body weight/day (kg) protein intake might be effective in improving tongue muscle strength [178]. Along with the daily protein intake, also the daily caloric intake should be strictly monitored in elderly patients given the high risk of malnutrition in these subjects, especially in dysphagic ones [26,179]. In more detail, it has been suggested that a caloric intake ≥ 35 kcal/IBW/day (kg) is needed to adequately treat patients with sarcopenic dysphagia [150]. Furthermore, it should be noted that the reaching of an optimal energy and protein intake could be extremely challenging in these patients not only for the well-known swallowing impairment but also for the high prevalence of concomitant age-related disabling conditions [174]. Therefore, a specific therapeutic approach should be tailored to the patient's needs and enteral or parenteral nutrition might be considered especially in post-acute patients [103]. However, conflicting data were reported for both enteral and parenteral nutrition solutions and oral feeding should be preferred if possible [180,181]. In this scenario, food texture modifications might be used to reduce the risk of inhalation and should be adapted to the swallowing deficiencies [182]. Moreover, an adequate nutritional supplementation might provide significant improvements in both macronutrients and micronutrients intake [183,184]. Indeed, promising results were reported in terms of vitamin D supplementation, which might have a crucial role not only on musculoskeletal health but also on immune system regulation with intriguing implications in several pathological conditions of the elderly [185,186].

To date, few studies assessed the effect of nutritional supplementation in patients with sarcopenic dysphagia reporting promising results [187–190]. However, it should be noted that nutritional supplements should be considered in an integrated multidisciplinary treatment including an adequate physical exercise [191–193]. In recent years, rehabilitation nutrition, a recent integrated approach aimed to counteract the effects of aging on the skeletal muscle system, has been proposed to optimize functional outcomes in the elderly [194]. It is based on a precise assessment of nutritional disorders, sarcopenia and potential deficits in nutritional intake [159]. More in detail, the close synergism between nutrition and rehabilitations has been deeply investigated in the past few decades [82,195]. Moreover, several papers supported the strong correlation between nutritional status and functional outcomes, and the greater improvement in these outcomes in sarcopenic patients obtained with combined nutritional and exercise interventions compared instead of single ones [196].

Despite these findings, good-quality clinical trials assessing the role of specific nutritional supplementation in sarcopenic dysphagic patients are still lacking. Moreover, there is still a gap of knowledge concerning the effect of physical exercise and nutritional supplementation in patients with sarcopenic dysphagia. Therefore, further research targeting these specific patients is still warranted to establish to guide clinicians in the management of frail subjects at risk of sarcopenic dysphagia.

7. Oropharyngeal Rehabilitation

Dysphagia and malnutrition are two major issues in the elderly with a negative impact on several pathological conditions, including cardiovascular disorders, cognitive status impairment, immune system downregulation, pressure ulcers, and skeletal muscle system worsening [197,198]. Therefore, effective interventions aimed at improving the nutritional intake and counter malnutrition are mandatory not only to prevent dysphagia-related complications (such as aspiration pneumonia) but also to improve the general health status and the HRQoL of older patients [199].

In this context, oropharyngeal rehabilitation is a relatively new concept in the complex multidisciplinary approach of dysphagia and swallowing disorders. This rehabilitative approach is characterized by several interventions including functional training, compensatory maneuvers, postural adjustments, swallowing maneuvers and diet modifications [156,200,201]. In more detail, postural adaptations might have a crucial role in airways closure and in reducing the risk of inhalations in order to improve the speed and safety of swallowing [201]. Thus, the posture of sitting upright and head/neck flexed should be adopted in sarcopenic dysphagic patients, because this is the optimal posture to improve swallowing performances in dysphagic patients [202]. Moreover, postural adjustments significantly improve self-perceived difficulties in swallowing maneuvers [202]. In more detail, an upright 90° seated position should be maintained at least 30 min after eating to reduce the risk of inhalation of unswallowed food [18].

Swallowing compensatory maneuvers represent not only a short-term compensation to provide immediate benefits in bolus flow but also a specific rehabilitative strategy to improve swallowing functional training [81]. In more detail, supra- and super-supraglottic swallow, Mendelsohn's maneuver and effortful swallow have been proposed to have a role in sarcopenic dysphagia.

Tongue-pressure resistance training (TPRT) is the most used strengthening exercise, and it has been proved to enable an improvement in hyoid bone movements, tongue pressure and width of the upper esophageal sphincter [203]. In 2020, Nagano et al. [178] reported an increased maximal tongue pressure in sarcopenic patients after 2-month physical and occupational therapy, without additional swallowing training. Therefore, these findings emphasized the role of a multitarget rehabilitative intervention focusing not only on swallowing training but including physical exercise combined with a rehabilitative nutrition approach to improve the overall well-being of older patients and consequent swallowing deficits related to a decrease of physical function and sarcopenia.

Lastly, compensatory strategies might include changes in the consistency of solid and/or liquid foods. In more detail, food texture represents one of the first therapeutic targets aimed at improving the safety and effectiveness of oral feeding and oral intake in dysphagic patients [81].

In accordance with the International Dysphagia Diet Standardization Initiative (IDDSI) framework [204], food texture can be categorized into eight different levels (0–7). The eight levels included both liquids (ranging from level 0 to level 4) and solids (ranging from level 3 to level 7). Therefore, levels 3 and 4 are characterized by a cross-over of both fluids and solids [204].

Based on these food texture levels, an IDDSI Functional Diet Scale [205] was introduced to standardize the food texture prescription based on the patient's characteristics. Despite the great consensus received by the IDDSI worldwide, there is still a large heterogeneity of standards of diet texture and fluid modifications in the different countries [156].

Functional training might provide long-term benefits in patients suffering from dysphagia, such as lingual resistance exercises, considering the recent evidence supporting the strict relationship between sarcopenic dysphagia and tongue strength [206]. Given that resistance exercise requires specific and progressive training, a multidisciplinary approach should be provided, involving not only speech-language pathologists but also nurses, caregivers, and the patients themselves [85]. Moreover, specific exercises such as "shaker exercise" and "masako" (tongue hold) maneuver might improve swallowing physiology promoting muscles mechanics and bolus flow [207]. In this context, a meta-analysis performed by Carnaby-Mann et al. [208] assessed the effects of transcutaneous neuromuscular electrical stimulations for swallowing muscles, underlining the benefits of this treatment in improving swallowing performances. Moreover, strength deficits seem to be considered the main responsible for dysphagia in sarcopenic patients, suggesting intriguing implications of this treatment in elderly patients [206].

Despite several studies [209–211] underlining the positive effects of swallowing muscle training in swallowing function, dysphagia-related morbidities prevention and swallowing physiology improvement, there are only a few low-quality studies [188,189,191,192] that supported this rehabilitative intervention in patients with sarcopenic dysphagia.

Taken together, these findings highlight the effectiveness of a comprehensive oral rehabilitation approach in dysphagic patients, suggesting positive implications in sarcopenic dysphagia too. In contrast, there is still low evidence supporting oropharyngeal rehabilitation in a specific cohort of patients suffering from sarcopenic dysphagia, emphasizing the needing for clinical trials assessing this specific intervention in these patients.

8. Oral Health Management for Older Subjects

Populations across the world are ageing and the average life expectancy is rising in developed and developing countries [212]. On a global scale, the World Health Organization identified oral health as a major public health problem [213,214]. Among the oral diseases, caries and periodontal diseases are the most prevalent ones, even because the damage due to both periodontitis and caries is quite irreversible and so cumulative over the lifetime. Moreover, aging might affect both diseases directly, through aging of the immune system as well as impaired wound healing, and indirectly via physical and cognitive impairment as well as reduced access to care [215,216]. Indeed, the age-related decline in terms of physical performance and cognitive functions could influence older people's ability to carry out an adequate oral hygiene, with a consequent higher prevalence of oral diseases (e.g., periodontal disease, caries, and oral mucosal inflammation) [129,217–219]. Moreover, as previously underlined, oral health status might be strictly linked to dysphagia and malnutrition with detrimental consequences in terms of the overall well-being of older adults.

In the literature, cognitive disorders have received growing attention for their possible link to oral diseases. In this context, studies have examined the effect of lower cognitive abilities on periodontal health, showing that reduced number of teeth, augmented alveolar bone loss, and increased pocket depth were associated with cognitive impairment [220,221]. If untreated, caries and periodontal diseases could lead to tooth loss, edentulism, reduction of the lower third of the face, poor esthetics, phonetic problems, loss of masticatory function, poor nutrition status, as well as loss of self-esteem, and reduced HRQoL [222,223]. Therefore, the treatment of caries, periodontitis, and replacement of teeth lost are the most used among the clinical approaches to improve masticatory function in older people and consequently might reduce the risk of malnutrition.

More in detail, the periodontal treatment aims to reduce the bacterial deposits with a reduction of the inflammatory response through the active therapy, which consists of full-mouth scaling (FMS) and full-mouth disinfection [224]. The scaling techniques allow the debridement of bacterial deposits coating the surface of the root, deep within the periodontal pocket. In addition, periodontal surgery is used when the depth of the periodontal pockets prevents adequate access for debridement. After causal therapy, a supportive periodontal therapy is employed to reduce the probability that the disease will flare up again, thus maintaining teeth without pain, excessive mobility, or persistent infection [225–227]. According to the American Academy of Periodontology, supportive periodontal therapy should include a periodontal re-evaluation and risk assessment, supragingival and subgingival removal of bacterial plaque and calculus, and re-treatment of any sites showing recurrent or persistent disease [225].

Frail and complex care needs elderly people suffered the most from oral dryness, which could lead to rapidly progressing caries and oral infections [113,228]. In this context, patients with xerostomia should be adequately treated to reduce dysgeusia, halitosis, burning mouth, oral pain, difficulty in chewing and swallowing, and speech impairment [120,121]. Salivary stimulation by means of systemic pharmacotherapies, such as pilocarpine, might be appropriate for use by patients with some degree of salivary gland function [115]. However, whereas the stimulation of saliva production could be effective, these drugs are associated with adverse effects and might be contraindicated in patients with existing chronic respiratory, cardiovascular and renal disease [229,230] in patients in whom drug therapy is contraindicated, non-pharmacological interventions, such as electrostimulation of the salivary glands, acupuncture or the application of low level laser therapy, have the potential to increase saliva production especially in patients with some residual salivary gland function [231].

The main goal of treatment of patients with co-morbidities or contraindications to pharmacological therapies remains the reduction of clinical symptoms to provide a short-term relief during daily hours [230]. Thus, the common therapy involves the topical application of salivary substitutes [231] or artificial saliva [232], including carboxymethylcellulose [233], herbal powder of Alcea digitata, and Malva sylvestris [234], and immunologically active saliva substitutes [235].

Replacement of teeth lost is conventionally addressed by replacing multiple missing teeth with prosthetic dental elements. Through the aid of partial or complete prosthesis (removable or fixed) it is possible to restore missing dental elements, both in patients who have the loss of some dental elements and in edentulous patients [236]. Techniques for replacing one or more missing teeth are removable dental prostheses, tooth and tooth-tissue supported, and fixed dental prostheses, tooth supported [237]. The use of complete removable dentures might induce clinical manifestations, such as stomatitis, traumatic ulcers, irritation-induced hyperplasia, and altered taste perception [237]. In this context, the implant-retained prostheses represent the new approach and a long-term therapeutic solution [238]. It is shown that prosthetic treatments could provide a better oral HRQoL in edentulous patients, and that the fixed implant-supported prostheses might also improve the patient satisfaction better than complete removable dentures treatment. These intriguing results might promote a significant improvement of masticatory function with possible implications in terms of oral intake and risk of malnutrition in older people.

It is important to highlight that the geriatric management should provide an interdisciplinary diagnostic and therapeutic process aimed at determining the psychophysical and functional problems of older people. Despite the significant progress in dental science and oral health prevention in recent years, chronic oral diseases are still common in older people [35].

Moreover, in geriatric subjects with serious illnesses and functional dependency, oral health problems are often underdiagnosed and untreated [239,240]. Increasing evidence also reveals significant interactions between oral health and general health that are unidirectional and often bidirectional [127,129,130,241,242]. It has been hypothesized that a strict correlation between oral health and quality of life, as reported by Hoeksema et al. [3] while assessing the oral health in community-living elderly, demonstrated that general health and HRQoL were higher in older people with remaining teeth and implant-supported dentures than the edentulous ones. Indeed, edentulous individuals with up to one denture were associated with higher risk of malnutrition, whereas in edentulous older persons with two complete dentures, a better nutritional status was observed [243].

Therefore, given that poor oral health has been recently identified as a determinant for malnutrition and sarcopenia [103], an adequate dental and oral screening might play a key role in a comprehensive management of older patients. Moreover, as suggested by the European Policy Recommendations on Oral Health in Older Adults [244], an adequate patient-tailored oral health rehabilitation program is crucial to prevent not only oral diseases but also malnutrition, particularly in the older people at high risk of sarcopenic dysphagia.

9. Study Limitations

We are aware that this study is not free from limitations. In particular, the narrative design severely limits the strength of the study results. However, it should be noted that considering the heterogeneity of pathological conditions and treatment assessed a systematic review was not possible according to the Cochrane Handbook for Systematic Review of Intervention (Ver, 6.1, 2020) [245].

10. Conclusions and Future Perspectives

This comprehensive review showed that there is a negative bond among sarcopenic dysphagia, malnutrition, and oral frailty in older people. These conditions share several risk factors some phenotypically overlapping features and should be adequately assessed and treated, particularly in the elderly.

A specific screening for sarcopenic dysphagia might be introduced in routine clinical practice for high-risk patients to promote early rehabilitative interventions preventing health-related consequences. Tailored treatment based on patient's characteristics should be proposed aiming at targeting not only sarcopenic dysphagia consequences but also the etiological causes including oral frailty, malnutrition, and sarcopenia. Moreover, a comprehensive intervention should be proposed to promote the synergic effects of different therapies in frail elderly subjects.

Therefore, an adequate management of older people should include oropharyngeal rehabilitation, oral health treatment, and nutritional supplementation to counteract the age-related functional decline and to improve the quality of life.

Despite these considerations, future studies are warranted to provide strong evidence supporting a transdisciplinary approach to sarcopenic dysphagic elderly patients.

Author Contributions: Conceptualization, A.d.S. and M.F.; methodology, A.d.S., M.I. and M.M.; investigation, L.L., F.A. and R.d.S.; writing—original draft preparation, A.d.S., M.F. and L.L.; writing—review and editing, M.I. and M.M.; visualization F.A., R.d.S., P.E.F., G.R. (Giuseppe Raguso), S.R., A.R. and G.R. (Gianpaolo Ronconi); supervision, A.d.S. and M.M. All authors have read and agreed to the published version of the manuscript.

Funding: This research received no external funding.

Institutional Review Board Statement: Not applicable.

Informed Consent Statement: Not applicable.

Data Availability Statement: Not applicable.

Conflicts of Interest: The authors declare no conflict of interest.

References

1. Abdullah, B.; Wolbring, G. Analysis of newspaper coverage of active aging through the lens of the 2002 World Health Organization Active Ageing Report: A Policy Framework and the 2010 Toronto Charter for Physical Activity: A Global Call for Action. *Int. J. Environ. Res. Public Health* **2013**, *10*, 6799–6819. [CrossRef]
2. Branca, S.; Bennati, E.; Ferlito, L.; Spallina, G.; Cardillo, E.; Malaguarnera, M.; Motta, M. The health-care in the extreme longevity. *Arch. Gerontol. Geriatr.* **2009**, *49*, 32–34. [CrossRef]
3. Hoeksema, A.R.; Spoorenberg, S.; Peters, L.L.; Meijer, H.; Raghoebar, G.M.; Vissink, A.; Visser, A. Elderly with remaining teeth report less frailty and better quality of life than edentulous elderly: A cross-sectional study. *Oral. Dis.* **2017**, *23*, 526–536. [CrossRef]
4. Kojima, G.; Liljas, A.E.M.; Iliffe, S. Frailty syndrome: Implications and challenges for health care policy. *Risk Manag. Healthc. Policy* **2019**, *12*, 23–30. [CrossRef]
5. De Sire, A.; Giachero, A.; De Santi, S.; Inglese, K.; Solaro, C. Screening dysphagia risk in 534 older patients undergoing rehabilitation after total joint replacement: A cross-sectional study. *Eur. J. Phys. Rehabil. Med.* **2021**, *57*, 131–136. [CrossRef]
6. Fan, Y.; Ni, S.; Zhang, H. Association between Healthy Eating Index-2015 total and component food scores with osteoporosis in middle-aged and older Americans: A cross-sectional study with U.S. National Health and Nutrition Examination Survey. *Osteoporos. Int.* **2021**, 1–9. [CrossRef]
7. Leigheb, M.; de Sire, A.; Colangelo, M.; Zagaria, D.; Grassi, F.A.; Rena, O.; Ferraro, E. Sarcopenia Diagnosis: Reliability of the Ultrasound Assessment of the Tibialis Anterior Muscle as an Alternative Evaluation Tool. *Diagnostics* **2021**, *11*, 2158. [CrossRef]
8. Palmer, K.; Onder, G.; Cesari, M. The geriatric condition of frailty. *Eur. J. Intern. Med.* **2018**, *56*, 1–2. [CrossRef]
9. Beard, J.R.; Officer, A.; de Carvalho, I.A.; Sadana, R.; Pot, A.M.; Michel, J.P.; Chatterji, S. The World report on ageing and health: A policy framework for healthy ageing. *Lancet* **2016**, *387*, 2145–2154. [CrossRef]
10. Hoogendijk, E.O.; Afilalo, J.; Ensrud, K.E.; Kowal, P.; Onder, G.; Fried, L.P. Frailty: Implications for clinical practice and public health. *Lancet* **2019**, *394*, 1365–1375. [CrossRef]
11. Di Monaco, M.; Castiglioni, C.; Bardesono, F.; Milano, E.; Massazza, G. Sarcopenic obesity and function in women with subacute hip fracture: A short-term prospective study. *Eur. J. Phys. Rehabil. Med.* **2021**, *57*, 940–947. [CrossRef] [PubMed]

12. Cruz-Jentoft, A.J.; Baeyens, J.P.; Bauer, J.M.; Boirie, Y.; Cederholm, T.; Landi, F.; Zamboni, M. Sarcopenia: European consensus on definition and diagnosis: Report of the European Working Group on Sarcopenia in Older People. *Age Ageing* **2010**, *39*, 412–423. [CrossRef] [PubMed]

13. Mayhew, A.J.; Amog, K.; Phillips, S.; Parise, G.; McNicholas, P.D.; de Souza, R.J.; Raina, P. The prevalence of sarcopenia in community-dwelling older adults, an exploration of differences between studies and within definitions: A systematic review and meta-analyses. *Age Ageing* **2019**, *48*, 48–56. [CrossRef]

14. Agostini, F.; Bernetti, A.; Di Giacomo, G.; Viva, M.G.; Paoloni, M.; Mangone, M.; Masiero, S. Rehabilitative Good Practices in the Treatment of Sarcopenia: A Narrative Review. *Am. J. Phys. Med. Rehabil.* **2021**, *100*, 280–287. [CrossRef] [PubMed]

15. Beaudart, C.; Rolland, Y.; Cruz-Jentoft, A.J.; Bauer, J.M.; Sieber, C.; Cooper, C.; Al-Daghri, N.; Araujo de Carvalho, I.; Bautmans, I.; Bernabei, R.; et al. Assessment of Muscle Function and Physical Performance in Daily Clinical Practice: A position paper endorsed by the European Society for Clinical and Economic Aspects of Osteoporosis, Osteoarthritis and Musculoskeletal Diseases (ESCEO). *Calcif. Tissue Int.* **2019**, *105*, 1–14. [CrossRef] [PubMed]

16. Cha, S.; Kim, W.S.; Kim, K.W.; Han, J.W.; Jang, H.C.; Lim, S.; Paik, N.J. Sarcopenia is an Independent Risk Factor for Dysphagia in Community-Dwelling Older Adults. *Dysphagia* **2019**, *34*, 692–697. [CrossRef] [PubMed]

17. Maeda, K.; Takaki, M.; Akagi, J. Decreased Skeletal Muscle Mass and Risk Factors of Sarcopenic Dysphagia: A Prospective Observational Cohort Study. *J. Gerontol. A Biol. Sci. Med. Sci.* **2017**, *72*, 1290–1294. [CrossRef] [PubMed]

18. Baijens, L.W.; Clavé, P.; Cras, P.; Ekberg, O.; Forster, A.; Kolb, G.F.; Walshe, M. European Society for Swallowing Disorders—European Union Geriatric Medicine Society white paper: Oropharyngeal dysphagia as a geriatric syndrome. *Clin. Interv. Aging* **2016**, *11*, 1403–1428. [CrossRef]

19. Dziewas, R.; Beck, A.M.; Clave, P.; Hamdy, S.; Heppner, H.J.; Langmore, S.E.; Wirth, R. Recognizing the Importance of Dysphagia: Stumbling Blocks and Stepping Stones in the Twenty-First Century. *Dysphagia* **2017**, *32*, 78–82. [CrossRef]

20. Wirth, R.; Dziewas, R.; Beck, A.M.; Clavé, P.; Hamdy, S.; Heppner, H.J.; Volkert, D. Oropharyngeal dysphagia in older persons—from pathophysiology to adequate intervention: A review and summary of an international expert meeting. *Clin. Interv. Aging* **2016**, *11*, 189–208. [CrossRef]

21. Kuroda, Y.; Kuroda, R. Relationship between thinness and swallowing function in Japanese older adults: Implications for sarcopenic dysphagia. *J. Am. Geriatr. Soc.* **2012**, *60*, 1785–1786. [CrossRef]

22. Wakabayashi, H. Presbyphagia and Sarcopenic Dysphagia: Association between Aging, Sarcopenia, and Deglutition Disorders. *J. Frailty Aging* **2014**, *3*, 97–103. [CrossRef] [PubMed]

23. Invernizzi, M.; Baricich, A.; Riso, S.; Lippi, L.; Cisari, C.; de Sire, A. Sarcopenic dysphagia: A narrative review. *Clin. Cases Miner. Bone Metab.* **2019**, *16*, 147–149.

24. Mann, T.; Heuberger, R.; Wong, H. The association between chewing and swallowing difficulties and nutritional status in older adults. *Aust. Dent. J.* **2013**, *58*, 200–206. [CrossRef]

25. N'Gom, P.I.; Woda, A. Influence of impaired mastication on nutrition. *J. Prosthet. Dent.* **2002**, *87*, 667–673. [CrossRef] [PubMed]

26. Veldee, M.S.; Peth, L.D. Can protein-calorie malnutrition cause dysphagia? *Dysphagia* **1992**, *7*, 86–101. [CrossRef] [PubMed]

27. Krishnamoorthy, Y.; Vijayageetha, M.; Kumar, S.G.; Rajaa, S.; Rehman, T. Prevalence of malnutrition and its associated factors among elderly population in rural Puducherry using mini-nutritional assessment questionnaire. *J. Fam. Med. Prim. Care* **2018**, *7*, 1429–1433. [CrossRef]

28. Lieu, P.K.; Chong, M.S.; Seshadri, R. The impact of swallowing disorders in the elderly. *Ann. Acad. Med. Singap.* **2001**, *30*, 148–154.

29. De Sire, A.; Baricich, A.; Ferrillo, M.; Migliario, M.; Cisari, C.; Invernizzi, M. Buccal hemineglect: Is it useful to evaluate the differences between the two halves of the oral cavity for the multidisciplinary rehabilitative management of right brain stroke survivors? A cross-sectional study. *Top. Stroke Rehabil.* **2020**, *27*, 208–214. [CrossRef]

30. De Sire, A.; Invernizzi, M.; Ferrillo, M.; Gimigliano, F.; Baricich, A.; Cisari, C.; Migliario, M. Functional status and oral health in patients with amyotrophic lateral sclerosis: A cross-sectional study. *NeuroRehabilitation* **2021**, *48*, 49–57. [CrossRef]

31. Kloukos, D.; Roccuzzo, A.; Stähli, A.; Sculean, A.; Katsaros, C.; Salvi, G.E. Effect of combined periodontal and orthodontic treatment of tilted molars and of teeth with intra-bony and furcation defects in stage-IV periodontitis patients: A systematic review. *J. Clin. Periodontol.* **2021**, *6*, 1–28. [CrossRef] [PubMed]

32. Toniazzo, M.P.; Amorim, P.S.; Muniz, F.; Weidlich, P. Relationship of nutritional status and oral health in elderly: Systematic review with meta-analysis. *Clin. Nutr.* **2018**, *37*, 824–830. [CrossRef] [PubMed]

33. Lee, K.H.; Plassman, B.L.; Pan, W.; Wu, B. Mediation Effect of Oral Hygiene on the Relationship Between Cognitive Function and Oral Health in Older Adults. *J. Gerontol. Nurs.* **2016**, *42*, 30–37. [CrossRef] [PubMed]

34. El Osta, N.; Hennequin, M.; Tubert-Jeannin, S.; Abboud Naaman, N.B.; El Osta, L.; Geahchan, N. The pertinence of oral health indicators in nutritional studies in the elderly. *Clin. Nutr.* **2014**, *33*, 316–321. [CrossRef]

35. Petersen, P.E.; Yamamoto, T. Improving the oral health of older people: The approach of the WHO Global Oral Health Programme. *Community Dent. Oral Epidemiol.* **2005**, *33*, 81–92. [CrossRef]

36. Lopez-Jornet, P.; Saura-Perez, M.; Llevat-Espinosa, N. Effect of oral health dental state and risk of malnutrition in elderly people. *Geriatr. Gerontol. Int.* **2013**, *13*, 43–49. [CrossRef]

37. Kaiser, M.J.; Bauer, J.M.; Ramsch, C.; Uter, W.; Guigoz, Y.; Cederholm, T.; Sieber, C.C. Validation of the Mini Nutritional Assessment short-form (MNA-SF): A practical tool for identification of nutritional status. *J. Nutr. Health Aging* **2009**, *13*, 782–788. [CrossRef]

38. Vellas, B.; Villars, H.; Abellan, G.; Soto, M.E.; Rolland, Y.; Guigoz, Y.; Garry, P. Overview of the MNA–Its history and challenges. *J. Nutr. Health Aging* **2006**, *10*, 456–463; discussion 455–463.
39. Rudnicka, E.; Napierała, P.; Podfigurna, A.; Męczekalski, B.; Smolarczyk, R.; Grymowicz, M. The World Health Organization (WHO) approach to healthy ageing. *Maturitas* **2020**, *139*, 6–11. [CrossRef]
40. Norman, K.; Haß, U.; Pirlich, M. Malnutrition in Older Adults-Recent Advances and Remaining Challenges. *Nutrients* **2021**, *13*, 2764. [CrossRef]
41. Cederholm, T.; Bosaeus, I.; Barazzoni, R.; Bauer, J.; Van Gossum, A.; Klek, S.; Singer, P. Diagnostic criteria for malnutrition—An ESPEN Consensus Statement. *Clin. Nutr.* **2015**, *34*, 335–340. [CrossRef]
42. Fleurke, M.; Voskuil, D.; Kolmer, D. The role of the dietitian in the management of malnutrition in the elderly: A systematic review of current practices. *Nutr. Diet.* **2019**, *77*, 60–75. [CrossRef] [PubMed]
43. Cereda, E.; Pedrolli, C.; Klersy, C.; Bonardi, C.; Quarleri, L.; Cappello, S.; Caccialanza, R. Nutritional status in older persons according to healthcare setting: A systematic review and meta-analysis of prevalence data using MNA(®). *Clin. Nutr.* **2016**, *35*, 1282–1290. [CrossRef] [PubMed]
44. Wojzischke, J.; van Wijngaarden, J.; van den Berg, C.; Cetinyurek-Yavuz, A.; Diekmann, R.; Luiking, Y.; Bauer, J. Nutritional status and functionality in geriatric rehabilitation patients: A systematic review and meta-analysis. *Eur. Geriatr. Med.* **2020**, *11*, 195–207. [CrossRef] [PubMed]
45. Landi, F.; Calvani, R.; Tosato, M.; Martone, A.M.; Ortolani, E.; Savera, G.; Marzetti, E. Anorexia of Aging: Risk Factors, Consequences, and Potential Treatments. *Nutrients* **2016**, *8*, 69. [CrossRef]
46. Naruishi, K.; Nishikawa, Y. Swallowing impairment is a significant factor for predicting life prognosis of elderly at the end of life. *Aging Clin. Exp. Res.* **2018**, *30*, 77–80. [CrossRef]
47. Hägglund, P.; Fält, A.; Hägg, M.; Wester, P.; Levring Jäghagen, E. Swallowing dysfunction as risk factor for undernutrition in older people admitted to Swedish short-term care: A cross-sectional study. *Aging Clin. Exp. Res.* **2019**, *31*, 85–94. [CrossRef]
48. Nishioka, S.; Okamoto, T.; Takayama, M.; Urushihara, M.; Watanabe, M.; Kiriya, Y.; Kageyama, N. Malnutrition risk predicts recovery of full oral intake among older adult stroke patients undergoing enteral nutrition: Secondary analysis of a multicentre survey (the APPLE study). *Clin. Nutr.* **2017**, *36*, 1089–1096. [CrossRef]
49. Saarela, R.K.; Soini, H.; Hiltunen, K.; Muurinen, S.; Suominen, M.; Pitkälä, K. Dentition status, malnutrition and mortality among older service housing residents. *J. Nutr. Health Aging* **2014**, *18*, 34–38. [CrossRef]
50. Anastassiadou, V.; Heath, M.R. Food choices and eating difficulty among elderly edentate patients in Greece. *Gerodontology* **2002**, *19*, 17–24. [CrossRef]
51. Joshipura, K.J.; Willett, W.C.; Douglass, C.W. The impact of edentulousness on food and nutrient intake. *J. Am. Dent. Assoc.* **1996**, *127*, 459–467. [CrossRef] [PubMed]
52. O'Connor, J.P.; Milledge, K.L.; O'Leary, F.; Cumming, R.; Eberhard, J.; Hirani, V. Poor dietary intake of nutrients and food groups are associated with increased risk of periodontal disease among community-dwelling older adults: A systematic literature review. *Nutr. Rev.* **2020**, *78*, 175–188. [CrossRef] [PubMed]
53. Kotsakis, G.A.; Chrepa, V.; Shivappa, N.; Wirth, M.; Hébert, J.; Koyanagi, A.; Tyrovolas, S. Diet-borne systemic inflammation is associated with prevalent tooth loss. *Clin. Nutr.* **2018**, *37*, 1306–1312. [CrossRef] [PubMed]
54. Van der Putten, G.J.; Vanobbergen, J.; De Visschere, L.; Schols, J.; de Baat, C. Association of some specific nutrient deficiencies with periodontal disease in elderly people: A systematic literature review. *Nutrition* **2009**, *25*, 717–722. [CrossRef]
55. Vellas, B.; Guigoz, Y.; Garry, P.J.; Nourhashemi, F.; Bennahum, D.; Lauque, S.; Albarede, J.L. The Mini Nutritional Assessment (MNA) and its use in grading the nutritional state of elderly patients. *Nutrition* **1999**, *15*, 116–122. [CrossRef]
56. Chapple, I.L.C.; Mealey, B.L.; Van Dyke, T.E.; Bartold, P.M.; Dommisch, H.; Eickholz, P.; Yoshie, H. Periodontal health and gingival diseases and conditions on an intact and a reduced periodontium: Consensus report of workgroup 1 of the 2017 World Workshop on the Classification of Periodontal and Peri-Implant Diseases and Conditions. *J. Periodontol.* **2018**, *89* (Suppl. S1), S74–S84. [CrossRef] [PubMed]
57. Ferguson, M.; Capra, S.; Bauer, J.; Banks, M. Development of a valid and reliable malnutrition screening tool for adult acute hospital patients. *Nutrition* **1999**, *15*, 458–464. [CrossRef]
58. Keller, H.H.; Goy, R.; Kane, S.L. Validity and reliability of SCREEN II (Seniors in the community: Risk evaluation for eating and nutrition, Version II). *Eur. J. Clin. Nutr.* **2005**, *59*, 1149–1157. [CrossRef]
59. Stratton, R.J.; King, C.L.; Stroud, M.A.; Jackson, A.A.; Elia, M. 'Malnutrition Universal Screening Tool' predicts mortality and length of hospital stay in acutely ill elderly. *Br. J. Nutr.* **2006**, *95*, 325–330. [CrossRef]
60. Wilson, M.M.; Thomas, D.R.; Rubenstein, L.Z.; Chibnall, J.T.; Anderson, S.; Baxi, A.; Morley, J.E. Appetite assessment: Simple appetite questionnaire predicts weight loss in community-dwelling adults and nursing home residents. *Am. J. Clin. Nutr.* **2005**, *82*, 1074–1081. [CrossRef]
61. Kondrup, J.; Rasmussen, H.H.; Hamberg, O.; Stanga, Z. Nutritional risk screening (NRS 2002): A new method based on an analysis of controlled clinical trials. *Clin. Nutr.* **2003**, *22*, 321–336. [CrossRef]
62. Bai, A.V.; Agostini, F.; Bernetti, A.; Mangone, M.; Fidenzi, G.; D'Urzo, R.; Masiero, S. State of the evidence about rehabilitation interventions in patients with dysphagia. *Eur. J. Phys. Rehabil. Med.* **2021**, *57*, 900–911. [CrossRef]
63. Eroğlu, A.G. Malnutrition and the heart. *Turk. Pediatri. Ars.* **2019**, *54*, 139–140. [CrossRef] [PubMed]

64. Raposeiras Roubín, S.; Abu Assi, E.; Cespón Fernandez, M.; Barreiro Pardal, C.; Lizancos Castro, A.; Parada, J.A.; Íñiguez Romo, A. Prevalence and Prognostic Significance of Malnutrition in Patients with Acute Coronary Syndrome. *J. Am. Coll. Cardiol.* **2020**, *76*, 828–840. [CrossRef] [PubMed]

65. Wells, J.C.; Sawaya, A.L.; Wibaek, R.; Mwangome, M.; Poullas, M.S.; Yajnik, C.S.; Demaio, A. The double burden of malnutrition: Aetiological pathways and consequences for health. *Lancet* **2020**, *395*, 75–88. [CrossRef]

66. Elmadfa, I.; Meyer, A.L. The Role of the Status of Selected Micronutrients in Shaping the Immune Function. *Endocr. Metab. Immune Disord. Drug Targets* **2019**, *19*, 1100–1115. [CrossRef]

67. Cantorna, M.T.; McDaniel, K.; Bora, S.; Chen, J.; James, J. Vitamin D, immune regulation, the microbiota, and inflammatory bowel disease. *Exp. Biol. Med.* **2014**, *239*, 1524–1530. [CrossRef]

68. Andrès, E.; Loukili, N.H.; Noel, E.; Kaltenbach, G.; Abdelgheni, M.B.; Perrin, A.E.; Blicklé, J.F. Vitamin B12 (cobalamin) deficiency in elderly patients. *Cmaj* **2004**, *171*, 251–259. [CrossRef]

69. Cunha, D.F.; Cunha, S.F.; Unamuno, M.R.; Vannucchi, H. Serum levels assessment of vitamin A, E, C, B2 and carotenoids in malnourished and non-malnourished hospitalized elderly patients. *Clin. Nutr.* **2001**, *20*, 167–170. [CrossRef]

70. Spinneker, A.; Sola, R.; Lemmen, V.; Castillo, M.J.; Pietrzik, K.; González-Gross, M. Vitamin B6 status, deficiency and its consequences—An overview. *Nutr. Hosp.* **2007**, *22*, 7–24.

71. Vaquero, M.P. Magnesium and trace elements in the elderly: Intake, status and recommendations. *J. Nutr. Health Aging* **2002**, *6*, 147–153. [PubMed]

72. Carmel, R. Nutritional anemias and the elderly. *Semin. Hematol.* **2008**, *45*, 225–234. [CrossRef] [PubMed]

73. Cruz-Jentoft, A.J.; Kiesswetter, E.; Drey, M.; Sieber, C.C. Nutrition, frailty, and sarcopenia. *Aging Clin. Exp. Res.* **2017**, *29*, 43–48. [CrossRef] [PubMed]

74. Rizzoli, R. Nutritional aspects of bone health. *Best Pract. Res. Clin. Endocrinol. Metab.* **2014**, *28*, 795–808. [CrossRef] [PubMed]

75. Gaffney-Stomberg, E.; Insogna, K.L.; Rodriguez, N.R.; Kerstetter, J.E. Increasing dietary protein requirements in elderly people for optimal muscle and bone health. *J. Am. Geriatr. Soc.* **2009**, *57*, 1073–1079. [CrossRef] [PubMed]

76. Rizzoli, R. Postmenopausal osteoporosis: Assessment and management. *Best Pract. Res. Clin. Endocrinol. Metab.* **2018**, *32*, 739–757. [CrossRef]

77. Bikle, D.D.; Tahimic, C.; Chang, W.; Wang, Y.; Philippou, A.; Barton, E.R. Role of IGF-I signaling in muscle bone interactions. *Bone* **2015**, *80*, 79–88. [CrossRef]

78. De Sire, A.; Invernizzi, M.; Baricich, A.; Lippi, L.; Ammendolia, A.; Grassi, F.A.; Leigheb, M. Optimization of transdisciplinary management of elderly with femur proximal extremity fracture: A patient-tailored plan from orthopaedics to rehabilitation. *World J. Orthop.* **2021**, *12*, 456–466. [CrossRef] [PubMed]

79. Marzetti, E.; Calvani, R.; Tosato, M.; Cesari, M.; Di Bari, M.; Cherubini, A.; Broccatelli, M.; Savera, G.; D'Elia, M.; Pahor, M.; et al. Physical activity and exercise as countermeasures to physical frailty and sarcopenia. *Aging Clin. Exp. Res.* **2017**, *29*, 35–42. [CrossRef]

80. Namasivayam, A.M.; Steele, C.M. Malnutrition and Dysphagia in long-term care: A systematic review. *J. Nutr. Gerontol. Geriatr.* **2015**, *34*, 1–21. [CrossRef]

81. Sura, L.; Madhavan, A.; Carnaby, G.; Crary, M.A. Dysphagia in the elderly: Management and nutritional considerations. *Clin. Interv. Aging* **2012**, *7*, 287–298. [CrossRef] [PubMed]

82. Damanti, S.; Azzolino, D.; Roncaglione, C.; Arosio, B.; Rossi, P.; Cesari, M. Efficacy of Nutritional Interventions as Stand-Alone or Synergistic Treatments with Exercise for the Management of Sarcopenia. *Nutrients* **2019**, *11*, 1991. [CrossRef] [PubMed]

83. Logrippo, S.; Ricci, G.; Sestili, M.; Cespi, M.; Ferrara, L.; Palmieri, G.F.; Blasi, P. Oral drug therapy in elderly with dysphagia: Between a rock and a hard place! *Clin. Interv. Aging* **2017**, *12*, 241–251. [CrossRef] [PubMed]

84. Siebens, H.; Trupe, E.; Siebens, A.; Cook, F.; Anshen, S.; Hanauer, R.; Oster, G. Correlates and consequences of eating dependency in institutionalized elderly. *J. Am. Geriatr. Soc.* **1986**, *34*, 192–198. [CrossRef] [PubMed]

85. Dellis, S.; Papadopoulou, S.; Krikonis, K.; Zigras, F. Sarcopenic Dysphagia. A Narrative Review. *J. Frailty Sarcopenia Falls* **2018**, *3*, 1–7. [CrossRef]

86. Feng, X.; Todd, T.; Lintzenich, C.R.; Ding, J.; Carr, J.J.; Ge, Y.; Butler, S.G. Aging-related geniohyoid muscle atrophy is related to aspiration status in healthy older adults. *J. Gerontol. A Biol. Sci. Med. Sci.* **2013**, *68*, 853–860. [CrossRef]

87. Nakao, Y.; Uchiyama, Y.; Honda, K.; Yamashita, T.; Saito, S.; Domen, K. Age-related composition changes in swallowing-related muscles: A Dixon MRI study. *Aging Clin. Exp. Res.* **2021**, *33*, 3205–3213. [CrossRef]

88. Miyashita, T.; Kikutani, T.; Nagashima, K.; Igarashi, K.; Tamura, F. The effects of sarcopenic dysphagia on the dynamics of swallowing organs observed on videofluoroscopic swallowing studies. *J. Oral Rehabil.* **2020**, *47*, 584–590. [CrossRef]

89. Kunieda, K.; Fujishima, I.; Wakabayashi, H.; Ohno, T.; Shigematsu, T.; Itoda, M.; Ogawa, S. Relationship Between Tongue Pressure and Pharyngeal Function Assessed Using High-Resolution Manometry in Older Dysphagia Patients with Sarcopenia: A Pilot Study. *Dysphagia* **2021**, *36*, 33–40. [CrossRef]

90. Nawaz, S.; Tulunay-Ugur, O.E. Dysphagia in the Older Patient. *Otolaryngol. Clin. N. Am.* **2018**, *51*, 769–777. [CrossRef]

91. Belafsky, P.C.; Mouadeb, D.A.; Rees, C.J.; Pryor, J.C.; Postma, G.N.; Allen, J.; Leonard, R.J. Validity and reliability of the Eating Assessment Tool (EAT-10). *Ann. Otol. Rhinol. Laryngol.* **2008**, *117*, 919–924. [CrossRef] [PubMed]

92. Cheney, D.M.; Siddiqui, M.T.; Litts, J.K.; Kuhn, M.A.; Belafsky, P.C. The Ability of the 10-Item Eating Assessment Tool (EAT-10) to Predict Aspiration Risk in Persons with Dysphagia. *Ann. Otol. Rhinol. Laryngol.* **2015**, *124*, 351–354. [CrossRef] [PubMed]

93. Tohara, H.; Saitoh, E.; Mays, K.A.; Kuhlemeier, K.; Palmer, J.B. Three tests for predicting aspiration without videofluorography. *Dysphagia* **2003**, *18*, 126–134. [CrossRef]
94. Yagi, N.; Oku, Y.; Nagami, S.; Yamagata, Y.; Kayashita, J.; Ishikawa, A.; Takahashi, R. Inappropriate Timing of Swallow in the Respiratory Cycle Causes Breathing-Swallowing Discoordination. *Front. Physiol.* **2017**, *8*, 676. [CrossRef] [PubMed]
95. Audag, N.; Goubau, C.; Toussaint, M.; Reychler, G. Screening and evaluation tools of dysphagia in adults with neuromuscular diseases: A systematic review. *Ther. Adv. Chronic. Dis.* **2019**, *10*, 2040622318821622. [CrossRef]
96. Crary, M.A.; Mann, G.D.; Groher, M.E. Initial psychometric assessment of a functional oral intake scale for dysphagia in stroke patients. *Arch. Phys. Med. Rehabil.* **2005**, *86*, 1516–1520. [CrossRef]
97. Kunieda, K.; Ohno, T.; Fujishima, I.; Hojo, K.; Morita, T. Reliability and validity of a tool to measure the severity of dysphagia: The Food Intake LEVEL Scale. *J. Pain Symptom Manag.* **2013**, *46*, 201–206. [CrossRef]
98. Giraldo-Cadavid, L.F.; Pantoja, J.A.; Forero, Y.; Gutierrez, H.M.; Bastidas, A. Aspiration in the Fiberoptic Endoscopic Evaluation of Swallowing Associated with an Increased Risk of Mortality in a Cohort of Patients Suspected of Oropharyngeal Dysphagia. *Dysphagia* **2019**, *35*, 369–377. [CrossRef]
99. Budtz-Jørgensen, E.; Chung, J.P.; Mojon, P. Successful aging—The case for prosthetic therapy. *J. Public Health Dent.* **2000**, *60*, 308–312. [CrossRef]
100. Avlund, K.; Schultz-Larsen, K.; Christiansen, N.; Holm-Pedersen, P. Number of Teeth and Fatigue in Older Adults. *J. Am. Geriatr. Soc.* **2011**, *59*, 1459–1464. [CrossRef]
101. Coleman, P. Improving oral health care for the frail elderly: A review of widespread problems and best practices. *Geriatr. Nurs.* **2002**, *23*, 189–199. [CrossRef] [PubMed]
102. Iwasaki, M.; Taylor, G.W.; Manz, M.C.; Yoshihara, A.; Sato, M.; Muramatsu, K.; Miyazaki, H. Oral health status: Relationship to nutrient and food intake among 80-year-old Japanese adults. *Community Dent. Oral Epidemiol.* **2014**, *42*, 441–450. [CrossRef] [PubMed]
103. Azzolino, D.; Passarelli, P.C.; De Angelis, P.; Piccirillo, G.B.; D'Addona, A.; Cesari, M. Poor Oral Health as a Determinant of Malnutrition and Sarcopenia. *Nutrients* **2019**, *11*, 2898. [CrossRef] [PubMed]
104. Veronese, N.; Punzi, L.; Sieber, C.; Bauer, J.; Reginster, J.Y.; Maggi, S.; the Task Finish Group on "Arthritis" of the European Geriatric Medicine Society. Sarcopenic osteoarthritis: A new entity in geriatric medicine? *Eur. Geriatr. Med.* **2018**, *9*, 141–148. [CrossRef] [PubMed]
105. Hussein, S.; Kantawalla, R.F.; Dickie, S.; Suarez-Durall, P.; Enciso, R.; Mulligan, R. Association of Oral Health and Mini Nutritional Assessment in Older Adults: A Systematic Review with Meta-analyses. *J. Prosthodont. Res.* **2021**. [CrossRef]
106. Iwasaki, M.; Motokawa, K.; Watanabe, Y.; Shirobe, M.; Inagaki, H.; Edahiro, A.; Awata, S. Association between Oral Frailty and Nutritional Status among Community-Dwelling Older Adults: The Takashimadaira Study. *J. Nutr. Health Aging* **2020**, *24*, 1003–1010. [CrossRef]
107. Lamy, M.; Mojon, P.; Kalykakis, G.; Legrand, R.; Butz-Jorgensen, E. Oral status and nutrition in the institutionalized elderly. *J. Dent.* **1999**, *27*, 443–448. [CrossRef]
108. Anil, S.; Vellappally, S.; Hashem, M.; Preethanath, R.S.; Patil, S.; Samaranayake, L.P. Xerostomia in geriatric patients: A burgeoning global concern. *J. Investig. Clin. Dent.* **2016**, *7*, 5–12. [CrossRef]
109. Liu, B.; Dion, M.R.; Jurasic, M.M.; Gibson, G.; Jones, J.A. Xerostomia and salivary hypofunction in vulnerable elders: Prevalence and etiology. *Oral Surg. Oral Med. Oral Pathol. Oral Radiol.* **2012**, *114*, 52–60. [CrossRef]
110. Ouanounou, A. Xerostomia in the Geriatric Patient: Causes, Oral Manifestations, and Treatment. *Compend. Contin. Educ. Dent.* **2016**, *37*, 306–311, quiz312.
111. Thomson, W.M.; Chalmers, J.M.; Spencer, A.J.; Williams, S.M. The Xerostomia Inventory: A multi-item approach to measuring dry mouth. *Community Dent. Health* **1999**, *16*, 12–17.
112. Nederfors, T.; Isaksson, R.; Mörnstad, H.; Dahlöf, C. Prevalence of perceived symptoms of dry mouth in an adult Swedish population–relation to age, sex and pharmacotherapy. *Community Dent. Oral. Epidemiol.* **1997**, *25*, 211–216. [CrossRef] [PubMed]
113. Aliko, A.; Wolff, A.; Dawes, C.; Aframian, D.; Proctor, G.; Ekström, J.; Vissink, A. World Workshop on Oral Medicine VI: Clinical implications of medication-induced salivary gland dysfunction. *Oral Surg. Oral Med. Oral Pathol. Oral Radiol.* **2015**, *120*, 185–206. [CrossRef] [PubMed]
114. Von Bültzingslöwen, I.; Sollecito, T.P.; Fox, P.C.; Daniels, T.; Jonsson, R.; Lockhart, P.B.; Schiødt, M. Salivary dysfunction associated with systemic diseases: Systematic review and clinical management recommendations. *Oral Surg. Oral Med. Oral Pathol. Oral Radiol. Endodontol.* **2007**, *103*, S57-e1. [CrossRef] [PubMed]
115. Porter, S.R.; Scully, C.; Hegarty, A.M. An update of the etiology and management of xerostomia. *Oral Surg. Oral Med. Oral Pathol. Oral Radiol. Endodontol.* **2004**, *97*, 28–46. [CrossRef]
116. Napeñas, J.J.; Brennan, M.T.; Fox, P.C. Diagnosis and treatment of xerostomia (dry mouth). *Odontology* **2009**, *97*, 76–83. [CrossRef]
117. Carrozzo, M. Oral diseases associated with hepatitis C virus infection. Part 1. sialadenitis and salivary glands lymphoma. *Oral Dis.* **2008**, *14*, 123–130. [CrossRef]
118. Humphrey, S.P.; Williamson, R.T. A review of saliva: Normal composition, flow, and function. *J. Prosthet. Dent.* **2001**, *85*, 162–169. [CrossRef]
119. Salles, C.; Chagnon, M.-C.; Feron, G.; Guichard, E.; Laboure, H.; Morzel, M.; Yven, C. In-mouth mechanisms leading to flavor release and perception. *Crit. Rev. Food Sci. Nutr.* **2011**, *51*, 67–90. [CrossRef]

120. Han, P.; Suarez-Durall, P.; Mulligan, R. Dry mouth: A critical topic for older adult patients. *J. Prosthodont. Res.* **2015**, *59*, 6–19. [CrossRef]

121. Muñoz-González, C.; Vandenberghe-Descamps, M.; Feron, G.; Canon, F.; Labouré, H.; Sulmont-Rossé, C. Association between Salivary Hypofunction and Food Consumption in the Elderlies. A Systematic Literature Review. *J. Nutr. Health Aging* **2017**, *22*, 407–419. [CrossRef] [PubMed]

122. Di Stasio, D.; Lauritano, D.; Minervini, G.; Paparella, R.S.; Petruzzi, M.; Romano, A.; Lucchese, A. Management of denture stomatitis: A narrative review. *J. Biol. Regul. Homeost. Agents* **2018**, *32* (Suppl. S1), 113–116. [PubMed]

123. Kaplan, I.; Zuk-Paz, L.; Wolff, A. Association between salivary flow rates, oral symptoms, and oral mucosal status. *Oral Surg. Oral Med. Oral Pathol. Oral Radiol. Endodontol.* **2008**, *106*, 235–241. [CrossRef]

124. Plemons, J.M.; Al-Hashimi, I.; Marek, C.L. Managing xerostomia and salivary gland hypofunction: Executive summary of a report from the American Dental Association Council on Scientific Affairs. *J. Am. Dent. Assoc.* **2014**, *145*, 867–873. [CrossRef] [PubMed]

125. Könönen, E.; Gursoy, M.; Gursoy, U.K. Periodontitis: A Multifaceted Disease of Tooth-Supporting Tissues. *J. Clin. Med.* **2019**, *8*, 1135. [CrossRef]

126. Sanz, M.; van Winkelhoff, A.J. Periodontal infections: Understanding the complexity–consensus of the Seventh European Workshop on Periodontology. *J. Clin. Periodontol.* **2011**, *38* (Suppl. S11), 3–6. [CrossRef] [PubMed]

127. Ferrillo, M.; Migliario, M.; Roccuzzo, A.; Molinero-Mourelle, P.; Falcicchio, G.; Umano, G.R.; de Sire, A. Periodontal Disease and Vitamin D Deficiency in Pregnant Women: Which Correlation with Preterm and Low-Weight Birth? *J. Clin. Med.* **2021**, *10*, 4578. [CrossRef]

128. Aimetti, M.; Romano, F.; Nessi, F. Microbiologic Analysis of Periodontal Pockets and Carotid Atheromatous Plaques in Advanced Chronic Periodontitis Patients. *J. Periodontol.* **2007**, *78*, 1718–1723. [CrossRef]

129. Carrizales-Sepúlveda, E.F.; Ordaz-Farías, A.; Vera-Pineda, R.; Flores-Ramírez, R. Periodontal Disease, Systemic Inflammation and the Risk of Cardiovascular Disease. *Heart Lung Circ.* **2018**, *27*, 1327–1334. [CrossRef]

130. Li, W.; Xu, J.; Zhang, R.; Li, Y.; Wang, J.; Zhang, X.; Lin, L. Is periodontal disease a risk indicator for colorectal cancer? A systematic review and meta-analysis. *J. Clin. Periodontol.* **2021**, *48*, 336–347. [CrossRef]

131. Chandra, R.K. Nutrition and the immune system: An introduction. *Am. J. Clin. Nutr.* **1997**, *66*, 460s–463s. [CrossRef] [PubMed]

132. Cunningham-Rundles, S. Analytical Methods for Evaluation of Immune Response in Nutrient Intervention. *Nutr. Rev.* **1998**, *56*, S27–S37. [CrossRef] [PubMed]

133. Dommisch, H.; Kuzmanova, D.; Jönsson, D.; Grant, M.; Chapple, I. Effect of micronutrient malnutrition on periodontal disease and periodontal therapy. *Periodontol. 2000* **2018**, *78*, 129–153. [CrossRef]

134. Džopalić, T.; Božić-Nedeljković, B.; Jurišić, V. The role of vitamin A and vitamin D in modulation of the immune response with a focus on innate lymphoid cells. *Cent. Eur. J. Immunol.* **2021**, *46*, 264–269. [CrossRef]

135. Meydani, S.N.; Meydani, M.; Blumberg, J.B.; Leka, L.S.; Siber, G.; Loszewski, R.; Stollar, B.D. Vitamin E supplementation and in vivo immune response in healthy elderly subjects. A randomized controlled trial. *JAMA* **1997**, *277*, 1380–1386. [CrossRef]

136. Boyd, L.D.; Madden, T.E. Nutrition, infection, and periodontal disease. *Dent. Clin. N. Am.* **2003**, *47*, 337–354. [CrossRef]

137. Hatta, K.; Ikebe, K. Association between oral health and sarcopenia: A literature review. *J. Prosthodont. Res.* **2021**, *65*, 131–136. [CrossRef]

138. Chang, H.R.; Bistrian, B. The role of cytokines in the catabolic consequences of infection and injury. *JPEN J. Parenter. Enteral Nutr.* **1998**, *22*, 156–166. [CrossRef]

139. Visser, M.; Pahor, M.; Taaffe, D.R.; Goodpaster, B.H.; Simonsick, E.M.; Newman, A.B.; Harris, T.B. Relationship of Interleukin-6 and Tumor Necrosis Factor-α With Muscle Mass and Muscle Strength in Elderly Men and Women: The Health ABC Study. *J. Gerontol. Ser. A* **2002**, *57*, M326–M332. [CrossRef]

140. Payette, H.; Roubenoff, R.; Jacques, P.F.; Dinarello, C.A.; Wilson, P.W.F.; Abad, L.W.; Harris, T. Insulin-like growth factor-1 and interleukin 6 predict sarcopenia in very old community-living men and women: The Framingham Heart Study. *J. Am. Geriatr. Soc.* **2003**, *51*, 1237–1243. [CrossRef]

141. Shiraishi, A.; Yoshimura, Y.; Wakabayashi, H.; Tsuji, Y. Prevalence of stroke-related sarcopenia and its association with poor oral status in post-acute stroke patients: Implications for oral sarcopenia. *Clin. Nutr.* **2018**, *37*, 204–207. [CrossRef] [PubMed]

142. Ortega, O.; Parra, C.; Zarcero, S.; Nart, J.; Sakwinska, O.; Clavé, P. Oral health in older patients with oropharyngeal dysphagia. *Age Ageing* **2014**, *43*, 132–137. [CrossRef] [PubMed]

143. Poisson, P.; Laffond, T.; Campos, S.; Dupuis, V.; Bourdel-Marchasson, I. Relationships between oral health, dysphagia and undernutrition in hospitalised elderly patients. *Gerodontology* **2016**, *33*, 161–168. [CrossRef]

144. Osterberg, T.; Tsuga, K.; Rothenberg, E.; Carlsson, G.E.; Steen, B. Masticatory ability in 80-year-old subjects and its relation to intake of energy, nutrients and food items. *Gerodontology* **2002**, *19*, 95–101. [CrossRef]

145. Hämäläinen, P.; Rantanen, T.; Keskinen, M.; Meurman, J.H. Oral health status and change in handgrip strength over a 5-year period in 80-year-old people. *Gerodontology* **2004**, *21*, 155–160. [CrossRef] [PubMed]

146. Sakai, K.; Nakayama, E.; Tohara, H.; Maeda, T.; Sugimoto, M.; Takehisa, T.; Ueda, K. Tongue Strength is Associated with Grip Strength and Nutritional Status in Older Adult Inpatients of a Rehabilitation Hospital. *Dysphagia* **2017**, *32*, 241–249. [CrossRef] [PubMed]

147. Yamaguchi, K.; Tohara, H.; Hara, K.; Nakane, A.; Kajisa, E.; Yoshimi, K.; Minakuchi, S. Relationship of aging, skeletal muscle mass, and tooth loss with masseter muscle thickness. *BMC Geriatr.* **2018**, *18*, 67. [CrossRef] [PubMed]
148. Picca, A.; Calvani, R.; Manes-Gravina, E.; Spaziani, L.; Landi, F.; Bernabei, R.; Marzetti, E. Bone-Muscle Crosstalk: Unraveling New Therapeutic Targets for Osteoporosis. *Curr. Pharm. Des.* **2017**, *23*, 6256–6263. [CrossRef]
149. Contaldo, M.; Itro, A.; Lajolo, C.; Gioco, G.; Inchingolo, F.; Serpico, R. Overview on Osteoporosis, Periodontitis and Oral Dysbiosis: The Emerging Role of Oral Microbiota. *Appl. Sci.* **2020**, *10*, 6000. [CrossRef]
150. Fujishima, I.; Fujiu-Kurachi, M.; Arai, H.; Hyodo, M.; Kagaya, H.; Maeda, K.; Yoshimura, Y. Sarcopenia and dysphagia: Position paper by four professional organizations. *Geriatr. Gerontol. Int.* **2019**, *19*, 91–97. [CrossRef]
151. Pizzoferrato, M.; de Sire, R.; Ingravalle, F.; Mentella, M.C.; Petito, V.; Martone, A.M.; Gasbarrini, A. Characterization of Sarcopenia in an IBD Population Attending an Italian Gastroenterology Tertiary Center. *Nutrients* **2019**, *11*, 2281. [CrossRef]
152. Larsson, L.; Degens, H.; Li, M.; Salviati, L.; Lee, Y.i.; Thompson, W.; Sandri, M. Sarcopenia: Aging-Related Loss of Muscle Mass and Function. *Physiol. Rev.* **2019**, *99*, 427–511. [CrossRef] [PubMed]
153. De Carvalho, F.G.; Justice, J.N.; Freitas, E.C.; Kershaw, E.E.; Sparks, L.M. Adipose Tissue Quality in Aging: How Structural and Functional Aspects of Adipose Tissue Impact Skeletal Muscle Quality. *Nutrients* **2019**, *11*, 2553. [CrossRef] [PubMed]
154. De Sire, A.; de Sire, R.; Petito, V.; Masi, L.; Cisari, C.; Gasbarrini, A.; Invernizzi, M. Gut-Joint Axis: The Role of Physical Exercise on Gut Microbiota Modulation in Older People with Osteoarthritis. *Nutrients* **2020**, *12*, 574. [CrossRef] [PubMed]
155. Nardone, O.M.; de Sire, R.; Petito, V.; Testa, A.; Villani, G.; Scaldaferri, F.; Castiglione, F. Inflammatory Bowel Diseases and Sarcopenia: The Role of Inflammation and Gut Microbiota in the Development of Muscle Failure. *Front. Immunol.* **2021**, *12*, 694217. [CrossRef]
156. Azzolino, D.; Damanti, S.; Bertagnoli, L.; Lucchi, T.; Cesari, M. Sarcopenia and swallowing disorders in older people. *Aging Clin. Exp. Res.* **2019**, *31*, 799–805. [CrossRef]
157. Molfenter, S.M.; Amin, M.R.; Branski, R.C.; Brumm, J.D.; Hagiwara, M.; Roof, S.A.; Lazarus, C.L. Age-Related Changes in Pharyngeal Lumen Size: A Retrospective MRI Analysis. *Dysphagia* **2015**, *30*, 321–327. [CrossRef]
158. Suzuki, M.; Koyama, S.; Kimura, Y.; Ishiyama, D.; Ohji, S.; Otobe, Y.; Yamada, M. Relationship between tongue muscle quality and swallowing speed in community-dwelling older women. *Aging Clin. Exp. Res.* **2019**, *32*, 2073–2079. [CrossRef]
159. Mizuno, S.; Wakabayashi, H.; Wada, F. Rehabilitation nutrition for individuals with frailty, disability, sarcopenic dysphagia, or sarcopenic respiratory disability. *Curr. Opin. Clin. Nutr. Metab. Care* **2022**, *25*, 29–36. [CrossRef]
160. Ogawa, N.; Mori, T.; Fujishima, I.; Wakabayashi, H.; Itoda, M.; Kunieda, K.; Ogawa, S. Ultrasonography to Measure Swallowing Muscle Mass and Quality in Older Patients with Sarcopenic Dysphagia. *J. Am. Med. Dir. Assoc.* **2017**, *19*, 516–522. [CrossRef]
161. Martone, A.M.; Marzetti, E.; Calvani, R.; Picca, A.; Tosato, M.; Santoro, L.; Landi, F. Exercise and Protein Intake: A Synergistic Approach against Sarcopenia. *Biomed. Res. Int.* **2017**, *2017*, 2672435. [CrossRef]
162. Matsuo, H.; Yoshimura, Y.; Fujita, S.; Maeno, Y. Dysphagia is associated with poor physical function in patients with acute heart failure: A prospective cohort study. *Aging Clin. Exp. Res.* **2020**, *32*, 1093–1099. [CrossRef] [PubMed]
163. Zhao, W.T.; Yang, M.; Wu, H.M.; Yang, L.; Zhang, X.M.; Huang, Y. Systematic Review and Meta-Analysis of the Association between Sarcopenia and Dysphagia. *J. Nutr. Health Aging* **2018**, *22*, 1003–1009. [CrossRef]
164. Mori, T.; Fujishima, I.; Wakabayashi, H.; Oshima, F.; Itoda, M.; Kunieda, K.; Ogawa, S. Development, reliability, and validity of a diagnostic algorithm for sarcopenic dysphagia. *JCSM Clin. Rep.* **2017**, *2*, 1–10. [CrossRef]
165. Sporns, P.B.; Muhle, P.; Hanning, U.; Suntrup-Krueger, S.; Schwindt, W.; Eversmann, J.; Dziewas, R. Atrophy of Swallowing Muscles Is Associated With Severity of Dysphagia and Age in Patients With Acute Stroke. *J. Am. Med. Dir. Assoc.* **2017**, *18*, 635.e1–635.e7. [CrossRef] [PubMed]
166. Can, B.; İsmagulova, N.; Enver, N.; Tufan, A.; Cinel, İ. Sarcopenic dysphagia following COVID-19 infection: A new danger. *Nutr. Clin. Pract.* **2021**, *36*, 828–832. [CrossRef] [PubMed]
167. Brodsky, M.B.; Gilbert, R.J. The Long-Term Effects of COVID-19 on Dysphagia Evaluation and Treatment. *Arch. Phys. Med. Rehabil.* **2020**, *101*, 1662–1664. [CrossRef]
168. Agostini, F.; Mangone, M.; Ruiu, P.; Paolucci, T.; Santilli, V.; Bernetti, A. Rehabilitation setting during and after Covid-19: An overview on recommendations. *J. Rehabil. Med.* **2021**, *53*, jrm00141. [CrossRef]
169. Roberts, S.; Collins, P.; Rattray, M. Identifying and Managing Malnutrition, Frailty and Sarcopenia in the Community: A Narrative Review. *Nutrients* **2021**, *13*, 2316. [CrossRef]
170. Kiss, N.; Bauer, J.; Boltong, A.; Brown, T.; Isenring, L.; Loeliger, J.; Findlay, M. Awareness, perceptions and practices regarding cancer-related malnutrition and sarcopenia: A survey of cancer clinicians. *Support. Care Cancer* **2020**, *28*, 5263–5270. [CrossRef]
171. Vellas, B.; Fielding, R.A.; Bens, C.; Bernabei, R.; Cawthon, P.M.; Cederholm, T.; Cesari, M. Implications of ICD-10 for Sarcopenia Clinical Practice and Clinical Trials: Report by the International Conference on Frailty and Sarcopenia Research Task Force. *J. Frailty Aging* **2018**, *7*, 2–9. [CrossRef] [PubMed]
172. Nagano, A.; Nishioka, S.; Wakabayashi, H. Rehabilitation Nutrition for Iatrogenic Sarcopenia and Sarcopenic Dysphagia. *J. Nutr. Health Aging* **2019**, *23*, 256–265. [CrossRef] [PubMed]
173. Chen, K.-C.; Jeng, Y.; Wu, W.-T.; Wang, T.-G.; Han, D.-S.; Özçakar, L.; Chang, K.-V. Sarcopenic Dysphagia: A Narrative Review from Diagnosis to Intervention. *Nutrients* **2021**, *13*, 4043. [CrossRef]

174. Shimizu, A.; Fujishima, I.; Maeda, K.; Wakabayashi, H.; Nishioka, S.; Ohno, T. The Japanese Working Group on Sarcopenic, D. Nutritional Management Enhances the Recovery of Swallowing Ability in Older Patients with Sarcopenic Dysphagia. *Nutrients* **2021**, *13*, 596. [CrossRef] [PubMed]

175. Nagano, A.; Maeda, K.; Shimizu, A.; Nagami, S.; Takigawa, N.; Ueshima, J.; Suenaga, M. Association of Sarcopenic Dysphagia with Underlying Sarcopenia Following Hip Fracture Surgery in Older Women. *Nutrients* **2020**, *12*, 1365. [CrossRef]

176. Volkert, D.; Beck, A.M.; Cederholm, T.; Cruz-Jentoft, A.; Goisser, S.; Hooper, L.; Bischoff, S.C. ESPEN guideline on clinical nutrition and hydration in geriatrics. *Clin. Nutr.* **2019**, *38*, 10–47. [CrossRef]

177. Bauer, J.; Biolo, G.; Cederholm, T.; Cesari, M.; Cruz-Jentoft, A.J.; Morley, J.E.; Boirie, Y. Evidence-based recommendations for optimal dietary protein intake in older people: A position paper from the PROT-AGE Study Group. *J. Am. Med. Dir. Assoc.* **2013**, *14*, 542–559. [CrossRef]

178. Nagano, A.; Maeda, K.; Koike, M.; Murotani, K.; Ueshima, J.; Shimizu, A.; Mori, N. Effects of Physical Rehabilitation and Nutritional Intake Management on Improvement in Tongue Strength in Sarcopenic Patients. *Nutrients* **2020**, *12*, 3104. [CrossRef]

179. Hudson, H.M.; Daubert, C.R.; Mills, R.H. The interdependency of protein-energy malnutrition, aging, and dysphagia. *Dysphagia* **2000**, *15*, 31–38. [CrossRef]

180. Harvey, S.E.; Parrott, F.; Harrison, D.A.; Bear, D.E.; Segaran, E.; Beale, R.; Rowan, K.M. Trial of the Route of Early Nutritional Support in Critically Ill Adults. *N. Engl. J. Med.* **2014**, *371*, 1673–1684. [CrossRef]

181. Lewis, S.R.; Schofield-Robinson, O.J.; Alderson, P.; Smith, A.F. Enteral versus parenteral nutrition and enteral versus a combination of enteral and parenteral nutrition for adults in the intensive care unit. *Cochrane Database Syst. Rev.* **2018**, *6*, Cd012276. [CrossRef] [PubMed]

182. Cichero, J.A.Y. Age-Related Changes to Eating and Swallowing Impact Frailty: Aspiration, Choking Risk, Modified Food Texture and Autonomy of Choice. *Geriatrics* **2018**, *3*, 69. [CrossRef] [PubMed]

183. Johnson, M.A.; Kimlin, M.G. Vitamin D, Aging, and the 2005 Dietary Guidelines for Americans. *Nutr. Rev.* **2006**, *64*, 410–421. [CrossRef] [PubMed]

184. Invernizzi, M.; de Sire, A.; D'Andrea, F.; Carrera, D.; Renò, F.; Migliaccio, S.; Cisari, C. Effects of essential amino acid supplementation and rehabilitation on functioning in hip fracture patients: A pilot randomized controlled trial. *Aging Clin. Exp. Res.* **2019**, *31*, 1517–1524. [CrossRef]

185. Iolascon, G.; Mauro, G.L.; Fiore, P.; Cisari, C.; Benedetti, M.G.; Panella, L.; Gimigliano, F. Can vitamin D deficiency influence muscle performance in postmenopausal women? A multicenter retrospective study. *Eur. J. Phys. Rehabil. Med.* **2018**, *54*, 676–682. [CrossRef]

186. Gimigliano, F.; Moretti, A.; de Sire, A.; Calafiore, D.; Iolascon, G. The combination of vitamin D deficiency and overweight affects muscle mass and function in older post-menopausal women. *Aging Clin. Exp. Res.* **2018**, *30*, 625–631. [CrossRef]

187. Hashida, N.; Shamoto, H.; Maeda, K.; Wakabayashi, H.; Suzuki, M.; Fujii, T. Rehabilitation and nutritional support for sarcopenic dysphagia and tongue atrophy after glossectomy: A case report. *Nutrition* **2017**, *35*, 128–131. [CrossRef]

188. Yamada, Y.; Shamoto, H.; Maeda, K.; Wakabayashi, H. Home-based Combined Therapy with Rehabilitation and Aggressive Nutrition Management for a Parkinson's Disease Patient with Sarcopenic Dysphagia: A Case Report. *Prog. Rehabil. Med.* **2018**, *3*, 20180019. [CrossRef]

189. Wakabayashi, H.; Uwano, R. Rehabilitation Nutrition for Possible Sarcopenic Dysphagia After Lung Cancer Surgery: A Case Report. *Am. J. Phys. Med. Rehabil.* **2016**, *95*, e84–e89. [CrossRef]

190. Borda, M.G.; Venegas-Sanabria, L.C.; Puentes-Leal, G.A.; Garcia-Cifuentes, E.; Chavarro-Carvajal, D.A.; Cano, C.A. Oropharyngeal dysphagia in older adults: The well-known tale. *Geriatr. Gerontol. Int.* **2017**, *17*, 1031–1033. [CrossRef]

191. Paolucci, T.; Cardarola, A.; Colonnelli, P.; Ferracuti, G.; Gonnella, R.; Murgia, M.; Mangone, M. Give me a kiss! An integrative rehabilitative training program with motor imagery and mirror therapy for recovery of facial palsy. *Eur. J. Phys. Rehabil. Med.* **2020**, *56*, 58–67. [CrossRef] [PubMed]

192. Maeda, K.; Akagi, J. Treatment of Sarcopenic Dysphagia with Rehabilitation and Nutritional Support: A Comprehensive Approach. *J. Acad. Nutr. Diet.* **2016**, *116*, 573–577. [CrossRef]

193. Nakayama, E.; Tohara, H.; Sato, M.; Hino, H.; Sakai, M.; Nagashima, Y.; Ooshima, M. Time Course and Recovery of the Movements of Hyoid Bone and Thyroid Cartilage During Swallowing in a Patient with Sarcopenic Dysphagia. *Am. J. Phys. Med. Rehabil.* **2019**, *99*, e64–e67. [CrossRef] [PubMed]

194. Wakabayashi, H.; Takahashi, R.; Murakami, T. The Prevalence and Prognosis of Sarcopenic Dysphagia in Patients Who Require Dysphagia Rehabilitation. *J. Nutr. Health Aging* **2019**, *23*, 84–88. [CrossRef] [PubMed]

195. Yamada, M.; Kimura, Y.; Ishiyama, D.; Nishio, N.; Otobe, Y.; Tanaka, T.; Arai, H. Synergistic effect of bodyweight resistance exercise and protein supplementation on skeletal muscle in sarcopenic or dynapenic older adults. *Geriatr. Gerontol. Int.* **2019**, *19*, 429–437. [CrossRef] [PubMed]

196. Yoshimura, Y.; Uchida, K.; Jeong, S.; Yamaga, M. Effects of Nutritional Supplements on Muscle Mass and Activities of Daily Living in Elderly Rehabilitation Patients with Decreased Muscle Mass: A Randomized Controlled Trial. *J. Nutr. Health Aging* **2016**, *20*, 185–191. [CrossRef]

197. Almeida, T.M.d.; Gomes, L.M.S.; Afonso, D.; Magnoni, D.; Mota, I.C.P.; França, J.Í.D.; Silva, R.G.d. Risk factors for oropharyngeal dysphagia in cardiovascular diseases. *J. Appl. Oral Sci. Rev. FOB* **2020**, *28*, e20190489. [CrossRef]

198. Neloska, L.; Damevska, K.; Nikolchev, A.; Pavleska, L.; Petreska-Zovic, B.; Kostov, M. The Association between Malnutrition and Pressure Ulcers in Elderly in Long-Term Care Facility. *Open Access Maced. J. Med. Sci.* **2016**, *4*, 423–427. [CrossRef]

199. Byeon, H. Predicting the Swallow-Related Quality of Life of the Elderly Living in a Local Community Using Support Vector Machine. *Int. J. Environ. Res. Public Health* **2019**, *16*, 4269. [CrossRef]

200. Wakabayashi, H.; Kishima, M.; Itoda, M.; Fujishima, I.; Kunieda, K.; Ohno, T.; Ogawa, S. Diagnosis and Treatment of Sarcopenic Dysphagia: A Scoping Review. *Dysphagia* **2021**, *36*, 523–531. [CrossRef]

201. Di Pede, C.; Mantovani, M.E.; Del Felice, A.; Masiero, S. Dysphagia in the elderly: Focus on rehabilitation strategies. *Aging Clin. Exp. Res.* **2016**, *28*, 607–617. [CrossRef] [PubMed]

202. Alghadir, A.H.; Zafar, H.; Al-Eisa, E.S.; Iqbal, Z.A. Effect of posture on swallowing. *Afr. Health Sci.* **2017**, *17*, 133–137. [CrossRef] [PubMed]

203. Namiki, C.; Hara, K.; Tohara, H.; Kobayashi, K.; Chantaramanee, A.; Nakagawa, K.; Minakuchi, S. Tongue-pressure resistance training improves tongue and suprahyoid muscle functions simultaneously. *Clin. Interv. Aging* **2019**, *14*, 601–608. [CrossRef] [PubMed]

204. Cichero, J.A.Y.; Lam, P.; Steele, C.M.; Hanson, B.; Chen, J.; Dantas, R.O.; Stanschus, S. Development of International Terminology and Definitions for Texture-Modified Foods and Thickened Fluids Used in Dysphagia Management: The IDDSI Framework. *Dysphagia* **2017**, *32*, 293–314. [CrossRef]

205. Steele, C.M.; Namasivayam-MacDonald, A.M.; Guida, B.T.; Cichero, J.A.; Duivestein, J.; Hanson, B.; Riquelme, L.F. Creation and Initial Validation of the International Dysphagia Diet Standardisation Initiative Functional Diet Scale. *Arch. Phys. Med. Rehabil.* **2018**, *99*, 934–944. [CrossRef]

206. Chen, K.-C.; Lee, T.-M.; Wu, W.-T.; Wang, T.-G.; Han, D.-S.; Chang, K.-V. Assessment of Tongue Strength in Sarcopenia and Sarcopenic Dysphagia: A Systematic Review and Meta-Analysis. *Front. Nutr.* **2021**, *8*, 684840. [CrossRef]

207. Vose, A.; Nonnenmacher, J.; Singer, M.L.; González-Fernández, M. Dysphagia Management in Acute and Sub-acute Stroke. *Curr. Phys. Med. Rehabil. Rep.* **2014**, *2*, 197–206. [CrossRef]

208. Carnaby, G.; Crary, M. Examining the Evidence on Neuromuscular Electrical Stimulation for Swallowing. *Arch. Otolaryngol.—Head Neck Surg.* **2007**, *133*, 564–571. [CrossRef]

209. Carnaby-Mann, G.; Crary, M.A.; Schmalfuss, I.; Amdur, R. "Pharyngocise": Randomized controlled trial of preventative exercises to maintain muscle structure and swallowing function during head-and-neck chemoradiotherapy. *Int. J. Radiat. Oncol. Biol. Phys.* **2012**, *83*, 210–219. [CrossRef]

210. Carnaby-Mann, G.D.; Crary, M.A. McNeill dysphagia therapy program: A case-control study. *Arch. Phys. Med. Rehabil.* **2010**, *91*, 743–749. [CrossRef]

211. Crary, M.A.; Carnaby, G.D.; LaGorio, L.A.; Carvajal, P.J. Functional and physiological outcomes from an exercise-based dysphagia therapy: A pilot investigation of the McNeill Dysphagia Therapy Program. *Arch. Phys. Med. Rehabil.* **2012**, *93*, 1173–1178. [CrossRef] [PubMed]

212. National Institute on Aging; National Institutes of Health; U.S. Department of Health and Human Services. Why Population. 2008. Available online: https://2001-2009.state.gov/documents/organization/81775.pdf (accessed on 25 January 2022).

213. Marcenes, W.; Kassebaum, N.J.; Bernabé, E.; Flaxman, A.; Naghavi, M.; Lopez, A.; Murray, C.J. Global burden of oral conditions in 1990–2010: A systematic analysis. *J. Dent. Res.* **2013**, *92*, 592–597. [CrossRef]

214. Petersen, P.E. Global policy for improvement of oral health in the 21st century–implications to oral health research of World Health Assembly 2007, World Health Organization. *Community Dent. Oral Epidemiol.* **2009**, *37*, 1–8. [CrossRef] [PubMed]

215. Preshaw, P.M.; Henne, K.; Taylor, J.J.; Valentine, R.A.; Conrads, G. Age-related changes in immune function (immune senescence) in caries and periodontal diseases: A systematic review. *J. Clin. Periodontol.* **2017**, *44* (Suppl. S18), S153–S177. [CrossRef] [PubMed]

216. López, R.; Smith, P.C.; Göstemeyer, G.; Schwendicke, F. Ageing, dental caries and periodontal diseases. *J. Clin. Periodontol.* **2017**, *44* (Suppl. S18), S145–S152. [CrossRef]

217. Azarpazhooh, A.; Leake, J.L. Systematic review of the association between respiratory diseases and oral health. *J. Periodontol.* **2006**, *77*, 1465–1482. [CrossRef] [PubMed]

218. Martinez-Herrera, M.; Silvestre-Rangil, J.; Silvestre, F.J. Association between obesity and periodontal disease. A systematic review of epidemiological studies and controlled clinical trials. *Med. Oral Patol. Oral Cir. Bucal.* **2017**, *22*, e708–e715. [CrossRef] [PubMed]

219. Dizdar, O.; Hayran, M.; Guven, D.C.; Yılmaz, T.B.; Taheri, S.; Akman, A.C.; Berker, E. Increased cancer risk in patients with periodontitis. *Curr. Med. Res. Opin.* **2017**, *33*, 2195–2200. [CrossRef]

220. Wu, B.; Fillenbaum, G.G.; Plassman, B.L.; Guo, L. Association Between Oral Health and Cognitive Status: A Systematic Review. *J. Am. Geriatr. Soc.* **2016**, *64*, 739–751. [CrossRef]

221. Tonsekar, P.P.; Jiang, S.S.; Yue, G. Periodontal disease, tooth loss and dementia: Is there a link? A systematic review. *Gerodontology* **2017**, *34*, 151–163. [CrossRef]

222. Zarb, G.A. The edentulous milieu. *J. Prosthet. Dent.* **1983**, *49*, 825–831. [CrossRef]

223. Niesten, D.; van Mourik, K.; van der Sanden, W. The impact of frailty on oral care behavior of older people: A qualitative study. *BMC Oral Health* **2013**, *13*, 61. [CrossRef]

224. Eberhard, J.; Jepsen, S.; Jervøe-Storm, P.M.; Needleman, I.; Worthington, H.V. Full-mouth treatment modalities (within 24 hours) for chronic periodontitis in adults. *Cochrane Database Syst. Rev.* **2015**, *4*, Cd004622. [CrossRef]

225. Manresa, C.; Sanz-Miralles, E.C.; Twigg, J.; Bravo, M. Supportive periodontal therapy (SPT) for maintaining the dentition in adults treated for periodontitis. *Cochrane Database Syst. Rev.* **2018**, *1*, Cd009376. [CrossRef]
226. Castro-Calderón, A.; Roccuzzo, A.; Ferrillo, M.; Gada, S.; González-Serrano, J.; Fonseca, M.; Molinero-Mourelle, P. Hyaluronic acid injection to restore the lost interproximal papilla: A systematic review. *Acta Odontol. Scand.* **2021**, *2*, 1–13. [CrossRef]
227. Roccuzzo, A.; Molinero-Mourelle, P.; Ferrillo, M.; Cobo-Vázquez, C.; Sanchez-Labrador, L.; Ammendolia, A.; de Sire, A. Type I Collagen-Based Devices to Treat Nerve Injuries after Oral Surgery Procedures. A Systematic Review. *Appl. Sci.* **2021**, *11*, 3927. [CrossRef]
228. Togni, L.; Mascitti, M.; Santarelli, A.; Contaldo, M.; Romano, A.; Serpico, R.; Rubini, C. Unusual Conditions Impairing Saliva Secretion: Developmental Anomalies of Salivary Glands. *Front. Physiol.* **2019**, *10*, 855. [CrossRef]
229. Davies, A.N.; Shorthose, K. Parasympathomimetic drugs for the treatment of salivary gland dysfunction due to radiotherapy. *Cochrane Database Syst. Rev.* **2007**, *3*, CD003782.
230. Fedele, S.; Wolff, A.; Strietzel, F.; López, R.M.; Porter, S.R.; Konttinen, Y.T. Neuroelectrostimulation in treatment of hyposalivation and xerostomia in Sjögren's syndrome: A salivary pacemaker. *J. Rheumatol.* **2008**, *35*, 1489–1494.
231. Sugiura, Y.; Soga, Y.; Yamabe, K.; Tsutani, S.; Tanimoto, I.; Maeda, H.; Takashiba, S. Total bacterial counts on oral mucosa after using a commercial saliva substitute in patients undergoing hematopoietic cell transplantation. *Support. Care Cancer* **2010**, *18*, 395–398. [CrossRef]
232. Assery, M.K.A. Efficacy of Artificial Salivary Substitutes in Treatment of Xerostomia: A Systematic Review. *J. Pharm. Bioallied Sci.* **2019**, *11* (Suppl. S1), S1–S12. [CrossRef] [PubMed]
233. Vadcharavivad, S.; Boonroung, T. Original article. Effects of two carboxymethylcellulose-containing saliva substitutes on post-radiation xerostomia in head and neck cancer patients related to quality of life. *Asian Biomed.* **2013**, *7*, 193–202.
234. Ameri, A.; Heydarirad, G.; Rezaeizadeh, H.; Choopani, R.; Ghobadi, A.; Gachkar, L. Evaluation of Efficacy of an Herbal Compound on Dry Mouth in Patients with Head and Neck Cancers: A Randomized Clinical Trial. *J. Evid. Based Complement. Altern. Med.* **2016**, *21*, 30–33. [CrossRef] [PubMed]
235. Montaldo, L.; Montaldo, P.; Papa, A.; Caramico, N.; Toro, G. Effects of saliva substitutes on oral status in patients with Type 2 diabetes. *Diabet. Med.* **2010**, *27*, 1280–1283. [CrossRef] [PubMed]
236. Abt, E.; Carr, A.B.; Worthington, H.V. Interventions for replacing missing teeth: Partially absent dentition. *Cochrane Database Syst. Rev.* **2012**, *2*, Cd003814. [CrossRef]
237. Marra, R.; Acocella, A.; Alessandra, R.; Ganz, S.D.; Blasi, A. Rehabilitation of Full-Mouth Edentulism: Immediate Loading of Implants Inserted with Computer-Guided Flapless Surgery Versus Conventional Dentures: A 5-Year Multicenter Retrospective Analysis and OHIP Questionnaire. *Implant. Dent.* **2017**, *26*, 54–58. [CrossRef]
238. Allen, P.F.; McMillan, A.S.; Walshaw, D. A patient-based assessment of implant-stabilized and conventional complete dentures. *J. Prosthet. Dent.* **2001**, *85*, 141–147. [CrossRef]
239. Ornstein, K.A.; DeCherrie, L.; Gluzman, R.; Scott, E.S.; Kansal, J.; Shah, T.; Soriano, T.A. Significant unmet oral health needs of homebound elderly adults. *J. Am. Geriatr. Soc.* **2015**, *63*, 151–157. [CrossRef]
240. Chen, X.; Kistler, C.E. Oral Health Care for Older Adults with Serious Illness: When and How? *J. Am. Geriatr. Soc.* **2015**, *63*, 375–378. [CrossRef]
241. Paquette, D.W. The periodontal infection-systemic disease link: A review of the truth or myth. *J. Int. Acad. Periodontol.* **2003**, *4*, 101–109.
242. Borgnakke, W.S.; Ylöstalo, P.V.; Taylor, G.W.; Genco, R.J. Effect of periodontal disease on diabetes: Systematic review of epidemiologic observational evidence. *J. Periodontol.* **2013**, *84* (Suppl. S4), S135–S152. [CrossRef]
243. Stoffel, L.M.B.; Muniz, F.W.M.G.; Colussi, P.R.G.; Rösing, C.K.; Colussi, E.L. Nutritional assessment and associated factors in the elderly: Apopulation-based cross-sectional study. *Nutrition* **2018**, *55–56*, 104–110. [CrossRef]
244. Kossioni, A.E.; Hajto-Bryk, J.; Maggi, S.; McKenna, G.; Petrovic, M.; Roller-Wirnsberger, R.E.; Müller, F. An Expert Opinion from the European College of Gerodontology and the European Geriatric Medicine Society: European Policy Recommendations on Oral Health in Older Adults. *J. Am. Geriatr. Soc.* **2018**, *66*, 609–613. [CrossRef]
245. Cumpston, M.; Li, T.; Page, M.J.; Chandler, J.; Welch, V.A.; Higgins, J.P.; Thomas, J. Updated guidance for trusted systematic reviews: A new edition of the Cochrane Handbook for Systematic Reviews of Interventions. *Cochrane Database Syst. Rev.* **2019**, *10*, ED000142. [CrossRef]

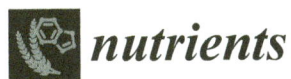 *nutrients*

Systematic Review

The Clinical, Microbiological, and Immunological Effects of Probiotic Supplementation on Prevention and Treatment of Periodontal Diseases: A Systematic Review and Meta-Analysis

Zohre Gheisary [1,†], Razi Mahmood [1,†], Aparna Harri shivanantham [1], Juxin Liu [2], Jessica R. L. Lieffers [3], Petros Papagerakis [4] and Silvana Papagerakis [1,*]

1   Laboratory of Oral, Head and Neck Cancer—Personalized Diagnostics and Therapeutics, College of Medicine, University of Saskatchewan, 107 Wiggins Road, Saskatoon, SK S7N 5E5, Canada; zog389@usask.ca (Z.G.); razi.mahmood@usask.ca (R.M.); eti908@mail.usask.ca (A.H.s.)
2   Department of Mathematics and Statistics, College of Arts and Science, University of Saskatchewan, 106 Wiggins Road, Saskatoon, SK S7N 5E6, Canada; jul086@mail.usask.ca
3   College of Pharmacy and Nutrition, University of Saskatchewan, 107 Wiggins Road, Saskatoon, SK S7N 5E5, Canada; jessica.lieffers@usask.ca
4   Laboratory of Precision Oral Health and Chronobiology, College of Dentistry, University of Saskatchewan, 107 Wiggins Road, Saskatoon, SK S7N 5E5, Canada; petros.papagerakis@usask.ca
*   Correspondence: silvana.papagerakis@usask.ca; Tel.: +1-3069661960
†   These authors contributed equally to this work.

Citation: Gheisary, Z.; Mahmood, R.; Harri shivanantham, A.; Liu, J.; Lieffers, J.R.L.; Papagerakis, P.; Papagerakis, S. The Clinical, Microbiological, and Immunological Effects of Probiotic Supplementation on Prevention and Treatment of Periodontal Diseases: A Systematic Review and Meta-Analysis. *Nutrients* 2022, 14, 1036. https://doi.org/10.3390/nu14051036

Academic Editors: Kirstin Vach and Johan Peter Woelber

Received: 12 January 2022
Accepted: 23 February 2022
Published: 28 February 2022

Publisher's Note: MDPI stays neutral with regard to jurisdictional claims in published maps and institutional affiliations.

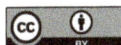
Abstract: (1) Background: Periodontal diseases are a global health concern. They are multi-stage, progressive inflammatory diseases triggered by the inflammation of the gums in response to periodontopathogens and may lead to the destruction of tooth-supporting structures, tooth loss, and systemic health problems. This systematic review and meta-analysis evaluated the effects of probiotic supplementation on the prevention and treatment of periodontal disease based on the assessment of clinical, microbiological, and immunological outcomes. (2) Methods: This study was registered under PROSPERO (CRD42021249120). Six databases were searched: PubMed, MEDLINE, EMBASE, CINAHL, Web of Science, and Dentistry and Oral Science Source. The meta-analysis assessed the effects of probiotic supplementation on the prevention and treatment of periodontal diseases and reported them using Hedge's g standardized mean difference (SMD). (3) Results: Of the 1883 articles initially identified, 64 randomized clinical trials were included in this study. The results of this meta-analysis indicated statistically significant improvements after probiotic supplementation in the majority of the clinical outcomes in periodontal disease patients, including the plaque index (SMD = 0.557, 95% CI: 0.228, 0.885), gingival index, SMD = 0.920, 95% CI: 0.426, 1.414), probing pocket depth (SMD = 0.578, 95% CI: 0.365, 0.790), clinical attachment level (SMD = 0.413, 95% CI: 0.262, 0.563), bleeding on probing (SMD = 0.841, 95% CI: 0.479, 1.20), gingival crevicular fluid volume (SMD = 0.568, 95% CI: 0.235, 0.902), reduction in the subgingival periodontopathogen count of *P. gingivalis* (SMD = 0.402, 95% CI: 0.120, 0.685), *F. nucleatum* (SMD = 0.392, 95% CI: 0.127, 0.658), and *T. forsythia* (SMD = 0.341, 95% CI: 0.050, 0.633), and immunological markers MMP-8 (SMD = 0.819, 95% CI: 0.417, 1.221) and IL-6 (SMD = 0.361, 95% CI: 0.079, 0.644). (4) Conclusions: The results of this study suggest that probiotic supplementation improves clinical parameters, and reduces the periodontopathogen load and pro-inflammatory markers in periodontal disease patients. However, we were unable to assess the preventive role of probiotic supplementation due to the paucity of studies. Further clinical studies are needed to determine the efficacy of probiotic supplementation in the prevention of periodontal diseases.

Keywords: probiotic; periodontal disease; gingivitis; periodontitis; oral health; clinical parameters; prevention; therapeutics

1. Introduction

Periodontal disease is a growing public health concern, affecting approximately 750 million individuals worldwide [1]. The burden of this disease is expected to continue to grow as the global population ages [2,3]. Periodontal disease is preventable and reversible in its early stages; however, it can progress to chronic, irreversible states with significant destruction of the tooth-supporting tissues [4]. The cause of periodontal disease is multifactorial with modifiable risk factors, including smoking, unhealthy diet (e.g., a western diet with high sugars and saturated fats), poor oral hygiene, hormonal changes, stress, various medications, and poorly managed comorbidities (e.g., type 2 diabetes), while non-modifiable risk factors include age, sex, and genetics [5]. Periodontal disease, when left untreated, can have local and/or systemic consequences, leading to poor oral and systemic health and quality of life [5,6]. The underlying link of periodontal disease with other chronic systemic diseases likely results from the dissemination of periodontopathogens into the bloodstream, endotoxin release, and the associated imbalanced inflammatory response to periodontopathogens [7,8].

Periodontal disease is an inflammatory progressive multi-stage disease of the periodontium (which includes the gingiva, periodontal ligament, alveolar bone, and cementum); this disease is triggered in response to periodontopathogens in the biofilm of the dental plaque on tooth surfaces located near the gingiva (Figure 1) [9–11]. The first stage and mildest form of periodontal disease is known as gingivitis [4]. Gingivitis is a reversible condition, and, if untreated, may progress to periodontitis, which is the advanced stage of periodontal disease [4,12,13]. Gingivitis is characterized by redness, swelling, mild irritation and inflammation of the gingival tissue, and mild bleeding on brushing or flossing, while periodontitis is characterized by deep inflammation and loss of alveolar bone and connective tissue between the gingiva and tooth root [9,14]. The progression of periodontal disease is associated with dynamic shifts in the subgingival bacterial counts and composition in the periodontal pocket [15–18].

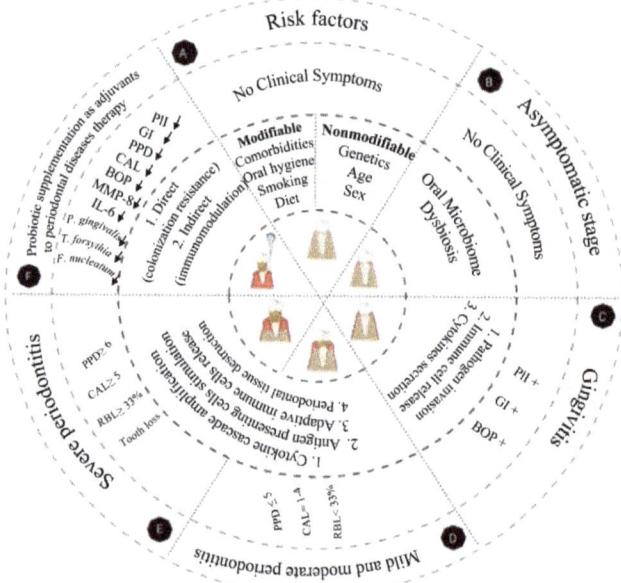

Figure 1. Etiology and pathogenesis of periodontal diseases. Periodontal disease is initiated by disrupting the commensal oral microbiome–host homeostasis. (**A**). Both modifiable and nonmodifiable risk factors impact the oral microbiome composition and disrupt homeostasis between the host

and microbiome. Modifiable risk factors include diet, smoking, oral hygiene, and comorbidities (such as type 2 diabetes), while genetics, age, and sex are nonmodifiable risk factors. (**B**). Disrupted homeostasis provides appropriate conditions for the growth of periodontopathogens and biofilm formation on the tooth surfaces extending sub-gingivally. There are no clinical symptoms in this stage. (**C**). These bacteria penetrate and grow in the gingival epithelium. Host–bacteria interactions cause a chemotactic gradient that attracts innate immune cells, including neutrophils, macrophages, and NK cells, to the affected sites. In addition, the outgrowth of bacteria progressively destroys the tissue and provides enough nutrients for more pathogen growth, followed by increased activity of innate immune cells and the secretion of pro-inflammatory cytokines, including IL-1, IL-8, and TNF. Early clinical symptoms in this stage are redness, swelling, mild inflammation, and bleeding of the gingiva, which are diagnosed by measuring the PlI, GI, and BOP. (**D**). Then, Antigen-Presenting Cells (APC), including dendritic cells, present bacterial antigens to lymphocytes and trigger adaptive immune system activity and antibody and cell-mediated immune responses, resulting in a pro-inflammatory response with high expression of IL-4, 6, 8, 10, 12, TGF-β, and IFN-γ. (**E**). High levels of these inflammatory mediators stimulate more inflammatory mediators, causing periodontal tissue destruction and leading to the loss of the gingival attachment to the tooth, and causing deep pockets around the teeth that provide appropriate conditions for the growth and colonization of other anaerobic periodontopathogens. Untreated, these pathophysiological changes can lead to alveolar bone resorption and, ultimately, tooth loss in the most advanced stage of the disease. (**F**). Probiotics may have therapeutic benefits in periodontal disease treatment when used as an adjuvant to standard periodontal care. Various mechanisms of action have been considered for the role of probiotics in periodontal disease improvement. Probiotics interact directly with periodontopathogens through colonization resistance, which includes competition for binding sites and nutrients, and the production of antibacterial agents inhibiting pathogen growth. Probiotics can play a role in periodontal disease improvement indirectly via the modulation of innate and adaptive immunity and through the gut–oral microbiome axis. PlI, Plaque Index; GI, Gingival Index; BOP, Bleeding on Probing; IL, Interleukin; TGF-β, Tumor Growth Factor-β; and IFN-γ, Interferon-γ.

1.1. Etiology of Periodontal Disease

The primary etiology of periodontal disease is an imbalanced subgingival microbiome population developing progressively over time due to an increasing relative abundance of periodontal disease-associated bacteria and a corresponding decrease in health-associated bacteria, leading to the disruption of the microbiota–host homeostasis [16,19–21]. This gradual phenomenon begins with the early adherence, growth, and colonization of Gram-negative and Gram-positive bacteria on the tooth surface extending sub-gingivally [22]. This provides appropriate conditions for the growth of and colonization by other anaerobic Gram-negative orange and red-complex bacteria [20]. The orange complex consists of *Prevotella intermedia*, *Parvimonas micra*, and *Fusobacterium nucleatum*, while *Porphyromonas gingivalis*, *Tanerella forsythia*, and *Treponema denticola* are components of the red complex [20]. These bacteria are highly pathogenic and have the ability to release bacterial collagenases and other proteases, leading to the stimulation of the pro-inflammatory response and periodontal tissue damage [9,10,20] (Figure 1).

1.2. Periodontal Disease Assessment, Diagnosis, and Therapy

The clinical assessment of periodontal disease includes the evaluation of patient-reported outcomes (i.e., bleeding while brushing or flossing, receding gums, halitosis, sensitive teeth, pain during mastication, and loose teeth) [4] and visual assessment of the distance between the base of the periodontal pocket and gingival margin or cementoenamel junction, the amount of plaque in the gingival margin on the tooth surface, and gingival bleeding [9,23]. All of these factors are measured by standard procedures and defined as specific indexes, including: the plaque index (PlI), gingival index (GI), periodontal pocket depth (PPD), clinical attachment level (CAL), bleeding on probing (BOP), gingival recession (REC), and gingival crevicular fluid (GCF) volume [23–27].

The clinical diagnosis of periodontal diseases is based on the periodontal exam, radiography, and patient's oral/dental and medical history [28]. The American Academy of Periodontology (AAP) classifies periodontitis into four stages based on severity, complexity, and extent (stage I, II, III, and IV) and three grades based on the evidence of the disease's progression and its rate (slow, moderate, and rapid) [29,30].

Periodontal therapy consists of the removal of the supra- and subgingival plaque from tooth surfaces using Scaling and Root Planing (SRP) [31,32]. To improve disease outcomes, SRP can be incorporated into surgical procedures or adjunctive antibiotics can be administered [3,31–33]. However, antibiotics may cause adverse side effects, or can be contraindicated in some situations; therefore, there is a need for alternative approaches [14].

1.3. Periodontal Diseases and Probiotics

Increasing attention has been devoted to probiotic supplementation as a therapeutic adjuvant/alternative to improve oral health [34]. Probiotics are live organisms (usually bacteria) administered to provide health benefits in the prevention or clinical management of different diseases [35,36]. Probiotics have been traditionally accepted in the medical field as an adjuvant treatment of gastrointestinal disorders [37]. Moreover, probiotics are recommended to patients who take antibiotics for the prevention and treatment of Antibiotics-Associated Diarrhea (AAD) [38]. They have also been considered in the clinical management of other conditions, including respiratory tract infections [39]. Furthermore, probiotics may have a therapeutic benefit in dental caries prevention by decreasing the number of cariogenic bacteria, such as *Streptococcus mutans* [40]. Probiotics may function through various mechanisms, including the production of antimicrobial metabolites, immunomodulation, mucosal barrier enhancement, and microbial flora shift through competition for cell adhesion with pathogenic strains [34,41]. The use of probiotics for the clinical management of periodontal diseases is an active area of research. There have been conflicting results based on several individual studies assessing the effects of probiotics on gingival inflammation [42,43]. Furthermore, previously published systematic reviews have had limited findings with conflicting results when examining the clinical efficacy of probiotics on periodontal diseases. For instance, Akram et al. showed no improvement in PlI and GI in patients with gingivitis after probiotic use, while other reviews concluded that probiotics could improve PlI and GI [44–46]. A previous systematic review was unable to assess the immunological benefits of probiotic supplementation due to limited studies; however, the included individual studies indicated an immunomodulatory effect of probiotics [47]. Microbiological findings suggested that probiotic supplementation reduced periodontopathogens in subgingival plaque samples [47]; however, there is conflicting evidence in the literature [48].

The purpose of our systematic review and meta-analysis was to combine results from randomized clinical trials involving adults with periodontal diseases or healthy volunteers receiving probiotic supplementation (control groups did not receive probiotic supplementation) to assess the effects on the clinical, microbiological, and immunological outcomes related to periodontal disease prevention and management.

2. Materials and Methods

2.1. Eligibility Criteria

Studies that were eligible for inclusion in this review satisfied the following criteria: 1. Randomized controlled trials with adults aged 18 years or older clinically diagnosed with either periodontal disease or healthy adults (without periodontal disease); 2. The study design consisted of intervention groups that received probiotics in any form (i.e., lozenge, capsule, tablet, powder, probiotic drink, probiotic-fortified food, toothpaste, mouthwash, spray, or subgingival delivery) and control groups (without probiotic, with a placebo, or with antibiotics); 3. Studies assessing any of the following: clinical, microbiological, or immunological outcomes. Clinical outcomes included: plaque index (PlI), gingival index (GI), probing pocket depth (PPD), clinical attachment level (CAL), bleeding on probing (BOP), gingival recession (REC), and gingival crevicular fluid (GCF) volume. Microbiological outcomes included the subgingival count of periodontopathogens, including: *Porphyromonas gingivalis* (*P. gingivalis*), *Fusobacterium nucleatum* (*F. nucleatum*), *Tannerella forsythia* (*T. forsythia*), *Prevotella intermedia* (*P. intermedia*), and *Aggregatibacter actinomycetemcomitans* (*A. actinomycetemcomitans*), and of commensal oral microbiota, such as *Streptococcus mutans* (*S. mutans*) and *Lactobacillus* species. Immunological outcomes included the GCF levels of matrix metalloproteinase-8 (MMP-8), interleukin-6 (IL-6), interleukin-1β (IL-1β), interleukin-8 (IL-8), interleukin-10 (IL-10), and tumor necrosis factor-α (TNF-α).

English language, peer-reviewed studies published since 2000, which were either open access or accessible to the researchers (via the University of Saskatchewan Library, inter-library loan, or through Google scholar), were included. Detailed information about the inclusion and exclusion criteria are available in Supplemental Table S1.

2.2. Information Sources, Search Strategy, and Study Selection

Six databases were searched without restrictions, including PubMed, MEDLINE, EMBASE, CINAHL, Web of Science, and Dentistry and Oral Science Source. A combination of keywords and MeSH terms related to the following search domains were used: 1. Periodontal diseases; 2. Clinical, microbiological, and immunological outcomes; 3. Probiotics. These three domains were combined with the "AND" operator. Details of the search strategy are included in the Supplementary Materials (Supplemental Table S2).

This systematic review and meta-analysis was registered with the International Prospective Register of Systematic Reviews (PROSPERO) (registration number: CRD42021249120).

After calibration, two screeners (ZG and AH) independently conducted dual screening (title and abstract, and full-text), and if consensus was not reached, a third author (RM) provided a tie-breaker vote.

2.3. Data Items and Collection Process

Two authors (ZG and AH) independently conducted data extraction, then compared the extracted data, and, in case of disagreement, they referred to the publication. The researchers used a Microsoft Excel (Microsoft Inc., Redmond, WA, USA) spreadsheet to record data pertaining to the study design, sample size, age of participants, health status, periodontal disease stage, dose and probiotic strain, treatment and follow-up durations, oral hygiene instructions, mode of probiotic delivery, clinical measurements (PlI, GI, PPD, CAL, BOP, GCF, and REC), oral bacterial count (*P. gingivalis*, *F. nucleatum*, *T. forsythia*, *P. intermedia*, *A. actinomycetemcomitans*, *S. mutans*, and *Lactobacillus species*), immunological outcomes (MMP-8, IL-6, IL-1β, IL-8, IL-10, and TNF-α), and key findings of each study.

2.4. Risk of Bias within Studies

The risk of bias within studies was assessed independently by two authors (ZG and AH) using the Cochrane risk–of–bias assessment tool version 2 designed for randomized trials [49]. This tool evaluates within-study bias by assessing the randomization process, deviations from intended interventions, missing outcome data, measurement of the outcome, and selection of the reported result. Studies were categorized as follows: low risk, some concerns, or high risk of bias.

2.5. Summary Measures and Synthesis of Results

Comprehensive meta-analysis version 3.3070 (Biostat Inc., Englewood, NJ, USA) was used for the meta-analysis. The meta-analysis was conducted using the mean and standard deviations from the studies at baseline until the immediate follow-up after the end of probiotic treatment. Hedge's g standardized mean difference (SMD) was calculated with a 95% confidence interval (CI) for each individual study and pooled in the meta-analysis using random-effects models. SMD can be interpreted as follows: a value of 0 indicates that there is no statistically significant difference in the effect of treatment compared to the control; values greater or less than 0 indicate a difference in effect. The strength of the effect can be roughly interpreted as small (SMD = 0.2), medium (SMD = 0.5), and large (SMD = 0.8) [50]. Heterogeneity was assessed using I^2, which can be interpreted as low (25%), moderate (50%), or high (75%) [51].

The meta-analysis used the following steps: 1. Pooled random-effects models examining the effect of probiotic supplementation on clinical, microbiological, and immunological outcomes in periodontal disease patients compared to controls (without probiotics); 2. Pooled random-effects models examining the potential preventive effect of probiotic use on clinical, microbiological, and immunological outcomes in healthy individuals (without periodontal diseases) compared to controls (without probiotics); 3. Subgroup analysis (see Section 2.7). The results of the meta-analysis were reported as the SMD, 95% CI, heterogeneity score (I^2), and *p*-value.

Studies lacking data on the mean, standard deviation, and sample size for treatment and/or control were excluded from the meta-analysis, unless these values could be calculated.

2.6. Risk of Bias across Studies

Publication bias and small study effects were evaluated using visual inspection of funnel plots and Egger's regression test. If publication bias/small study effects were detected, we used Duval and Tweedie's trim and fill methodology to correct for funnel plot asymmetry [52].

2.7. Additional Analysis (Subgroup Analysis and Investigation of Heterogeneity)

The following subgroup analyses were conducted: 1. Type of periodontal disease (gingivitis, periodontitis); 2. Disease severity; 3. Probiotic treatment duration; 4. Mode of probiotic delivery; 5. Type of probiotic strain; 6. Type of *lactobacillus* species; and 7. Oral hygiene instructions (yes/no). In addition, subgroup analyses assessed the effects of probiotics compared to a control group receiving antibiotics. Disease severity was categorized as moderate (PPD = 4–6 mm) or deep (PPD > 6 mm) periodontal pockets. The treatment duration was categorized as follows: 1. Up to one month; 2. More than one month to two months; or 3. More than two months. The mode of probiotic delivery was categorized as follows: 1. Oral (i.e., toothpaste, mouthwash, sachet applied orally, mouth spray, or oil drops); 2. Oral and ingestion (i.e., lozenges, tablets, or chewing gum); 3. Ingestion (i.e., sachet dissolved in water to drink, capsules, yogurt, or fermented milk/Yakult); or 4. Local application (i.e., subgingival delivery as a paste or gel). The type of probiotic strain was classified as follows: 1. *Lactobacillus* (*Lactobacillus* species only); 2. Mixed (*Lactobacillus* species and other bacterial species); and 3. Other (not *lactobacillus* species). The type of *Lactobacillus* was classified as follows: 1. *Lactobacillus Reuteri*; and 2. Other *Lactobacillus* spp. (any *Lactobacillus* species other than *L. Reuteri*). The oral hygiene instructions were categorized as follows: 1. Yes (when providing specific oral hygiene instructions); or 2. No (when asking participants to maintain their regular oral hygiene habits).

3. Results

3.1. Study Selection

A total of 1883 publications were identified through the electronic search of the six databases. After removing duplicates, two reviewers conducted title and abstract screening on 994 publications, and 890 were excluded. In the next step, 104 publications underwent full-text screening. Finally, 64 publications remained for the systematic review and 47 were included in the meta-analysis (17 studies were removed due to insufficient/incompatible data for meta-analysis) (Figure 2).

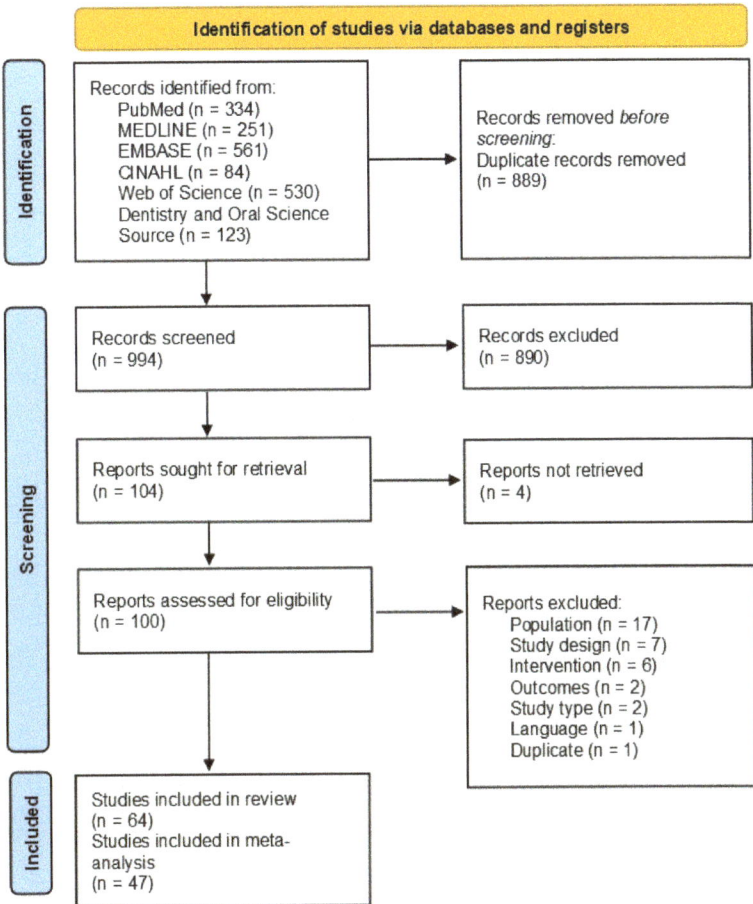

Figure 2. Preferred Reporting Items for Systematic Reviews and Meta-Analyses (PRISMA) flow diagram detailing the study selection.

3.2. Study Characteristics

There was a total of 64 studies eligible for the systematic review and 47 studies for the meta-analysis. Table 1 presents the detailed individual study characteristics including: periodontal disease status, sample size, probiotic strain, treatment duration and immediate follow-up, mode of probiotic delivery, other treatments, oral hygiene instructions, outcomes investigated, and key findings. The probiotic treatment duration varied from one day to four months. The sample sizes varied from 10 to 120 individuals. The most common probiotic formulation was composed of *Lactobacillus reuteri*. The majority of studies had periodontitis patients.

Table 1. Characteristics of the studies included in the systematic review and meta-analysis.

Author, Year, Country	Study Sample Characteristics			Probiotic Formulation	Treatment Duration/ Immediate Follow-Up	Mode of Probiotic Delivery	Other Treatments	Oral Hygiene Instructions	Outcomes Investigated	Key Findings
	Disease Status	Sample Size								
		Probiotic	Control							
Alkaya, 2016 [53] Turkey	Gingivitis	20	20	B. megaterium, B. pumilus, B. subtilis	8 weeks / 8 weeks	Toothpaste, mouth rinse, and toothbrush	Supragingival scaling and/or oral prophylaxis	Yes	PII*, GI*, PPD*, BOP*	No statistically significant difference attributed to probiotic use in gingivitis patients.
Alshareef, 2020 [54] Saudi Arabia	Periodontitis	15	10	B. bifidum, L. acidophilus, L. casei, L. rhamnosus, L. salivarius	30 days / 30 days	Lozenge	SRP	Yes	PII*, CAL*, PPD*, GBI+, GCF*, MMP-8*	Statistically significant improvement in GBI and greater improvement in GCF with probiotic use.
Bazyar, 2020 [55] Iran	Periodontitis	23	24	Bifidobacterium, B. longum, L. acidophilus, L. bulgaricus, L. casei, L. rhamnosus, S. thermophilus	8 weeks / 8 weeks	Capsule	NSPT	No	PII+, CAL+, BOP+, PPD*, IL1β+, MDA+, TAC+, SOD+, CAT, GPx+	Probiotic supplementation and NSPT in type 2 diabetes patients with chronic periodontitis may improve antioxidant, anti-inflammatory, and periodontal parameters.
Bollero, 2017 [56] Italy	Gingivitis	19	21	B. animalis, B. bifidum, L. acidophilus, L. delbrueckii, L. plantarum, L. reuteri, L. lactis, S. thermophilus	1 week / 1 week	Mouthwash	None	Not mentioned	BOP+, PCR+	Probiotic mouthwash may serve as an additional prophylactic to standard oral hygiene procedures.
Boyeena, 2019 [57] India	Periodontitis	10	10	B. bifidum, B. longum, L. acidophilus, L. rhamnosus	Once / 45 days	Paste	1) SRP + tetracycline fibers 2) SRP + tetracycline fibers + Probiotic	Yes	PII*, PPD*, SBI*, total bacteria*	Probiotic and tetracycline may act synergistically in the treatment of periodontitis.
Chandra, 2016 [58] India	Periodontitis	28	27	S. boulardii	Once / 1 week	Paste	SRP	Yes	PI, MGI*, CAL+, PPD+	S. boulardii and SRP significantly improved periodontal disease parameters compared to SRP alone.
Deshmukh, 2017 [59] India	Healthy	15	15	Bifidobacterium, Lactobacillus, S. Boulardii	14 days / 14 days	Sachet	Supragingival scaling + chlorhexidine mouthwash control	Yes	PII*, GI*	Probiotic mouthwashes have similar efficacy to chlorhexidine and are a potential alternative with fewer side effects.
Dhaliwal, 2017 [60] India	Periodontitis	14	13	B. mesentericus, C. butyricum, L. sporogenes, S. faecalis	21 days / 30 days	Lozenge	SRP	Not mentioned	PII*, GI*, PPD*, RAL*, A. actinomycetemcomitans, P. gingivalis+, P. intermedia	Probiotics may be used as an adjunctive treatment for the management of chronic periodontitis.
Duarte, 2019 [61] United Arab Emirates	Gingivitis	5	5	S. oralis, S. rattus, S. uberis	30 days / 30 days	Mouthwash	1) SRP 2) SRP + chlorhexidine mouthwash	Yes	GI*, OHI+, PI*	Changes may be attributed to type and duration of intervention. Probiotics showed similar efficacy to chlorhexidine and better results compared to SRP alone.

Table 1. *Cont.*

Author, Year, Country	Study Sample Characteristics — Disease Status	Sample Size — Probiotic	Sample Size — Control	Probiotic Formulation	Treatment Duration/Immediate Follow-Up	Mode of Probiotic Delivery	Other Treatments	Oral Hygiene Instructions	Outcomes Investigated	Key Findings
Elsadek, 2020 [62] Saudi Arabia	Periodontitis	19	19	*L. reuteri*	3 weeks/12 weeks	Lozenge	1) RSD + Photodynamic therapy 2) RSD alone	Yes	CAL *, BOP *, PPD *, PS*, *P. gingivalis* +, *T. Forsythia* +, *T. denticola* +	Photodynamic therapy showed greater benefits for deeper periodontal pockets. Probiotics reduced bacterial counts more than RSD alone.
Ercan, 2020 [63] Turkey	Gingivitis	40	40	*B. lactis, B. longum, E. faecium, L. acidophilus, L. plantarum, S. thermophilus,*	1 month/1 month	Chewing tablet	SRP	Yes	PlI *, GI *, GCF *, IL-6 +, IL8 +, IL10 +	Adjunct synbiotics improved clinical and immunological outcomes in gingivitis patients, irrespective of smoking status.
Grusovin, 2019 [64] Italy	Periodontitis	10	10	*L. reuteri*	3 months, 3-month washout, 3 months/3 months, 9 months	Lozenge	FM-GBT	Yes	BOP +, PPD +, PAL +, tooth survival	Probiotics improved clinical parameters with periodontal maintenance therapy.
Hallström, 2013 [42] Sweden	Healthy	9	9	*L. reuteri*	3 weeks/3 weeks	Lozenge	None	No	PI, GI, BOP, GCF, IL-1β *, IL6, IL8 *, IL10, IL-18 *, MIP-1β *, TNF-α, *A. actinomycetemcomitan, A. naeslundii, C. rectus, F. alocis, F. nucleatum *, L. reuteri, L. fermentum, P. micra, P. endodontis, P. intermedia, P. gingivalis, S. intermedia, S. mutans, S. oralis *, S. sanguinis, T. forsythia, T. denticola, V. parvula *	Probiotic supplementation did not significantly affect plaque accumulation, inflammatory reactions in the gingiva, and the microbiological composition in healthy individuals with experimental gingivitis.
Ikram, 2018 [65] Pakistan	Periodontitis	15	15	*L. reuteri*	3 months/4 months	Sachet	SRP + amoxicillin + metronidazole	Yes	PlI *, CAL +, BOP *, PPD *	Probiotics showed similar efficacy in the improvement of periodontal clinical outcomes as antibiotics.
Ikram, 2019 [66] Pakistan	Periodontitis	14	14	*L. reuteri*	12 weeks/12 weeks	Sachet	SRP	Yes	PlI *, CAL +, BOP +, PPD +	Probiotics may be used as an adjunctive treatment with SRP to treat chronic periodontitis.
Ince, 2015 [67] Turkey	Periodontitis	15	15	*L. reuteri*	3 weeks/3 weeks	Lozenge	SRP	Yes	PlI +, GI +, BOP +, PPD +, CAL +, GCF *, MMP-8 +, TIMP-1 +	Adjunct probiotic treatment improved clinical and immunological outcomes in periodontitis patients.

Table 1. *Cont.*

Author, Year, Country	Study Sample Characteristics			Probiotic Formulation	Treatment Duration/ Immediate Follow-Up	Mode of Probiotic Delivery	Other Treatments	Oral Hygiene Instructions	Outcomes Investigated	Key Findings
	Disease Status	Sample Size								
		Probiotic	Control							
Iniesta, 2012 [43] Spain	Gingivitis	20	20	*L. reuteri*	4 weeks/ 4 weeks	Chewing tablet	None	No	PlI, GI, *Lactobacillus* spp., *A. actinomycetemcomitan*, *C. rectus*, *Capnocytophaga* spp., *E. corrodens*, *F. nucleatum*, *P. micra*, *P. intermedia*, *P. gingivalis*, *Tannerella forsythia*, total bacteria	Probiotic administration reduced subgingival periodontopathogen count.
Invernici, 2018 [68] Brazil	Periodontitis	20	21	*B. lactis*	30 days/ 30 days	Lozenge	SRP	Yes	PlI +, CAL +, PPD +, BOP +, REC, IL-1β +, IL-8 +, IL-10 +, *B. animalis* +,	Probiotic supplementation in addition to SRP may improve clinical, microbiological, and immunological outcomes in generalized chronic periodontitis patients.
Iwasakia, 2016 [69] Japan	Periodontitis	19	17	*L. plantarum*	12 weeks/ 12 weeks	Capsule	SPT	Not mentioned	PlI, GI, BOP, PPD	Chronic periodontitis patients with adjunctive probiotic treatment may lead to improvements in periodontal pockets.
Jagadeesh, 2017 [70] India	Gingivitis	15	15	*B. coagulans*	3 weeks/ 3 weeks	Chewing tablet	None	Not mentioned	PlI, GI +, BOP +, GPx	Probiotic use led to a statistically significant decrease in BOP.
Jäsberg, 2018 [71] Finland	Healthy	29	31	*B. animalis*, *L. rhamnosus*	4 weeks/ 4 weeks	Lozenge	None	Not mentioned	PlI +, GI +, MMP-8, MMP-9 +, TIMP-1 +, *S. mutans*, *lactobacilli*	Probiotics may immunomodulate the oral cavity.
Keller, 2018 [72] Denmark	Gingivitis	23	24	*L. curvatus*, *L. rhamnosus*	4 weeks/ 4 weeks	Tablet	None	No	PlI +, BOP + GCF +, IL-1β, IL-6, IL-8, IL-10, TNF-α	Probiotic use may improve gingival health without affecting the oral microbiome and immune response.
Krasse, 2005 [73] Sweden	Gingivitis	20	18	*L. reuteri*	14 days/ 14 days	Chewing gum	None	Yes	PlI +, GI +, *L. reuteri* +, Total *lactobacillus* +	*L. reuteri* can reduce PlI and GI in gingivitis patients.
Kuka, 2019 [74] Turkey	Periodontitis	18	18	*L. reuteri*	3 weeks/ 12 weeks	Tablet	IPT	Yes	BOP +, PPD +, GCF +, NO +	Probiotics may be an adjunct to IPT. NO in GCF is a potential inflammatory marker in periodontal diseases.

Table 1. Cont.

Author, Year, Country	Study Sample Characteristics			Probiotic Formulation	Treatment Duration/ Immediate Follow-Up	Mode of Probiotic Delivery	Other Treatments	Oral Hygiene Instructions	Outcomes Investigated	Key Findings
	Disease Status	Sample Size								
		Probiotic	Control							
Kuru, 2017 [75] Turkey	Healthy	26	25	B. animalis	4 weeks/ 4 weeks	Yogurt	None	Yes	PII+, GI+, BOP+, PPD+, GCF+, IL-1β+	Probiotics improved clinical and immunological outcomes compared to controls after a 5-day non-brushing period.
Laleman, 2015 [76] Turkey	Periodontitis	24	24	S. oralis, S. rattus, S. uberis	12 weeks/ 12 weeks	Tablet	SRP	Not mentioned	CAL*, BOP*, PPD*, REC*, F. nucleatum*, P. gingivalis*, P. intermedia+, T. forsythia*	Probiotic formulation used did not show statistically significant improvements in clinical or microbiological outcomes.
Laleman, 2019 [77] Belgium	Periodontitis	19	20	L. reuteri	12 weeks/ 12 weeks	Lozenge	NSPT	Yes	PII+, CAL*, BOP PPD+, REC*, A. actinomycetemcomitans, F. nucleatum, P. intermedia, P. gingivalis	Adjunctive use of probiotics after NSPT reduced PPD and the percentage of sites in need of surgery.
Lee, 2015 [78] Korea	Healthy	14	16	L. brevis	14 days/ 14 days	Lozenge	Scaling and polishing	Yes	PII+, GI+, BOP*, NO, MMP-8, PGE2*	Probiotic supplementation may decrease inflammatory cascades through NO and PGE2.
Mayanagi, 2009 [79] Japan	Periodontitis	34	32	L. salivarius	8 weeks/ 8 weeks	Tablet	None	No	A. actinomycetemcomitans, P. intermedia, P. gingivalis, T. forsythia+, T. denticola, total bacteria*	Probiotics decreased the subgingival T. forsythia count at 4 and 8 weeks and the total bacteria count at 4 weeks.
Meenakshi, 2018 [80] India	Periodontitis	10	10	L. casei	1 month/ 1 month	Drink	SRP	No	PII+, GI+, CAL+, PPD+, total bacteria+	Probiotics as an adjunct to SRP improved clinical outcomes and reduced total bacterial count.
Mitic, 2017 [81] Macedonia	Periodontitis	15	15	B. bifidum, B. coagulans, L. acidophilus, L. bulgaricus, S. thermophilus	15 days/ 1 month	Lozenge	SRP	Yes	PII+, GI+, GBI+, CAL+, PPD+, anaerobic bacterial count+	Probiotics may improve clinical outcomes and bacterial count in periodontitis patients.
Montero, 2017 [14] Spain	Gingivitis	30	29	L. brevis, L. plantarum, P. acidilactici	6 weeks/ 6 weeks	Chewing tablet	PMPR	Yes	PII*, GI*, AngBs+, A. actinomycetemcomitans*, C. rectus, Fusobacterium spp., P. gingivalis, T. forsythia*	Decreased number of sites with severe inflammation compared to placebo group in gingivitis patients. Decreased T. forsythia count.
Morales, 2016 [82] Chile	Periodontitis	14	14	L. rhamnosus	3 months/ 3 months	Sachet	SRP	Yes	CAL*, PII*, BOP, PPD*	Probiotic use improved clinical symptoms similar to SRP alone.

Table 1. *Cont.*

Author, Year, Country	Study Sample Characteristics	Sample Size		Probiotic Formulation	Treatment Duration/ Immediate Follow-Up	Mode of Probiotic Delivery	Other Treatments	Oral Hygiene Instructions	Outcomes Investigated	Key Findings
	Disease Status	Probiotic	Control							
Morales, 2017 [10] Chile	Periodontitis	16	15	*L. rhamnosus*	3 months/ 9 months	Sachet	1) SRP 2) SRP + Antibiotic	Yes	CAL *, BOP, PPD *, PA *, *A. actinomycetemcomitans*, *P. gingivalis* *, *T. forsythia*, total bacteria *	Probiotic and antibiotic groups had similar clinical and microbiological improvements to placebo.
Nadkerny, 2015 [83] India	Gingivitis	15	15	*B. longum*, *L. acidophilus*, *L. rhamnosus*, *L. sporogenes*, *S. boulardii*	4 weeks/ 4 weeks	Sachet	Scaling and polishing 1) Chlorhexidine 2) Normal saline	Yes	PII +, GI +, OHI-S +	Probiotic mouthwash effectively reduced plaque accumulation and gingival inflammation.
Nasry, 2018 [84] Egypt	Gingivitis	20	20	*L. rhamnosus*	2 weeks/ 2 weeks	Spray	Scaling and polishing	Yes	PII +, GI +, SI +	Miswak and probiotic formulation led to the greatest reduction in plaque and gingival indices.
Pelekos, 2019 [34] Hong Kong	Periodontitis	21	20	*L. reuteri*	28 days/ 90 days	Lozenge	NSPT	Yes	CAL *, BOP *, PPD *	Adjunctive use of probiotics did not show increased effectiveness compared to control.
Pelekos, 2020 [85] Hong Kong	Periodontitis	20	20	*L. reuteri*	28 days/ 90 days	Lozenge	NSPT	Yes	CAL *, BOP *, PPD +	Probiotic supplementation improved periodontal pockets ≥ 5 mm and CAL.
Penala, 2015 [86] India	Periodontitis	15	14	*L. reuteri*, *L. salivarius*	15 days/ 3 months	Capsule & Mouthwash	SRP	Yes	PII +, MGI +, GBI +, PPD *, CAL *, BANA, ORG	Probiotic use improved clinical outcomes and oral malodor parameters.
Pudgar, 2020 [87] Slovenia	Periodontitis	20	20	*L. brevis*, *L. plantarum*	Once (gel) 3 months (lozenge)/ 3 months	Local gel & Lozenge	SRP	Yes	DS *, PII *, CAL *, BOP *, PPD *, REC*, GBI *	Probiotic and control groups both had significant clinical improvements, but there was no statistically significant difference between the two groups.
Sabatini, 2017 [88] Italy	Gingivitis	40	40	*L. reuteri*	30 days/ 30 days	Tablet	None	Yes	PII +, BOP +	Probiotics were effective in reducing plaque and BOP in type 2 diabetes patients with gingivitis.
Sajedinejad, 2017 [89] Iran	Periodontitis	10	10	*L. salivarius*	4 weeks/ 4 weeks	Mouthwash	SRP	Yes	PII, GI +, BOP +, PPD *, *A. actinomycetemcomitans* +	Probiotic use improved clinical and microbiological outcomes.
Scariya, 2015 [90] India	Gingivitis and Periodontitis	14	14	*S. salivarius*	30 days/ 30 days	Tablet	None	Yes	PII +, GI +, SBI +, PPD+	Probiotic use improved clinical outcomes compared to controls.

Table 1. Cont.

| Author, Year, Country | Study Sample Characteristics | | | Probiotic Formulation | Treatment Duration/ Immediate Follow-Up | Mode of Probiotic Delivery | Other Treatments | Oral Hygiene Instructions | Outcomes Investigated | Key Findings |
| | Disease Status | Sample Size | | | | | | | | |
		Probiotic	Control							
Schlagenhauf, 2018 [91] Germany	Gingivitis	24	21	L. reuteri	Within 2 days after delivery (41.9 ± 16.0 days)	Lozenge	None	No	PlI⁺, GI⁺, TNF-α	Probiotics may be a useful adjunct for pregnancy-related gingivitis.
Schlagenhauf, 2020 [92] Germany	Gingivitis & Periodontitis	33	35	L. reuteri	42 days/ 42 days	Lozenge	None	No	PCR⁺, GI⁺, BOP⁺, PAL⁺, PPD⁺	Probiotic use improved all clinical outcomes compared to controls.
Shah, 2013 [93] India	Periodontitis	10	10 (Control) 10 (Antibiotic)	L. brevis	2 weeks/ 2 months	Tablet	SRP 1) Probiotic + Doxycycline 2) Doxycycline alone	No	PlI*, GI*, CAL*, PPD*, lactobacilli*, A. actinomycetemcomitans*	Probiotic use decreased clinical and microbiological parameters when used alone or in combination with doxycycline.
Shah, 2017 [94] India	Periodontitis	6	6	L. brevis	14 days/ 5 months	Lozenge	SRP 1) Probiotics + Doxycycline 2) Doxycycline alone	No	GI⁺, PlI, PPD, CAL, A. actinomycetemcomitans, Lactobacillus spp.	No synergy at 5 months when probiotics and doxycycline were both given. No statistically significant difference between antibiotic and probiotic supplementation.
Shetty, 2020 [95] India	Periodontitis	60	60	B. mesentericus, C. butyricum, L. sporogenes. S. faecalis	Once (local)/ 3 months	Local	SRP	Not mentioned	PlI*, GI*, PPD*, IL-6⁺, ALP*, P.Gingivalis*, P. intermedia*	Synbiotic treatment may improve clinical, microbiological, and immunological outcomes in patients with chronic periodontitis.
Shimauchi, 2008 [96] Japan	Healthy	34	32	L. salivarius	8 weeks/ 8 weeks	Tablet	None	No	PlI*, GI*, BOP*, PPD*, L. salivarius⁺, Lactoferritin* (Saliva)	Probiotics may be useful for maintenance and/or improvement of oral health in individuals at risk of periodontal diseases.
Sinkiewicz, 2010 [97] Sweden	Healthy	11	12	L. reuteri	12 weeks/ 12 weeks	Chewing gum	None	No	PlI, A. naeslundii*, A. actinomycetemcomitans*, C. rectus*, F. alocis*, F. nucleatum*, L. acidophilus, L. fermentum*, L. reuteri*, P. micra, P. gingivalis*, P. endodontalis*, P. intermedia*, T. forsythia*, T. denticola*, S. intermedia, S. mutans*, S. oralis, S. sanguinis*, V. parvula*	There was a statistically significant increase in plaque in the controls, but not the probiotics group. No changes between probiotics and control groups in the oral microbiota.
Slawik, 2011 [98] Germany	Healthy	11	17	L. casei	14 days/ 14 days	Drink	None	No	PlI*, GI*, BOP⁺, GCF⁺	Probiotics may have an anti-inflammatory effect.

Table 1. Cont.

Author, Year, Country	Study Sample Characteristics — Disease Status	Sample Size — Probiotic	Sample Size — Control	Probiotic Formulation	Treatment Duration/ Immediate Follow-Up	Mode of Probiotic Delivery	Other Treatments	Oral Hygiene Instructions	Outcomes Investigated	Key Findings
Snulingga, 2020 [99] Indonesia	Periodontitis	8	8	L. reuteri	14 days/ 14 days	Lozenge	SRP	Not mentioned	CAL+, IL-4	Probiotic use as an adjunct decreased CAL and increased IL-4.
Staab, 2009 [100] Germany	Healthy	25	25	L. casei	8 weeks/ 8 weeks	Drink	None	No	PlI+, PBI*, MPO+, MMP-3+, Elastase*	Probiotics may improve periodontal health through immunomodulation.
Suzuki, 2012 [101] Japan	Periodontitis	20	22	L. salivarius	2 weeks/ 2 weeks	Oil drops	None	No	BOP+, PPD*, Ubiquitous bacteria*, F. nucleatum, P. gingivalis, L. salivarius*, P. intermedia, S. mutans, T. forsythia, T. denticola	Probiotics improved BOP and had a decreased periodontopathogen count compared to controls.
Tekce, 2015 [41] Turkey	Periodontitis	20	20	L. reuteri	3 weeks/ 3 weeks	Lozenge	SRP	Yes	PlI+, GI+, BOP+, PPD+, RAL*, Anaerobic bacteria+, TVC+	Probiotics as an adjuvant can improve clinical and microbiological outcomes.
Teughels, 2013 [102] Turkey	Periodontitis	15	15	L. reuteri	12 weeks/ 12 weeks	Lozenge	SRP	Yes	PlI*, CAL+, GBI+, BOP+, PPD+, REC, A. actinomycetemcomitans*, F. nucleatum*, T. forsythia*, P. gingivalis+, P. intermedia*, Total bacteria*	Probiotics as an adjuvant can improve clinical and microbiological outcomes.
Theodoro, 2019 [103] Brazil	Periodontitis	14	14	L. reuteri	21 days/ 90 days	Chewing tablet	SRP	Yes	BOP+, CAL, PPD+, REC	Adjuvant use of probiotics to treat chronic periodontitis in smokers reduced gingival inflammation.
Tobita, 2018 [104] Japan	Healthy	8	8	L. crispatus	4 weeks/ 4 weeks	Tablet	None	No	PS+, A. actinomycetemcomitans, F. nucleatum*, T. forsythia, P. gingivalis+, P. intermedia, T. denticola.	Probiotic use can improve the oral environment and hence may help prevent periodontal disease.
Toiviainen, 2015 [105] Finland	Healthy	29	31	B. lactis, L. rhamnosus	4 weeks/ 4 weeks	Lozenge	None	Not mentioned	PlI*, GI*, Lactobacillus, S. mutans	Probiotics improved clinical outcomes but not microbiological.
Twetman, 2009 [106] Denmark	Gingivitis	14	13	L. reuteri	2 weeks/ 2 weeks	Chewing gum	None	Yes	BOP*, IL-1β, TNF-α, GCF*, IL-6*, IL-8*, IL-10	Probiotics are beneficial to gingival health in a dose dependent manner.
Vicario, 2013 [107] Spain	Periodontitis	10	9	L. reuteri	1 month/ 1 month	Tablet	None	Yes	PlI*, BOP*, PPD*	Probiotic supplementation can improve inflammatory and clinical outcomes in patients with mild to moderate periodontitis.

Table 1. Cont.

Author, Year, Country	Disease Status	Sample Size Probiotic	Sample Size Control	Probiotic Formulation	Treatment Duration/ Immediate Follow-Up	Mode of Probiotic Delivery	Other Treatments	Oral Hygiene Instructions	Outcomes Investigated	Key Findings
Vivekananda, 2010 [108] India	Periodontitis	15	15	L. reuteri	21 days/ 42 days	Lozenge	1) SRP 2) Without SRP	Yes	PlI*, GI*, GBI*, CAL*, PPD*, A. actinomycetemcomitans*, P. gingivalis*, P. intermedia	Probiotic use can improve periodontal health through plaque inhibition, anti-inflammatory and antimicrobial effects.
Vohra, 2019 [109] Saudi Arabia	Periodontitis	31	32	L. reuteri	21 days/ 3 months	Lozenge	SRP	Yes	PlI*, CAL*, BOP*, PPD*	Probiotic use is not an effective adjunct to SRP in chronic periodontitis patients.
Yuki, 2019 [110] Japan	Periodontal disease	12	11	L. rhamnosus	90 days/ 90 days	Yogurt	None	Yes	GI*, PPD*, PMA*	Probiotic use improved clinical parameters under study.

Note: * Indicates a statistically significant difference within the probiotic group from baseline to follow-up. + Indicates a statistically significant difference between the probiotic and control groups. Abbreviations: Clinical—AngBs, Angulated bleeding score; BOP, Bleeding on probing; CAL, Clinical attachment level; DS, Disease sites defined as probing pocket depth > 4 mm and BOP; GBI, Gingival bleeding index; GCF, Gingival crevicular fluid; GI, Gingival index; MGI, Modified gingival index; OHI, Oral hygiene index; OHI-S, Oral hygiene index simplified; PAL, Probing attachment level; PCR, Plaque control record; PI, Periodontal index; PA, Plaque accumulation; PBI, Papillary bleeding index; PlI, Plaque index; PMA, Papillary-marginal-attached index; PPD, Probing pocket depth; PS, Plaque score; RAL, Relative attachment level; REC, Gingival recession; SBI, Sulcular bleeding index; SI, Stain index; Microbiological—A. actinomycetemcomitans, Aggregatibacter actinomycetemcomitans; A. naeslundii, Actinomyces naeslundii; B. subtilis, Bacillus subtilis; B. megaterium, Bacillus megaterium; B. mesentericus, Bacillus mesentericus; B. pumulus, Bacillus pumulus; B. animalis, Bifidobacterium animalis; B. bifidum, Bifidobacterium bifidum; B. coagulans, Bacillus coagulans; B. lactis, Bifidobacterium lactis; B. longum, Bifidobacterium longum; C. rectus, Campylobacter rectus; C. butyricum, Clostridium butyricum; E. corrodens, Eikenella corrodens; E. faccium, Enterococcus faccium; F. alocis, Filifactor alocis; F. nucleatum, Fusobacterium nucleatum; L. acidophilus, Lactobacillus acidophilus; L. brevis, Lactobacillus brevis; L. bulgaricus, Lactobacillus bulgaricus; L. casei, Lactobacillus casei; L. crispatus, Lactobacillus crispatus; L. curvatus, Lactobacillus curvatus; L. delbrueckii, Lactobacillus delbrueckii; L. fermentum, Lactobacillus fermentum; L. plantarum, Lactobacillus plantarum; L. rhamnosus, Lactobacillus rhamnosus; L. reuteri, Lactobacillus reuteri; L. salivarius, Lactobacillus salivarius; L. sporogenes, Lactobacillus sporogenes; L. lactis, Lactococcus lactis; P. acidilactici, Pediococcus acidilactici; P. endodontalis, Porphyromonas endodontalis; P. gingivalis, Porphyromonas gingivalis; P. intermedia, Prevotella intermedia; P. micra, Parvimonas micra; S. faecalis, Streptococcus faecalis; S. intermedia, Streptococcus intermedia; S. mutans, Streptococcus mutans; S. oralis, Streptococcus oralis; S. rattus, Streptococcus rattus; S. salivarius, Streptococcus salivarius; S. sanguinis, Streptococcus sanguinis; S. thermophilus, Streptococcus thermophilus; S. uberis, Streptococcus uberis; S. boulardii, Saccharomyces boulardii; T. forsythia, Tannerella forsythia; T. denticola, Treponema denticola; V. parvula, Veillonella parvula; Immunological—CAT, Catalase; GPx, Glutathione peroxidase; IL, Interleukin; MDA, Malondialdehyde; MIP-1β, Macrophage inflammatory protein 1 beta; MMP-8, matrix metalloproteinase-8; MPO, myeloperoxidase; NO, Nitric oxide; SOD, Super-oxide dismutase; TAC, Total antioxidant capacity; TIMP-1, Tissue inhibitor of metalloproteinase; TNF-α, Tumor necrosis factor alpha; Other—BANA, N-benzoyl-DL-arginine-naphthylamide; ORG, Halitosis assessment with organoleptic scores; FM-GBT, Full mouth guided biofilm therapy; IPT, Initial periodontal therapy; NSPT, Non-surgical periodontal therapy; PMPR, Professional manual plaque removal; RSD, Root surface debridement; SPT, Supporting periodontal therapy; SRP, Scaling and root planing; TVC, Total viable count.

3.3. Risk of Bias within Studies

Using the Cochrane risk–of–bias assessment tool version 2, the majority of studies included were classified as having a low risk of bias (n = 38). Additionally, 13 studies were classified as having some concerns, and another 13 studies were classified as having a high risk of bias. The majority of concerns were due to questions related to the randomization process domain. There were minimal concerns regarding the missing outcome data domain. The results are presented in Supplemental Table S3.

3.4. Synthesis of Results

This meta-analysis used the Hedge's g standardized mean difference (SMD) to report effect sizes. Forest plots depicting the pooled meta-analysis examining the effects of probiotic supplementation on clinical, microbiological, and immunological outcomes are presented in Figures 3–5, respectively. The overall measures of effect are summarized in Supplemental Table S4. The results of subgroup analysis are presented in Table 2 with additional information available in the Supplemental File. The forest plots for the subgroup analysis of clinical parameters are depicted in Supplemental Figure S1.

Table 2. Subgroup analysis examining the effects of probiotic supplementation on clinical outcomes.

Clinical Outcomes	Subgroup	Level of Subgroup	SMD	95% CI	I^2	*p*-Value	Sample Size Probiotic	Control
Plaque index (PlI)	Type of periodontal disease	Gingivitis	0.153	−0.152, 0.457	20.906	0.281	108	99
		Periodontitis	0.736	0.267, 1.206	71.842	**0.001**	136	135
	Type of probiotic strain	*Lactobacillus*	0.639	0.169, 1.110	75.533	**<0.001**	154	151
		Mixed	0.280	−0.159, 0.719	0.000	0.523	42	36
		Other	0.185	−0.212, 0.582	0.000	0.431	48	47
	Type of *Lactobacillus* species	*L. Reuteri*	0.707	0.034, 1.381	80.976	**<0.001**	98	95
		Other	0.590	−0.456, 1.636	81.557	**0.004**	42	42
	Treatment duration	≤1 month	0.615	0.146, 1.084	75.448	**<0.001**	154	153
		>1 to 2 months	0.328	−0.006, 0.661	0.000	0.406	73	64
		> 2 months	0.053	−0.603, 0.710	0.000	1.000	17	17
	Mode of delivery	Ingestion	0.952	−0.894, 2.797	89.037	**0.003**	27	27
		Local	0.323	−0.202, 0.847	0.000	1.000	28	27
		Oral	0.239	−0.302, 0.780	0.251	0.251	34	34
		Oral and Ingestion	0.495	0.061, 0.930	0.001	**<0.001**	155	146
	Oral hygiene instructions	Yes	0.622	0.204, 1.040	66.923	**0.006**	145	138
		No	0.665	−0.415, 1.746	85.436	**<0.001**	54	51
Mean plaque percentage (MPP)	Type of periodontal disease	Gingivitis	1.279	−0.905, 3.463	96.629	**<0.001**	63	64
		Periodontitis	0.681	0.072, 1.290	82.212	**<0.001**	130	130
	Type of probiotic strain	*Lactobacillus*	1.037	0.391, 1.683	88.278	**<0.001**	195	198
		Mixed	0.112	−0.728, 0.952	0.000	1.000	10	10
		Other	0.199	−0.396, 0.794	0.000	1.000	21	21
	Type of *Lactobacillus* species	*L. Reuteri*	1.458	0.724, 2.191	86.723	**<0.001**	148	150
		Other	0.193	−0.200, 0.586	0.000	0.889	47	48
	Treatment duration	≤1 month	0.937	0.076, 1.798	90.960	**<0.001**	145	146
		>1 to 2 months	1.560	1.022, 2.099	0.000	1.000	33	35
		> 2 months	0.460	0.008, 0.912	21.718	0.279	48	48

Table 2. *Cont.*

Clinical Outcomes	Subgroup	Level of Subgroup	SMD	95% CI	I^2	*p*-Value	Sample Size	
							Probiotic	Control
Gingival index (GI)	Mode of delivery	Ingestion	0.969	−0.506, 2.445	94.211	**<0.001**	77	78
		Oral	0.537	−0.348, 1.423	59.024	0.118	24	24
		Oral and Ingestion	0.942	0.159, 1.725	87.844	**<0.001**	125	127
	Oral hygiene instructions	Yes	0.880	0.197, 1.564	88.210	**<0.001**	170	170
		No	0.865	−0.502, 2.232	91.878	**<0.001**	56	59
	Type of periodontal disease	Gingivitis	0.298	−0.089, 0.684	49.985	0.092	108	99
		Periodontitis	1.069	0.296, 1.841	86.299	**<0.001**	116	112
	Type of probiotic strain	*Lactobacillus*	1.236	0.574, 1.897	87.366	**<0.001**	178	174
		Mixed	0.101	−0.333, 0.535	0.000	0.949	43	36
		Other	0.329	−0.070, 0.729	0.000	0.354	48	47
	Type of *Lactobacillus* species	*L. Reuteri*	1.621	0.648, 2.595	89.871	**<0.001**	112	111
		Other	0.817	0.018, 1.616	79.137	0.001	66	63
	Treatment duration	≤1 month	0.949	0.270, 1.628	85.079	**<0.001**	132	130
		>1 to 2 months	0.900	−0.116, 1.915	91.498	**<0.001**	106	99
		>2 months	0.888	−0.920, 2.696	89.949	0.002	31	28
Pocket probing depth (PPD)	Mode of delivery	Ingestion	1.258	−0.169, 2.686	87.547	**<0.001**	41	38
		Local	0.494	−0.035, 1.023	0.000	1.000	28	27
		Oral	0.189	−0.305, 0.682	0.000	0.674	30	30
		Oral and Ingestion	1.051	0.306, 1.797	89.846	**<0.001**	170	162
	Oral hygiene instructions	Yes	1.051	0.327, 1.775	86.466	**<0.001**	134	126
		No	1.344	0.261, 2.427	89.898	**<0.001**	87	86
	Type of periodontal disease	Gingivitis	0.997	−0.853, 2.848	92.406	**<0.001**	35	38
		Periodontitis	0.578	0.355, 0.801	62.720	**<0.001**	442	434
	Type of probiotic strain	*Lactobacillus*	0.674	0.386, 0.962	69.524	**<0.001**	330	329
		Mixed	0.387	0.045, 0.729	0.000	0.740	67	62
		Other	0.379	−0.037, 0.795	51.535	0.103	92	92
	Type of *Lactobacillus* species	*L. Reuteri*	0.677	0.315, 1.040	74.541	**<0.001**	249	252
		Other	0.657	0.169, 1.144	56.911	0.041	81	77
	Treatment duration	≤1 month	0.737	0.430, 1.044	66.736	**<0.001**	270	264
		>1 to 2 months	0.514	−0.030, 1.059	65.160	0.057	76	79
		> 2 months	0.326	0.015, 0.636	43.082	0.080	143	140
	Mode of delivery	Ingestion	0.514	0.106, 0.922	47.870	0.088	94	91
		Local	0.919	0.370, 1.468	0.000	1.000	28	27
		Oral	0.918	−0.071, 1.907	79.291	0.008	44	44
		Oral and Ingestion	0.525	0.251, 0.800	66.577	**<0.001**	323	321
	Oral hygiene instructions	Yes	0.592	0.343, 0.841	63.935	**<0.001**	366	360
		No	0.953	0.308, 1.597	65.707	0.054	66	69
	Disease severity	Deep	0.735	0.209, 1.261	73.585	0.002	112	114
		Moderate	0.499	0.043, 0.955	66.202	0.011	112	114

Table 2. *Cont.*

Clinical Outcomes	Subgroup	Level of Subgroup	SMD	95% CI	I²	p-Value	Sample Size Probiotic	Sample Size Control
Clinical attachment level (CAL)	Type of probiotic strain	*Lactobacillus*	0.417	0.225, 0.609	8.881	0.355	229	228
		Mixed	0.395	−0.066, 0.855	0.000	0.401	38	34
		Other	0.415	0.076, 0.755	7.610	0.339	72	72
	Type of *Lactobacillus* species	*L. Reuteri*	0.416	0.201, 0.631	12.027	0.330	189	189
		Other	0.445	−0.086, 0.975	31.016	0.235	40	39
	Treatment duration	≤1 month	0.388	0.185, 0.592	0.000	0.547	186	181
		>1 to 2 months	0.789	0.236, 1.343	34.507	0.217	41	41
		> 2 months	0.330	0.071, 0.588	0.000	0.571	112	112
	Mode of delivery	Ingestion	0.464	0.116, 0.812	0.276	0.390	63	63
		Local	0.696	0.159, 1.233	0.000	1.000	28	27
		Oral	0.887	0.132, 1.643	0.000	1.000	14	14
		Oral and Ingestion	0.339	0.159, 0.520	0.000	0.543	234	230
	Oral hygiene instructions	Yes	0.351	0.178, 0.523	0.000	0.789	256	251
		No	0.835	0.437, 1.233	0.000	0.376	51	51
	Disease severity	Deep	0.373	0.088, 0.657	0.000	0.690	92	94
		Moderate	0.422	0.137, 0.706	0.000	0.886	92	94
Bleeding on probing (BOP)	Type of periodontal disease	Gingivitis	0.685	−0.438, 1.808	93.899	**<0.001**	117	120
		Periodontitis	0.749	0.404, 1.094	72.526	**<0.001**	260	257
	Type of probiotic strain	*Lactobacillus*	0.878	0.442, 1.313	85.057	**<0.001**	314	312
		Mixed	0.035	−0.574, 0.643	0.000	1.000	19	21
		Other	0.202	−0.210, 0.613	0.000	0.640	44	44
	Type of *Lactobacillus* species	*L. Reuteri*	1.054	0.485, 1.622	86.818	**<0.001**	217	217
		Other	0.502	−0.078, 1.081	74.262	**0.002**	97	95
	Treatment duration	≤1 month	1.024	0.454, 1.595	88.021	**<0.001**	236	238
		>1 to 2 months	0.095	−0.513, 0.703	0.000	1.000	20	20
		> 2 months	0.402	0.020, 0.785	55.314	**0.037**	121	119
	Mode of delivery	Ingestion	0.742	−0.391, 1.876	93.499	**<0.001**	112	110
		Oral	1.166	−0.037, 2.370	89.525	**<0.001**	63	65
		Oral and Ingestion	0.616	0.296, 0.936	60.339	**0.005**	202	202
	Oral hygiene instructions	No	0.054	−0.508, 0.617	0.000	1.000	23	24
		Yes	0.966	0.478, 1.454	86.250	**<0.001**	277	276
Gingival crevicular fluid (GCF)	Type of periodontal disease	Gingivitis	0.626	0.162, 1.091	0.000	0.392	36	36
		Periodontitis	0.507	0.027, 0.986	0.000	0.496	33	33

Subgroup analysis assessing the effects of probiotic supplementation compared to a control on clinical outcomes in periodontal diseases using a random-effects model based on the: 1. Type of periodontal disease; 2. Type of probiotic strain; 3. Type of *Lactobacillus* species; 4. Treatment duration; 5. Mode of probiotic delivery; and 6. Oral hygiene instruction. Note: Bold indicates statistically significant findings (p-value ≤ 0.05). SMD, Hedge's g standardized mean difference. I², Measure of heterogeneity.

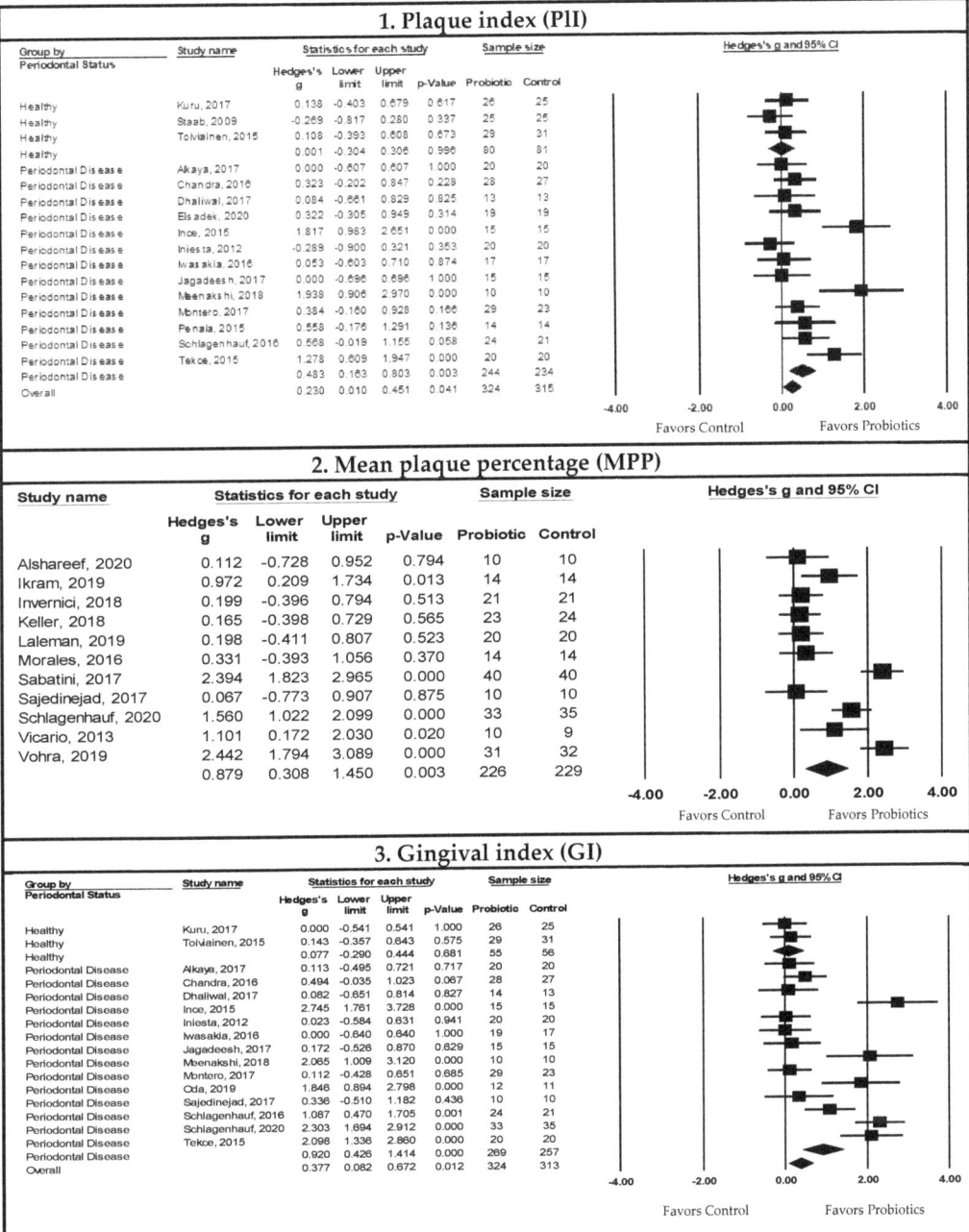

Figure 3. *Cont.*

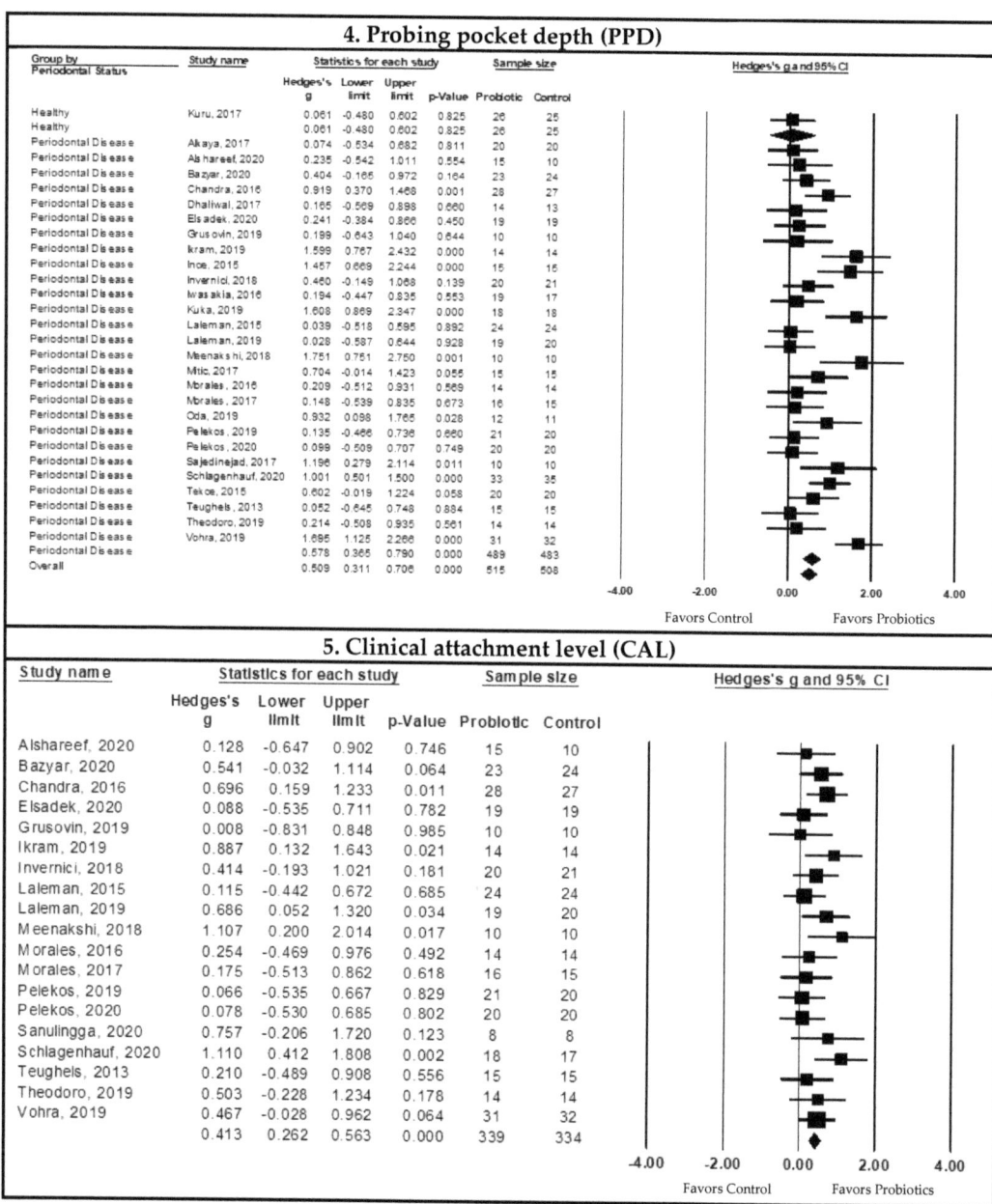

Figure 3. *Cont.*

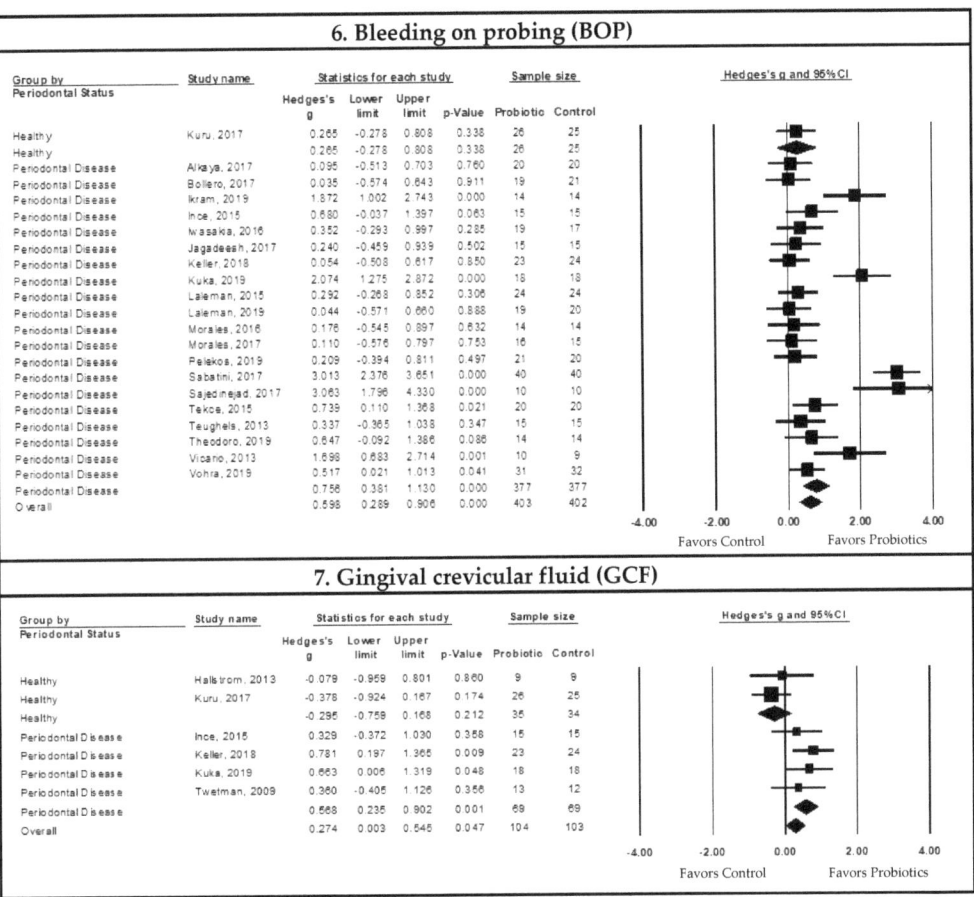

Figure 3. Pooled meta-analysis examining the effects of probiotic supplementation on clinical outcomes. 1. Forest plot of the Hedge's g SMD comparing the effects of probiotic supplementation to control groups on the plaque index (P1I) using a random-effects model. Note that we detected publication bias and/or small study effects, and the adjusted Hedge's g SMD = 0.557, 95% CI: 0.228, 0.885, and p-value ≤ 0.05 [14,41,43,53,58,60,62,67,69,70,80,86,91,105]. 2. Forest plot of the Hedge's g SMD comparing the effects of probiotic supplementation to control groups on the mean plaque percentage (MPP) using a random-effects model [54,66,68,72,77,82,88,89,92,107,109]. 3. Forest plot of the Hedge's g SMD comparing the effects of probiotic supplementation to control groups on the gingival index (GI) using a random-effects model [14,41,43,53,58,60,69,70,75,80,89,91,92,105,110]. 4. Forest plot of the Hedge's g SMD comparing the effects of probiotic supplementation to control groups on the probing pocket depth (PPD) using a random-effects model [10,34,41,53–55,58,60,62,64,66–69,74–77,80–82,85,89,92,102,103,109,110]. 5. Forest plot of the Hedge's g SMD comparing the effects of probiotic supplementation to control groups on the clinical attachment level (CAL) using a random-effects model [10,34,54,58,62,66,68,76,77,80,82,85,92,102,103,109]. 6. Forest plot of the Hedge's g SMD comparing the effects of probiotic supplementation to control groups on bleeding on probing (BOP) using a random-effects model. Note that we detected publication bias and/or small study effects, and the adjusted Hedge's g SMD = 0.841, 95% CI: 0.479, 1.200, and p-value ≤ 0.05 [10,34,41,53,56,66,67,69,70,72,74,76,77,88,89,102,103,107,109]. 7. Forest plot of the Hedge's g SMD comparing the effects of probiotic supplementation to control groups on the gingival crevicular fluid (GCF) using a random-effects model [42,67,72,74,75,106].

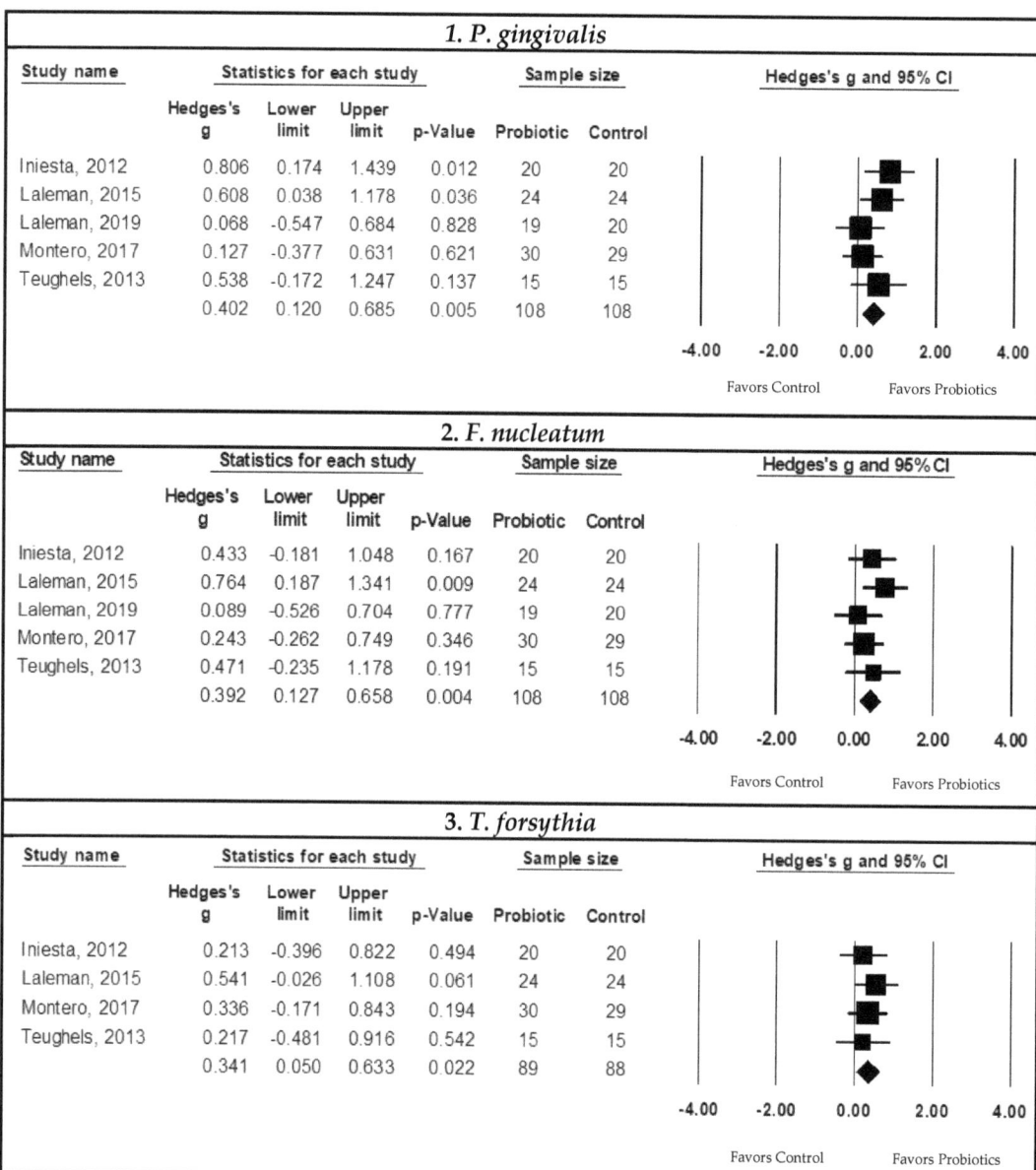

Figure 4. Pooled meta-analysis examining the effects of probiotic supplementation on microbiological outcomes in periodontal disease patients. 1. Forest plot of the Hedge's g SMD comparing the effects of probiotic supplementation to control groups on the subgingival *P. gingivalis* bacterial count using a random-effects model [14,43,76,77,102]. 2. Forest plot of the Hedge's g SMD comparing the effects of probiotic supplementation to control groups on the subgingival *F. nucleatum* bacterial count using a random-effects model [14,43,76,77,102]. 3. Forest plot of the Hedge's g SMD comparing the effects of probiotic supplementation to control groups on the subgingival *T. forsythia* bacterial count using a random-effects model [14,43,76,102].

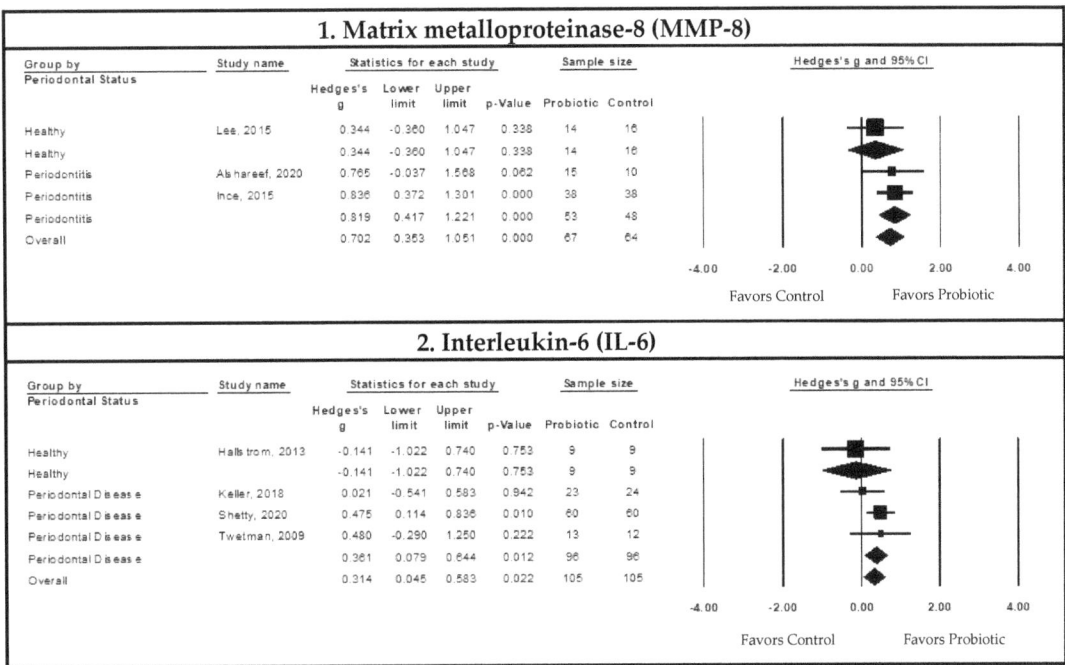

Figure 5. Pooled meta-analysis examining the effects of probiotic supplementation on immunological outcomes in periodontal disease patients; 1. Forest plot of the Hedge's g SMD comparing the effects of probiotic supplementation to control groups on the gingival crevicular fluid (GCF) level of matrix metalloproteinase-8 (MMP-8) using a random-effects model [59,67,78]. 2. Forest plot of the Hedge's g SMD comparing the effects of probiotic supplementation to control groups on the GCF level of interleukin-6 (IL-6) using a random-effects model [42,72,95,106].

3.4.1. Associations between Probiotic Supplementation and Clinical Outcomes in Periodontal Disease Patients

Pooled Meta-Analysis Examining the Effects of Probiotics on Plaque Index (PlI)

The effect of probiotic supplementation on the plaque index (PlI) indicated a statistically significant decrease with probiotic supplementation compared to controls in patients with periodontal diseases (SMD = 0.483, 95% CI: 0.163, 0.803, I^2 = 67.044, p-value $\leq$ 0.05, and n = 13 studies). Upon visual inspection of the funnel plot and confirmation through Egger's regression test (p-value = 0.040), there was evidence of publication bias/small study effects. Duval and Tweedie's trim and fill method gave an adjusted pooled estimate (SMD = 0.557, 95% CI: 0.228, 0.885, I^2 = 75.716, p-value $\leq$ 0.05, and n = 13 studies) (Figure 3).

Pooled Meta-Analysis Examining the Effects of Probiotics on Mean Plaque Percentage (MPP)

A change in the mean plaque percentage (MPP) was reported in 11 studies. The pooled SMD showed a statistically significant decrease in the MPP with probiotic supplementation compared to controls (SMD = 0.879, 95% CI: 0.308, 1.450, I^2 = 87.544, p-value $\leq$ 0.05, and n = 11 studies). There was no evidence of publication bias or small study effects upon visual inspection of the funnel plot and confirmation through Egger's regression test (p-value > 0.05) (Figure 3).

Pooled Meta-Analysis Examining the Effects of Probiotics on Gingival Index (GI)

The pooled SMD using data from patients with periodontal disease indicated a statistically significant reduction in the gingival index (GI) with probiotic supplementation compared to controls (SMD = 0.920, 95% CI: 0.426, 1.414, I^2 = 86.027, p-value $\leq$ 0.05, and n = 14 studies). There was no evidence of publication bias or small study effects upon visual inspection of the funnel plot and confirmation through Egger's regression test (p-value > 0.05) (Figure 3).

Pooled Meta-Analysis Examining the Effects of Probiotics on Probing Pocket Depth (PPD)

The pooled SMD indicated a statistically significant decrease in the probing pocket depth (PPD) with probiotic supplementation in patients with periodontal disease compared to controls (SMD = 0.578, 95% CI: 0.365, 0.790, I^2 = 62.840, p-value $\leq$ 0.05, and n = 27 studies). There was no evidence of publication bias or small study effect upon visual inspection of the funnel plot, and this was confirmed by Egger's regression test (p-value > 0.05) (Figure 3).

Pooled Meta-Analysis Examining the Effects of Probiotics on Clinical Attachment Level (CAL)

The pooled meta-analysis of the effect of probiotic supplementation on the clinical attachment level (CAL) was assessed in patients with periodontitis (n = 19 studies). Meta-analysis was not conducted to assess the effects of probiotics on CAL in healthy participants and those with gingivitis due to a lack of studies.

The pooled SMD indicates that there was a statistically significant CAL gain with probiotic supplementation compared to controls in patients with periodontitis (SMD = 0.413, 95% CI: 0.262, 0.563, I^2 < 0.001, p-value $\leq$ 0.05, and n = 19 studies). There was no evidence of publication bias and small study effects upon visual inspection of the funnel plot, which was confirmed by Egger's regression test (p-value > 0.05) (Figure 3).

Pooled Meta-Analysis Examining the Effects of Probiotics on Bleeding on Probing (BOP)

The effect of probiotic supplementation on bleeding on probing (BOP) indicated a statistically significant decrease with probiotic supplementation compared to controls in patients with periodontal disease (SMD = 0.756, 95% CI: 0.381, 1.130, I^2 = 83.699, p-value $\leq$ 0.05, and n = 20 studies). Inspection of the funnel plot for potential publication bias or small study effects suggested a right skew. This was confirmed by Egger's regression test (p-value = 0.020). After adjusting with Duval and Tweedie's trim and fill method, the adjusted SMD remained significant with high heterogeneity (SMD = 0.841, 95% CI: 0.479, 1.20; and I^2 = 86.750) (Figure 3).

Pooled Meta-Analysis Examining the Effects of Probiotics on Gingival Crevicular Fluid (GCF)

The effect of probiotic supplementation on the gingival crevicular fluid (GCF) volume indicated a statistically significant decrease in the GCF with probiotic supplementation compared to controls in patients with periodontal disease (SMD = 0.568, 95% CI: 0.235, 0.902, I^2 < 0.001, p-value $\leq$ 0.05, and n = four studies). There was no evidence of publication bias or small study effects upon visual inspection of the funnel plot and confirmation by Egger's regression test (p-value > 0.05) (Figure 3).

Pooled Meta-Analysis Examining the Effects of Probiotics on Gingival Recession (REC)

There was no statistically significant evidence that probiotic supplementation improved gingival recession (REC) compared to controls in patients with periodontitis (p-value = 0.741, and n = 5 studies). There was no evidence of publication bias or small study effects upon visual inspection of the funnel plot and confirmation by Egger's regression test (p-value > 0.05).

3.4.2. Associations between Probiotic Supplementation and Microbiological Outcomes in Periodontal Disease Patients

Pooled Meta-Analysis Examining the Effects of Probiotics on Subgingival *Porphyromonas Gingivalis* Count

The pooled SMD indicated a statistically significant decrease in the subgingival *P. gingivalis* count with probiotic supplementation compared to controls in patients with periodontal disease (SMD = 0.402, 95% CI: 0.120, 0.685, I^2 = 10.769, p-value $\leq$ 0.05, and n = five studies). There was no evidence of publication bias or small study effects through visual funnel plot inspection and Egger's regression test (p-value > 0.05) (Figure 4).

Pooled Meta-Analysis Examining the Effects of Probiotics on Subgingival *Fusobacterium nucleatum* Count

The pooled SMD using data from periodontal disease patients indicated a statistically significant decrease in the subgingival *F. nucleatum* count with probiotic supplementation compared to controls (SMD = 0.392, 95% CI: 0.127, 0.658, I^2 < 0.001, p-value $\leq$ 0.05, and n = 5 studies). There was no evidence of publication bias or small study effects through visual inspection of the funnel plot and Egger's regression test (p-value > 0.05) (Figure 4).

Pooled Meta-Analysis Examining the Effects of Probiotic on Subgingival *Tannerella forsythia* Count

The pooled SMD indicated a statistically significant decrease in the subgingival *T. forsythia* count with probiotic supplementation compared to controls in patients with periodontal disease (SMD = 0.341, 95% CI: 0.050, 0.633, I^2 < 0.001, p-value $\leq$ 0.05, and n = four studies). There was no evidence of publication bias or small study effects upon visual inspection of the funnel plot and with Egger's regression test (p-value > 0.05) (Figure 4).

Pooled Meta-Analysis Examining the Effects of Probiotics on Subgingival Counts of Other periodonthopathogenes

The meta-analyses conducted to assess the effects of probiotic supplementation on the subgingival bacterial counts of *P. intermedia* (p-value = 0.193, and n = four studies) and *A. actinomycetemcomitans* (p-value = 0.164, and n = 5 studies) were not statistically significant when compared to controls.

3.4.3. Associations between Probiotic Supplementation and Immunological Outcomes in Periodontal Disease Patients

Pooled Meta-Analysis Examining the Effects of Probiotics on Matrix Metalloproteinase-8 (MMP-8) Levels in the Gingival Crevicular Fluid (GCF)

The pooled SMD indicated a statistically significant decrease in the GCF MMP-8 levels with probiotic supplementation compared to the controls in patients with periodontal disease (SMD = 0.819, 95% CI: 0.417, 1.221, I^2 < 0.001, p-value $\leq$ 0.05, and n = two studies) (Figure 5).

Pooled Meta-Analysis Examining the Effects of Probiotics on Interleukin-6 (IL-6) Levels in the Gingival Crevicular Fluid

The GCF Interleukin-6 (IL-6) levels showed statistically significant decreases with probiotic supplementation compared to controls in patients with periodontal disease (SMD = 0.361, 95% CI: 0.079, 0.644, I^2 < 0.001, p-value $\leq$ 0.05, and n = three studies). There was no evidence of publication bias or small study effects through visual funnel plot inspection and Egger's regression test (p-value > 0.05) (Figure 5).

Pooled Meta-Analysis Examining the Effects of Probiotics on Other Immunological Biomarkers in the Gingival Crevicular Fluid (GCF)

The meta-analyses conducted to assess the effects of probiotic supplementation on GCF levels of IL-1β (p-value = 0.393 and n = three studies), IL-8 (p-value = 0.434 and n = two studies), IL-10 (p-value = 0.902 and n = two studies), and TNF-α (p-value = 0.495

and *n* = three studies) in periodontal disease patients were not statistically significant when compared to controls.

4. Discussion

The aim of this systematic review and meta-analysis was to examine if probiotic supplementation is associated with preventive and therapeutic benefits in terms of improvement of clinical, microbiological, and immunological outcomes in patients with periodontal disease. In summary, the findings of this analysis are promising and indicate that probiotic supplementation significantly improved clinical outcomes, decreased certain periodontopathogen counts, and reduced the levels of specific pro-inflammatory biomarkers in patients with periodontal disease.

The overall results of this meta-analysis showed statistically significant improvements in all clinical parameters (PlI, MPP, GI, PPD, CAL, BOP, and GCF volume) in patients with periodontal disease after probiotic supplementation compared to control groups who did not receive probiotics. When examining the microbiological outcomes, the subgingival periodontopathogen counts of *P. gingivalis*, *F. nucleatum*, and *T. forsythia* showed statistically significant reductions with probiotic supplementation. Furthermore, there was a statistically significant reduction in the GCF levels of inflammatory mediators (MMP-8 and IL-6) with probiotic supplementation.

In addition to the pooled meta-analysis, the effects of probiotic supplementation on clinical outcomes were further assessed through subgroup analysis based on:

1. Type of periodontal disease, which indicated that probiotic supplementation improved clinical outcomes in patients with periodontitis, but not in those with gingivitis or healthy individuals. However, the GCF volume had statistically significant reductions in both gingivitis and periodontitis patients;
2. Probiotic formulations consisting of *Lactobacillus* species and, more specifically, *L. reuteri* were associated with statistically significant improvements in all clinical outcomes in patients with periodontal disease;
3. Probiotic treatment duration, which showed that probiotic supplementation resulted in statistically significant improvements in the clinical outcomes after one month of supplementation in periodontal disease patients;
4. Mode of probiotic delivery, which indicated that probiotic supplementation through the "oral and ingestion" mode was associated with statistically significant improvements in all clinical outcomes in periodontal disease patients.
5. Oral hygiene instructions along with probiotic supplementation improved PlI and BOP, while GI, PPD, and CAL improved with probiotic supplementation, irrespective of the presence or absence of oral hygiene instructions.

Periodontal disease stability refers to a state of successful treatment where clinical indicators do not progress in severity and is characterized by a minimized BOP score and improved PPD and CAL scores [111,112]. The results of our meta-analysis suggest that probiotic supplementation is a promising adjuvant to the current standard of care (SRP) to improve prognosis and clinical outcomes in patients with periodontitis. Given the improvements in the clinical, immunological, and microbiological outcomes in periodontal disease patients, it seems plausible that probiotics may contribute to reaching periodontal stability.

4.1. Probiotics and Severity of Periodontal Disease

Our subgroup analysis did not have significant findings in gingivitis patients, which may be partially attributed to: 1. Gingivitis being an early stage of periodontal disease, and, therefore, the clinical aspects of disease and consequently the effects of probiotic supplementation may be less notable; 2. Some studies on gingivitis did not use probiotics along with the standard of care; and 3. These results could be due to the lack of eligible studies and the moderate to high levels of heterogeneity in our analysis. However, the statistically significant improvements that our meta-analysis found in all clinical parameters at the late/severe disease stages (periodontitis) adds evidence to the existing literature on the clinical benefits of probiotic supplementation in the management of periodontal disease.

4.2. Probiotics vs. Antibiotics

The current non-surgical standard of care for periodontal disease includes SRP, which is sometimes followed by antibiotic treatment [31,33]. However, previous studies have reported that antibiotic use, particularly long-term administration, may increase the risk of oral and gut dysbiosis, antibiotic-resistant bacteria, allergic reactions, and other side effects [42]. Probiotics are a promising adjuvant/alternative approach that can be taken safely for longer periods of time. Our meta-analysis comparing probiotic supplementation to antibiotics as adjuvants to SRP did not show any statistically significant differences in CAL and PPD in periodontitis patients. (Note: The other clinical outcomes were not assessed due to insufficient studies). This finding suggests that probiotic supplementation-may be as effective as antibiotics in improving clinical outcomes. Previous studies found similar results when either one is administered as an adjuvant to SRP [61,83]. Furthermore, a more recent study concluded that probiotics are a more effective adjuvant with SRP than antibiotics [113]. However, there is evidence indicating that, when probiotics or antibiotics were administered independently, neither one was more efficacious than SRP alone [10,61]. Although these conclusions warrant more research, our meta-analysis indicated improved clinical outcomes, and it is plausible from a mechanistic perspective that probiotic supplementation as an adjuvant to SRP may be a safer and more effective long-term therapeutic option in the management of periodontal disease compared to antibiotics.

4.3. Probiotic Formulation and Duration

Our findings also indicated that probiotic formulation and the type of probiotic strain have clinical relevance. Specifically, our subgroup analysis examining the type of probiotic strain indicated that *Lactobacillus* probiotic formulations improved all clinical outcomes. Further analysis into the types of *Lactobacillus* species identified that *L. reuteri*-containing probiotic formulations improved all clinical outcomes. *Lactobacillus* species may play a role in plaque control through direct interaction via colonization resistance, which includes competition for binding sites and nutrients or antimicrobial agent production to inhibit other oral bacteria [114]. Additional evidence suggests that *L. reuteri* may also influence the composition of the oral microbiome and is correlated with reduced periodontopathogens, including *F. nucleatum* [115,116]. As oral microbiome dysbiosis is one of the root causes of periodontal disease, the shift induction by *L. reuteri* may result in improvements in periodontal disease clinical outcomes. The only study without *Lactobacillus* included in our meta-analysis with statistically significant reduction of PPD and CAL, but not PlI, used the subgingival delivery of *Saccharomyces Boulardii* [58]. *S. Bouldarii* is a yeast probiotic that is non-colonizing [117], which likely caused nonsignificant changes in plaque accumulation [58]. However, the improvements in other clinical parameters (PPD and CAL) may be due to its role in immunomodulation [118].

Two out of eleven studies with *L. reuteri* probiotic formulations in patients with periodontitis did not result in significant reductions in plaque accumulation [62,119]. Elsadek et al. recruited periodontitis patients with type 2 diabetes, and the most immediate follow-up data available for our analysis was nine weeks after ending the probiotic treatment [62]. Non-significant plaque reduction could be due to the fast turnover of the oral microbiome after probiotic treatment completion [116], although a recent meta-analysis conducted to assess the long-term efficacy of probiotics found that clinical improvements persisted for up to eleven months after the completion of probiotic treatment [47]. Our subgroup analysis based on probiotic treatment duration suggested that the beneficial effects of probiotics on clinical outcomes may occur within a month. However, the optimal treatment duration cannot be inferred from our meta-analysis because there were few studies of participants with a treatment duration of more than one month to two months.

4.4. Probiotic Mode of Delivery

Studies have suggested that probiotics may have different mechanisms of action to improve periodontal disease, including direct interaction with oral bacteria and/or indirect action in the oral cavity through the modulation of innate and adaptive immunity [114] and the gut–oral microbiome axis [120]. It has also been suggested that probiotics need to have enough contact time with the oral environment to become part of the biofilm and fight against pathogens through competition for binding sites, nutrients, and the production of anti-microbial substances [114,121]. Probiotics can also interact with immune cells, altering the production of inflammatory mediators, thereby modulating the immune response in the oral cavity [114]. Probiotics are also often administered to balance the gut microbiome [122]. A well-balanced gut microbiome regulates overall immune homeostasis [123,124]. The high count of periodontopathogens in periodontal disease may translocate to the gut resulting in gut microbiome dysbiosis [120]. Thus, it is plausible that probiotic supplementation may improve periodontal disease severity, at least in part, via this indirect mechanism linking the gut and oral microbiomes. Therefore, different modes of probiotic delivery may improve clinical outcomes based on the type of administration (oral, ingestion, or a combination of both). Interestingly, our meta-analysis indicated that probiotic administration via 'ingestion' only improved signs of tissue destruction (PPD and CAL). However, all clinical outcomes showed improvements with 'oral and ingestion' probiotic administration, potentially due to the combined direct and indirect mechanisms of action.

4.5. Probiotic Supplementation and Oral Hygiene Instructions

Poor oral hygiene leads to periodontal disease progression, recurrence, and treatment failure [125]. Oral hygiene instructions (OHI) play a key role in all stages of periodontal disease management. Educating patients on the importance of oral hygiene practices and techniques to ensure motivation to adhere to oral hygiene routines are critical components of OHI [125]. Our analysis showed that, irrespective of the oral hygiene instructions, probiotic supplementation improved GI, PPD, and CAL, but not plaque accumulation. Poor plaque control is a key determinant of periodontal disease [126]. Effective OHI can control and reduce plaque accumulation and improve the gingival health status, independent of professional prophylactic care [127,128]. Supporting this evidence, our findings indicated that probiotic supplementation combined with OHI resulted in statistically significant improvements in all clinical outcomes, including plaque accumulation. This suggests that probiotics may synergistically improve clinical outcomes with OHI, stressing the importance of OHI in effectively preventing/reducing plaque accumulation.

4.6. Probiotic Supplementation and GCF Volume

In the healthy gingival sulcus, the GCF flow and volume are lower compared to those of the inflamed gingival sulcus [25]. Increased GCF flow is a host defense mechanism to flush bacteria and their metabolites from the gingival sulcus [25]. Furthermore, the GCF content, including the microbial composition and concentration of inflammatory mediators, differs between periodontal disease and healthy individuals, as well as during disease progression and during and after treatment [129]. This is in line with findings from a study by Teles et al., who found a greater GCF volume and inflammatory mediators when comparing clinically healthy oral sites in periodontitis patients compared to healthy individuals. Their results suggested a higher risk of periodontal disease initiation and progression from healthy sites in patients with periodontitis [130]. Altogether, these findings indicate the potential clinical importance of the GCF volume and its level of inflammatory mediators as an early diagnostic test for periodontal disease prior to the onset of clinical manifestations. Based on our findings, the GCF volume was significantly decreased after probiotic supplementation in both gingivitis and periodontitis patients, and other clinical outcomes also improved in these patients [67,72,74,106]. Although our study did not find statistically significant differences between probiotic supplementation and GCF volume in healthy participants, it should be noted that each individual study included in our analysis reported that the GCF volume increased without probiotic supplementation, but not with probiotic supplementation [42,78]. Probiotics may potentially be of therapeutic value for the prevention and early treatment of periodontal disease. Due to the limited number of studies included in our analysis, our results need to be interpreted with caution until further studies fully ascertain the preventive role of probiotics in periodontal disease.

4.7. Probiotic Supplementation and Microbiological Outcomes

Our meta-analysis examined the effects of probiotic supplementation on subgingival bacterial counts in periodontal disease. Our results found statistically significant reductions in the periodontopathogens *P. gingivalis* and *T. forsythia* from the red complex and *F. nucleatum* from the orange complex after probiotic supplementation. Teles et al. reported that subgingival plaque samples from healthy sites in patients with periodontitis had a higher proportion of orange and red-complex bacteria compared to healthy individuals (without periodontitis), suggesting a higher risk for these sites to be colonized by periodontopathogens [130]. Hence, probiotics, by reducing periodontopathogens, may be beneficial in inhibiting the progression of periodontal diseases to healthy sites. Orange-complex bacteria create favorable conditions for colonization by red-complex bacteria, which are strictly anaerobic [131]. *F. nucleatum* plays a crucial role as a bridging organism between early and late colonizers, including red-complex bacteria [132]. Red-complex pathogens are higher in number in plaques found in deeper periodontal pockets and advanced lesions [20]. Although, in our meta-analysis, probiotic supplementation resulted in statistically significant improvements in PPD for both moderate and deep pockets, this improvement was more pronounced in deeper pockets. These findings and their potential ramifications may imply that probiotic supplementation has the potential to alter the relative abundance of orange and red-complex bacteria, thus reducing oral tissue destruction and leading to conditions favoring periodontal healing/stability.

4.8. Probiotic Supplementation and Immunological Outcomes

Our analysis of the effects of probiotic supplementation on immunological outcomes indicated that the GCF levels of MMP-8 and IL-6 were reduced after probiotic supplementation in patients with periodontal disease. Previously, MMP-8 and IL-6 were identified as salivary biomarkers that increased in periodontitis [133,134]. MMP-8 is the main collagenase involved in periodontal disease, with the highest collagenolytic activity in GCF [135]. A recent meta-analysis reported significantly higher levels of salivary MMP-8 in periodontitis patients compared to healthy participants [135]. Similarly, a study found that the GCF in the healthy sites of periodontitis patients had elevated inflammatory mediators, including MMP-8, when compared to healthy individuals [130], suggesting that inflammatory mechanisms may occur before they are clinically diagnosed or symptomatic. Moreover, additional evidence indicates that higher GCF levels of MMP-8 may predict periodontal disease progression [136], and that MMP-8 can also be measured as a grading biomarker to classify disease stage and progression in periodontitis [137].

IL-6 is an inflammatory mediator induced by pathogens and other pro-inflammatory cytokines, and has been reported to be elevated in periodontitis [138]. A recent meta-analysis concluded that the GCF levels of IL-6 are significantly increased in patients with chronic periodontitis [139]. However, there is conflicting evidence in the literature, with other studies suggesting that there is no correlation between the IL-6 levels and periodontal disease [140,141]. The proposed role of IL-6 in periodontal disease pathogenesis is through the stimulation of MMP production and the activation of pathways involved in inflammation [142]. Accordingly, there may be a link between the IL-6 levels and clinical parameters of periodontal disease. The pooled results of our meta-analysis showed statistically significant reductions in the GCF levels of IL-6 after probiotic supplementation, despite individual studies having differing results. Twetman et al. indicated that the use of *L. reuteri* probiotic gum reduced the GCF levels of IL-6 and numbers of sites with bleeding on probing [106]. Keller et al. did not observe any significant change in the GCF levels of IL-6 with other strains of *Lactobacillus* probiotics; however, BOP improved significantly compared to the baseline in both the probiotic and control groups [72]. Shetty et al. found a significant reduction in the GCF levels of IL-6 after non-*Lactobacillus*-containing probiotic supplementation in periodontitis patients compared to controls, but not clinical outcomes [95]. Further research is required to determine the potential effects of different probiotic formulations on inflammatory molecular pathways and their impact on the clinical aspects of periodontal diseases.

4.9. Probiotic Supplementation and Periodontal Disease Prevention

When examining the potential preventive role of probiotic supplementation in periodontal disease in healthy individuals, the results of our meta-analysis did not find any statistically significant improvements in PlI and GI after probiotic supplementation. There were insufficient studies to analyze the effects of probiotic supplementation on other outcomes in healthy participants to clearly assess the preventive potential of probiotics in periodontal diseases.

4.10. Strengths and Limitations

This is the first study examining the influence of probiotic formulation, mode of delivery, treatment duration, and the impact of oral hygiene instructions on periodontal diseases using subgroup analysis. Another strength of this study is that it used an up–to–date analysis of the literature, used a systematic approach, and examined emerging factors that may assist in the prevention, diagnosis, and treatment of periodontal diseases.

A limitation of this meta-analysis was that the number of studies examining microbiological and immunological outcomes was scarce; thus, some of the results need to be interpreted with caution. We used Hedge's g standardized mean difference to provide better accounting for small study sample sizes. A further limitation was that, due to the aggregated data, we were unable to examine the effects of probiotic supplementation on periodontal diseases stratified by risk factors, such as sex, age, smoking status, and comorbidities. We were also unable to investigate the correlation between periodontopathogens and inflammatory biomarkers before and after probiotic treatment.

5. Conclusions

This systematic review and meta-analysis highlights the potential therapeutic benefits of probiotic supplementation in the treatment of periodontal disease. The results indicate that probiotic supplementation improved the clinical parameters, reduced the subgingival bacterial counts of specific periodontopathogens, and reduced the GCF levels of some proinflammatory mediators in periodontal disease patients. The impact of probiotic supplementation on clinical outcomes is affected by the probiotic formulation, mode of delivery, treatment duration, and the type of periodontal disease. More research is needed to better assess the therapeutic and preventive value of probiotic supplementation in patients with gingivitis (early disease), as well as in healthy (without periodontal disease) individuals.

Supplementary Materials: The following supporting information can be downloaded at: https://www.mdpi.com/article/10.3390/nu14051036/s1, Supplemental Table S1. Inclusion and exclusion criteria, Supplemental Table S2. Search terms and strategy, Supplemental Table S3: Risk of bias within studies, Supplemental Table S4. Overall measure of effects of probiotic supplementation on clinical, immunological, and microbiological outcomes. Subgroup analysis of the associations between probiotic supplementation and clinical outcomes in periodontal diseases patients. Supplemental Figure S1. Subgroup analysis—forest plots examining the effects of probiotic supplementation on clinical outcomes: 1. Plaque Index (PlI); 2. Mean Plaque Percentage (MPP); 3. Gingival Index (GI); 4. Probing Pocket Depth (PPD); 5. Clinical Attachment Level (CAL); 6. Bleeding on Probing (BOP); and 7. Gingival Crevicular Fluid (GCF).

Author Contributions: Conceptualization, Z.G., R.M., S.P., P.P. and J.R.L.L.; methodology, Z.G., A.H.s. and R.M.; Data collection and data analysis, Z.G., R.M., A.H.s. and S.P., writing—original draft, Z.G., R.M. and A.H.s.; writing—review and editing, Z.G., R.M., A.H.s., J.R.L.L., J.L., P.P. and S.P.; Supervision, S.P. and J.R.L.L. All authors have read and agreed to the published version of the manuscript.

Funding: The authors would like to acknowledge the funding support from the Patient-oriented Research Leadership Grant (S.P.) supported by the Saskatchewan Centre for Patient Oriented Research (SCPOR) and the Saskatchewan Health Research Foundation (SHRF); Saskatchewan Centre for Patient Oriented Research Graduate (Z.G.; A.H.) and Postdoctoral Fellowships (R.M.); University of Saskatchewan College of Medicine CoMGRAD Graduate Student Fellowship (Z.G.); University of Saskatchewan Department of Biochemistry, Microbiology and Immunology Devolved Scholarship (Z.G.); Saskatchewan Innovation and Opportunity Scholarship (Z.G.); University of Saskatchewan College of Dentistry start-up funds (P.P.); and University of Saskatchewan Centennial Enhancement Chair in One Health Research (P.P.).

Institutional Review Board Statement: Not applicable.

Informed Consent Statement: Not applicable.

Acknowledgments: The authors would like to thank Janice Michael, MBA, CPA, CGA, Research Facilitator of the Colleges of Dentistry and Public Health at the University of Saskatchewan, for the English editing of this manuscript. Figure 1 made in BioRender.com (accessed on 19 December 2021).

Conflicts of Interest: The authors declare no conflict of interest.

Abbreviations

Plaque Index (PlI)	The plaque index is a clinical indicator of oral hygiene status that measures the level and rate of microbial plaque formation on the gingival margin of the tooth's surface. PlI is also used to estimate the potential therapeutic or preventive roles of oral care products [24].
Gingival Index (GI)	The gingival index is a numeric scoring system that assesses inflammation and structural changes in gingival tissue [27].
Pocket Probing Depth (PPD)	The probing depth is the distance between the gingival margin and base of the periodontal pocket, providing one of the most accurate parameters for the clinical diagnosis of periodontal disease [23].
Clinical Attachment Level (CAL)	CAL is measured between the fixed point of the cemento-enamel junction of the tooth and the base of the periodontal pocket. The CAL is one of the most accurate and widely used measures for the clinical diagnosis of periodontal disease [23].
Bleeding on Probing (BOP)	BOP is a reliable indicator of gingival inflammation and refers to the bleeding of gingival tissue upon gentle probing [143].
Gingival crevicular fluid (GCF)	GCF is an inflammatory exudate that permits non-invasive sampling from the oral cavity and is composed of serum, leukocytes, and structural cells from the periodontium and oral bacteria. It is found in the periodontal sulcus between the tooth and marginal gingiva. The GCF flow rate and volume is used as an indicator of gingival inflammation, which can be used to assess periodontal disease severity [25].
Gingival recession (REC)	REC is a clinical measurement of the distance between the cemento-enamel junction and the free gingival margin measured in millimeters (mm) during periodontal probing [26].

References

1. GBD 2016 Disease and Injury Incidence and Prevalence Collaborators. Global, regional, and national incidence, prevalence, and years lived with disability for 328 diseases and injuries for 195 countries, 1990–2016: A systematic analysis for the Global Burden of Disease Study 2016. *Lancet* **2017**, *390*, 1211–1259. [CrossRef]
2. Nazir, M.; Al-Ansari, A.; Al-Khalifa, K.; Alhareky, M.; Gaffar, B.; Almas, K. Global Prevalence of Periodontal Disease and Lack of Its Surveillance. *Sci. World J.* **2020**, *2020*, 2146160. [CrossRef] [PubMed]

3. Seminario-Amez, M.; Lopez-Lopez, J.; Estrugo-Devesa, A.; Ayuso-Montero, R.; Jane-Salas, E. Probiotics and oral health: A systematic review. *Med. Oral Patol. Oral Cir. Bucal* **2017**, *22*, E282–E288. [CrossRef] [PubMed]
4. Gasner, N.S.; Schure, R.S. Periodontal Disease. In *StatPearls [Internet]*; StatPearls Publishing: Treasure Island, FL, USA, 2021.
5. Nazir, M.A. Prevalence of periodontal disease, its association with systemic diseases and prevention. *Int. J. Health Sci.* **2017**, *11*, 72–80.
6. Ferreira, M.C.; Dias-Pereira, A.C.; Branco-de-Almeida, L.S.; Martins, C.C.; Paiva, S.M. Impact of periodontal disease on quality of life: A systematic review. *J. Periodontal Res.* **2017**, *52*, 651–665. [CrossRef] [PubMed]
7. Hajishengallis, G.; Chavakis, T. Local and systemic mechanisms linking periodontal disease and inflammatory comorbidities. *Nat. Rev. Immunol.* **2021**, *21*, 426–440. [CrossRef] [PubMed]
8. Cardoso, E.M.; Reis, C.; Manzanares-Céspedes, M.C. Chronic periodontitis, inflammatory cytokines, and interrelationship with other chronic diseases. *Postgrad. Med.* **2018**, *130*, 98–104. [CrossRef]
9. Pihlstrom, B.L.; Michalowicz, B.S.; Johnson, N.W. Periodontal diseases. *Lancet* **2005**, *366*, 1809–1820. [CrossRef]
10. Morales, A.; Gandolfo, A.; Bravo, J.; Carvajal, P.; Silva, N.; Godoy, C.; Garcia-Sesnich, J.; Hoare, A.; Diaz, P.; Gamonal, J. Microbiological and clinical effects of probiotics and antibiotics on nonsurgical treatment of chronic periodontitis: A randomized placebocontrolled trial with 9-month follow-up. *J. Appl. Oral Sci.* **2018**, *26*, e20170075. [CrossRef]
11. Könönen, E.; Gursoy, M.; Gursoy, U.K. Periodontitis: A Multifaceted Disease of Tooth-Supporting Tissues. *J. Clin. Med.* **2019**, *8*, 1135. [CrossRef]
12. Williams, R.C. Periodontal Disease. *N. Engl. J. Med.* **1990**, *322*, 373–382. [CrossRef] [PubMed]
13. Laudenbach, J.M.; Simon, Z. Common Dental and Periodontal Diseases: Evaluation and Management. *Med. Clin. N. Am.* **2014**, *98*, 1239–1260. [CrossRef] [PubMed]
14. Montero, E.; Iniesta, M.; Rodrigo, M.; Marín, M.J.; Figuero, E.; Herrera, D.; Sanz, M. Clinical and microbiological effects of the adjunctive use of probiotics in the treatment of gingivitis: A randomized controlled clinical trial. *J. Clin. Periodontol.* **2017**, *44*, 708–716. [CrossRef]
15. Shi, B.; Chang, M.; Martin, J.; Mitreva, M.; Lux, R.; Klokkevold, P.; Sodergren, E.; Weinstock, G.M.; Haak, S.K.; Lia, H. Dynamic changes in the subgingival microbiome and their potential for diagnosis and prognosis of periodontitis. *MBio* **2015**, *6*, e01926-14. [CrossRef]
16. Abusleme, L.; Dupuy, A.K.; Dutzan, N.; Silva, N.; Burleson, J.A.; Strausbaugh, L.D.; Gamonal, J.; Diaz, P.I. The subgingival microbiome in health and periodontitis and its relationship with community biomass and inflammation. *ISME J.* **2013**, *7*, 1016–1025. [CrossRef]
17. Griffen, A.L.; Beall, C.J.; Campbell, J.H.; Firestone, N.D.; Kumar, P.S.; Yang, Z.K.; Podar, M.; Leys, E.J. Distinct and complex bacterial profiles in human periodontitis and health revealed by 16S pyrosequencing. *ISME J.* **2012**, *6*, 1176–1185. [CrossRef] [PubMed]
18. Liu, B.; Faller, L.L.; Klitgord, N.; Mazumdar, V.; Ghodsi, M.; Sommer, D.D.; Gibbons, T.R.; Treangen, T.J.; Chang, Y.C.; Li, S.; et al. Deep sequencing of the oral microbiome reveals signatures of periodontal disease. *PLoS ONE* **2012**, *7*, e37919. [CrossRef]
19. Curtis, M.A.; Diaz, P.I.; Van Dyke, T.E. The role of the microbiota in periodontal disease. *Periodontol. 2000* **2020**, *83*, 14–25. [CrossRef]
20. Mohanty, R.; Asopa, S.J.; Joseph, M.D.; Singh, B.; Rajguru, J.P.; Saidath, K.; Sharma, U. Red complex: Polymicrobial conglomerate in oral flora: A review. *J. Fam. Med. Prim. Care* **2019**, *8*, 3480–3486. [CrossRef]
21. Kinane, D.F.; Stathopoulou, P.G.; Papapanou, P.N. Periodontal diseases. *Nat. Rev. Dis. Primers* **2017**, *3*, 17038. [CrossRef]
22. Lamont, R.J.; Koo, H.; Hajishengallis, G. The oral microbiota: Dynamic communities and host interactions. *Nat. Rev. Microbiol.* **2018**, *16*, 745–759. [CrossRef] [PubMed]
23. Armitage, G.C. The complete periodontal examination. *Periodontol. 2000* **2004**, *34*, 22–33. [CrossRef] [PubMed]
24. Joiner, A.C. 4—The Cleaning of Teeth. In *Handbook for Cleaning/Decontamination of Surfaces*; Johansson, I., Somasundaran, P., Eds.; Elsevier Science B.V.: Amsterdam, The Netherlands, 2007; pp. 371–405, ISBN 978-0-444-51664-0.
25. Subbarao, K.C.; Nattuthurai, G.S.; Sundararajan, S.K.; Sujith, I.; Joseph, J.; Syedshah, Y.P. Gingival Crevicular Fluid: An Overview. *J. Pharm. Bioallied Sci.* **2019**, *11*, S135–S139. [CrossRef] [PubMed]
26. Handelman, C.S.; Eltink, A.P.; BeGole, E. Quantitative measures of gingival recession and the influence of gender, race, and attrition. *Prog. Orthod.* **2018**, *19*, 5. [CrossRef] [PubMed]
27. Rebelo, M.A.B.; de Queiroz, A.C. Gingival Indices: State of Art. In *Gingival Diseases—Their Aetiology, Prevention and Treatment*; Panagakos, F.S., Davies, R.M., Eds.; IntechOpen: Rijeka, Croatia, 2011; Chapter 3.
28. Sweeting, L.A.; Davis, K.; Cobb, C.M. Periodontal Treatment Protocol (PTP) for the general dental practice. *J. Dent. Hyg. JDH* **2008**, *82* (Suppl. 3), 16–26. [PubMed]
29. Tonetti, M.S.; Greenwell, H.; Kornman, K.S. Staging and grading of periodontitis: Framework and proposal of a new classification and case definition. *J. Clin. Periodontol.* **2018**, *45*, S149–S161. [CrossRef]
30. Tonetti, M.S.; Sanz, M. Implementation of the new classification of periodontal diseases: Decision-making algorithms for clinical practice and education. *J. Clin. Periodontol.* **2019**, *46*, 398–405. [CrossRef]
31. Comprehensive Periodontal Therapy: A Statement by the American Academy of Periodontology. *J. Periodontol.* **2011**, *82*, 943–949. [CrossRef]
32. Mirbod, S.; Matthews, D.C.; Ellis, L.; Marquez, I.C. Point of Care. *JCDA* **2007**, *73*, 137–147.

33. Hung, H.-C.; Douglass, C.W. Meta-Analysis of the effect of scaling and root planing, surgical treatment and antibiotic therapies on periodontal probing depth and attachment loss. *J. Clin. Periodontol.* **2002**, *29*, 975–986. [CrossRef]
34. Pelekos, G.; Ho, S.N.; Acharya, A.; Leung, W.K.; McGrath, C. A double-blind, paralleled-arm, placebo-controlled and randomized clinical trial of the effectiveness of probiotics as an adjunct in periodontal care. *J. Clin. Periodontol.* **2019**, *46*, 1217–1227. [CrossRef]
35. Saini, K.; Minj, J. Multifunctional Aspects of Probiotics and Prebiotics in Health Management: An Overview BT. In *Dairy Processing: Advanced Research to Applications*; Minj, J., Sudhakaran, V.A., Kumari, A., Eds.; Springer: Singapore, 2020; pp. 119–131, ISBN 978-981-15-2608-4.
36. Palai, S.; Derecho, C.M.P.; Kesh, S.S.; Egbuna, C.; Onyeike, P.C. Prebiotics, Probiotics, Synbiotics and Its Importance in the Management of Diseases BT. In *Functional Foods and Nutraceuticals: Bioactive Components, Formulations and Innovations*; Egbuna, C., Dable Tupas, G., Eds.; Springer International Publishing: Cham, Switzerland, 2020; pp. 173–196, ISBN 978-3-030-42319-3.
37. McFarland, L.V.; Surawicz, C.M.; Greenberg, R.N.; Fekety, R.; Elmer, G.W.; Moyer, K.A.; Melcher, S.A.; Bowen, K.E.; Cox, J.L.; Noorani, Z.; et al. A Randomized Placebo-Controlled Trial of Saccharomyces boulardii in Combination with Standard Antibiotics for Clostridium difficile Disease. *JAMA* **1994**, *271*, 1913–1918. [CrossRef] [PubMed]
38. Rodgers, B.; Kirley, K.; Mounsey, A.; Ewigman, B. Prescribing an antibiotic? Pair it with probiotics. *J. Fam. Pract.* **2013**, *62*, 148–150. [PubMed]
39. Rondanelli, M.; Faliva, M.A.; Perna, S.; Giacosa, A.; Peroni, G.; Castellazzi, A.M. Using probiotics in clinical practice: Where are we now? A review of existing meta-analyses. *Gut Microbes* **2017**, *8*, 521–543. [CrossRef] [PubMed]
40. Çaglar, E.; Cildir, S.K.; Ergeneli, S.; Sandalli, N.; Twetman, S. Salivary mutans streptococci and lactobacilli levels after ingestion of the probiotic bacterium *Lactobacillus reuteri* ATCC 55730 by straws or tablets. *Acta Odontol. Scand.* **2006**, *64*, 314–318. [CrossRef]
41. Tekce, M.; Ince, G.; Gursoy, H.; Ipci, S.D.; Cakar, G.; Kadir, T.; Yılmaz, S. Clinical and microbiological effects of probiotic lozenges in the treatment of chronic periodontitis: A 1-year follow-up study. *J. Clin. Periodontol.* **2015**, *42*, 363–372. [CrossRef]
42. Hallström, H.; Lindgren, S.; Yucel-Lindberg, T.T.; Dahlén, G.; Renvert, S.; Twetman, S. Effect of probiotic lozenges on inflammatory reactions and oral biofilm during experimental gingivitis. *Acta Odontol. Scand.* **2013**, *71*, 828–833. [CrossRef]
43. Iniesta, M.; Herrera, D.; Montero, E.; Zurbriggen, M.; Matos, A.R.; Marín, M.J.; Sánchez-Beltrán, M.C.; Llama-Palacio, A.; Sanz, M. Probiotic effects of orally administered *Lactobacillus reuteri*-containing tablets on the subgingival and salivary microbiota in patients with gingivitis. A randomized clinical trial. *J. Clin. Periodontol.* **2012**, *39*, 736–744. [CrossRef]
44. Yanine, N.; Araya, I.; Brignardello-Petersen, R.; Carrasco-Labra, A.; Gonzalez, A.; Preciado, A.; Villanueva, J.; Sanz, M.; Martin, C. Effects of probiotics in periodontal diseases: A systematic review. *Clin. Oral Investig.* **2013**, *17*, 1627–1634. [CrossRef]
45. Akram, Z.; Shafqat, S.S.; Aati, S.; Kujan, O.; Fawzy, A. Clinical efficacy of probiotics in the treatment of gingivitis: A systematic review and meta-analysis. *Aust. Dent. J.* **2020**, *65*, 12–20. [CrossRef]
46. Vives-Soler, A.; Chimenos-Kustner, E. Effect of probiotics as a complement to non-surgical periodontal therapy in chronic periodontitis: A systematic review. *Med. Oral Patol. Oral Cir. Bucal* **2020**, *25*, e161–e167. [CrossRef] [PubMed]
47. Ho, S.N.; Acharya, A.; Sidharthan, S.; Li, K.Y.; Leung, W.K.; McGrath, C.; Pelekos, G. A Systematic Review and Meta-analysis of Clinical, Immunological, and Microbiological Shift in Periodontitis After Nonsurgical Periodontal Therapy with Adjunctive Use of Probiotics. *J. Evid. Based Dent. Pract.* **2020**, *20*, 101397. [CrossRef] [PubMed]
48. Villafuerte, K.R.V.; Martinez, C.J.H.; Nobre, A.V.V.; Maia, L.P.; Tirapelli, C. What are microbiological effects of the adjunctive use of probiotics in the treatment of periodontal diseases? A systematic review. *Benef. Microbes* **2021**, *12*, 307–319. [CrossRef] [PubMed]
49. Sterne, J.A.C.; Savović, J.; Page, M.J.; Elbers, R.G.; Blencowe, N.S.; Boutron, I.; Cates, C.J.; Cheng, H.-Y.; Corbett, M.S.; Eldridge, S.M.; et al. RoB 2: A revised tool for assessing risk of bias in randomised trials. *BMJ* **2019**, *366*, l4898. [CrossRef]
50. Faraone, S.V. Interpreting estimates of treatment effects: Implications for managed care. *Pharm. Ther.* **2008**, *33*, 700–711.
51. Higgins, J.P.T.; Thompson, S.G.; Deeks, J.J.; Altman, D.G. Measuring inconsistency in meta-analyses. *Br. Med. J.* **2003**, *327*, 557–560. [CrossRef] [PubMed]
52. Duval, S.; Tweedie, R. Trim and Fill: A Simple Funnel-Plot–Based Method of Testing and Adjusting for Publication Bias in Meta-Analysis. *Biometrics* **2000**, *56*, 455–463. [CrossRef]
53. Alkaya, B.; Laleman, I.; Keceli, S.; Ozcelik, O.; Haytac, M.C.; Teughels, W. Clinical effects of probiotics containing Bacillus species on gingivitis: A pilot randomized controlled trial. *J. Periodontal Res.* **2017**, *52*, 497–504. [CrossRef]
54. Alshareef, A.; Attia, A.; Almalki, M.; Alsharif, F.; Melibari, A.; Mirdad, B.; Azab, E.; Youssef, A.R.; Dardir, A. Effectiveness of Probiotic Lozenges in Periodontal Management of Chronic Periodontitis Patients: Clinical and Immunological Study. *Eur. J. Dent.* **2020**, *14*, 281–287. [CrossRef]
55. Bazyar, H.; Maghsoumi-Norouzabad, L.; Yarahmadi, M.; Gholinezhad, H.; Moradi, L.; Salehi, P.; Haghighi-Zadeh, M.H.; Zare Javid, A. The impacts of synbiotic supplementation on periodontal indices and biomarkers of oxidative stress in type 2 diabetes mellitus patients with chronic periodontitis under non-surgical periodontal therapy. A double-blind, placebo-controlled trial. *Diabetes Metab. Syndr. Obes. Targets Ther.* **2020**, *13*, 19–29. [CrossRef]
56. Bollero, P.; Di Renzo, L.; Franco, R.; Rampello, T.; Pujia, A.; Merra, G.; De Lorenzo, A.; Docimo, R. Effects of new probiotic mouthwash in patients with diabetes mellitus and cardiovascular diseases. *Eur. Rev. Med. Pharmacol. Sci.* **2017**, *21*, 5827–5836. [PubMed]
57. Boyeena, L.; Koduganti, R.R.; Panthula, V.R.; Jammula, S.P. Comparison of efficacy of probiotics versus tetracycline fibers as adjuvant to scaling and root planing. *J. Indian Soc. Periodontol.* **2019**, *23*, 539–544. [PubMed]

58. Chandra, R.V.; Swathi, T.; Reddy, A.A.; Chakravarthy, Y.; Nagarajan, S.; Naveen, A. Effect of a Locally Delivered Probiotic-Prebiotic Mixture as an Adjunct to Scaling and Root Planing in the Management of Chronic Periodontitis. *J. Int. Acad. Periodontol.* **2016**, *18*, 67–75. [PubMed]

59. Deshmukh, M.A.; Dodamani, A.S.; Karibasappa, G.; Khairnar, M.R.; Naik, R.G.; Jadhav, H.C. Comparative Evaluation of the Efficacy of Probiotic, Herbal and Chlorhexidine Mouthwash on Gingival Health: A Randomized Clinical Trial. *J. Clin. Diagn. Res.* **2017**, *11*, ZC13–ZC16. [CrossRef] [PubMed]

60. Dhaliwal, P.K.; Grover, V.; Malhotra, R.; Kapoor, A. Clinical and Microbiological Investigation of the Effects of Probiotics Combined with Scaling and Root Planing in the Management of Chronic Periodontitis: A Randomized, Controlled Study. *J. Int. Acad. Periodontol.* **2017**, *19*, 101–108. [PubMed]

61. Duarte, C.; Al-Yaqoob, A.; Al-Ani, A. Efficacy of probiotics used as a periodontal treatment aid: A pilot study. *Saudi Dent. J.* **2019**, *31*, 143–147. [CrossRef] [PubMed]

62. Elsadek, M.F.; Ahmed, B.M.; Alkhawtani, D.M.; Zia Siddiqui, A. A comparative clinical, microbiological and glycemic analysis of photodynamic therapy and *Lactobacillus reuteri* in the treatment of chronic periodontitis in type-2 diabetes mellitus patients. *Photodiagn. Photodyn. Ther.* **2020**, *29*, 101629. [CrossRef]

63. Ercan, N.; Olgun, E.; Kisa, U.; Yalim, M. Effect of synbiotics in the treatment of smokers and nonsmokers with gingivitis: Randomized controlled trial. *Aust. Dent. J.* **2020**, *65*, 210–219. [CrossRef]

64. Grusovin, M.G.; Bossini, S.; Calza, S.; Cappa, V.; Garzetti, G.; Scotti, E.; Gherlone, E.F.; Mensi, M. Clinical efficacy of Lactobacillus reuteri-containing lozenges in the supportive therapy of generalized periodontitis stage III and IV, grade C: 1-year results of a double-blind randomized placebo-controlled pilot study. *Clin. Oral Investig.* **2020**, *24*, 2015–2024. [CrossRef]

65. Ikram, S.; Hassan, N.; Baig, S.; Ansari, S.A.; Borges, K.J.J.; Raffat, M.A. Clinical Efficacy of Probiotics as An Adjunct to Scaling and Root Planning in The Treatment of Chronic Periodontitis. *Ann. Abbasi Shaheed Hosp. Karachi Med. Dent. Coll.* **2019**, *24*, 31–37.

66. Ikram, S.; Hassan, N.; Baig, S.; Borges, K.J.J.; Raffat, M.A.; Akram, Z. Effect of local probiotic (*Lactobacillus reuteri*) vs systemic antibiotic therapy as an adjunct to non-surgical periodontal treatment in chronic periodontitis. *J. Investig. Clin. Dent.* **2019**, *10*, e12393. [CrossRef] [PubMed]

67. İnce, G.; Gürsoy, H.; İpçi, Ş.D.; Cakar, G.; Emekli-Alturfan, E.; Yılmaz, S. Clinical and Biochemical Evaluation of Lozenges Containing *Lactobacillus reuteri* as an Adjunct to Non-Surgical Periodontal Therapy in Chronic Periodontitis. *J. Periodontol.* **2015**, *86*, 746–754. [CrossRef] [PubMed]

68. Invernici, M.M.; Salvador, S.L.; Silva, P.H.F.; Soares, M.S.M.; Casarin, R.; Palioto, D.B.; Souza, S.L.S.; Taba, M.; Novaes, A.B.; Furlaneto, F.A.C.; et al. Effects of Bifidobacterium probiotic on the treatment of chronic periodontitis: A randomized clinical trial. *J. Clin. Periodontol.* **2018**, *45*, 1198–1210. [CrossRef] [PubMed]

69. Iwasaki, K.; Maeda, K.; Hidaka, K.; Nemoto, K.; Hirose, Y.; Deguchi, S. Daily intake of heat-killed *Lactobacillus plantarum* L-137 decreases the probing depth in patients undergoing supportive periodontal therapy. *Oral Health Prev. Dent.* **2016**, *14*, 207–214. [CrossRef]

70. Jagadeesh K., M.; Shenoy, N.; Talwar, A.; Shetty, S. Clinical effect of pro-biotic containing Bacillus coagulans on plaque induced gingivitis: A randomized clinical pilot study. *J. Health Allied Sci. NU.* **2017**, *7*, 7–12. [CrossRef]

71. Jäsberg, H.; Tervahartiala, T.; Sorsa, T.; Söderling, E.; Haukioja, A. Probiotic intervention influences the salivary levels of Matrix Metalloproteinase (MMP)-9 and Tissue Inhibitor of metalloproteinases (TIMP)-1 in healthy adults. *Arch. Oral Biol.* **2018**, *85*, 58–63. [CrossRef]

72. Keller, M.K.; Brandsborg, E.; Holmstrom, K.; Twetman, S. Effect of tablets containing probiotic candidate strains on gingival inflammation and composition of the salivary microbiome: A randomised controlled trial. *Benef. Microbes* **2018**, *9*, 487–494. [CrossRef]

73. Krasse, P.; Carlsson, B.; Dahl, C.; Paulsson, A.; Nilsson, A.; Sinkiewicz, G. Decreased gum bleeding and reduced gingivitis by the probiotic *Lactobacillus reuteri*. *Swed. Dent. J.* **2006**, *30*, 55–60.

74. Kuka, G.I.; Gursoy, H.; Emekli-Alturfan, E.; Ustundag, U.V.; Kuru, B. Evaluation of nitric oxide levels in chronic periodontitis patients treated with initial periodontal therapy and probiotic food supplements: A double blind, randomized controlled clinical trial. *Biotechnol. Biotechnol. Equip.* **2019**, *33*, 974–979. [CrossRef]

75. Kuru, B.E.; Laleman, I.; Yalnızoğlu, T.; Kuru, L.; Teughels, W. The Influence of a Bifidobacterium animalis Probiotic on Gingival Health: A Randomized Controlled Clinical Trial. *J. Periodontol.* **2017**, *88*, 1115–1123. [CrossRef]

76. Laleman, I.; Yilmaz, E.; Ozcelik, O.; Haytac, C.; Pauwels, M.; Herrero, E.R.; Slomka, V.; Quirynen, M.; Alkaya, B.; Teughels, W. The effect of a streptococci containing probiotic in periodontal therapy: A randomized controlled trial. *J. Clin. Periodontol.* **2015**, *42*, 1032–1041. [CrossRef] [PubMed]

77. Laleman, I.; Pauwels, M.; Quirynen, M.; Teughels, W. A dual-strain *Lactobacilli reuteri* probiotic improves the treatment of residual pockets: A randomized controlled clinical trial. *J. Clin. Periodontol.* **2020**, *47*, 43–53. [CrossRef] [PubMed]

78. Lee, J.-K.; Kim, S.-J.; Ko, S.-H.; Ouwehand, A.C.; Ma, D.S. Modulation of the host response by probiotic *Lactobacillus brevis* CD2 in experimental gingivitis. *Oral Dis.* **2015**, *21*, 705–712. [CrossRef] [PubMed]

79. Mayanagi, G.; Kimura, M.; Nakaya, S.; Hirata, H.; Sakamoto, M.; Benno, Y.; Shimauchi, H. Probiotic effects of orally administered *Lactobacillus salivarius* WB21-containing tablets on periodontopathic bacteria: A double-blinded, placebo-controlled, randomized clinical trial. *J. Clin. Periodontol.* **2009**, *36*, 506–513. [CrossRef]

80. Swarna Meenakshi, S.; Varghese, S. Adjunctive effect of probiotic (*Lactobacillus casei* Shirota) to scaling and root planing in the management of chronic periodontitis. *Drug Invent. Today* **2018**, *10*, 1381–1386.

81. Mitic, K.A. Probiotics and Oral Health Research. *Res. J. Pharm. Biol. Chem. Sci.* **2017**, *8*, 1021–1029.

82. Morales, A.; Carvajal, P.; Silva, N.; Hernandez, M.; Godoy, C.; Rodriguez, G.; Cabello, R.; Garcia-Sesnich, J.; Hoare, A.; Diaz, P.I.; et al. Clinical Effects of *Lactobacillus rhamnosus* in Non-Surgical Treatment of Chronic Periodontitis: A Randomized Placebo-Controlled Trial With 1-Year Follow-Up. *J. Periodontol.* **2016**, *87*, 944–952. [CrossRef]

83. Nadkerny, P.V.; Ravishankar, P.L.; Pramod, V.; Agarwal, L.A.; Bhandari, S. A comparative evaluation of the efficacy of probiotic and chlorhexidine mouthrinses on clinical inflammatory parameters of gingivitis: A randomized controlled clinical study. *J. Indian Soc. Periodontol.* **2015**, *19*, 633–639. [CrossRef]

84. De Luca, P.; Carvalho, G.; Franco, A.; Kreve, S.; Avila, G.; Dias, S. Zirconia-Reinforced Lithium Silicate Biocompatibility Polished in Different Stages–An In Vitro Study. *J. Int. Dent. Med. Res.* **2018**, *11*, 759–764.

85. Pelekos, G.; Acharya, A.; Eiji, N.; Hong, G.; Leung, W.K.; McGrath, C. Effects of adjunctive probiotic *L. reuteri* lozenges on S/RSD outcomes at molar sites with deep pockets. *J. Clin. Periodontol.* **2020**, *47*, 1098–1107. [CrossRef]

86. Penala, S.; Kalakonda, B.; Pathakota, K.; Jayakumar, A.; Koppolu, P.; Lakshmi, B.; Pandey, R.; Mishra, A. Efficacy of local use of probiotics as an adjunct to scaling and root planing in chronic periodontitis and halitosis: A randomized controlled trial. *J. Res. Pharm. Pract.* **2016**, *5*, 86. [CrossRef] [PubMed]

87. Pudgar, P.; Povšič, K.; Čuk, K.; Seme, K.; Petelin, M.; Gašperšič, R. Probiotic strains of *Lactobacillus brevis* and *Lactobacillus plantarum* as adjunct to non-surgical periodontal therapy: 3-month results of a randomized controlled clinical trial. *Clin. Oral Investig.* **2021**, *25*, 1411–1422. [CrossRef] [PubMed]

88. Tomasello, G.; Tralongo, P.; Amoroso, F.; Damiani, P.; Sinagra, E.; Noto, M.; Arculeo, V.M.; Zein, R.J.; Saad, W.; Jurjus, A.; et al. Dysmicrobism, Inflammatory Bowel Disease and Thyroiditis: Analysis of the Literature. *J. Biol. Regul. Homeost. Agents* **2015**, *29*, 265–272. [PubMed]

89. Sajedinejad, N.; Paknejad, M.; Houshmand, B.; Sharafi, H.; Jelodar, R.; Zahiri, H.S.; Noghabi, K.A. *Lactobacillus salivarius* NK02: A Potent Probiotic for Clinical Application in Mouthwash. *Probiotics Antimicrob. Proteins* **2018**, *10*, 485–495. [CrossRef]

90. Scaryia, L.; Nagarathna, D.V.; Varghese, M. Probiotics in periodontal therapy. *Int. J. Pharma Bio Sci.* **2015**, *6*, 242–250.

91. Schlagenhauf, U.; Jakob, L.; Eigenthaler, M.; Segerer, S.; Jockel-Schneider, Y.; Rehn, M. Regular consumption of *Lactobacillus reuteri*-containing lozenges reduces pregnancy gingivitis: An RCT. *J. Clin. Periodontol.* **2016**, *43*, 948–954. [CrossRef]

92. Schlagenhauf, U.; Rehder, J.; Gelbrich, G.; Jockel-Schneider, Y. Consumption of *Lactobacillus reuteri*-containing lozenges improves periodontal health in navy sailors at sea: A randomized controlled trial. *J. Periodontol.* **2020**, *91*, 1328–1338. [CrossRef]

93. Shah, M.P.; Gujjari, S.K.; Chandrasekhar, V.S. Evaluation of the effect of probiotic (inersan(R)) alone, combination of probiotic with doxycycline and doxycycline alone on aggressive periodontitis—A clinical and microbiological study. *J. Clin. Diagn. Res.* **2013**, *7*, 595–600. [CrossRef]

94. Shah, M.P.; Gujjari, S.K.; Chandrasekhar, V.S. Long-term effect of *Lactobacillus brevis* CD2 (Inersan((R))) and/or doxycycline in aggressive periodontitis. *J. Indian Soc. Periodontol.* **2017**, *21*, 341–343. [CrossRef]

95. Shetty, S.; Srigiri, S.K.; Sheikh, K.H. A Comparative Clinical, Microbiological and Biochemical Evaluation of Guided Periodontal Pocket Recolonisation (GPR) using Synbiotics as an Adjunct to Scaling and Root Planing in Patients with Chronic Periodontitis: A Pilot Project. *Int. J. Med. Res. Health Sci.* **2020**, *9*, 20–32. [CrossRef]

96. Shimauchi, H.; Mayanagi, G.; Nakaya, S.; Minamibuchi, M.; Ito, Y.; Yamaki, K.; Hirata, H. Improvement of periodontal condition by probiotics with *Lactobacillus salivarius* WB21: A randomized, double-blind, placebo-controlled study. *J. Clin. Periodontol.* **2008**, *35*, 897–905. [CrossRef] [PubMed]

97. Sinkiewicz, G.; Cronholm, S.; Ljunggren, L.; Dahlen, G.; Bratthall, G. Influence of dietary supplementation with *Lactobacillus reuteri* on the oral flora of healthy subjects. *Swed. Dent. J.* **2010**, *34*, 197–206.

98. Slawik, S.; Staufenbiel, I.; Schilke, R.; Nicksch, S.; Weinspach, K.; Stiesch, M.; Eberhard, J. Probiotics affect the clinical inflammatory parameters of experimental gingivitis in humans. *Eur. J. Clin. Nutr.* **2011**, *65*, 857–863. [CrossRef] [PubMed]

99. Sinulingga, R.T.N.; Soeroso, Y.; Lessang, R.; Sastradipura, D.F.S. Probiotic *Lactobacillus reuteri* effect's on the levels of interleukin-4 in periodontitis patients after scaling and root planing. *Int. J. Appl. Pharm.* **2020**, *12*, 66–68. [CrossRef]

100. Staab, B.; Eick, S.; Knöfler, G.; Jentsch, H. The influence of a probiotic milk drink on the development of gingivitis: A pilot study. *J. Clin. Periodontol.* **2009**, *36*, 850–856. [CrossRef]

101. Suzuki, N.; Tanabe, K.; Takeshita, T.; Yoneda, M.; Iwamoto, T.; Oshiro, S.; Yamashita, Y.; Hirofuji, T. Effects of oil drops containing *Lactobacillus salivarius* WB21 on periodontal health and oral microbiota producing volatile sulfur compounds. *J. Breath Res.* **2012**, *6*, 017106. [CrossRef]

102. Teughels, W.; Durukan, A.; Ozcelik, O.; Pauwels, M.; Quirynen, M.; Haytac, M.C. Clinical and microbiological effects of *Lactobacillus reuteri* probiotics in the treatment of chronic periodontitis: A randomized placebo-controlled study. *J. Clin. Periodontol.* **2013**, *40*, 1025–1035. [CrossRef]

103. Theodoro, L.H.; Claudio, M.M.; Nuernberg, M.A.A.; Miessi, D.M.J.; Batista, J.A.; Duque, C.; Garcia, V.G. Effects of *Lactobacillus reuteri* as an adjunct to the treatment of periodontitis in smokers: Randomised clinical trial. *Benef. Microbes* **2019**, *10*, 375–384. [CrossRef]

104. Tobita, K.; Watanabe, I.; Tomokiyo, M.; Saito, M. Effects of heat-treated *Lactobacillus crispatus* KT-11 strain consumption on improvement of oral cavity environment: A randomised double-blind clinical trial. *Benef. Microbes* **2018**, *9*, 585–592. [CrossRef]

105. Toiviainen, A.; Jalasvuori, H.; Lahti, E.; Gursoy, U.; Salminen, S.; Fontana, M.; Flannagan, S.; Eckert, G.; Kokaras, A.; Paster, B.; et al. Impact of orally administered lozenges with Lactobacillus rhamnosus GG and Bifidobacterium animalis subsp. lactis BB-12 on the number of salivary mutans streptococci, amount of plaque, gingival inflammation and the oral microbiome in healthy adults. *Clin. Oral Investig.* **2015**, *19*, 77–83. [CrossRef]

106. Twetman, S.; Derawi, B.; Keller, M.; Ekstrand, K.; Yucel-Lindberg, T.; Stecksén-Blicks, C. Short-term effect of chewing gums containing probiotic Lactobacillus reuteri on the levels of inflammatory mediators in gingival crevicular fluid. *Acta Odontol. Scand.* **2009**, *67*, 19–24. [CrossRef]

107. Vicario, M.; Santos, A.; Violant, D.; Nart, J.; Giner, L. Clinical changes in periodontal subjects with the probiotic Lactobacillus reuteri Prodentis: A preliminary randomized clinical trial. *ACTA Odontol. Scand.* **2013**, *71*, 813–819. [CrossRef]

108. Vivekananda, M.R.; Vandana, K.L.; Bhat, K.G. Effect of the probiotic Lactobacilli reuteri (Prodentis) in the management of periodontal disease: A preliminary randomized clinical trial. *J. Oral Microbiol.* **2010**, *2*, 5344. [CrossRef]

109. Vohra, F.; Bukhari, I.A.; Sheikh, S.A.; Albaijan, R.; Naseem, M.; Hussain, M. Effectiveness of scalling and root plannng with and without adjunct probiotic therapy. *J. Periodontol.* **2020**, *91*, 1177–1185. [CrossRef] [PubMed]

110. Oda, Y.; Furutani, C.; Mizota, Y.; Wakita, A.; Mimura, S.; Kihara, T.; Ohara, M.; Okada, Y.; Okada, M.; Nikawa, H. Effect of bovine milk fermented with lactobacillus rhamnosus l8020 on periodontal disease in individuals with intellectual disability: A randomized clinical trial. *J. Appl. Oral Sci.* **2019**, *27*, 1–9. [CrossRef]

111. Corbet, E.; Smales, R. Oral diagnosis and treatment planning: Part 6. Preventive and treatment planning for periodontal disease. *Br. Dent. J.* **2012**, *213*, 277–284. [CrossRef] [PubMed]

112. Lang, N.P.; Bartold, P.M. Periodontal health. *J. Periodontol.* **2018**, *89*, S9–S16. [CrossRef]

113. Butera, A.; Gallo, S.; Maiorani, C.; Molino, D.; Chiesa, A.; Preda, C.; Esposito, F.; Scribante, A. Probiotic alternative to chlorhexidine in periodontal therapy: Evaluation of clinical and microbiological parameters. *Microorganisms* **2021**, *9*, 69. [CrossRef]

114. Allaker, R.P.; Stephen, A.S. Use of Probiotics and Oral Health. *Curr. Oral Health Rep.* **2017**, *4*, 309–318. [CrossRef] [PubMed]

115. Mu, Q.; Tavella, V.J.; Luo, X.M. Role of *Lactobacillus reuteri* in Human Health and Diseases. *Front. Microbiol.* **2018**, *9*, 757. [CrossRef]

116. Romani Vestman, N.; Chen, T.; Lif Holgerson, P.; Öhman, C.; Johansson, I. Oral Microbiota Shift after 12-Week Supplementation with *Lactobacillus reuteri* DSM 17938 and PTA 5289; A Randomized Control Trial. *PLoS ONE* **2015**, *10*, e0125812. [CrossRef]

117. Narwal, A. Probiotics in Dentistry—A Review. *J. Nutr. Food Sci.* **2011**, *1*. [CrossRef]

118. Bartlett, A.; Gullickson, R.G.; Singh, R.; Ro, S.; Omaye, S.T. The link between oral and gut microbiota in inflammatory bowel disease and a synopsis of potential salivary biomarkers. *Appl. Sci.* **2020**, *10*, 6421. [CrossRef]

119. Laleman, I.; Pauwels, M.; Quirynen, M.; Teughels, W. The usage of a lactobacilli probiotic in the non-surgical therapy of peri-implantitis: A randomized pilot study. *Clin. Oral Implant. Res.* **2020**, *31*, 84–92. [CrossRef]

120. Olsen, I.; Yamazaki, K. Can oral bacteria affect the microbiome of the gut? *J. Oral Microbiol.* **2019**, *11*, 1586422. [CrossRef]

121. Çaglar, E.; Kargul, B.; Tanboga, I. Bacteriotherapy and probiotics' role on oral health. *Oral Dis.* **2005**, *11*, 131–137. [CrossRef]

122. Kim, S.-K.; Guevarra, R.B.; Kim, Y.-T.; Kwon, J.; Kim, H.; Cho, J.H.; Kim, H.B.; Lee, J.-H. Role of Probiotics in Human Gut Microbiome-Associated Diseases. *J. Microbiol. Biotechnol.* **2019**, *29*, 1335–1340. [CrossRef]

123. Belkaid, Y.; Harrison, O.J. Homeostatic Immunity and the Microbiota. *Immunity* **2017**, *46*, 562–576. [CrossRef]

124. Wu, H.-J.; Wu, E. The role of gut microbiota in immune homeostasis and autoimmunity. *Gut Microbes* **2012**, *3*, 4–14. [CrossRef]

125. Carra, M.C.; Detzen, L.; Kitzmann, J.; Woelber, J.P.; Ramseier, C.A.; Bouchard, P. Promoting behavioural changes to improve oral hygiene in patients with periodontal diseases: A systematic review. *J. Clin. Periodontol.* **2020**, *47* (Suppl. S2), 72–89. [CrossRef]

126. Bouchard, P.; Carra, M.C.; Boillot, A.; Mora, F.; Rangé, H. Risk factors in periodontology: A conceptual framework. *J. Clin. Periodontol.* **2017**, *44*, 125–131. [CrossRef] [PubMed]

127. Singla, S.; Gupta, P.; Lehl, G.; Talwar, M. Effects of Reinforced Oral Hygiene Instruction Program With and Without Professional Tooth Cleaning on Plaque Control and Gingival Health of Orthodontic Patients Wearing Multibracket Appliances. *J. Indian Orthod. Soc.* **2019**, *53*, 272–277. [CrossRef]

128. Newton, J.T.; Asimakopoulou, K. Managing oral hygiene as a risk factor for periodontal disease: A systematic review of psychological approaches to behaviour change for improved plaque control in periodontal management. *J. Clin. Periodontol.* **2015**, *42*, S36–S46. [CrossRef] [PubMed]

129. Barros, S.P.; Williams, R.; Offenbacher, S.; Morelli, T. Gingival crevicular fluid as a source of biomarkers for periodontitis. *Periodontol. 2000* **2016**, *70*, 53–64. [CrossRef]

130. Teles, R.; Sakellari, D.; Teles, F.; Konstantinidis, A.; Kent, R.; Socransky, S.; Haffajee, A. Relationships among gingival crevicular fluid biomarkers, clinical parameters of periodontal disease, and the subgingival microbiota. *J. Periodontol.* **2010**, *81*, 89–98. [CrossRef]

131. Bourgeois, D.; Inquimbert, C.; Ottolenghi, L.; Carrouel, F. Periodontal Pathogens as Risk Factors of Cardiovascular Diseases, Diabetes, Rheumatoid Arthritis, Cancer, and Chronic Obstructive Pulmonary Disease-Is There Cause for Consideration? *Microorganisms* **2019**, *7*, 424. [CrossRef]

132. Brennan, C.A.; Garrett, W.S. Fusobacterium nucleatum—Symbiont, opportunist and oncobacterium. *Nat. Rev. Microbiol.* **2019**, *17*, 156–166. [CrossRef]

133. Javed, F.; Ahmed, H.B.; Saeed, A.; Mehmood, A.; Bain, C. Whole Salivary Interleukin-6 and Matrix Metalloproteinase-8 Levels in Patients with Chronic Periodontitis With and Without Prediabetes. *J. Periodontol.* **2014**, *85*, e130–e135. [CrossRef]

134. Ebersole, J.L.; Dawson, D.R.; Morford, L.A.; Peyyala, R.; Miller, C.S.; Gonzaléz, O.A. Periodontal disease immunology: "Double indemnity" in protecting the host. *Periodontol. 2000* **2013**, *62*, 163–202. [CrossRef]
135. Zhang, L.; Li, X.; Yan, H.; Huang, L. Salivary matrix metalloproteinase (MMP)-8 as a biomarker for periodontitis: A PRISMA-compliant systematic review and meta-analysis. *Medicine* **2018**, *97*, e9642. [CrossRef]
136. Al-Majid, A.; Alassiri, S.; Rathnayake, N.; Tervahartiala, T.; Gieselmann, D.-R.; Sorsa, T. Matrix Metalloproteinase-8 as an Inflammatory and Prevention Biomarker in Periodontal and Peri-Implant Diseases. *Int. J. Dent.* **2018**, *2018*, 7891323. [CrossRef]
137. Sorsa, T.; Alassiri, S.; Grigoriadis, A.; Räisänen, I.T.; Pärnänen, P.; Nwhator, S.O.; Gieselmann, D.-R.; Sakellari, D. Active MMP-8 (aMMP-8) as a Grading and Staging Biomarker in the Periodontitis Classification. *Diagnostics* **2020**, *10*, 61. [CrossRef]
138. Pan, W.; Wang, Q.; Chen, Q. The cytokine network involved in the host immune response to periodontitis. *Int. J. Oral Sci.* **2019**, *11*, 30. [CrossRef] [PubMed]
139. Stadler, A.F.; Angst, P.D.M.; Arce, R.M.; Gomes, S.C.; Oppermann, R.V.; Susin, C. Gingival crevicular fluid levels of cytokines/chemokines in chronic periodontitis: A meta-analysis. *J. Clin. Periodontol.* **2016**, *43*, 727–745. [CrossRef] [PubMed]
140. Teles, R.P.; Likhari, V.; Socransky, S.S.; Haffajee, A.D. Salivary cytokine levels in subjects with chronic periodontitis and in periodontally healthy individuals: A cross-sectional study. *J. Periodontal Res.* **2009**, *44*, 411–417. [CrossRef]
141. Goutoudi, P.; Diza, E.; Arvanitidou, M. Effect of periodontal therapy on crevicular fluid interleukin-6 and interleukin-8 levels in chronic periodontitis. *Int. J. Dent.* **2012**, *2012*, 362905. [CrossRef]
142. Ross, J.H.; Hardy, D.C.; Schuyler, C.A.; Slate, E.H.; Mize, T.W.; Huang, Y. Expression of periodontal interleukin-6 protein is increased across patients with neither periodontal disease nor diabetes, patients with periodontal disease alone and patients with both diseases. *J. Periodontal Res.* **2010**, *45*, 688–694. [CrossRef] [PubMed]
143. Checchi, L.; Montevecchi, M.; Checchi, V.; Zappulla, F. The Relationship Between Bleeding on Probing and Subgingival Deposits. An Endoscopical Evaluation. *Open Dent. J.* **2009**, *3*, 154–160. [CrossRef]

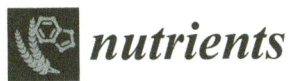

nutrients

MDPI

Article

The Suitability of Questionnaires for Exploring Relations of Dietary Behavior and Tooth Wear

Maximiliane Amelie Schlenz [1], Moritz Benedikt Schlenz [1], Bernd Wöstmann [1], Alexandra Jungert [2], Anna Sophia Glatt [3] and Carolina Ganss [3,*]

[1] Department of Prosthodontics, Dental Clinic, Justus Liebig University, Schlangenzahl 14, 35392 Giessen, Germany; maximiliane.a.schlenz@dentist.med.uni-giessen.de (M.A.S.); moritz.schlenz@dentist.med.uni-giessen.de (M.B.S.); bernd.woestmann@dentist.med.uni-giessen.de (B.W.)

[2] Biometry and Population Genetics, Institute of Agronomy and Plant Breeding II, Interdisciplinary Research Center for Biosystems, Land Use and Dietary (IFZ), Justus Liebig University, Heinrich-Buff-Ring 26-32, 35392 Giessen, Germany; alexandra.jungert@ernaehrung.uni-giessen.de

[3] Department of Conservative and Preventive Dentistry, Dental Clinic, Justus Liebig University, Schlangenzahl 14, 35392 Giessen, Germany; anna.s.glatt@dentist.med.uni-giessen.de

* Correspondence: carolina.ganss@dentist.med.uni-giessen.de; Tel.: +49-641-9946171

Abstract: Tooth wear is a relevant oral health problem, especially at a young age. Although ongoing acid exposures may contribute to tooth wear, the role of acidic dietary components in this context remains unclear. To date, in tooth wear studies, dietary behavior has been assessed using traditional questionnaires, but the suitability of this approach has not been investigated so far. In our longitudinal study, we followed 91 participants (21.0 ± 2.2 years) over a period of 1 year (373 ± 19 days) and monitored tooth wear with an intraoral scanner. At baseline (T0) and at the end (T1), we assessed dietary behavior with questionnaires asking about the consumption frequencies of acidic dietary components and the acid taste preferences. Complete data were available from 80 subjects. The consumption frequencies of T0 and T1 correlated weakly to moderately. Taste preferences seem to be a more consistent measure, but there was predominantly no significant correlation with the corresponding consumption frequencies. None of the dietary parameters showed a significant relation with tooth wear. The suitability of dietary questionnaires to assess tooth-relevant dietary behavior seems to be limited.

Keywords: diet; oral health; questionnaires; erosion; young adults; tooth wear; dentistry

Citation: Schlenz, M.A.; Schlenz, M.B.; Wöstmann, B.; Jungert, A.; Glatt, A.S.; Ganss, C. The Suitability of Questionnaires for Exploring Relations of Dietary Behavior and Tooth Wear. *Nutrients* **2022**, *14*, 1165. https://doi.org/10.3390/nu14061165

Academic Editors: Kirstin Vach, Johan Peter Woelber and Bernadette P. Marriott

Received: 4 February 2022
Accepted: 9 March 2022
Published: 10 March 2022

Publisher's Note: MDPI stays neutral with regard to jurisdictional claims in published maps and institutional affiliations.

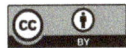
1. Introduction

Tooth wear is a type of dental hard tissue loss that occurs due to the effects of physical and chemical factors. Physical factors include forces due to tooth-to-tooth contact (attrition) that can appear as parafunctions, such as tooth grinding. Furthermore, physical factors can also be so-called foreign objects (abrasion), for example, oral hygiene may play a role. Chemical factors include acid exposure of any kind that does not originate from bacterial metabolism (erosion) [1]. These factors affect the dental hard tissue throughout the entire functional period of the dentition and cause irreversible and, therefore, cumulative dental hard tissue loss.

Enamel is a very densely mineralized avital tissue with considerable hardness and wear resistance [2]. However, acid impacts are able to demineralize enamel relatively easily, which can significantly reduce its microhardness. As a result, subsequent physical impacts may increase dental hard tissue loss [3]. All these factors interact with the multiple functions of the oral cavity. When acid impacts are prominent, it is referred to as erosive tooth wear [1].

That a variety of food and drinks are capable of demineralizing enamel is well known from laboratory experiments [4]. These include, for example, fruit juices, soft drinks, wines, fruit, vinegar, and pickles. It is, therefore, plausible to assume that an acidic diet can contribute to tooth wear. However, epidemiological studies show only weak associations, if any, between acid impacts from the diet and the prevalence and severity of tooth wear. For example, a systematic review that included more than fifty cross-sectional studies had very heterogeneous and contradictory results, with the majority of studies showing no association between dietary acid impacts and tooth wear [5].

While cross-sectional studies can, at best, show associations, longitudinal surveys are more capable of identifying causal or risk factors, but well-conducted studies are sparse. A Dutch study [6] included 656 children aged 10–12 years, of whom 572 were followed up 3 years later. The only risk factors identified were frequent consumption of alcoholic mixed drinks and acidic vegetables. However, the strength of the association was weak (alcoholic mixed drinks OR = 1.82; acidic vegetables OR = 1.16). A recent Brazilian study [7] included 801 12-year-olds; 680 could be followed up after 2 and a half years. Dietary behavior was not a risk factor in this study.

Generally, in such studies, the dietary data are collected only once, in longitudinal studies at the beginning of the study period. Furthermore, the consumption frequencies of individual items or individual classes (e.g., soft drinks or fruit juices) are usually considered, which means that the total amount of daily acid impacts, regardless of their source, is not taken into account. To the best of the authors' knowledge, only two studies also included a measure for the total amount of acidic drinks consumed [8,9].

Even if these methodological aspects can, at least, partially explain the heterogeneous study results, the question remains: why it is so difficult to establish associations between dietary behavior and tooth wear, even though the potential demineralizing properties of acidic food have been clearly demonstrated? It is conceivable that questionnaires do not adequately reflect actual eating behavior, that a cross-sectional observation of diet is not very representative of dietary behavior over a longer period of time, or that dietary behavior is so variable that individual surveys generally have little significance when it comes to processes that only manifest themselves in longer contexts.

For this reason, we have modified the above-mentioned mostly used procedure for collecting dietary data. When such data are collected at the beginning of a longitudinal study, it is assumed that these data will reflect dietary behavior over the course of the observation period. However, since this assumption cannot be easily substantiated, we conducted a second survey at the end of the observation period. Furthermore, we did not only collect data on the consumption frequencies of acidic food and drinks but also the taste preferences of our study participants.

The main aim of our study was to investigate to what extent the dietary habits reported at baseline are related to those reported at the end of the observation period and whether the reported taste preferences reflect the reported consumption frequencies. A further but subordinate aim was to explore how these results relate to tissue loss values measured with an intraoral scanner in the corresponding observation period.

2. Participants, Materials and Methods

2.1. Study Group

The study was conducted in accordance with the principles of the Declaration of Helsinki [2] and approved by the Ethics Committee of the medical faculty of the Justus Liebig University Giessen (ref. no. 148/18). The procedure and methodology of the study have been described earlier [10] as part of the project "Intraoral scanner-based monitoring of tooth wear in young adults". The data for this publication were based on the data set from [10].

Between the end of 2018 and the beginning of 2020, a total of 91 participants (mean age at the start of the study: 21.0 ± 2.2 years) were included. Inclusion criteria were defined as age between 18 and 25 years, a lower first molar without caries and clinically visible plaque, as well as without any restoration or one whose extent did not exceed one-third of the occlusal width. The same criteria were defined for the occluding antagonist.

Exclusion criteria were determined as severe disease [11], ongoing orthodontic treatment, and maxillary crowns or bridges.

2.2. Questionnaire

The questionnaire regarding dietary behavior was designed by an experienced nutritionist (A.J.) and provided in paper form. In advance of this study, cognitive pre-tests using the technique of thinking aloud were applied, and expert interviews were conducted. The survey contained questions about the frequency of consumption of specific drinks and food items in order to calculate the acid impacts per day. To this end, for each frequency category, the mean value of the given range was determined and subsequently converted in frequencies per day. As an example: for the consumption frequency "1–4× per week", the mean would be 2.5× per week, converted to the day this would result in 0.36. The values of all items (or those related to food or drinks separately) were summed and constituted the total number of daily acid impacts (or acid impacts from drinks and food, respectively).

Furthermore, a five-point Likert scale was used to ask about the taste preference for drinks and food. The abstention of answers was allowed, and questionnaires were evaluated anonymously. The items of the questionnaire that were analyzed here can be found in the Appendix A. Participants completed a dietary questionnaire twice: at baseline (T0) and at follow-up after one year (T1; mean observation time 373 ± 19 d).

Please also see further information in the Appendix A.

Re-Test of Questionnaire

To investigate the reliability of the questionnaire, a re-test was conducted independently of the main study procedure with a group of 28 participants (12 female, 16 male; age 25.8 ± 4.6 years) not involved in the clinical study. Participants were asked to fill out the questionnaire twice at a 1-week interval.

The intra class coefficient (ICC) estimates and their 95% confident intervals (95% CI) for the acidic impacts at both survey times were calculated based on a single-rating, absolute-agreement, 2-way mixed-effects model. The following ICCs (95% CI) were found: acid impacts from drinks: ICC = 0.795 (0.605;0.900, $p \leq 0.001$), acid impacts from food: ICC = 0.653 (0.381;0.822, $p \leq 0.001$), all acid impacts: ICC = 0.809 (0.629;0.906, $p \leq 0.001$), indicating a moderate to good reliability [12].

The kappa value for "I like to drink acidic drinks" at both survey times was 0.441 ($p \leq 0.01$), and for "I like to eat acidic food" was 0.408 ($p \leq 0.01$), indicating a moderate agreement [13] for both items (the combined Likert categories, see Section 2.4).

2.3. Tooth Wear Monitoring

Besides investigating the dietary behavior with a survey, tooth wear of one lower first molar (study tooth) was analyzed using an intraoral scanner (Trios 3, 3Shape, Copenhagen, Denmark). An experienced investigator (M.A.S.) scanned the study tooth at T0 and T1. To determine tooth wear, datasets of T0 and T1 were superimposed in an external 3D software (GOM Inspect, version V8 SR1, GOM GmbH, Braunschweig, Germany) using the established best-fit alignment with the iterative closest point technique for the measurement of the maximum vertical tissue loss in micrometer. The 3D measurements were conducted by a second investigator (M.B.S.) to avoid bias, and this investigator was blinded to dietary data.

2.4. Statistics

Of the 91 participants, 11 had some missing dietary data, and these were therefore not included. In total, the 80 complete datasets were analyzed here. For the quantitative data (tissue loss and the number of acid impacts), significant deviations from the Gaussian distribution were found (Kolmogorov–Smirnov test); therefore, these are given as the median and 95% confidence interval (after bootstrapping). Non-parametric test procedures were used for the analysis.

For taste preferences, the five-point Likert scale items were combined into three categories. For this purpose, the categories "I do not agree at all" and "I rather disagree" were pooled into "disagree", and "I tend to agree" and "I fully agree" were pooled into "agree". "Neither" remained a category of its own. In addition, the participants were divided into two groups according to the number of acid impacts per day (low acid impacts: <4 acid impacts per day; high acid impacts: $\geq$4 acid impacts per day) [14].

All statistical procedures were done with IBM SPSS Statistics version 27 (IBM Germany GmbH, Ehningen, Germany).

2.4.1. Comparison of Dietary Data T0 to T1

The intra class coefficient (ICC) estimates and their 95% confidence intervals for the number of acidic impacts at T0 and T1 were calculated based on a single-rating, absolute agreement, 2-way mixed-effects model. The relation of taste preferences at T0 and T1 was analyzed using Kappa statistics.

2.4.2. Comparison of the Number of Acid Impacts and Taste Preferences

The relation between the number of acid impacts and taste preferences at both T0 and T1 was analyzed using the Kruskal–Wallis test for independent samples.

2.4.3. Comparison of Dietary Data with Tissue Loss Values

Qualitative data on dietary behavior and quantitative data on tissue loss values at both T0 and T1 were examined using the Kruskal–Wallis test for independent samples. Furthermore, Spearman's rank correlation was computed to assess the relationship between acid impacts and tissue loss.

3. Results

3.1. Comparison of Dietary Data T0 to T1

Table 1 describes the acid impacts at the two observation time points (T0 and T1).

Table 1. Descriptive data of the number of acid impacts from different sources at the beginning (T0) and at the end (T1) of the observation period. Acid impacts from drinks included wine.

	Median	95% CI	Minimum;Maximum
Acid impacts from drinks T0	1.0	0.7;1.3	0.1;5.2
Acid impacts from drinks T1	0.9	0.7;1.1	0;11.7
Acid impacts from food T0	1.4	1.1;1.7	0.1;5.4
Acid impacts from food T1	1.5	1.3;1.9	0.1;6.2
Total acid impacts T0	2.5	2.3;3.0	0.4;7.9
Total acid impacts T1	2.7	2.3;3.0	0.6;12.0

The ICC for the comparison of the number of acid impacts from food, drinks, and overall at T0 and T1 was 0.387 (0.187;0.557, $p \leq 0.001$), 0.068 ($-0.154;0.284$, $p = 0.274$), and 0.175 ($-0.042;0.377$, $p = 0.057$), respectively, indicating a fair relation for the first (Figure 1) and no significant relation for the others.

Kappa coefficients for "I like to eat acidic food" and "I like to drink acidic drinks" at T0 and T1 were 0.408 ($p \leq 0.01$) and 0.403 ($p \leq 0.01$), respectively, indicating a moderate relation. The comparison of the two items with each other resulted in a Kappa coefficient for T0 of 0.149 ($p \leq 0.05$) and for T1 of 0.205 ($p \leq 0.05$), indicating a slight relation.

At T0, 63 participants were in the low acid impacts group, and 17 were in the high acid impacts group; at T1, there were 62 and 18 subjects, respectively; 63.7% of the par-ticipants remained in the low acid impacts and 7.5% in the high acid impacts group, but 28.7% switched between groups. Figure 2 shows all participants ranked by the number of acid impacts per day at T0 and the corresponding data at T1.

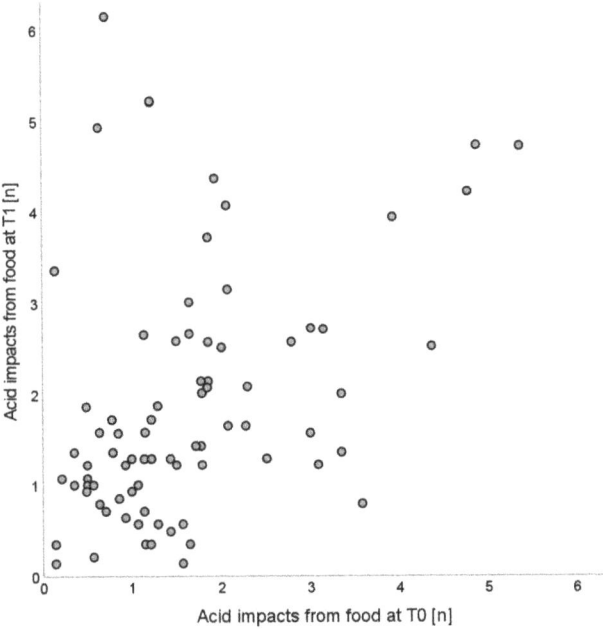

Figure 1. Scatterplot of acid impacts from food per day at baseline (T0) and at the end of the observation period after one year (T1).

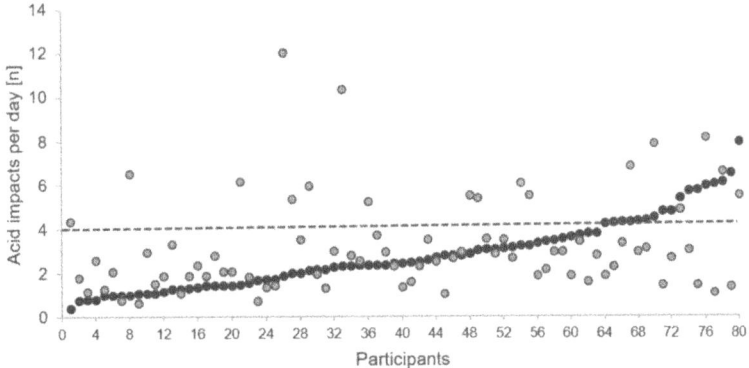

Figure 2. Scatterplot of acid impacts per day at T0 and T1, participants were ranked by their acid impacts at T0. The dotted line indicates the threshold for low and high acid impact groups; black dots indicate the number of acid impacts per day at T0 and the grey dots the corresponding values at T1.

3.2. Comparison of the Taste Preferences and Consumption Frequencies

Most items addressing taste preferences did not show a significant relation to the corresponding acidic impacts. Table 2 shows that those agreeing with the statement "I like to eat acidic food" did not have significantly more acid impacts from acidic food than those who were undecided or disagreed with this statement. This was true for both observation time points. In contrast, taste preferences regarding drinks had a significant effect on acid impacts, but this was only the case at T1.

Table 2. The number of acid impacts per day (median, 95% confidence interval, and range) in the different categories of taste preferences at baseline (T0) and follow-up after one year (T1) (* = Kruskal–Wallis test $p \leq 0.001$). Drinks include wine.

	Disagree	Neither	Agree
	Acid impacts from food T0		
I like to eat acidic food T0	$n = 27$ 1.2 (0.8;1.8) range 5.0	$n = 15$ 1.2 (0.9;2.3) range 4.7	$n = 38$ 1.5 (1.2;1.8) range 4.2
	Acid impacts from food T1		
I like to eat acidic food T1	$n = 18$ 1.3 (0.9;2.1) range 4.6	$n = 20$ 1.5 (0.8;2.1) range 5.0	$n = 42$ 1.6 (1.3;2.2) range 5.8
	Acid impacts from drinks T0		
I like to drink acidic drinks T0	$n = 50$ 0.9 (0.6;1.2) range 5.1	$n = 14$ 1.1 (0.6;1.6) range 2.2	$n = 16$ 1.5 (0.7;1.9) range 3.4
	Acid impacts from drinks T1		
I like to drink acidic drinks T1 *	$n = 45$ 0.7 (0.5;0.9) range 5.1	$n = 14$ 0.9 (0.6;1.1) range 2.7	$n = 21$ 1.4 (1.2;1.7) range 11.2

3.3. Comparison of Dietary Data with Tissue Loss Values

The median tissue loss was 42.5 (38.0;49.0) μm with a range of 183 μm.

There was no significant correlation between acid impacts and tissue loss, regardless of whether the source of the acids (from drinks, food, or total) or the time point of the survey were considered. At T0, the correlation coefficients were 0.114 ($p = 0.315$), -0147 ($p = 0.966$), and -0.058 ($p = 0.612$), respectively, and at T1, they were 0.082 ($p = 0.469$), 0.005 ($p = 0.966$), and 0.018 ($p = 0.871$), respectively.

There was also no significant relationship between taste preferences for drinks and food and tissue loss. A numerical relationship was found between tissue loss and preference for acidic drinks at baseline. The tissue loss values were 39.0 (36.0;47.5), 44.5 (33.0;54.5), and 51 (38.0;67.9) μm for those who disagreed, were undecided, or agreed, but these differences did not reach statistical significance ($p = 0.088$).

4. Discussion

We investigated a new approach to shed light on the role of questionnaires in analyzing the relationship between diet and progression of tooth wear.

First of all, in the present context, there is no generally accepted questionnaire to fall back on. For this reason, we developed a new one and included some novel aspects. In this questionnaire, we collected the consumption frequencies of potentially erosive food and drinks that are frequently queried in the literature. In contrast to the usual analyses of individual drink or food categories with regard to their effect on tooth wear, we used the consumption frequencies only to determine the frequency of acid impacts overall. This approach seems more meaningful to us because the erosive potential of products in a category can vary greatly [15] (for example, different brands within the soft drink class), thus categories such as "soft drinks" or "fruit juices" do not represent an entity to which one could assign an independent erosive potential.

Dietary habits are multidimensional, of course, and self-reported frequencies may be biased in various ways, for example, in terms of recall, or social desirability [16]. We, therefore, included not only consumption frequencies but also qualitative aspects of diet and asked about taste preferences. We assumed that such questions could provide an indicator of basic preferences and general dietary behavior and might be more meaningful for our research question than consumption frequencies. In another context, food (taste) preferences have, indeed, been identified as an important factor in food choice [17].

Finally, we coupled our one-year wear observation period with two dietary surveys to obtain both a prospective and a retrospective dimension of dietary behavior in relation to the observation period.

With regard to the measurement of tissue loss, we focused on a single tooth observation, although tooth wear naturally can occur across the entire dentition. However, measuring tissue loss with intraoral scanners is less accurate when looking at larger sections of the jaw [18]. For this reason, we have only collected loss values for the first lower molar. This was well suited for our purpose because it is the tooth where tooth wear manifests itself earliest and has the highest progression rates [9,19,20].

First of all, we were interested in how consistent the data from the questionnaires were. With regard to the acid impacts from drinks and food, similar numbers were found at the beginning (T0) and at the end of the study (T1), but at the individual level, their correlation was low. That this was not due to random errors is indicated by the comparison with the results of the retest of our questionnaire, which showed a very good correlation with the consumption frequencies. This variability in the consumption frequencies is also reflected in the classification of the participants into the low and high acid impacts groups, as almost 30% of them were classified differently depending on whether the data from the beginning or the end of the studies were used.

Self-reported dietary data are subject to a variety of influencing factors, including memory, social desirability [7,16], and behavioral changes due to participation in a study. While the first two aspects mean that the actual dietary behavior differs from the reported one, the last aspect would imply an actual change in consumption. It is quite conceivable that our study participants, based on their knowledge of the study objective, have informed themselves about the reasons for tooth wear and the role of diet and have adapted their diet accordingly. This could have led to a reduction in reported acid impacts over time, but our data do not confirm this. That knowledge about a healthy diet only has a limited effect on behavioral change has also been shown in other contexts [21].

Eating habits are also a very strongly socially influenced construct [22], and it is quite conceivable that a dynamic social environment, as is possibly assumed especially in younger adults, could lead to variable and changing dietary behavior. Especially for the age group studied here, there seem to be many potential factors that determine eating behavior [23]. Among these factors are also taste preferences, and this factor is perhaps one for which a certain continuity can be assumed and which could have a certain basic influence on dietary behavior. It was, indeed, shown that those who agreed with the statement "I like the taste of most fruits" in fact ate more fruit than those who did not [24]. Furthermore, taste preferences and eating habits seem to be consistently associated with each other over a longer period of time [24]. In our study, taste preferences for both food and drinks at T0 and T1 were at least moderately consistent, in contrast to consumption frequencies. Contrary to what might be assumed, taste preference for drinks and food does not seem to be always in the same direction because those who liked to consume acidic drinks did not necessarily consume acidic food. Interestingly, taste preference was, except for acid drinks, only by trend associated with a corresponding frequency of consumption, which seems to contradict the results of the study mentioned above. However, it certainly depends on how the question is framed. In the context of erosive tooth wear, questionnaire items focus on drinks and food that are acidic in the chemical sense. However, low pH does not necessarily reflect taste sensation. For example, it was shown that participants rated the sweetness intensity of two commercial soft drinks with a sugar content of about 10% comparably high, even though the pH value of one drink was 6.3 and that of the other 2.1 [25]. It would, therefore, be interesting to investigate in further studies whether taste or consumption preferences can be found that have a better predictive value for tissue loss than the simple question about acidic taste sensations. Furthermore, the nutrient content and pH value may largely differ within a food category or even within a food item, and food items are often combined (e.g., fruits and yoghurt), which may influence the erosive potential. Finally, not only the original pH value of food is relevant for the erosive potential of food, but also the buffering capacity [26]. Moreover, human saliva has protective properties, thus a low pH value of food does not lead automatically to a low intraoral pH [26].

Our data show that, on the one hand, the participants reported a wide range in consumption of acidic food and drinks, and, on the other hand, they also experienced considerable tissue loss. This is similar to our first, very basic analysis, where we only looked at the dietary data reported at T0 [10]. However, neither the consumption frequencies of potentially erosive drinks or food nor the taste preferences at both time points could provide an explanation for the tissue loss. Accordingly, the classification of four or more acid impacts per day as a risk indicator for erosive tooth wear proposed by Lussi and Hellwig [14] could not be confirmed with our data; this is all the more so because about one-third of the participants changed this classification, depending on whether the data at T0 or T1 were taken into account. Thus, our study basically confirms the results of the two longitudinal studies mentioned at the beginning [6,7], which used a clinical index to assess tissue loss. Such indices represent a rather crude measure of tissue loss, and we had assumed that an objective and quantitative measure would be better suited to detect etiological factors attributable to diet. However, if we consider the heterogeneity of the dietary data at the two points in time of our study, it can be assumed that the dietary behavior, at least in the phase of life in which our participants found themselves, might be too variable to be grasped via only two data collection points. Thus, a cross-sectional survey of factors that can be attributed to diet might be generally unsuitable for explaining phenomena that manifest themselves over a longer period of time. A longer study period with multiple data collection points could shed light on this. Finally, however, the fundamental question can be asked whether and to what extent self-reported dietary habits have anything at all to do with real dietary behavior, and the relevance of dietary data collected on the basis of memory-based dietary assessment methods has generally been questioned [27]. As the relationship between diet and (oral) health remains an important area of research, it would be valuable to think about novel methods for assessing dietary behavior [28,29].

A strength of our study is that we have objectively quantified tissue loss with a digital measurement method that can represent tissue loss very sensitively. However, this relatively complex measurement method also means a limit to the number of test persons. The relatively small group of people is a limitation. Therefore, further studies must show how generalizable our results are. It could be regarded as a further limitation that other factors, such as oral hygiene behavior or bruxism, that could affect tooth wear were not included. Since it was not the aim of the present study to clarify which factors, in general, could be responsible for the wear that we found in our group of individuals, however, this limitation rather draws attention to methodological aspects for epidemiological studies in the field as a whole. If we consider bruxism, for example, as a possible factor for wear, studies show that self-reported behavior, collected with questionnaires, may also be less reliable in this context than one might presume [30]. It would, therefore, be an important research perspective to look at the research methodology for analytical, epidemiological questions on tooth wear from a broader perspective.

5. Conclusions

Considering the duration of longitudinal studies on tooth wear, it is important to note that the dietary behavior reported at intervals of only one year was only partially consistent. Although taste preferences seem to be more consistent over a longer period of time than consumption frequencies, it remains unclear to what extent these also reflect acid exposure from food and drinks. None of the dietary parameters showed a significant relation with tissue loss. The suitability of dietary questionnaires seems to be limited, and new survey methods may be needed to clarify the role of diet in the context of tooth wear.

Author Contributions: Conceptualization, M.A.S., C.G., A.J.; methodology, M.A.S., C.G., A.J. and M.B.S.; validation, M.A.S., M.B.S. and C.G.; formal analysis, M.A.S. and C.G.; investigation, M.A.S., M.B.S. and A.S.G.; resources, B.W.; data curation, M.A.S., A.J. and C.G.; writing—original draft preparation, C.G.; writing—review and editing, M.A.S., A.J., A.S.G., M.B.S., B.W. and C.G.; visualization, C.G.; supervision, M.A.S. and C.G.; project administration, M.A.S. and M.B.S. All authors have read and agreed to the published version of the manuscript.

Funding: This research received no external funding.

Institutional Review Board Statement: The study was conducted according to the guidelines of the Declaration of Helsinki and approved by the local ethics committee of the medical faculty of the Justus Liebig University Giessen (ref. no. 148/18, date of approval: 5 October 2018).

Informed Consent Statement: Informed consent was obtained from all participants involved in the study.

Data Availability Statement: The datasets of this article are available from the corresponding author on a reasonable request.

Acknowledgments: We would like to thank our study participants for their patience and time.

Conflicts of Interest: The authors declare no conflict of interest.

Appendix A

Questionnaire items

1. Frequencies

To investigate the number of acid impacts per day, the consumption of the following drinks and food was enquired in the questionnaire. The participants were asked to reflect on the last four weeks before answering the questions.

Non-alcoholic drinks:

- Energy drinks
- Lemonade
- Cola/cola mixed drinks
- Soft drinks other than cola and lemonade
- Light soft drinks
- Fruit juices
- Smoothies
- Iced tea
- Isotonic sports drinks
- Fruit tea

Food:

- Citrus fruits
- Soft fruits
- Stone fruits
- Pome fruits
- Pineapple
- Sour pickled food
- Salad dressings with vinegar
- Sour sweets

The following answer options were available, which were considered equivalent to the acid impacts per day in brackets:

- Never/rarely (0)
- 1–3x per month (0.07)
- 1–4x per week (0.36)
- 5–6x per week (0.79)
- 1–2x daily (1.5)

- 3–4x daily (3.5)
- $\geq$5x daily (5)

In addition, the consumption of wine was enquired with the following answer options available, which were considered equivalent to the acid impacts per day in brackets:

- Never (0)
- $\leq$1x per month (0.02)
- 2–3x per month (0.08)
- 1–3x per week (0.29)
- 4–6x per week (0.71)
- 1x daily (1)
- $\geq$2x daily (2)

The values of all items (or those related to food or drinks separately) were summed and constituted the total number of daily acid impacts (or acid impacts from drinks and food, respectively).

Example:

Consumption frequencies of a subject:

i.   Energy drinks (1–4x per week)
ii.   Smoothies (5–6x per week)
iii.   Fruit tea (1–2x per day)
iv.   Wine (4–6x per week)
v.   Citrus fruits (1–2x daily)
vi.   Soft fruits (1–2x daily)
vii.   Salad dressings with vinegar (5–6x per week)
viii. Sour sweets (1–4x per week)

Calculation (addition of corresponding acid impacts):

i.   0.36
ii.   0.79
iii.   1.5
iv.   0.71
v.   1.5
vi.   1.5
vii.   0.79
viii. 0.36

Total: 7.51 acid impacts per day.

2   Taste preference

The answers to the questions were related to dietary behavior during the last four weeks.

1.   I like to eat acidic food.
2.   I like to drink acidic drinks.

The following answers could be chosen:

- I do not agree at all.
- I rather disagree.
- Neither.
- I tend to agree.
- I fully agree.

References

1. Schlueter, N.; Amaechi, B.T.; Bartlett, D.; Buzalaf, M.A.R.; Carvalho, T.S.; Ganss, C.; Hara, A.T.; Huysmans, M.; Lussi, A.; Moazzez, R.; et al. Terminology of erosive tooth wear: Consensus report of a workshop organized by the ORCA and the Cariology Research Group of the IADR. *Caries Res.* **2020**, *54*, 2–6. [CrossRef] [PubMed]
2. Wilmers, J.; Bargmann, S. Nature's design solutions in dental enamel: Uniting high strength and extreme damage resistance. *Acta Biomater.* **2020**, *107*, 1–24. [CrossRef] [PubMed]
3. Attin, T.; Koidl, U.; Buchalla, W.; Schaller, H.G.; Kielbassa, A.M.; Hellwig, E. Correlation of microhardness and wear in differently eroded bovine dental enamel. *Arch. Oral Biol.* **1997**, *42*, 243–250. [CrossRef]
4. Barbour, M.E.; Lussi, A.; Shellis, R.P. Screening and prediction of erosive potential. *Caries Res.* **2011**, *45* (Suppl. S1), 24–32. [CrossRef]
5. Chan, A.S.; Tran, T.T.K.; Hsu, Y.H.; Liu, S.Y.S.; Kroon, J. A systematic review of dietary acids and habits on dental erosion in adolescents. *Int. J. Paediatr. Dent.* **2020**, *30*, 713–733. [CrossRef] [PubMed]
6. El Aidi, H.; Bronkhorst, E.M.; Huysmans, M.C.; Truin, G.J. Multifactorial analysis of factors associated with the incidence and progression of erosive tooth wear. *Caries Res.* **2011**, *45*, 303–312. [CrossRef] [PubMed]
7. Brusius, C.D.; Alves, L.S.; Susin, C.; Maltz, M. Dental erosion among South Brazilian adolescents: A 2.5-year longitudinal study. *Community Dent. Oral Epidemiol.* **2018**, *46*, 17–23. [CrossRef]
8. Sovik, J.B.; Skudutyte-Rysstad, R.; Tveit, A.B.; Sandvik, L.; Mulic, A. Sour sweets and acidic beverage consumption are risk indicators for dental erosion. *Caries Res.* **2015**, *49*, 243–250. [CrossRef]
9. Hasselkvist, A.; Johansson, A.; Johansson, A.K. A 4 year prospective longitudinal study of progression of dental erosion associated to lifestyle in 13–14 year-old Swedish adolescents. *J. Dent.* **2016**, *47*, 55–62. [CrossRef]
10. Schlenz, M.A.; Schlenz, M.B.; Wöstmann, B.; Jungert, A.; Ganss, C. Intraoral scanner-based monitoring of tooth wear in young adults: 12-month results. *Clin. Oral Investig.* **2022**, *26*, 1869–1878. [CrossRef] [PubMed]
11. Institute of Medicine (US) Committee on Serious and Complex Medical Conditions. *Definition of Serious and Complex Medical Conditions*; 1. Introduction; National Academic Press: Washington, DC, USA, 1999. Available online: https://www.ncbi.nlm.nih.gov/books/NBK224968/ (accessed on 20 January 2022).
12. Koo, T.K.; Li, M.Y. A guideline of selecting and reporting intraclass correlation coefficients for reliability research. *J. Chiropr. Med.* **2016**, *15*, 155–163. [CrossRef] [PubMed]
13. Landis, J.R.; Koch, G.G. The measurement of observer agreement for categorical data. *Biometrics* **1977**, *33*, 159–174. [CrossRef] [PubMed]
14. Lussi, A.; Hellwig, E. Risk assessment and causal preventive measures. *Monogr. Oral Sci.* **2014**, *25*, 220–229. [CrossRef]
15. Lussi, A.; Megert, B.; Shellis, R.P.; Wang, X. Analysis of the erosive effect of different dietary substances and medications. *Br. J. Nutr.* **2012**, *107*, 252–262. [CrossRef]
16. Kirkpatrick, S.I.; Baranowski, T.; Subar, A.F.; Tooze, J.A.; Frongillo, E.A. Best practices for conducting and interpreting studies to validate self-report dietary assessment methods. *J. Acad. Nutr. Diet.* **2019**, *119*, 1801–1816. [CrossRef]
17. Deliens, T.; Clarys, P.; De Bourdeaudhuij, I.; Deforche, B. Determinants of eating behaviour in university students: A qualitative study using focus group discussions. *BMC Public Health* **2014**, *14*, 53. [CrossRef]
18. Keul, C.; Güth, J.F. Accuracy of full-arch digital impressions: An in vitro and in vivo comparison. *Clin. Oral Investig.* **2020**, *24*, 735–745. [CrossRef]
19. Ganss, C.; Klimek, J.; Giese, K. Dental erosion in children and adolescents—A cross-sectional and longitudinal investigation using study models. *Community Dent. Oral Epidemiol.* **2001**, *29*, 264–271. [CrossRef]
20. El Aidi, H.; Bronkhorst, E.M.; Huysmans, M.C.; Truin, G.J. Dynamics of tooth erosion in adolescents: A 3-year longitudinal study. *J. Dent.* **2010**, *38*, 131–137. [CrossRef]
21. Thakur, S.; Mathur, P. Nutrition knowledge and its relation with dietary behaviour in children and adolescents: A systematic review. *Int. J. Adolesc. Med. Health* **2021**. [CrossRef]
22. Suwalska, J.; Bogdanski, P. Social modeling and eating behavior-a narrative review. *Nutrients* **2021**, *13*, 1209. [CrossRef] [PubMed]
23. Stok, F.M.; Renner, B.; Clarys, P.; Lien, N.; Lakerveld, J.; Deliens, T. Understanding eating behavior during the transition from adolescence to young adulthood: A literature review and perspective on future research directions. *Nutrients* **2018**, *10*, 667. [CrossRef]
24. Larson, N.I.; Neumark-Sztainer, D.R.; Harnack, L.J.; Wall, M.M.; Story, M.T.; Eisenberg, M.E. Fruit and vegetable intake correlates during the transition to young adulthood. *Am. J. Prev. Med.* **2008**, *35*, 33–37. [CrossRef] [PubMed]
25. Odake, S. Sweetness intensity in low-carbonated beverages. *Biomol. Eng.* **2001**, *17*, 151–156. [CrossRef]
26. Loke, C.; Lee, J.; Sander, S.; Mei, L.; Farella, M. Factors affecting intra-oral pH—A review. *J. Oral Rehabil.* **2016**, *43*, 778–785. [CrossRef]
27. Archer, E.; Pavela, G.; Lavie, C.J. The inadmissibility of What We Eat in America and NHANES dietary data in nutrition and obesity research and the scientific formulation of national dietary guidelines. *Mayo Clin. Proc.* **2015**, *90*, 911–926. [CrossRef] [PubMed]
28. Archundia Herrera, M.C.; Chan, C.B. Narrative review of new methods for assessing food and energy intake. *Nutrients* **2018**, *10*, 1064. [CrossRef]

29. Ravelli, M.N.; Schoeller, D.A. Traditional self-reported dietary instruments are prone to inaccuracies and new approaches are needed. *Front. Nutr.* **2020**, *7*, 90. [CrossRef] [PubMed]
30. Casett, E.; Reus, J.C.; Stuginski-Barbosa, J.; Porporatti, A.L.; Carra, M.C.; Peres, M.A.; de Luca Canto, G.; Manfredini, D. Validity of different tools to assess sleep bruxism: A meta-analysis. *J. Oral Rehabil.* **2017**, *44*, 722–734. [CrossRef]

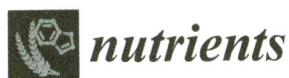

Article

How to Measure Adherence to a Mediterranean Diet in Dental Studies: Is a Short Adherence Screener Enough? A Comparative Analysis

Valentin Bartha [1,2,*], Lea Exner [2], Anna-Lisa Meyer [3], Maryam Basrai [3], Daniela Schweikert [4], Michael Adolph [4], Thomas Bruckner [5], Christian Meller [2], Johan Peter Woelber [6,†] and Diana Wolff [1,†]

1   Department for Conservative Dentistry, University Hospital of Heidelberg, Im Neuenheimer Feld 400, 69120 Heidelberg, Germany; diana.wolff@med.uni-heidelberg.de
2   Department for Conservative Dentistry, University Hospital Tuebingen, Osianderstraße 2-8, 72076 Tübingen, Germany; exner.lea@gmx.de (L.E.); christian.meller@med.uni-tuebingen.de (C.M.)
3   Institute of Nutritional Medicine, University of Hohenheim, Fruwirthstr. 12, 70599 Stuttgart, Germany; anna94.meyer@yahoo.de (A.-L.M.); m.basrai@uni-hohenheim.de (M.B.)
4   Department of Nutrition Management and Nutrition Support Team, University Hospital Tuebingen, Hoppe-Seyler-Straße, 72076 Tübingen, Germany; daniela.schweikert@med.uni-tuebingen.de (D.S.); michael.adolph@med.uni-tuebingen.de (M.A.)
5   Institute of Medical Biometry, Faculty of Medicine, University of Heidelberg, Im Neuenheimer Feld 130.3, 69120 Heidelberg, Germany; bruckner@imbi.uni-heidelberg.de
6   Department of Operative Dentistry and Periodontology, Faculty of Medicine, University of Freiburg, Hugstetter Str. 55, 79106 Freiburg, Germany; johan.woelber@uniklinik-freiburg.de
*   Correspondence: valentin.bartha@med.uni-heidelberg.de
†   These authors contributed equally to this work.

Citation: Bartha, V.; Exner, L.; Meyer, A.-L.; Basrai, M.; Schweikert, D.; Adolph, M.; Bruckner, T.; Meller, C.; Woelber, J.P.; Wolff, D. How to Measure Adherence to a Mediterranean Diet in Dental Studies: Is a Short Adherence Screener Enough? A Comparative Analysis. *Nutrients* 2022, 14, 1300. https://doi.org/10.3390/nu14061300

Academic Editor: Antoni Pons

Received: 13 February 2022
Accepted: 16 March 2022
Published: 19 March 2022
Corrected: 28 April 2022

Publisher's Note: MDPI stays neutral with regard to jurisdictional claims in published maps and institutional affiliations.

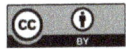

Abstract: This study aimed to evaluate the Mediterranean Diet Adherence Screener (MEDAS) in a study investigating the anti-inflammatory effect of a 6-week Mediterranean diet intervention on periodontal parameters. Data from a randomized clinical trial were analyzed for correlations between the MEDAS score and oral inflammatory parameters (bleeding on probing (BOP), gingival index (GI), and periodontal inflamed surface area (PISA)) and select nutrient intakes estimated by a food frequency questionnaire (FFQ) and a 24-h dietary recall (24dr). A mixed model, calculations of Spearman ϱ, Lin's Concordance Coefficient (CC), and Mann–Whitney U test were used for the statistical analyses. The MEDAS score was significantly negatively correlated with periodontal inflammation (BOP: CoE -0.391, $p < 0.001$; GI -0.407, $p < 0.001$; PISA -0.348, $p = 0.001$) and positively correlated with poly unsaturated fatty acids/total fat, vitamin C, and fiber intake estimates obtained from the FFQ and 24dr (ϱ 0.38–0.77). The FFQ and 24dr produced heterogeneously comparable intake results for most nutrients (CC 0–0.79, Spearman ϱ 0.16–0.65). Within the limitations of this study, the MEDAS was able to indicate nutritional habits associated with different levels of periodontal inflammation. Accordingly, the MEDAS can be a sufficient and useful diet screener in dental studies. Due to its correlation with oral inflammatory parameters, the MEDAS might also be useful in dental practice.

Keywords: dentistry; gingivitis; inflammation; Mediterranean diet; periodontology

1. Introduction

Increasing evidence has shown that the Mediterranean diet (MedD) is associated with lower morbidity and mortality and a lower likelihood of developing certain chronic diseases [1–3]. The MedD is characterized by an increased consumption of vegetables, fruits, and herbs, with fatty sea fish and olive oil as the main fat sources [4]. Caries, the most common oral disease, are mainly caused by nutritional behaviors, and an increasing number of studies have indicated that malnutrition is also an important risk factor for oral inflammatory diseases such as gingivitis and periodontitis [5–7]. However, in dentistry, there is a lack of interventional studies on this topic; consequently, there is little evidence supporting dietary-based prevention and treatment concepts [5,8]. Thus, current periodontitis therapy guidelines require further evidence for nutritional interventions [8]. In the last decade, nutritional studies in the field of periodontology have gained increasing attention after it was found that nutrition has a beneficial effect on oral inflammation. By replacing Western dietary habits with dietary concepts found in the MedD, several nutritional interventions have shown impressive results in the reduction of oral inflammation. These dietary concepts (such as a paleolithic diet, the consumption of lettuce juice, a nitrate-rich diet, and a mainly plant-based whole foods diet) were able to reduce inflammation even though the participants had higher or constant plaque values [9–12]. Our group recently investigated the MedD in a 6-week randomized clinical trial and found comparable results to the studies above [13]. The findings of that study were in accordance with a cross-sectional study that reported lower odds of periodontitis when the participants adhered to the MedD [14]. Accordingly, the MedD offers advantages both for general and oral health and should therefore be recommended to dental patients.

However, to the best of our knowledge, how to optimally and relevantly assess the diet of dental patients with regard to the MedD remains unclear. This assessment could be in regards to diet adherence or to analyze food or nutrient intake [15,16]. When the goal is to monitor general dietary habits or adherence to recommendations, short and easy evaluable assessment screeners might be sufficient, such as the Mediterranean Diet Assessment Screener (MEDAS), which covers 14 items [16,17]. Typical food groups are queried for a minimum consumption and the result is given as a score. A score of ≥ 10 has been suggested to indicate sufficient adherence to the MedD [18]. MEDAS has been recently used in numerous diet studies, and negative correlations between the MEDAS score and cardiovascular diseases (CVD), symptoms of depression, odds for mobility limitations in seniors, unhealthy anthropometric parameters, occurrence of gestational diabetes, and mortality were reported [19–24]. Moreover, the MEDAS score was positively correlated with higher levels of education, nutritional knowledge, and physical activity [25–27]. So far, no similar study has focused on periodontal inflammatory parameters. However, the MEDAS does not allow for detailed nutrient or food analyses. The 24-h diet recall (24dr) and food frequency questionnaires (FFQs) provide the ability to analyze the consumption of certain foods or nutrient intake levels. The 24dr might demand a more intense cooperation of study participants, possibly influencing adherence and the return rate. This might lower the use of the 24dr in a dental practice compared with clinical research. The results of FFQs and the 24dr have generally been shown to agree [15,28]. The assessment of nutrient intake demands detailed documentation of one's diet, with the consequent conversion into nutrient amounts per day prior to data analysis [29]. In studies with small sample sizes, data agreement between these methods, as well as differences between study groups, might be less valid [30]. Hence, a determination of diet adherence without the need for detailed nutrient analysis could be a beneficial alternative for those studies. Moreover, screeners such as the MEDAS might correlate positively or negatively with clinical dental parameters when there is an association between the investigated diet and oral inflammation. Consequently, in addition to the goal of low plaque levels, traditionally used in dental medicine [31,32], an increased screener score might be an additional goal of periodontal therapy. Monitoring diet adherence with an easy and efficient evaluation tool without the use of detailed nutrient analysis might facilitate study implementation and increase data validity.

Therefore, the present study aimed to determine the validity of the MEDAS using the framework and data of a recent study [13] that investigated the effect of a 6-week MedD intervention in patients with gingival inflammation. The MEDAS score was correlated with clinical data and nutritional parameters obtained from an FFQ and 24dr. The nutrient analysis results of the FFQ and 24dr were also analyzed for their correlation.

2. Materials and Methods

2.1. Study Design

The data used in the correlative analysis were from a clinical trial that investigated the effect of the MedD on gingivitis (Bartha et al., 2021). The trial was designed in accordance with the CONSORT statement for clinical trials (Figure 1). The study protocol was approved by the University of Tübingen Ethics Committee (745/2019BO2) and registered in the German Clinical Trials Register (DRKS 00025103).

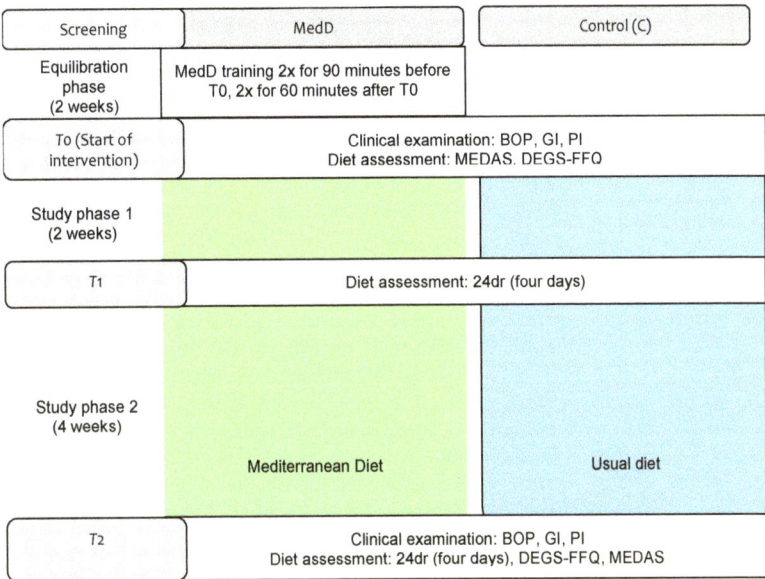

Figure 1. Study flow chart [13] PI = plaque index, GI = gingival index, BOP = bleeding on probing, PD = pocket depth, 24dr = 24-h dietary recall, FFQ = food frequency questionnaire, MEDAS = Mediterranean Diet Adherence Screener.

2.2. Inclusion Criteria

Patients were included if they met all of the following criteria: had generalized gingivitis defined as >30% of sites around the teeth exhibiting bleeding on probing (BOP) [33]; $\geq$20 present teeth; aged 18 to 49; a BMI of 18–30 kg/m^2; self-reported Western diet defined as a daily intake of processed carbohydrates, sugar, animal protein, saturated fatty acids, or other Western diet characteristics [34] elicited by verbal anamnesis.

2.3. Exclusion Criteria

Patients were excluded for any of the following reasons: periodontitis defined as a Community Periodontal Index of Treatment Needs (Ainamo et al., 1982) score > 2; smoker; severe illnesses (e.g., HIV, chronic hepatitis, cancer, illnesses of the salivary glands or the gastrointestinal tract, diabetes mellitus); pregnancy or breastfeeding; intake of antibiotics within 6 months prior to or during study; intake of anti-inflammatory drugs; treatment with medication affecting gingival bleeding; intake of probiotics; strict vegetarian, vegan, low-carb, or paleo diet; dislike or intolerance of fish, milk, or milk products; allergic to fish, fruits, or nuts; eating disorder (anorexia nervosa, bulimia, binge eating, or fasting). Those who missed more than one structured MedD training were also excluded from the study.

2.4. Patient Recruitment and Allocation

After recruitment through social media and institutional emails and flyers, applicants were comprehensively informed about the study and gave written consent. Eligibility screening was conducted at the Department of Conservative Dentistry, University Hospital Tübingen, Germany.

The included participants were pseudonymized and allocated to either the Mediterranean diet group (MedDG) or control group (CG) using minimalization according to gender and age (JMP, SAS Institute, Heidelberg, Germany).

2.5. Diet Intervention

Aiming to harmonize the clinical conditions before the start of the intervention, all participants continued their usual diet for the first 2 weeks. Furthermore, at-home dental care was equalized by asking all participants to refrain from using interdental cleaning tools and mouthwashes [11,13]. During the subsequent 6 weeks, the MedDG changed their diet to conform to a MedD. They also participated in four nutrition classes in groups of up to five participants: two sessions before starting the MedD and two meetings during the intervention period (Figure 1). Further information can be found in [13].

The Institute of Nutritional Medicine of the University of Hohenheim, Germany, provided the diet training material.

The nutrition classes were conducted by a dietician and a dentist who were specialized in the field of nutrient medicine. The first session consisted of a short lecture and group discussion on the background of the MedD and its health effects, including information on the MedD food pyramid and meal planning. Training material was distributed, and ten training tasks were set such as online research and grocery shopping; recommendations for books and apps were also given. The second session repeated much of the information and discussed selected training tasks, the MedD when eating out, canteen and restaurant menus and their agreement with the MedD, and easy preparations of MedD snacks and meals. The third session included a discussion of the first experiences with the MedD and a lecture about fat and fatty acids. Also discussed were MedD recipes and how to prepare typical Western diet meals using MedD ingredients. In the fourth session, there were further discussions about adhering to the MedD when eating out and implementation difficulties.

2.6. Diet Assessment and Clinical Examinations

Diet was evaluated at three time points: at week 2, near the start of the MedD intervention (*T0*); 2 weeks after *T0* (*T1*), and at the end of the dietary intervention, 6 weeks after *T0* (*T2*). The assessment tools used were the MEDAS, the German Health Interview and Examination Survey for Adults Food Frequency Questionnaire (DEGS-FFQ, Robert Koch Institute, Berlin, Germany), and the German Society of Nutrition 24-h dietary recall (24dr). The MEDAS is a 14-item questionnaire that queries the habitual intake of 12 typical MedD food components. The items are scored as 0 for nonadherence or 1 for adherence to the particular component [17]. A value of 10 or greater indicates MedD adherence. The DEGS-FFQ consists of 53 food items and is a reflection of one's daily intake frequency during the previous 4 weeks. For each component, consumption frequency is answered as: one serving per month; two to three servings per month; one to two, three to four, or five to six servings per week; or one, two, three, four to five, or more than five servings per day [15]. The daily nutrient intake can then be calculated based on reference tables. For the 24dr, participants reported their food consumption and portion size at each time point.

The assessments were filled out close to each time point.

T0: MEDAS and DEGS-FFQ; *T1*: 24dr; *T2*: 24dr, DEGS-FFQ, and MEDAS

At *T0* and *T2*, clinical examinations were conducted by a blinded examiner. The clinical examination used is described in Bartha et al. (2021).

2.7. Study Outcomes

The primary outcome was the correlation of the MEDAS score with the oral inflammatory parameters BOP, GI, and PISA. In addition, the MEDAS score was analyzed for correlations with the following nutrient intakes as evaluated by the 24dr and DEGS-FFQ: relative proportion of polyunsaturated fatty acids (PUFA) to total fat (PUFA/fat), vitamin C, and dietary fiber. The 24dr and DEGS-FFQ results at *T2* were compared for daily intake levels of total energy (E), carbohydrates (CH), protein (P), fat (F), PUFA, saturated fatty acids (SFA), cholesterol (CHOL), glucose (GLUC), fructose (FRUC), alcohol (ALC), vitamin C (ASC), vitamin E (TOC), carotin (CAR), and fiber (FB). Additionally, for each tool, the daily nutrient intake levels were compared between the two study groups at *T2*. The results were descriptively analyzed regarding their intragroup comparison results. Changes in the MEDAS score between *T0* and *T2* were calculated and compared between the two groups.

2.8. Statistical Methods

The DEGS-FFQ data were evaluated according to the recommendations of the Robert Koch Institute. The clinical data and the nutrient analysis data obtained from the DEGS-FFQ and 24dr were analyzed using Ebis Pro (University of Hohenheim, Stuttgart, Germany). Correlations between MEDAS and clinical parameters including all timepoints were calculated using a mixed model for data with repeated measures [35]. Due to the lack of a normal distribution (Anderson–Darling test $p < 0.05$), the *T2* intergroup comparisons were performed using the nonparametric Mann–Whitney U test. Lin´s Concordance correlation coefficient (CC) and the Spearman rank correlation between the 24dr and DEGS-FFQ was used to assess correlations between the 24dr and DEGS-FFQ. Additionally, Spearman rank correlation was used to assess correlations between the MEDAS score and nutrient intake. SAS 9.4WIN (SAS Institute, Cary, NC, USA) was used for calculation of the mixed model, Excel 16.57 (Microsoft, Redmond, WA, USA) with Real Statistics Using Excel Resource Pack for Mac, Release 8.1 (https://www.real-statistics.com, accessed on 14 March 2022) was used for calculation of CC, and JMP16.0 (SAS Institute, Cary, NC, USA) for all other statistical analyses.

3. Results

Of the 42 participants who met the inclusion criteria, 37 completed the study; 17 men and 20 women (Figure 2), with no difference in mean age between MedDG and CG. All participants completed the MEDAS and DEGS-FFQ at *T0* and *T2*, except one missing MEDAS at *T2*. In total, 24 participants completed the 24dr at *T2* (Table 1). The clinical data from our previous study are presented in Table 2. Between *T1* and *T2*, there were statistically significant improvements in the BOP, GI, and PISA in the MedDG. The plaque values did not change in either group, while the MEDAS score significantly improved in the MedDG (Table 2). For further details see [13].

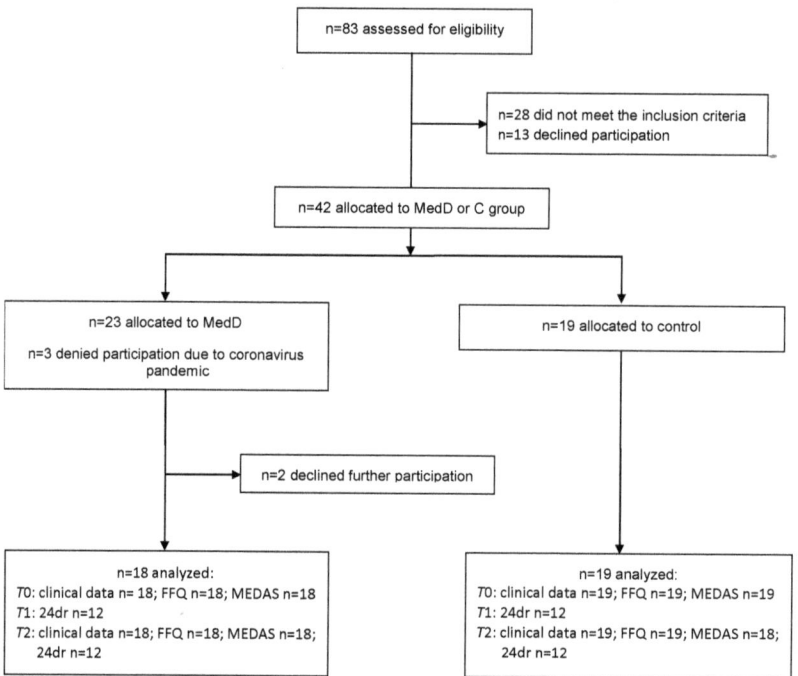

Figure 2. CONSORT flow diagram, modified according to [13], 24dr = 24-h dietary recall, FFQ = food frequency questionnaire, MEDAS = Mediterranean Diet Adherence Screener.

Table 1. Baseline characteristics of MedDG and CG.

	MedDG	CG	Intergroup *p*-Value
Men	10	7	0.2536
Women	8	12	
Age (years)	32.71 ± 8.87	29.21 ± 7.17	0.198

Note: MedDG = Mediterranean diet group; CG = Control group. The data are from [13].

Table 2. Clinical data with mean values and standard deviations, * paired *t*-test, PI = plaque index, GI = gingival index, BOP = bleeding on probing, PD = pocket depth, PISA = periodontal inflamed surface area.

	T1		T2			
	MedDG, T1	CG, T1	MedDG, T2	CG, T2	MedDG T1-T2 Intra *p*-Value *	CG T1-T2 Intra *p*-Value *
PI	1.51 ± 0.21	1.37 ± 0.38	1.49 ± 0.24	1.39 ± 0.24	0.560	0.823
GI	1.3 ± 0.25	1.11 ± 0.42	0.99 ± 0.22	0.97 ± 0.27	<0.001	0.093
BOP [%]	51.00 ± 14.65	43.21 ± 14.25	39.93 ± 13.74	39.74 ± 11.0	<0.001	0.151
PD [mm]	2.26 ± 0.18	2.29 ± 0.18	2.36 ± 0.17	2.36 ± 0.18	0.008	0.044
PISA [mm^2]	616.33 ± 201.39	528.94 ± 173.48	512.02 ± 205.83	514.26 ± 148.79	0.004	0.589
MEDAS Score	5.55 ± 3.01	6.52 ± 2.17	11.89 ± 1.90	7.22 ± 2.88	<0.001	0.310

Note: The data are from [13].

3.1. The MEDAS Score Was Negatively Correlated with Periodontal Inflammation and Positively Correlated with the Intake of MedD-Associated Nutrients

Analyzing all available data of MEDAS and the clinical examinations (T0 and T2), the mixed model revealed statistically significant negative correlations between the MEDAS score and BOP (correlation estimate (CoE) = −0.391, $p < 0.001$), GI (−0.407, $p < 0.001$), PISA (−0.348, $p = 0.001$), and PI (−0.23, $p = 0.045$) (Figure 3). Furthermore, using Spearman correlation analysis, the MEDAS score was positively correlated with the intake results of both detailed assessment methods (FFQ and 24dr at *T2*) for dietary fiber, vitamin C, and the relative fraction of PUFA in the daily total fat intake. The results were statistically significant for all correlations ($p < 0.01$) except 24dr vitamin C vs. MEDAS ($p = 0.069$) (Figure 4).

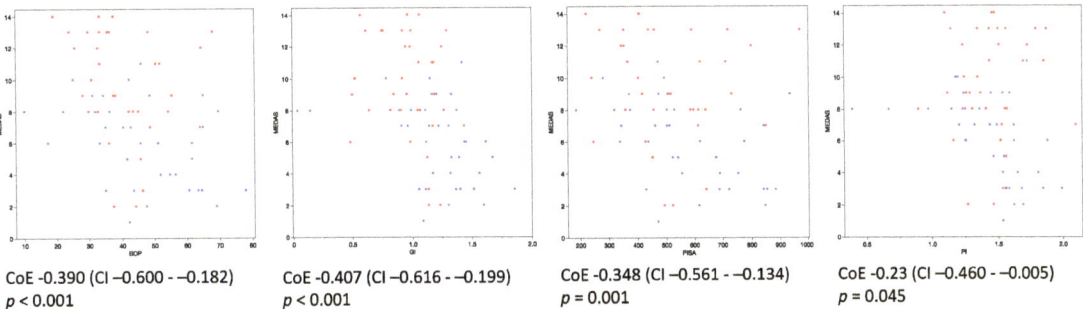

CoE -0.390 (CI −0.600 - −0.182)
$p < 0.001$

CoE -0.407 (CI −0.616 - −0.199)
$p < 0.001$

CoE -0.348 (CI −0.561 - −0.134)
$p = 0.001$

CoE -0.23 (CI −0.460 - −0.005)
$p = 0.045$

Figure 3. Correlation between the MEDAS score and clinical parameters (BOP, GI, PISA and PI). Scatterplots; data from *T0* 0 (blue) and *T2* (red) for both groups (*n* = 73). MEDAS = Mediterranean Diet Adherence Screener, BOP = bleeding on probing, GI = gingival index, PISA = periodontal inflammation surface area, PI = plaque index, CoE = correlation estimate, CI = 95% confidence interval.

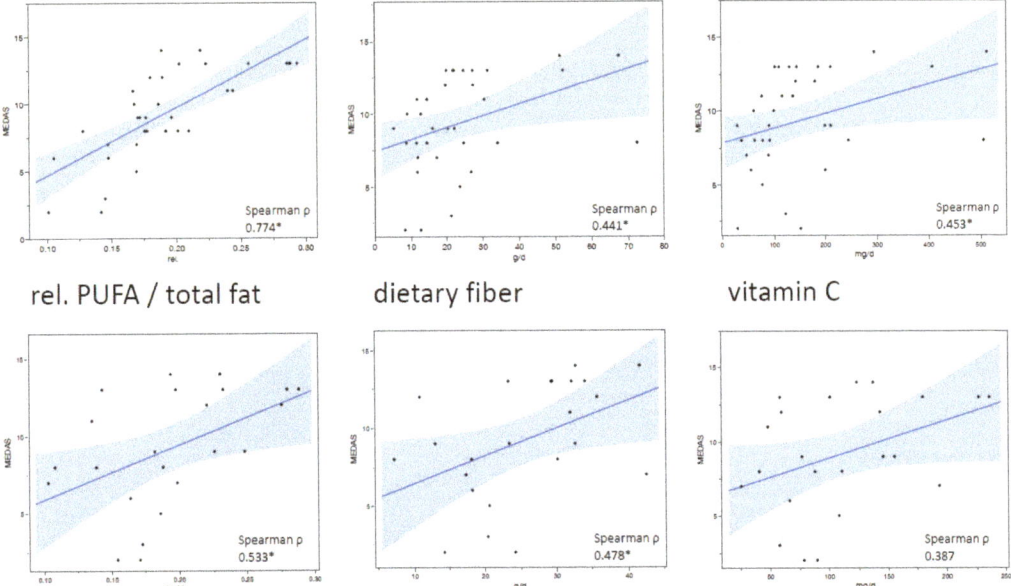

Figure 4. Correlations between the MEDAS score and MedD-associated nutrients. Scatterplots with regression lines and 95% confidence intervals; data from *T2* for both groups (FFQ, *n* = 36; 24dr, *n* = 23). * $p < 0.05$, MEDAS = Mediterranean Diet Adherence Screener, PUFA = polyunsaturated fatty acids.

Nutrients **2022**, *14*, 1300

3.2. DEGS-FFQ and 24dr Nutrient Intake Results Were Heterogeneous Comparable

Calculating the concordance coefficient, the 24dr and DEGS-FFQ results showed values between 0.00 and 0.79, most pronounced for CHO (0.79). The additionally calculated nonparametric Spearman ϱ displayed values from 0.16–0.65 with values less than 0.20 for CH and GLUC (Figure 5).

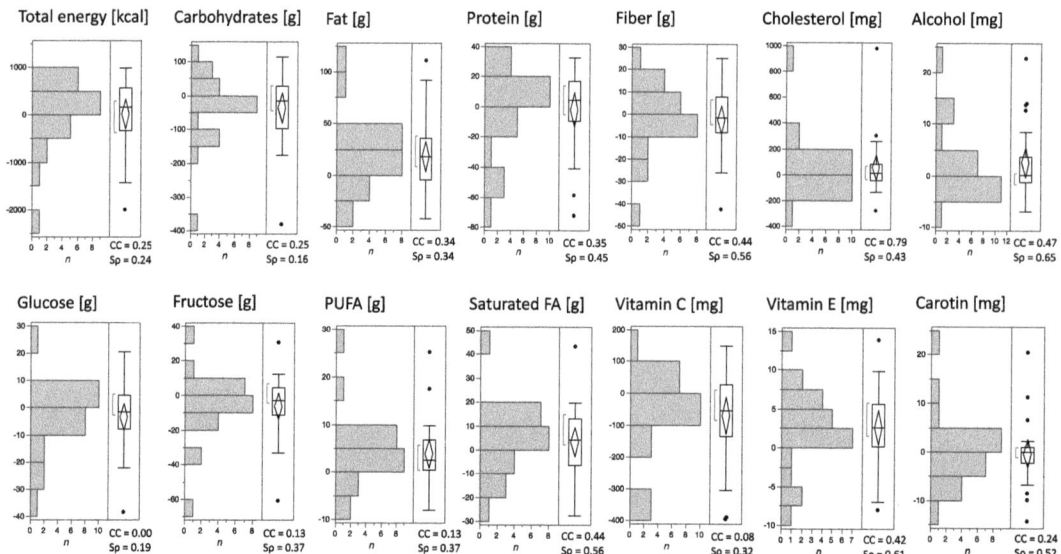

Figure 5. Concordances and differences between 24dr and DEGS-FFQ nutrient intake estimates for total energy, certain nutrients, and dietary fiber. Values of the calculated concordance and Spearman correlation; the data are from both groups at *T2* (n = 24). PUFA = polyunsaturated fatty acids, FA = fatty acids, n = number, 24dr = 24 h dietary recall, FFQ = DEGS Food Frequency Questionnaire.

At *T2*, there were significant differences in daily nutrient intake levels between the two groups for several nutrients. By comparing the statistical results of each assessment method, matching significant results were found for dietary fiber and all macronutrients except carbohydrates, which was significantly higher in the CG in the 24dr analysis. Similarly, the CG cholesterol intake was significantly higher than the MedDG in the 24dr analysis. The micronutrient and alcohol intake of the MedDG was significantly higher than that of the CG in the FFQ analysis (Table 3).

Table 3. Intergroup comparisons at *T2* from both assessment methods. Mean values and standard deviations are given; *p*-values from the Mann–Whitney U test. Matching results of intragroup comparisons are marked (+). The Spearman rank correlation and concordance correlation coefficient (CC) is shown for the 24dr and FFQ values of both groups.

	MedD Group		C Group		24dr Inter-*p*-Value *	FFQ Inter-*p*-Value *	Matching Results Regarding Both Intragroup Comparisons	Spearman ϱ: 24dr and FFQ	CC: 24dr and FFQ
	24dr (*n* = 12)	FFQ (*n* = 18)	24dr (*n* = 12)	FFQ (*n* = 19)					
Energy [kcal/d]	1647.21 ± 394.61	1769.11 ± 650.52	1963.00 ± 474.25	1785.46 ± 830.00	0.112	0.885		0.24	0.25 (−0.11–0.56)
Total carbohydrates [g]	160.03 ± 35.11	219.53 ± 74.74	210.39 ± 52.30	223.29 ± 146.51	0.030	0.507	+	0.16	0.25 (−0.03–0.49)
Total fat [g]	70.13 ± 24.65	52.83 ± 29.08	84.96 ± 44.54	64.84 ± 24.63	0.312	0.215		0.34	0.34 (0.01–0.60)
Total protein [g]	71.70 ± 19.90	82.06 ± 32.61	72.03 ± 18.51	65.04 ± 22.34	0.977	0.157	+	0.45	0.35 (−0.01–0.63)
Fibre [g]	29.29 ± 8.28	33.87 ± 15.24	20.40 ± 8.29	20.45 ± 17.05	0.026	0.003	+	0.56	0.44 (0.13–0.67)
Cholesterol	184.55 ± 102.15	205.10 ± 118.70	481.52 ± 609.69	341.62 ± 340.60	0.002	0.090		0.43	0.79 (0.69–0.86)
Glucose [g]	12.98 ± 9.90	18.80 ± 8.63	15.57 ± 5.31	16.36 ± 13.15	0.125	0.312	+	0.19	0.00 (−0.28–0.27)
Fructose [g]	16.38 ± 4.85	26.35 ± 12.75	19.46 ± 9.77	21.55 ± 21.73	0.624	0.126	+	0.37	0.13 (−0.15–0.38)
Polyunsaturated fatty acids [g]	15.16 ± 5.65	11.37 ± 5.22	14.08 ± 9.78	9.93 ± 4.28	0.370	0.471	+	0.34	0.32 (0.02–0.56)
Satured fatty acids [g]	21.74 ± 6.77	20.32 ± 13.06	35.38 ± 17.52	29.73 ± 11.73	0.005	0.046	+	0.56	0.44 (0.07–0.70)
Total alcohol [g]	10.60 ± 7.51	8.48 ± 5.28	6.91 ± 8.65	3.84 ± 4.05	0.126	0.020		0.65	0.47 (0.16–0.69)
Vitamin C [mg]	129.79 ± 62.71	228.47 ± 123.64	89.75 ± 45.86	128.33 ± 129.74	0.126	0.009		0.32	0.08 (−0.16–0.32)
Vitamine E [mg]	15.15 ± 5.35	12.57 ± 5.93	11.50 ± 3.09	8.82 ± 5.06	0.133	0.035		0.61	0.42 (0.08–0.67)
Carotin [mg]	6.99 ± 5.17	9.37 ± 5.81	5.32 ± 6.23	3.41 ± 2.43	0.285	0.002		0.52	0.24 (−0.17–0.58)

Note: MedDG = Mediterranean diet group, CG = control group, 24dr = 24-h dietary recall, FFQ = DEGS-Food Frequency Questionnaire, CC = concordance coefficient, * by U test.

4. Discussion

This study aimed to evaluate correlations between the MEDAS score and oral inflammatory parameters after a 6-week Mediterranean diet intervention and its comparability with the results of the DEGS-FFQ and 24dr. We found that the MEDAS score showed significant negative correlations with all assessed oral inflammatory parameters (GI, BOP, and PISA). The negative correlation was weaker, but still significant, between the MEDAS score and PI. The MEDAS score showed significant positive correlations with the intake levels of PUFA/total fat and fiber for both of the more detailed assessment methods. There were comparable values for nutrient intake as assessed by the 24dr and DEGS-FFQ.

Although the MEDAS has been evaluated for correlations with many medical and anthropometric parameters, no study has investigated its ability to assess MedD adherence within a diet intervention study in patients with gingivitis. The significant negative correlations between the MEDAS score and oral inflammatory parameters indicate the following: (i) adherence to the MedD is associated with decreased gingival inflammation and (ii) the MEDAS can be used as a dietary screening tool that can be related to the level of gingival inflammation. This tool can be recommended in research and in clinical practice, since it is easy to use by patients, and instantly interpreted by users. An explanation for the observed weak but significant correlation between the MEDAS score and PI could be that a higher adherence to a healthy diet might be associated with a higher awareness of healthy habits in general, as reported in some recent studies [25,27,36]. Alternatively, it might reflect a lower level of biofilm formation, as was seen in studies looking at sugar restriction [37,38]. In dentistry, plaque scores are traditionally used to monitor patients´ adherence to anti-inflammatory therapeutic concepts [31,32,39]. Investigating the diet in clinical studies and including dietary counseling in therapeutic concepts both require the evaluation of diet adherence. Thus, an easy evaluable form like the MEDAS might be suitable for these applications. Our results confirm the findings of Altun et al. (2021). In their cross-sectional study, they found a lower risk for periodontal disease when adherence to the MedD was increased, and they used the MEDAS as an evaluation tool [14].

The observed positive correlations between the MEDAS score and the FFQ and 24dr intake estimates for PUFA/total fat, vitamin C, and dietary fiber are comparable with the results of previous validation studies of the German and English versions of the MEDAS [17,29]. Additionally, recent studies have used the MEDAS to assess MedD adherence or adherence to healthy diets in general. In many cases, a lower MEDAS score was correlated with the presence of disease and an unhealthy lifestyle. It also correlated with the plasma metabolome profile and metabolic signature, which were able to predict the risk for CVD incidents in patients of the "Prevention with Mediterranean Diet" (PREDIMED) study [40]. In patients with depression, the occurrence of symptoms was negatively associated with the MEDAS score [23,41]. Zhao et al. found a reduced occurrence of gestational diabetes with higher MEDAS scores and with increased olive oil and pistachio consumption [24]. In summary, our results, together with those of Altun et al., are in line with previous studies that have investigated the correlations between the MEDAS score (and therefore MedD adherence) and parameters of numerous other diseases. Some studies additionally evaluated the relation between low consumption of certain food groups and lower MEDAS scores. In these studies, mostly olive oil, nuts, seafood, legumes, wine, and vegetables were the reduced food groups and the consumption of red meat and carbonated beverages was increased [23,27].

We used the DEGS-FFQ and a 24dr for the analysis of food groups and nutrient intake estimation. The nutrient and energy intake estimates from the 24dr and DEGS-FFQ at *T*2 showed significant differences for all parameters except for PUFA, SFA, ASC, and TOC. Concordance analysis revealed values ranging between 0 and 0.79. Additionally, the nonparametric Spearman correlation coefficient ranged from 0.15 to 0.65, with most values above 0.30. These results are comparable to those of validation studies of the DEGS-FFQ and other FFQs, with correlation coefficients ranging between 0.14 and 0.90 [15,28,42–44].

Nutrients **2022**, *14*, 1300

Haftenberger concluded that in cases where there are differences between the FFQ and 24dr, there is no evidence indicating which one reflects the most realistic food consumption.

In general, energy (and therefore nutrient intake) seems to be underestimated by both the 24dr and the FFQ. This underestimation has been shown in validation studies using the double-labeled water technique [45–47] and in comparisons of estimated sodium intake and sodium excretion in 24-h urine samples [48]. Furthermore, underestimation seems to be more pronounced with increasing BMI, especially at BMI values $\geq$30 [47,49]. We additionally compared the two methods regarding their ability to produce matching results when the estimated *T2* nutrient intake was tested for statistically significant differences. Intragroup comparisons of the 24dr and DEGS-FFQ showed matching results for all macronutrients except total carbohydrates and cholesterol. Differences between the groups for micronutrients and total alcohol were shown by only one of the two assessment methods. Regarding micronutrients, all estimated differences were found to be significant in the DEGS-FFQ analysis only. This again underlines the question as to which method produces the more accurate result. As the 24dr captures the diet for only one day, the results could be susceptible to intake fluctuations, especially when it is used to display diet for a longer time period. This might also be the case if 24drs are used for more than one day. For FFQs, inaccuracies can arise because individual foods are grouped into food groups, and participants have to remember a period of 4 or more weeks. The evaluated food groups might contain foods with variable nutrient contents [50]. Thus, both tools have advantages and disadvantages. The bias resulting from the short time period covered by the 24dr could be mitigated by increasing the number of 24dr days within the study period. However, more days requires a higher degree of participant compliance, again leading to possible bias.

When monitoring diet adherence is the only goal, we find the MEDAS to be an easy to use tool for monitoring MedD adherence in a dental study. European scientific societies for periodontal diseases and caries recommend the inclusion of dietary counseling in therapeutic concepts [33]. The S3 treatment guidelines for stage I–III periodontitis suggest dietary counseling for the control of HbA1c in patients suffering from diabetes mellitus [8]. Both publications mention the need for further randomized controlled trials on this topic. Future studies should try to confirm the correlation of easy evaluation screening tools such as the MEDAS with oral inflammatory parameters to provide adherence evaluation tools for use in clinical research and clinical practice. Although the diet affects inflammation [9–13], the common dental therapeutic goal of low plaque values may be oversimplified because it does not address possible malnutrition, which can also lead to other nonoral diseases. Plaque scores are regularly discussed with patients and are used to motivate patients to increase oral hygiene procedures. Plaque value documentation might be supplemented with dietary scores such as the MEDAS. Like the plaque score, a dietary score could serve as a motivational approach to increase and monitor patients' adherence to healthy diets, such as the MedD. In the context of a study with low participant numbers, an FFQ or a 24dr might be a supplement to the MEDAS, because these tools give at least an overview of the participants' food and nutrient intake. In the current study, comparable results for the two methods were found, implicating a sufficient reflection of dietary behavior. The lower return rate of the 24dr might indicate that the FFQ was more acceptable. Future studies should evaluate whether a 24dr or an FFQ are applicable in digital forms, such as a smartphone app.

Our study had some limitations. The main limitation was the low number of participants, which decreased the statistical power of the FFQ and 24dr analysis. The reason for the low number of participants was that the main outcome parameter was the percentage of BOP; hence, the calculated number of participants was based on a predicted change in this parameter. Another limitation was that at the beginning of the study, the FFQ and 24dr had to be filled out at different time points. The 24dr was used to monitor diet adherence in the MedDG during the first 2 weeks and during the final week of the intervention. This schedule limited the number of comparable FFQs and 24drs because the tools could only be compared at the final time point. Moreover, not all participants returned or filled out their 24dr at the end of the study, leading to an even lower number of analyzable cases. This might have resulted from decreasing motivation towards the end of the study and reflected that a 24dr demands a more intense cooperation.

5. Conclusions

In this study, the MEDAS was sufficiently able to monitor adherence to a Mediterranean diet throughout the study period. The MEDAS score was negatively correlated with the oral inflammatory parameters BOP, GI, and PISA, but was positively correlated with nutrient intake levels as assessed by both the FFQ and 24dr. These findings indicate that in situations where diet adherence (but not nutrient intake assessment) is concerned, the MEDAS is a suitable and easy evaluation tool for use in dental practice. The MEDAS score was correlated with the observed reduction of gingival inflammation in a MedD intervention.

Author Contributions: All authors contributed substantially through drafting, data interpretation, and critical revision of the paper. L.E. recruited and examined the participants; V.B., M.B., C.M., L.E. and J.P.W. conceived the study design; D.S. and V.B. conducted the Mediterranean diet group training and designed the didactic concept, supported by M.B. and T.B.; V.B. and L.E. analyzed the data; M.A. supported the diet group training; A.-L.M. and L.E. analyzed the nutritional data; V.B. wrote the manuscript with support from J.P.W. and D.W. All authors have read and agreed to the published version of the manuscript.

Funding: This research received no external funding.

Institutional Review Board Statement: The study was conducted according to the guidelines of the Declaration of Helsinki. The study protocol was approved by the University of Tübingen Ethics Committee (745/2019BO2) and is registered in DRKS (00025103). All participants provided written informed consent before participation.

Informed Consent Statement: Informed consent was obtained from all participants involved in the study.

Data Availability Statement: The data that support the findings of this study are available from the corresponding author upon reasonable request.

Conflicts of Interest: All authors declare that they have no conflict of interest.

References

1. Dinu, M.; Pagliai, G.; Casini, A.; Sofi, F. Mediterranean diet and multiple health outcomes: An umbrella review of meta-analyses of observational studies and randomised trials. *Eur. J. Clin. Nutr.* **2018**, *72*, 30–43. [CrossRef] [PubMed]
2. Machowicz, A.; Hall, I.; de Pablo, P.; Rauz, S.; Richards, A.; Higham, J.; Poveda-Gallego, A.; Imamura, F.; Bowman, S.J.; Barone, F.; et al. Mediterranean diet and risk of Sjögren's syndrome. *Clin. Exp. Rheumatol.* **2020**, *38* (Suppl. 126), 216–221.
3. Sofi, F.; Macchi, C.; Abbate, R.; Gensini, G.F.; Casini, A. Mediterranean diet and health status: An updated meta-analysis and a proposal for a literature-based adherence score. *Public Health Nutr.* **2014**, *17*, 2769–2782. [CrossRef] [PubMed]
4. Willett, W.C.; Sacks, F.; Trichopoulou, A.; Drescher, G.; Ferro-Luzzi, A.; Helsing, E.; Trichopoulos, D. Mediterranean diet pyramid: A cultural model for healthy eating. *Am. J. Clin. Nutr.* **1995**, *61*, 1402S–1406S. [CrossRef] [PubMed]
5. Chapple, I.L.C.; Bouchard, P.; Cagetti, M.G.; Campus, G.; Carra, M.-C.; Cocco, F.; Nibali, L.; Hujoel, P.; Laine, M.L.; Lingström, P.; et al. Interaction of lifestyle, behaviour or systemic diseases with dental caries and periodontal diseases: Consensus report of group 2 of the joint EFP/ORCA workshop on the boundaries between caries and periodontal diseases. *J. Clin. Periodontol.* **2017**, *44* (Suppl. 18), S39–S51. [CrossRef] [PubMed]
6. Hujoel, P. Dietary Carbohydrates and Dental-Systemic Diseases. *J. Dent. Res.* **2009**, *88*, 490–502. [CrossRef]
7. Woelber, J.P.; Tennert, C. Chapter 13: Diet and Periodontal Diseases. *Monogr. Oral Sci.* **2020**, *28*, 125–133. [CrossRef]
8. Sanz, M.; Herrera, D.; Kebschull, M.; Chapple, I.; Jepsen, S.; Berglundh, T.; Sculean, A.; Tonetti, M.S.; Aass, A.M.; Aimetti, M.; et al. Treatment of stage I-III periodontitis-The EFP S3 level clinical practice guideline. *J. Clin. Periodontol.* **2020**, *47* (Suppl. 22), 4–60. [CrossRef]
9. Baumgartner, S.; Imfeld, T.; Schicht, O.; Rath, C.; Persson, R.E.; Persson, G.R. The Impact of the Stone Age Diet on Gingival Conditions in the Absence of Oral Hygiene. *J. Periodontol.* **2009**, *80*, 759–768. [CrossRef]

10. Jockel-Schneider, Y.; Goßner, S.K.; Petersen, N.; Stölzel, P.; Hägele, F.; Schweiggert, R.M.; Haubitz, I.; Eigenthaler, M.; Carle, R.; Schlagenhauf, U. Stimulation of the nitrate-nitrite-NO-metabolism by repeated lettuce juice consumption decreases gingival inflammation in periodontal recall patients: A randomized, double-blinded, placebo-controlled clinical trial. *J. Clin. Periodontol.* **2016**, *43*, 603–608. [CrossRef] [PubMed]

11. Woelber, J.P.; Gärtner, M.; Breuninger, L.; Anderson, A.; König, D.; Hellwig, E.; Al-Ahmad, A.; Vach, K.; Dötsch, A.; Ratka-Krüger, P.; et al. The influence of an anti-inflammatory diet on gingivitis. A randomized controlled trial. *J. Clin. Periodontol.* **2019**, *46*, 481–490. [CrossRef]

12. Woelber, J.P.; Bremer, K.; Vach, K.; König, D.; Hellwig, E.; Ratka-Krüger, P.; Al-Ahmad, A.; Tennert, C. An oral health optimized diet can reduce gingival and periodontal inflammation in humans—A randomized controlled pilot study. *BMC Oral Health* **2016**, *17*, 28. [CrossRef]

13. Bartha, V.; Exner, L.; Schweikert, D.; Woelber, J.P.; Vach, K.; Meyer, A.; Basrai, M.; Bischoff, S.C.; Meller, C.; Wolff, D. Effect of the Mediterranean diet on gingivitis. A randomized controlled trial. *J. Clin. Periodontol.* **2021**, *49*, 111–122. [CrossRef]

14. Altun, E.; Walther, C.; Borof, K.; Petersen, E.; Lieske, B.; Kasapoudis, D.; Jalilvand, N.; Beikler, T.; Jagemann, B.; Zyriax, B.-C.; et al. Association between Dietary Pattern and Periodontitis-A Cross-Sectional Study. *Nutrients* **2021**, *13*, 4167. [CrossRef]

15. Haftenberger, M.; Heuer, T.; Heidemann, C.; Kube, F.; Krems, C.; Mensink, G.B. Relative validation of a food frequency questionnaire for national health and nutrition monitoring. *Nutr. J.* **2010**, *9*, 36. [CrossRef]

16. Schröder, H.; Fitó, M.; Estruch, R.; Martínez-González, M.A.; Corella, D.; Salas-Salvadó, J.; Lamuela-Raventós, R.; Ros, E.; Salaverría, I.; Fiol, M.; et al. A Short Screener Is Valid for Assessing Mediterranean Diet Adherence among Older Spanish Men and Women. *J. Nutr.* **2011**, *141*, 1140–1145. [CrossRef]

17. Papadaki, A.; Johnson, L.; Toumpakari, Z.; England, C.; Rai, M.; Toms, S.; Penfold, C.; Zazpe, I.; Martínez-González, M.A.; Feder, G. Validation of the English Version of the 14-Item Mediterranean Diet Adherence Screener of the PREDIMED Study, in People at High Cardiovascular Risk in the UK. *Nutrients* **2018**, *10*, 138. [CrossRef]

18. Vieira, L.M.; Gottschall, C.B.A.; Vinholes, D.B.; Martinez-Gonzalez, M.A.; Marcadenti, A. Translation and cross-cultural adaptation of 14-item Mediterranean Diet Adherence Screener and low-fat diet adherence questionnaire. *Clin. Nutr. ESPEN* **2020**, *39*, 180–189. [CrossRef]

19. Abu-Saad, K.; Endevelt, R.; Goldsmith, R.; Shimony, T.; Nitsan, L.; Shahar, D.R.; Keinan-Boker, L.; Ziv, A.; Kalter-Leibovici, O. Adaptation and predictive utility of a Mediterranean diet screener score. *Clin. Nutr.* **2019**, *38*, 2928–2935. [CrossRef]

20. Ballesteros, J.-M.; Struijk, E.A.; Rodríguez-Artalejo, F.; López-García, E. Mediterranean diet and risk of falling in community-dwelling older adults. *Clin. Nutr.* **2020**, *39*, 276–281. [CrossRef]

21. Giacalone, D.; Frøst, M.B.; Rodríguez-Pérez, C. Reported Changes in Dietary Habits During the COVID-19 Lockdown in the Danish Population: The Danish COVIDiet Study. *Front. Nutr.* **2020**, *7*, 592112. [CrossRef]

22. Jacobs, D.R.; Petersen, K.; Svendsen, K.; Ros, E.; Sloan, C.B.; Steffen, L.M.; Tapsell, L.C.; Kris-Etherton, P. Considerations to facilitate a US study that replicates PREDIMED. *Metab. -Clin. Exp.* **2018**, *85*, 361–367. [CrossRef]

23. Young, C.L.; Mohebbi, M.; Staudacher, H.; Berk, M.; Jacka, F.N.; O'Neil, A. Assessing the feasibility of an m-Health intervention for changing diet quality and mood in individuals with depression: The My Food & Mood program. *Int. Rev. Psychiatry* **2021**, *33*, 266–279. [CrossRef]

24. Zhao, L.; Zhang, P.; Zheng, Q.; Deka, A.; Choudhury, R.; Rastogi, S. Does a MediDiet with additional extra virgin olive oil (EVOO) and pistachios reduce the incidence of gestational diabetes? *Endocr. Pract.* **2021**, *28*, 135–141. [CrossRef]

25. Bottcher, M.R.; Marincic, P.Z.; Nahay, K.L.; Baerlocher, B.E.; Willis, A.W.; Park, J.; Gaillard, P.; Greene, M.W. Nutrition knowledge and Mediterranean diet adherence in the southeast United States: Validation of a field-based survey instrument. *Appetite* **2017**, *111*, 166–176. [CrossRef]

26. Cobo-Cuenca, A.I.; Garrido-Miguel, M.; Soriano-Cano, A.; Ferri-Morales, A.; Martínez-Vizcaíno, V.; Martín-Espinosa, N.M. Adherence to the Mediterranean Diet and Its Association with Body Composition and Physical Fitness in Spanish University Students. *Nutrients* **2019**, *11*, 2830. [CrossRef]

27. Mieziene, B.; Emeljanovas, A.; Fatkulina, N.; Stukas, R. Dietary Pattern and Its Correlates among Lithuanian Young Adults: Mediterranean Diet Approach. *Nutrients* **2020**, *12*, 2025. [CrossRef]

28. Pala, V.; Sieri, S.; Palli, D.; Salvini, S.; Berrino, F.; Bellegotti, M.; Frasca, G.; Tumino, R.; Sacerdote, C.; Fiorini, L.; et al. Diet in the Italian Epic Cohorts: Presentation of Data and Methodological Issues. *Tumori* **2003**, *89*, 594–607. [CrossRef]

29. Hebestreit, K.; Yahiaoui-Doktor, M.; Engel, C.; Vetter, W.; Siniatchkin, M.; Erickson, N.; Halle, M.; Kiechle, M.; Bischoff, S.C. Validation of the German version of the Mediterranean Diet Adherence Screener (MEDAS) questionnaire. *BMC Cancer* **2017**, *17*, 341. [CrossRef]

30. Lenth, R.V. Statistical power calculations. *J. Anim. Sci.* **2007**, *85*, E24–E29. [CrossRef]

31. Axelsson, P.; Lindhe, J. The significance of maintenance care in the treatment of periodontal disease. *J. Clin. Periodontol.* **1981**, *8*, 281–294. [CrossRef]

32. Reiniger, A.P.P.; Maier, J.; Wikesjö, U.M.E.; Moreira, C.H.C.; Kantorski, K.Z. Correlation between dental plaque accumulation and gingival health in periodontal maintenance patients using short or extended personal oral hygiene intervals. *J. Clin. Periodontol.* **2021**, *48*, 834–842. [CrossRef]

33. Chapple, I.L.C.; Mealey, B.L.; Van Dyke, T.E.; Bartold, P.M.; Dommisch, H.; Eickholz, P.; Geisinger, M.L.; Genco, R.J.; Glogauer, M.; Goldstein, M.; et al. Periodontal health and gingival diseases and conditions on an intact and a reduced periodontium: Consensus report of workgroup 1 of the 2017 World Workshop on the Classification of Periodontal and Peri-Implant Diseases and Conditions. *J. Periodontol.* **2018**, *89*, S74–S84. [CrossRef]

34. Cena, H.; Calder, P.C. Defining a Healthy Diet: Evidence for The Role of Contemporary Dietary Patterns in Health and Disease. *Nutrients* **2020**, *12*, 334. [CrossRef]

35. Irimata, K.; Li, X. Estimation of Correlation Coefficient in Data with Repeated Measures. *Proc. SAS Glob. Forum* **2018**, *2018*, 8–11.

36. Lobo, E.; Tamayo, M.; Sanclemente, T. Nutrition Literacy and Healthy Diet: Findings from the Validation of a Short Seniors-Oriented Screening Tool, the Spanish Myths-NL. *Int. J. Environ. Res. Public Health* **2021**, *18*, 12107. [CrossRef]

37. Harjola, U.; Liesmaa, H. Effects of poly of and sucrose candies on plaque, gingivitis and lactobacillus index scores: Observations on Helsinki school children. *Acta Odontol. Scand.* **1978**, *36*, 237–242. [CrossRef]

38. Rateitschak-Plüss, E.M.; Guggenheim, B. Effects of a carbohydrate-free diet and sugar substitutes on dental plaque accumulation. *J. Clin. Periodontol.* **1982**, *9*, 239–251. [CrossRef]

39. Teles, R.; Teles, F.; Frias-Lopez, J.; Paster, B.; Haffajee, A. Lessons learned and unlearned in periodontal microbiology: Lessons learned and unlearned in periodontal microbiology. *Periodontol. 2000* **2013**, *62*, 95–162. [CrossRef]

40. Li, J.; Guasch-Ferré, M.; Chung, W.; Ruiz-Canela, M.; Toledo, E.; Corella, D.; Bhupathiraju, S.N.; Tobias, D.K.; Tabung, F.K.; Hu, J.; et al. The Mediterranean diet, plasma metabolome, and cardiovascular disease risk. *Eur. Heart J.* **2020**, *41*, 2645–2656. [CrossRef]

41. Oliván-Blázquez, B.; Aguilar-Latorre, A.; Motrico, E.; Gómez-Gómez, I.; Zabaleta-Del-Olmo, E.; Couso-Viana, S.; Clavería, A.; Maderuelo-Fernandez, J.; Recio-Rodríguez, J.; Moreno-Peral, P.; et al. The Relationship between Adherence to the Mediterranean Diet, Intake of Specific Foods and Depression in an Adult Population (45–75 Years) in Primary Health Care. A Cross-Sectional Descriptive Study. *Nutrients* **2021**, *13*, 2724. [CrossRef]

42. Bohlscheid-Thomas, S.; Hoting, I.; Boeing, H.; Wahrendorf, J. Reproducibility and relative validity of food group intake in a food frequency questionnaire developed for the German part of the EPIC project. European Prospective Investigation into Cancer and Nutrition. *Int. J. Epidemiol.* **1997**, *26* (Suppl. 1), S59–S70. [CrossRef]

43. Deschamps, V.; de Lauzon-Guillain, B.; Lafay, L.; Borys, J.-M.; Charles, M.A.; Romon, M. Reproducibility and relative validity of a food-frequency questionnaire among French adults and adolescents. *Eur. J. Clin. Nutr.* **2009**, *63*, 282–291. [CrossRef]

44. Paalanen, L.; Männistö, S.; Virtanen, M.J.; Knekt, P.; Räsänen, L.; Montonen, J.; Pietinen, P. Validity of a food frequency questionnaire varied by age and body mass index. *J. Clin. Epidemiol.* **2006**, *59*, 994–1001. [CrossRef]

45. Hill, R.J.; Davies, P.S.W. The validity of self-reported energy intake as determined using the doubly labelled water technique. *Br. J. Nutr.* **2001**, *85*, 415–430. [CrossRef]

46. Mahabir, S.; Baer, D.J.; Giffen, C.; Subar, A.; Campbell, W.; Hartman, T.J.; Clevidence, B.; Albanes, D.; Taylor, P.R. Calorie intake misreporting by diet record and food frequency questionnaire compared to doubly labeled water among postmenopausal women. *Eur. J. Clin. Nutr.* **2006**, *60*, 561–565. [CrossRef]

47. Praxedes, D.R.S.; Pureza, I.R.O.M.; Vasconcelos, L.G.L.; Júnior, A.E.D.S.; Macena, M.D.L.; Florêncio, T.M.D.M.T.; de Melo, I.S.V.; Bueno, N.B. Association between energy intake under-reporting and previous professional nutritional counselling in low-income women with obesity: A cross-sectional study. *Nutr. Bull.* **2021**, *46*, 310–320. [CrossRef]

48. McLean, R.M.; Farmer, V.L.; Nettleton, A.; Cameron, C.M.; Cook, N.R.; Woodward, M.; Campbell, N.R.C.; TRUE Consortium (in Ternational Consortium for Quality Research on Dietary Sodium/Salt). Twenty-Four-Hour Diet recall and Diet records compared with 24-hour urinary excretion to predict an individual's sodium consumption: A Systematic Review. *J. Clin. Hypertens.* **2018**, *20*, 1360–1376. [CrossRef]

49. Wehling, H.; Lusher, J. People with a body mass index ≥30 under-report their dietary intake: A systematic review. *J. Health Psychol.* **2019**, *24*, 2042–2059. [CrossRef]

50. Willett, W. *Nutritional Epidemiology*; Oxford University Press: Oxford, UK, 2012.

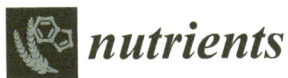

Correction

Correction: Bartha et al. How to Measure Adherence to a Mediterranean Diet in Dental Studies: Is a Short Adherence Screener Enough? A Comparative Analysis. *Nutrients* 2022, *14*, 1300

Valentin Bartha [1,2,*], Lea Exner [2], Anna-Lisa Meyer [3], Maryam Basrai [3], Daniela Schweikert [4], Michael Adolph [4], Thomas Bruckner [5], Christian Meller [2], Johan Peter Woelber [6,†] and Diana Wolff [1,†]

1   Department for Conservative Dentistry, University Hospital of Heidelberg, Im Neuenheimer Feld 400, 69120 Heidelberg, Germany; diana.wolff@med.uni-heidelberg.de
2   Department for Conservative Dentistry, University Hospital Tuebingen, Osianderstraße 2-8, 72076 Tübingen, Germany; exner.lea@gmx.de (L.E.); christian.meller@med.uni-tuebingen.de (C.M.)
3   Institute of Nutritional Medicine, University of Hohenheim, Fruwirthstr. 12, 70599 Stuttgart, Germany; anna94.meyer@yahoo.de (A.-L.M.); m.basrai@uni-hohenheim.de (M.B.)
4   Department of Nutrition Management and Nutrition Support Team, University Hospital Tuebingen, Hoppe-Seyler-Straße, 72076 Tübingen, Germany; daniela.schweikert@med.uni-tuebingen.de (D.S.); michael.adolph@med.uni-tuebingen.de (M.A.)
5   Institute of Medical Biometry, Faculty of Medicine, University of Heidelberg, Im Neuenheimer Feld 130.3, 69120 Heidelberg, Germany; bruckner@imbi.uni-heidelberg.de
6   Department of Operative Dentistry and Periodontology, Faculty of Medicine, University of Freiburg, Hugstetter Str. 55, 79106 Freiburg, Germany; johan.woelber@uniklinik-freiburg.de
*   Correspondence: valentin.bartha@med.uni-heidelberg.de
†   These authors contributed equally to this work.

Citation: Bartha, V.; Exner, L.; Meyer, A.-L.; Basrai, M.; Schweikert, D.; Adolph, M.; Bruckner, T.; Meller, C.; Woelber, J.P.; Wolff, D. Correction: Bartha et al. How to Measure Adherence to a Mediterranean Diet in Dental Studies: Is a Short Adherence Screener Enough? A Comparative Analysis. *Nutrients* 2022, *14*, 1300. *Nutrients* 2022, *14*, 1845. https://doi.org/10.3390/nu14091845

Received: 30 March 2022
Accepted: 24 April 2022
Published: 28 April 2022

Publisher's Note: MDPI stays neutral with regard to jurisdictional claims in published maps and institutional affiliations.

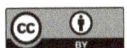
Error in Figures

The authors would like to make a correction in a recently published paper [1]. There were errors in Figures 1, 2 and 4. In the original Figures, there are missing lines, arrows, boxes, colours and confidence intervals due to the incompatibilities between different computer operating systems.

Original Figure 1:

Screening	MedD	Control (C)
Equilibration phase (2 weeks)	MedD training 2x for 90 minutes before T0, 2x for 60 minutes after T0	
T0 (Start of intervention)	Clinical examination: BOP, GI, PI Diet assessment: MEDAS, DEGS-FFQ	
Study phase 1 (2 weeks)		
T1	Diet assessment: 24dr (four days)	
Study phase 2 (4 weeks)		
	Mediterranean Diet	Usual diet
T2	Clinical examination: BOP, GI, PI Diet assessment: 24dr (four days), DEGS-FFQ, MEDAS	

We would like it to be corrected as shown below.
New Figure 1:

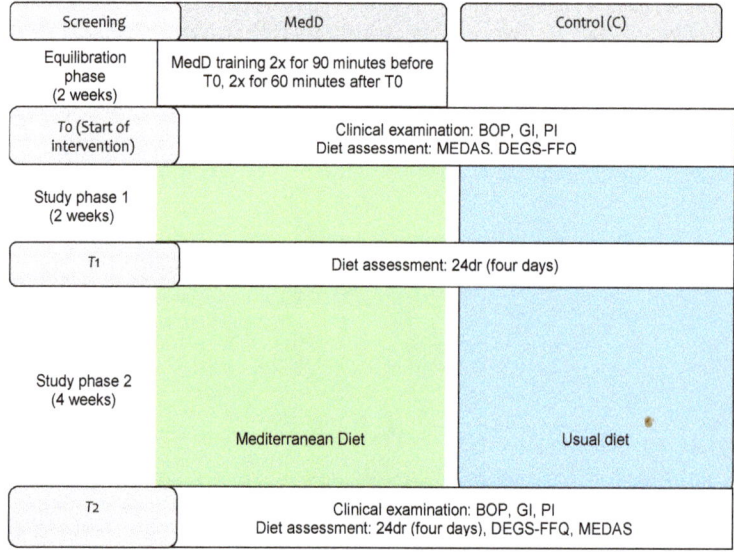

Original Figure 2:

n=83 assessed for eligibility

n=28 did not meet the inclusion criteria
n=13 declined participation

n=42 allocated to MedD or C group

n=23 allocated to MedD   n=19 allocated to control

n=3 denied participation due to coronavirus
pandemic

n=2 declined further participation

n=18 analyzed: n=19 analyzed:
T0: clinical data n= 18; FFQ n=18; MEDAS n=18   T0: clinical data n=19; FFQ n=19; MEDAS n=19
T1: 24dr n=12   T1: 24dr n=12
T2: clinical data n=18; FFQ n=18; MEDAS n=18;   T2: clinical data n=19; FFQ n=19; MEDAS n=18;
   24dr n=12   24dr n=12

New Figure 2:

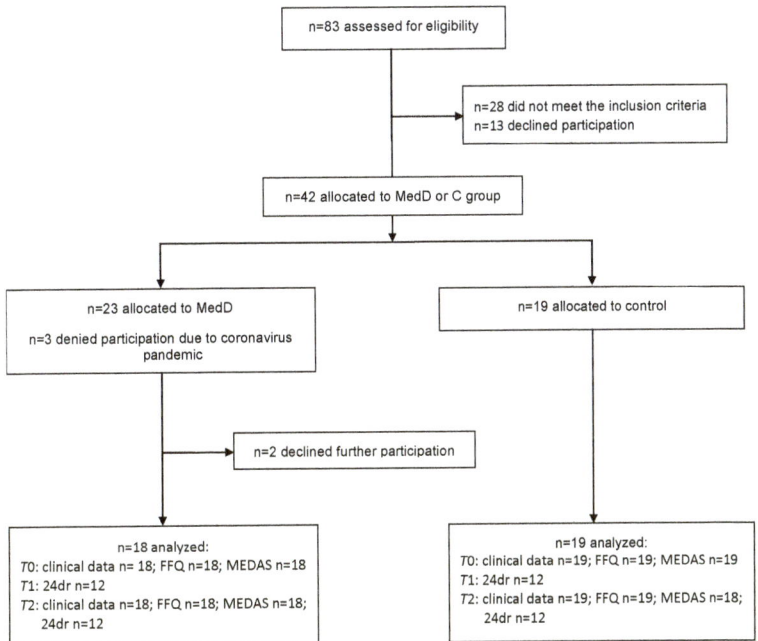

Original Figure 4:

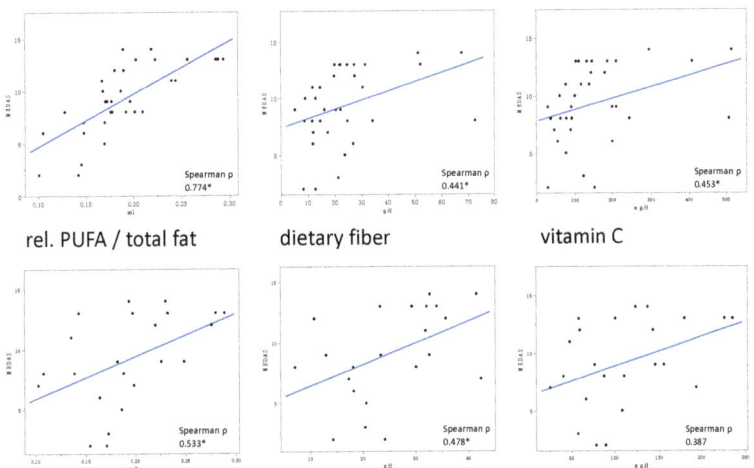

rel. PUFA / total fat   dietary fiber   vitamin C

New Figure 4:

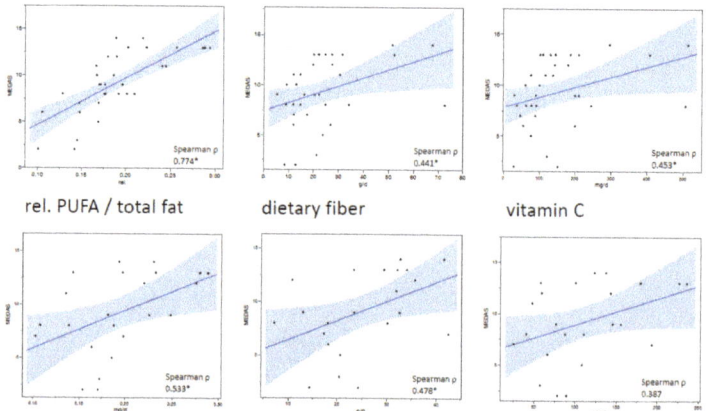

<table>
<tr><td>rel. PUFA / total fat</td><td>dietary fiber</td><td>vitamin C</td></tr>
</table>

The authors apologize for any inconvenience caused and state that the scientific conclusions are unaffected. The original publication has also been updated.

Reference

1. Bartha, V.; Exner, L.; Meyer, A.-L.; Basrai, M.; Schweikert, D.; Adolph, M.; Bruckner, T.; Meller, C.; Woelber, J.P.; Wolff, D. How to Measure Adherence to a Mediterranean Diet in Dental Studies: Is a Short Adherence Screener Enough? A Comparative Analysis. *Nutrients* **2022**, *14*, 1300. [CrossRef] [PubMed]

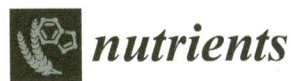

Article

A Healthier Smile in the Past? Dental Caries and Diet in Early Neolithic Farming Communities from Central Germany

Nicole Nicklisch [1,*], Vicky M. Oelze [2], Oliver Schierz [3], Harald Meller [4] and Kurt W. Alt [1,5]

1   Center for Natural and Cultural History of Man, Faculty of Medicine/Dentistry, Danube Private University, Förthofstraße 2, 3500 Krems, Austria; kurt.alt@dp-uni.ac.at
2   Anthropology Department, University of California at Santa Cruz, 1156 High Street, Santa Cruz, CA 96064, USA; voelze@ucsc.edu
3   Department of Prosthodontics and Materials Science, University of Leipzig, Liebig Str. 12, 04103 Leipzig, Germany; oliver.schierz@medizin.uni-leipzig.de
4   State Office for Heritage Management and Archaeology Saxony-Anhalt and State Museum of Prehistory, Richard-Wagner Str. 9, 06114 Halle, Germany; hmeller@lda.stk.sachsen-anhalt.de
5   Institute of Prehistory and Archaeological Science, Department of Environmental Sciences, University of Basel, Spalenring 145, 4055 Basel, Switzerland
*   Correspondence: nicole.nicklisch@dp-uni.ac.at; Tel.: +43-676-842-419-395

Citation: Nicklisch, N.; Oelze, V.M.; Schierz, O.; Meller, H.; Alt, K.W. A Healthier Smile in the Past? Dental Caries and Diet in Early Neolithic Farming Communities from Central Germany. *Nutrients* 2022, 14, 1831. https://doi.org/10.3390/nu14091831

Academic Editors: Kirstin Vach, Johan Peter Woelber and Gunter G.C. Kuhnle

Received: 27 February 2022
Accepted: 25 April 2022
Published: 27 April 2022

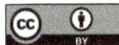
Abstract: Dental health is closely linked to an individual's health and diet. This bioarcheological study presents dental caries and stable isotope data obtained from prehistoric individuals ($n = 101$) from three Early Neolithic sites (c. 5500-4800 BCE) in central Germany. Dental caries and ante-mortem tooth loss (AMTL) were recorded and related to life history traits such as biological sex and age at death. Further, we correlate evidence on caries to carbon and nitrogen isotope data obtained from 83 individuals to assess the relationship between diet and caries. In 68.3% of the adults, carious lesions were present, with 10.3% of teeth affected. If AMTL is considered, the values increase by about 3%. The prevalence of subadults (18.4%) was significantly lower, with 1.8% carious teeth. The number of carious teeth correlated significantly with age but not sex. The isotopic data indicated an omnivorous terrestrial diet composed of domestic plants and animal derived protein but did not correlate with the prevalence of carious lesions. The combined evidence from caries and isotope analysis suggests a prevalence of starchy foods such as cereals in the diet of these early farmers, which aligns well with observations from other Early Neolithic sites but contrasts to Late Neolithic and Early Bronze Age populations in Germany.

Keywords: caries; nutrition; oral health; stable isotope analysis; bioarcheology

1. Introduction

In modern-day societies, caries is the most widespread non-communicable disease [1]. The nature of dental caries and its association with diet and oral hygiene are well understood [2,3]. Once the homeostasis of the physiological oral microbiome is disturbed, this may favour the colonization and multiplication of pathogenic bacteria [4,5]. *Streptococcus mutans* is the main representative of caries-promoting pathogens, which have the ability to metabolize low-molecular-weight carbohydrates such as sugars quite rapidly, producing organic acids such as lactic acid. An excess of acid-producing bacteria leads to the demineralization of tooth enamel, which can ultimately result in failure of the overall tooth structure and tooth loss. The bacterial infection can even spread to the jawbone and lead to so-called periapical alterations or abscesses, thus causing further complications [6]. Dental caries is a multifactorial disease in which individual dietary habits (food, processing, texture), oral hygiene, genetic factors (e.g., enamel thickness, microstructure, tooth morphology, saliva composition), and underlying pathological conditions may also play a role [2,4,7]. As dental health has an impact on a physiological and socio-cultural level, age- and sex-specific associations with caries have been described [8,9].

In the past, a sharp increase in dental caries correlated significantly with fundamental changes in human subsistence strategies and diet [9]. The first important event was the adoption of agricultural practices to procure food in the Neolithic period. Particularly the cultivation of several species of cereal provided a readily available and, thus, secure source of food. The higher starch and, hence, carbohydrate content in this novel diet and the way food was processed resulted in a higher prevalence of caries [9,10]. With the availability of cane and beet sugars in the 18th and 19th centuries, caries occurrence and frequency increased significantly [10]. However, in many industrialized Western nations, dental health has improved in the past few decades, especially among children and adolescents. The main elements are new concepts for prevention and treatment and the desire for wellbeing [3]. Nevertheless, the incidence of caries is still much higher in Western industrialized nations than in most African and Asian populations [11].

In archeological and forensic contexts, teeth can still provide information even when other tissue structures have already been destroyed by taphonomic processes [12,13]. Analyses of pathophysiological changes in dental hard tissue provide information on the frequency and severity of dental disease within a population, as well as information on individual and population-specific behaviors and dietary habits [9,14,15]. In addition, it is possible to visualize spatial and chronological trends in oral health in human history through comparative analysis of dental pathology data [8,10,16,17].

Our study provides an insight into the dental health of the earliest farmers of central Europe, who had their genetic origins in the Near East and settled in central Germany approximately 7000 years ago [18,19]. In addition to a (1) detailed survey of dental caries and ante-mortem tooth loss (AMTL) in three burial communities, this study puts the occurrence of dental caries in relation to stable isotope data obtained from human bone collagen, assessing the possible relationship between diet and dental disease [20]. Stable isotope analysis of carbon and nitrogen can provide information on the main source of dietary proteins and carbohydrates and allows us to differentiate between herbivore, omnivore, carnivore, and piscivore diets [21,22]. We expect to find (2) lower frequencies of dental caries in individuals with slightly higher nitrogen isotope values and, hence, higher amounts of animal protein (milk, meat) in their diet [20]. Another question is (3) how biological sex and (4) age relate to the prevalence of dental caries and AMTL in these populations. Gender-based differences in diet have been described for several Neolithic sites in Europe, with male individuals tending to show isotopic evidence of more frequent animal protein consumption than female individuals [23].

2. Materials and Methods

2.1. Material

This bioarcheological study includes data from the three Early Neolithic sites of Halberstadt-Sonntagsfeld, Derenburg-Meerenstieg II, and Karsdorf-Steigra in the Middle Elbe-Saale region (MES) of central Germany (Figure 1). Based on its characteristic ceramic ornamentation, the archaeological culture is referred to as linear pottery culture (Linearbandkeramik = LBK) [24]. The MES is bordered in the west and south by low mountain ranges (Harz, Thuringian Forest, and Ore Mountains) and in the east by glacial landscapes. The area is interspersed with fertile loess soils, which offered favorable conditions for settling and farming in prehistoric times [25,26]. In the western regions of the MES in particular, the lime-rich soils support the preservation of bones. The human remains sampled in this study were radiocarbon-dated to the period between 5450 and 4775 cal BC [27].

Two of the sites, Derenburg-Meerenstieg II (DEB) and Halberstadt-Sonntagsfeld (HBS), are located in the foothills of the northern Harz region (Nordharzvorland, Harz district, Saxony-Anhalt), at a distance of less than 10 km from each other. With its 47 burials, DEB can be defined as a cemetery. In contrast, the 41 skeletons from HBS were found in so-called settlement burials, i.e., grouped together close to the remains of wooden longhouse structures. Single burials dominated at HBS and DEB, but a few double burials were also found. More than half of the burials contained grave goods such as pottery, earth pigments, and spondylus shells [28]. The third site, Karsdorf-Steigra (KAR) in the Unstrut Valley (Burgenland), is located approximately 100 km from the other sites. As at HBS, the burials at KAR were also found within the settlement. The 30 individuals were grouped primarily to the west of the longhouse structures. All deceased were buried in individual grave pits, and the number of grave goods can be described as low compared to the other sites [29].

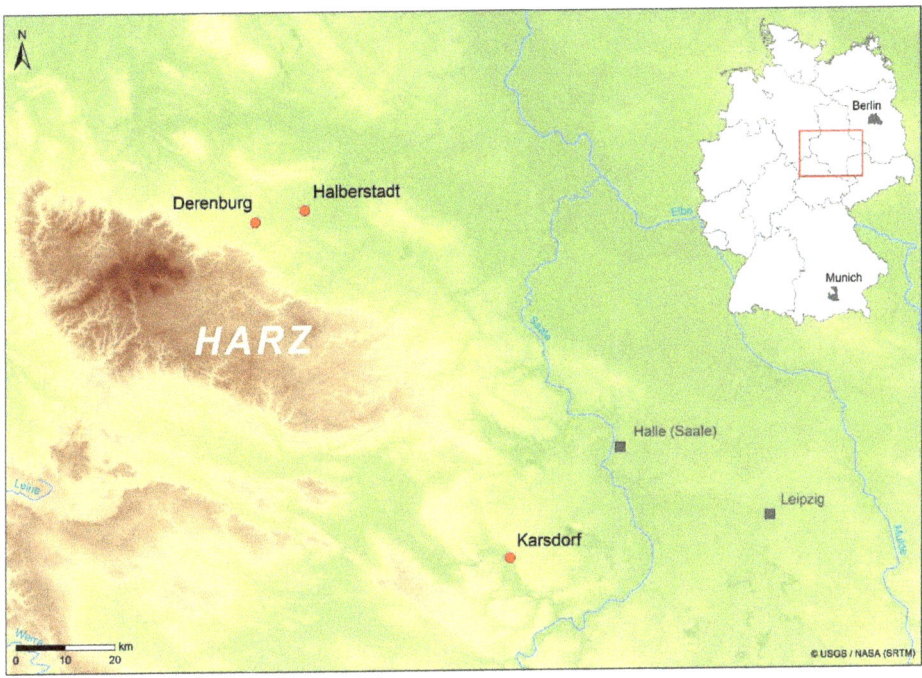

Figure 1. Location of the three sites in the Middle Elbe-Saale region, Saxony-Anhalt, central Germany (LDA, Halle/Saale).

2.2. Methods

2.2.1. Age and Sex Determination

Following international recommendations, a broad range of morphometric methods were used for age and sex determination of the skeletal remains [30,31]. The age determination in adult individuals (>20 years) was based on the assessment of the cranial suture closure [32], changes in the auricular surface [33,34], and the pubic symphysis [35]. In children and adolescents (<20 years = subadults), age determination was based on the tooth development and eruption [36], long-bone lengths [37], and ossification patterns of epiphyses and apophyses [38]. The sex was determined on the basis of morphological and metric criteria in adults only [38–40]. Age determinations were made according to the following classification [41]: *infans* I (0–6 years), *infans* II (7–14 years), *juvenis* (15–20 years), *adultas* (21–40 years), *maturitas* (41–60 years), *senilis* (≥61 years).

2.2.2. Morphological Examination of the Teeth

Assessment of the dental status was based on the designation standards of the Fédération Dentaire Internationale (FDI) [42]. Adapted to the bioarcheological evaluation of dental caries, the following two quotients were defined: (a) caries frequency (or prevalence) in percent (CF = number of affected individuals × 100/number of assessable individuals), (b) caries experience in percent (CE = number of affected teeth × 100/number of assessed teeth) [43–45]. Carious lesions (dental cavities) were divided into five stages:

caries superficialis (1), *caries media* (2), *caries profunda* without *pulpa aperta* (3), *caries profunda* with *pulpa aperta* (4), *radix relicta* (5) [12]. So-called "white spots" and "brown spots" were not part of this evaluation.

DMF scores are not appropriate for archeological investigations, because teeth may be missing due to periodontal disease, trauma, or heavy tooth wear, and teeth lost post-mortem (PMTL) may also have been carious [43,46]. Nevertheless, in the present study ante-mortem tooth loss (AMTL) was assessed and combined with carious lesions in relation to the assessable alveolar sockets (dental alveoli). AMTL was considered if the alveolus was completely remodeled or at least showed signs of remodeling. The number of assessable dental alveoli is composed of the number of preserved teeth, AMTL, and PMTL.

2.2.3. Digital Volume Tomography (DVT)

For a more detailed dental analysis of some individuals (n = 13), radiological images were taken at the Department of Prosthodontics and Materials Science, Leipzig University using digital volume tomography (DVT, Morita 3D Accuitomo 170), with a slice thickness of 1 mm and a voxel size of 0.250 (tube voltage: 80 kV; tube current: 2.0 mA).

2.2.4. Stable Isotope Data

To assess whether the occurrence and prevalence of carious lesions can be associated with dietary patterns in the three study populations, stable carbon and nitrogen isotope data, δ^{13}C and δ^{15}N, respectively, previously published by Oelze and colleagues [20], were also taken into account. Depending on the state of preservation, the bones used for isotope analysis were mainly ribs, but a few long bones and skull fragments were also sampled. Stable isotopes in collagen samples were extracted following the procedure outlined by Richards and Hedges [47] and analyzed in a Flash EA 2112 coupled to a DeltaXP isotope ratio mass spectrometer (Thermo-Finnigan, Bremen, Germany) at the Max Planck Institute for Evolutionary Anthropology in Leipzig, Germany. The δ^{13}C and δ^{15}N values are reported here in ‰ following the international standards vPDB and AIR. The analytical error was better than 0.2‰ (1σ) for both isotope systems [20]. Collagen quality was affirmed by inspecting %nitrogen, %carbon, and the atomic C:N ratios for each sample following the recommendations by Ambrose [48].

2.2.5. Statistical Data Analysis

To compare the prevalence of caries with life history parameters and stable isotope data in this archeological population with post-mortem tooth loss, we calculated percent caries (caries%) as the number of teeth affected by caries divided by the number of teeth present per individual. This allows us to assess dental caries in light of age, sex, site, and dietary patterns across individuals. We ran two linear regression models in R (version R 4.1.1, [49]) with the alpha level set to 0.05. One model was run using the full dataset (n = 83), thus testing the effect of age (average value in years), site (3 levels: DEB, HBS, KAR), and δ^{13}C and δ^{15}N values on the percentage of teeth affected by caries per individual (%caries/individual). Log1p transformations were conducted to remove the zeros from the response variable %caries/individual in both models. The fixed effect of sex was also included in the second model, having excluded all subadult individuals and those of undetermined sex from the dataset (n = 64). In the full dataset model, the possible interaction between δ^{13}C and δ^{15}N was initially tested; this, however, was not significant (χ^2 = 0.0, df = 76, p = 0.958) and was subsequently dropped from the full model. The interaction between isotopes was not considered in the second model.

Model diagnostics were carried out on both models by visually inspecting histograms, qq-plots, and residuals plotted against fitted values, all of which confirmed normally distributed and homogeneous residuals. Testing variance inflation factors in both models found no evidence for collinearity (vifs around 1–1.2). The final results were obtained by comparing both full models with a null model each, which only contained the fixed effect of site, using chi-square independence tests.

3. Results

Out of a total of 116 skeletons recovered from the three Neolithic sites, the dentitions of 101 individuals could be examined for this study (Table 1). These comprised 63 adults and 38 subadults (<20 years) with 1910 permanent and 277 deciduous teeth (Appendix A Table A1). For a total of 83 individuals, we can report both dental caries and isotope analysis results.

Table 1. Archeological sites, number (N) of excavated individuals separated in adults and subadults, and number of individuals with preserved teeth separated in adults and subadults.

Archeological Sites	N Excavated Individuals	N Adults	N Subadults	N Individuals with Teeth	N Adults with Teeth	N Subadults with Teeth
DEB	47	32	15	40	28	12
HBS	38	18	20	33	17	16
KAR	31	20	11	28	18	10
Total	116	70	46	101	63	38

The model testing the effects of age, site, and $\delta^{13}C$ and $\delta^{15}N$ values in relation to the percentage of carious teeth per individual ($n = 83$) was highly significant ($\chi^2 = 65.4$, df = 77, $p < 0.000$). However, as shown in Figure 2, this was driven exclusively by the effect of age ($p < 0.000$). Interestingly, none of the other predictors had any impact on the percentage of caries per individual (site: $p = 0.878$, $\delta^{13}C$: $p = 0.594$, $\delta^{15}N$: $p = 0.433$). A similar pattern emerged from the second model which included the fixed effect of sex in a subset of all adult individuals. Here too the full model was highly significant ($\chi^2 = 43.2$, df = 57, $p < 0.000$), exclusively driven by the effect of age ($p < 0.000$) and not by site ($p = 0.613$), sex ($p = 0.733$) or $\delta^{13}C$ ($p = 0.669$), and $\delta^{15}N$ ($p = 0.431$) values.

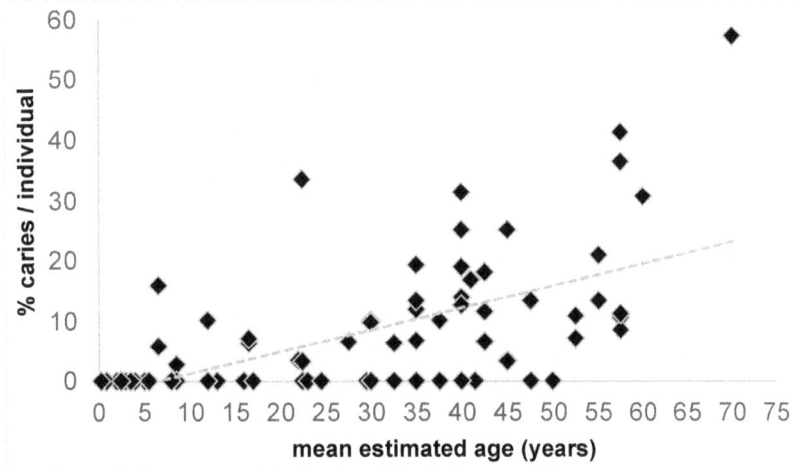

Figure 2. Scatterplot showing the significant relationship between the mean estimates of age in years and the percentage of caries per individual.

3.1. Age-Specific Differences

Table 2 summarizes the caries frequencies (CF) and caries experience (CE) for all adult and subadult individuals in this study. At DEB, 18 out of the 28 adults (64.3%) were affected by caries. The CF in the adults from HBS (12/17, 70.6%) and KAR (13/18, 72.2%) were slightly higher, but the number of assessable individuals was lower. A CF of 68.3% (43/63) can be determined for all three groups taken together. When considering CE, the adults from HBS exhibited the highest number of carious teeth (12.0%), followed by the group from KAR, with a CE of 10.9%. The adult group from DEB showed the lowest CE rate of

8.6%. Combining all three LBK sites, a CE value of 10.3% can be determined. In most cases, a small number of individuals were characterized by particularly severe dental cavities. AMTL could only be detected in adult individuals. Of 63 adults, 14 are affected (22.2%). Individuals from KAR are most frequently affected by AMTL; in relation to the assessable dental alveoli, HBS is in the lead. In total, two adults show AMTL but no carious lesions, which raises the combined frequency (AMTL + caries) by individuals to 71.4%. Looking at the combined data in relation to the assessable alveolar sockets, the average frequency increases by 3%.

Table 2. Caries frequency (CF) and caries experience (CE) in adult and subadult individuals for each site and in total. Information on AMTL and AMTL combined with caries is given by adult individuals and assessable alveolar sockets.

Site	Adults		Subadults	
	Individuals	CF %	Individuals	CF %
DEB	18/28	64.3	2/12	16.7
HBS	12/17	70.6	2/16	12.5
KAR	13/18	72.2	3/10	30.0
total	43/63	68.3	7/38	18.4
	Teeth	CE %	Teeth	CE %
DEB	52/594	8.8	4/255	1.6
HBS	49/409	12.0	4/281	1.4
KAR	52/477	10.9	5/171	2.9
total	153/1480	10.3	13/707	1.8
Adults with AMTL				
	AMTL by individuals	%	AMTL by alveolar sockets	%
DEB	5/28	17.9	9/625	1.4
HBS	3/17	17.6	23/453	5.1
KAR	6/18	33.3	23/517	4.4
total	14/63	22.2	55/1595	3.4
	AMTL + caries by individuals	%	AMTL + caries by alveolar sockets	%
DEB	19/28	67.9	61/625	9.8
HBS	12/17	70.6	72/453	15.9
KAR	14/18	77.8	75/517	14.5
total	45/63	71.4	208/1595	13.0

Among the subadults, the CF value was highest at KAR with 30% (Table 2). At DEB, two out of 12 (16.7%) and at HBS two out of 16 subadults (12.5%) were affected. Overall, seven of 38 subadult individuals (18.4%) had carious lesions. With 4–5 affected teeth, the CE values in the subadults of all three sites were low. At KAR, 2.9% of the preserved teeth were affected and at DEB, 1.6%. The lowest CE rate (1.4%) can be determined for the subadult group from HBS. Combining the data of the subadult individuals from all three LBK sites results in a CE rate of 1.8%. AMTL was not observed among the subadult group.

A closer look at all adult individuals by age group (Table 3) suggests an increase in both CF and CE with advancing age. The same tendency can be described for AMTL and AMTL combined with caries, both at the individual level and by alveolar sockets. However, the oldest age group (>61) is only represented by a single individual.

Table 3. Caries frequency (CF) and caries experience (CE) in subadult and adult individuals from all sites by age group, with data on permanent teeth and deciduous teeth affected. Data on AMTL and AMTL combined with caries are given by adult individuals and assessable alveolar sockets.

Age (Years)	Indidviduals	%	Permanent Teeth/Alveolar Sockets	%	Deciduous Teeth	%
	Caries (CF)		Caries by teeth (CE)			
0–6	0/19	0.0	0/105	0.0	0/188	0.0
7–14	5/13	38.5	2/194	1.0	8/87	9.2
15–20	2/6	33.3	3/131	2.3	0/2	0.0
21–40	22/37	59.5	75/873	8.6	—	—
41–60	20/25	80.0	66/586	11.3	—	—
>61	1/1	100	12/21	57.1	—	—
	AMTL		AMTL by alveolar sockets			
21–40	3/37	8.1	13/917	1.4	—	—
41–60	10/25	40.0	37/652	5.7	—	—
>61	1/1	100	5/26	19.2	—	—
all adults	14/63	22.2	55/1595	3.4	—	—
	AMTL + caries		AMTL + caries by alveolar sockets			
21–40	22/37	59.5	88/917	9.6	—	—
41–60	22/25	84.0	103/652	15.8	—	—
>61	1/1	100	17/26	65.4	—	—
all adults	45/63	71.4	208/1595	13.0	—	—

The subadults affected are exclusively children of the *infans* II age group (7–14 years) and juvenile individuals. Carious deciduous teeth were observed in the *infans* II group. Carious lesions are detectable in the permanent molars of an approximately 12-year-old child and two juvenile individuals (15–20 years). No carious lesions were found in the *infans* I group (0–6 years).

3.2. Sex-Related Differences

The results of our statistical data analysis show no significant effect of sex on the percentage of carious teeth per individual among all adults from the three Neolithic sites. However, although the sample sizes per archeological site are small, we can describe some trends in our dataset. At DEB and KAR, females (81.3% and 83.3%) tend to be more frequently affected by dental caries than males (40.0% and 63.6%) (Table 4). At HBS, the situation is different: all six male individuals show evidence of dental cavities, but only six out of 11 females (54.5%) have carious lesions. Overall, CF appears slightly higher for females (72.7%) than for males (63.0%). At the individual level AMTL is slightly higher in females, but the combined data from AMTL and caries do not lead to any significant changes.

Similar results occur when looking at the CE values. Again, males from DEB and KAR (5.9% and 4.9%, respectively) seem less affected by carious teeth than the females (10.2% and 21.6%). At HBS, males (13.7%) tend to show more carious lesions than females (11.5%). The female individuals from KAR show the highest CE with 21.6%. AMTL is more common in females than in males. In comparison, the combined data from AMTL and caries show a small but non-significant increase in frequencies.

Table 4. Sex-specific differences in caries frequency (CF), caries experience (CE). Data on AMTL and AMTL combined with caries are given by individuals and assessable alveolar sockets.

Site	Male	%	Female	%	Male	%	Female	%
	Caries by individuals (CF)				Caries by teeth (CE)			
DEB	4/10	40.0	13/16	81.3	13/221	5.9	38/365	10.4
HBS	6/6	100	6/11	54.5	24/175	13.7	27/234	11.5
KAR	7/11	63.6	5/6	83.3	14/285	4.9	35/162	21.6
Total	17/27	63.0	24/33	72.7	51/682	7.5	100/761	13.1
	AMTL by individuals				AMTL by alveolar sockets			
DEB	0/10	0.0	5/16	31.2	0/224	0.0	9/393	2.3
HBS	1/6	16.7	2/11	18.2	6/185	3.2	17/268	6.3
KAR	3/11	27.3	3/6	50.0	12/313	3.8	11/174	6.3
Total	4/27	14.8	10/33	30.3	18/722	2.5	37/835	4.4
	AMTL + caries by individuals				AMTL + caries by alveolar sockets			
DEB	4/10	40.0	14/16	87.5	13/224	5.8	47/393	12.0
HBS	6/6	100	6/11	54.5	28/185	15.1	44/268	16.4
KAR	8/11	72.7	5/6	83.3	26/313	8.3	46/174	26.4
Total	18/27	66.7	25/33	75.7	67/722	9.3	137/835	16.4

3.3. Affected Tooth Types

The adult individuals from all three sites are summarized in Table 5. The distribution shows a clear trend, whereby the post-canine teeth are clearly more affected by carious lesions than the anterior teeth. The first molar (tooth 16; 22.4%) and the second premolar (tooth 15; 20.4%) are most affected in the right maxilla. In the left maxilla, the most dental cavities are found on the second molar (tooth 27; 33.3%), followed by the first molar (tooth 26; 22.9%). In the right and left mandibles, most defects are evenly distributed among the molars, with third molars being slightly more affected.

Table 5. Distribution of carious lesions in the dentition of adult individuals from all sites with information on the number of assessable (N teeth) and carious teeth (N affected). The teeth were named according to the FDI system.

	Right Jaw														Left Jaw					
Upper Jaw	18	17	16	15	14	13	12	11		21	22	23	24	25	26	27	28		
N teeth	31	49	49	49	49	51	44	42		45	47	47	47	51	48	48	27		
N affected	4	7	11	10	8	4	2	1		1	1	2	2	6	11	16	5		
% affected	12.9	14.3	22.4	20.4	16.3	7.8	4.5	2.4		2.2	2.1	4.3	4.3	11.8	22.9	33.3	18.5		
Lower Jaw	48	47	46	45	44	43	42	41		31	32	33	34	35	36	37	38		
N teeth	35	50	49	51	48	51	47	45		40	47	49	51	53	49	51	40		
N affected	6	7	7	5	2	1	0	1		0	1	1	1	4	9	9	8		
% affected	17.1	14.0	14.3	9.8	4.2	2.0	0.0	2.2		0.0	2.1	2.0	2.0	7.5	18.4	17.6	20.0		

Due to the low prevalence in the subadults, a tabular presentation was omitted. A total of 13 teeth, eight deciduous teeth and five permanent teeth, are affected. The affected deciduous teeth are seven molars and one canine. The affected permanent teeth are four second molars and one first molar.

3.4. Severity of Caries Lesions

When looking at the adult individuals from all sites, most teeth affected by caries show only minor lesions in the form of *caries superficialis* (grade 1) and *caries media* (grade 2) (Table 6). These two forms of caries represent approximately 60% of all defects. Deeper structural defects, such as *caries profunda* without (grade 3) or with opened pulp cavity (grade 4), are less frequently observed considering the total number of affected teeth. There are differences between the sites: at DEB, the proportion of grade 4 cavities (25%) is higher, whereas, at KAR, the proportion of grade 3 (19.2%) and grade 5 (21.2%) is higher. HBS also shows a higher proportion of grade 5 defects (20.4%), which are associated with the complete destruction of the dental crowns.

Table 6. Degree of caries in adult individuals: number of affected teeth (N teeth) by severity of carious lesion (grade 1–5).

Grade	DEB		HBS		KAR		Total	
	N Teeth	%	N Teeth	%	N Teeth	%	N Teeth	%
1	11	21.2	20	40.8	19	36.5	50	32.7
2	24	46.2	9	18.4	9	17.3	42	27.5
3	3	5.8	7	14.3	10	19.2	20	13.1
4	13	25.0	3	6.1	3	5.8	19	12.4
5	1	1.9	10	20.4	11	21.2	22	14.4
Total	52	100	49	100	52	100	153	100

In the subadult individuals, the severity does not exceed grade 3. Of the eight deciduous teeth, two show grade 3, four teeth show grade 2, and two show grade 1. Of the five permanent teeth, three exhibit grade 1, one shows grade 2, and two show grade 3.

3.5. Stable Isotope Ratios and Diet

The stable isotope ratios for carbon and nitrogen for the three study populations have been reported and discussed previously by Oelze and colleagues [20]. No significant differences in stable isotope values were found between the sites. The stable isotope values in all fully weaned individuals (estimated age older than 5 years) cluster tightly in δ^{13}C with an average value of -19.8‰ (± 0.3‰ 1σ). The δ^{15}N values for these individuals show slightly more variation with an average value of 8.8‰ (± 0.7‰ 1σ). Subadults tend to have higher δ^{13}C and even higher δ^{15}N values than adult individuals.

4. Discussion

This paper presents the dental caries profiles and matching stable isotope records of three early Neolithic farming populations to describe the nuanced relationship between diet and dental heath in one of the earliest agricultural societies of central Europe. The comparison between HBS, DEB, and KAR is problematic due to the small number of individuals per burial community. Our statistic model did not pick up any differences between sites in the percentage of caries per individual, and the three sites were also found to be almost indistinguishable isotopically [20]. This suggests that, in respect of their dental health, we can treat all individuals sampled as one study population. The marginal differences between sites, such as the lower CF and CE of the adult individuals from DEB or the higher caries burden in the males from HBS, are of limited significance. The combined data of AMTL and caries show a relatively small, non-significant increase in the frequencies of age- and sex-specific differences. Overall, the three LBK populations show a rather moderate degree of dental cavities in which the milder forms of caries such as caries superficialis and caries media dominate. The results can be discussed under various aspects, with nutrition playing an essential role.

4.1. The Influence of Nutrition

The δ^{13}C data point to a dependence on domesticated C3-plants for these early farmers, whereas the possibility of prevalent wild plant foods and C4-plant cultivation can be excluded [20,50,51]. The δ^{15}N values suggest that this domestic plant-based diet was low in leguminous plants which fix nitrogen directly from the soil [21] and was mixed with considerable amounts of animal-derived protein, most likely meat from domestic cattle, sheep, goats, and pigs [20]. A previous comparison of human δ^{15}N values with those of domestic animals from each site suggested that individuals from DEB may have had slightly less animal protein in their everyday diet than the inhabitants of the two other sites [20]. If that is the case, we would predict that the plant and, hence, possibly cereal proportion of the diet might have been higher for DEB community members. However, this assumption does not align with the CF and CE values of the DEB individuals, which are very similar to those of the other two sites.

Based on the genetic evidence from several individuals from DEB, we can say that these people were likely not lactase-persistent and, hence, could not digest lactose from unfermented milk after reaching maturity [52]. As expected, children younger than five years ($n = 13$) have slightly elevated δ^{13}C and δ^{15}N values compared to older individuals, as their isotope values are influenced by the tropic level increase associated with human breastmilk consumption [20,53]. Isotopic differences between adult males and females are insignificant and do not suggest that men had considerably better access to meat than women. Overall, the isotopic evidence indicates that all individuals led an agricultural lifestyle with a mixed diet of domesticated plants (cereals and small amounts of legumes) and animal products [20].

Cereals occupied an important position in the diet of Early Neolithic farming cultures. The geographic region studied offered rich loess soils and, thus, optimal conditions for cereal cultivation. Archeological investigations show that the LBK people preferred to settle in these loess areas [24,25]. The cultivation of cereals increased the proportion of carbohydrate-rich food. New food processing techniques made starch and sugar easily accessible to bacteria of the oral cavity, thus promoting the development of caries [10]. Studies indicate that early farmers suffered an increase in caries prevalence compared to hunter-gatherers [9]. In addition to diet, genetic factors also affect the quality of tooth structure and saliva production [2,4]. Nevertheless, an essential role in cariogenesis can be attributed to the starch and sugar content in the diet [2,54]. Epidemiological studies suggest an increased caries risk when starch is combined with sugar [55]. In the European Early Neolithic, fruits and honey can be assumed as sweet foods. Genetic analyses of dental calculus samples from different time periods demonstrate that the composition of the oral flora from the Neolithic to the Middle Ages was more diverse than that of recent populations [56]. This trend can be attributed to continuous changes in the human diet.

4.2. Age-Specific Differences and Caries Localisation

At 68.3%, the CF was significantly higher in the adults than in the subadult individuals, at 18.4%. The difference in CE was also very clear, where the proportion of affected teeth was 5.7 times higher in adults than in children and adolescents. In principle, young children between 0 and 6 years of age were not affected. Only in the older children and adolescents a few carious teeth were found, including some deciduous teeth. The nutritional data indicated that children older than three years were weaned. Before that, there does not seem to have been any risk of dental caries, e.g., by feeding premasticated food.

The data confirm that the risk of dental caries increased significantly with age. Within the dentition, caries was almost exclusively found in the post-canine teeth. Few cavities in the anterior teeth were found in older group members who were severely affected by caries. The carious lesions seem to have originated predominantly on the approximal surfaces of the interdental space. An impressive example is the dentition of a 35–45-year-old male individual (ID 484) from DEB (Figure 3a–d). The morphological examination shows pronounced carious lesions on a total of five teeth, three maxillary molars (teeth 16, 26, 27), and two premolars (teeth 15, 44). In the three maxillary molars, the carious lesions originate on the approximal surfaces (Figure 3a). Severe wear is noticeable on the occlusal surfaces and is particularly pronounced in the anterior region (Figure 3a,c). Periapical changes resulting from deep caries lesions with opening of the pulp cavity are visible on teeth 26, 27, and 44 (Figure 3a,d). These periapical lesions can be clearly localized in DVT images of the maxilla and mandible (Figure 4a,b). Due to the osteolytic processes in the jaw bones, it is very likely that the man suffered from recurrent inflammatory reactions. Without medical intervention, chronic oral infections can spread to the adjacent tissue and the entire body [57–60].

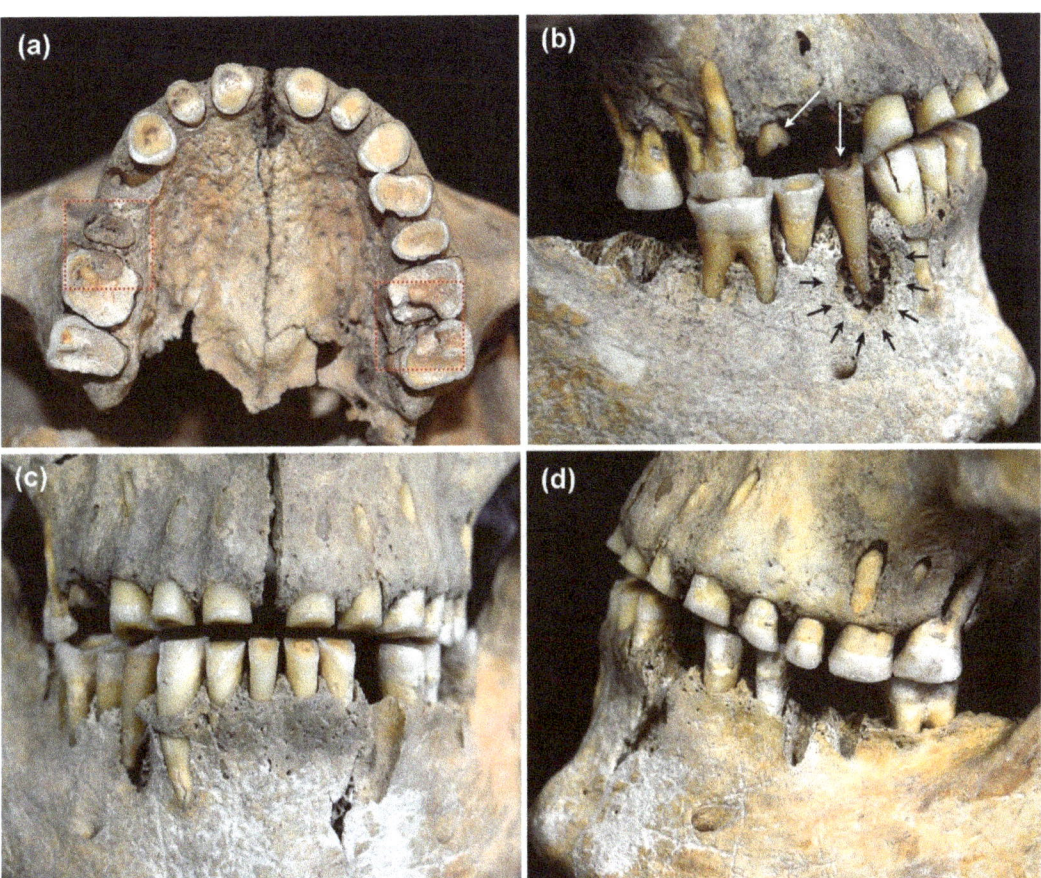

Figure 3. (**a**–**d**). Dentition of an adult male individual (ID 484) from DEB (**a**) In the upper molars (teeth 16, 26, 27), the carious lesions appear to originate in the interdental spaces (approximal caries; red rectangles). (**b**) In the two premolars (teeth 15, 44) in the right upper and lower jaw (white arrows), the crowns are destroyed, and the origin of the carious lesion cannot be reconstructed. The area around the first mandibular premolar (tooth 44) shows traces of an abscess (black arrows). (**c**) Dental wear is particularly pronounced in the anterior dentition. Incisors and canines of both maxilla and mandible show formation of secondary dentin (cf. (**a**)). (**d**) There is evidence of periapical changes on molars 26 and 27. Teeth 33, 36, and 47 were taken for DNA analyses, tooth 14 was lost post-mortem (DEB 484, 35–45 years, male).

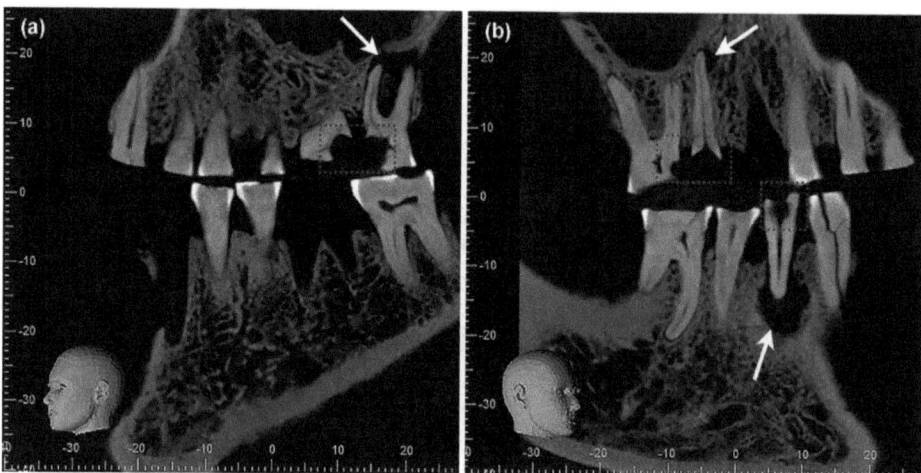

Figure 4. (**a**,**b**) The DVT images show that the dental cavities in some teeth (red rectangles) have led to periapical changes in the bone (white arrows): (**a**) in the left maxilla, the second molar (tooth 27) is affected; (**b**) in the right maxilla, there is a small lesion on the second premolar (tooth 15); and on the canine of the left mandible (tooth 33), there is a larger cavity that can be identified as a possible cyst due to its size. The latter has led to a vestibular abscess (cf. (**b**); DEB 484, 35–45 years, male).

4.3. Sex-Related Differences

In the present study, females had a slightly higher CF (72.7%) than males (63.0%). The difference was even more pronounced for CE. Although this difference is not statistically significant, female individuals had more carious teeth, with a CE of 13.1%, than male individuals with 7.5%. The same trend can be observed considering AMTL.

Differences between the sexes are not uncommon in archeological and ethnological contexts, and a higher carious burden is often reported in females [9,61,62]. This is usually explained by a difference in diet, with females consuming less animal protein than males. It is supposed that females consume more carbohydrate-rich foods to meet their primary caloric needs [16,63,64]. However, a higher proportion of animal protein in the diet has a more beneficial effect on dental health [10]. The proteins found in dairy products, especially casein, reduce caries activity by inhibiting bacterial attachment to enamel as well as decreasing the solubility of hydroxyapatite, thus counteracting demineralization [65–67]. However, it cannot be ruled out that women preferred foods with a higher starch or sugar content, such as porridge, fruits, and honey.

In addition to dietary habits, hormonal differences between the sexes can also play a role [63,68]. For example, females show lower salivary flow rates than males [69,70]. Furthermore, high estrogen levels during pregnancy have a negative effect on the quantity and composition of saliva [71,72]. This favors the colonization of cariogenic bacteria and the development of periodontal diseases, which indirectly affects tooth loss. This explains the observed higher number of AMTL in females in the present study and the correlation between births and tooth loss in other studies [73–75].

4.4. Influence of Dental Wear

Occlusal wear protects against occlusal caries to a certain extent by preventing plaque from adhering to the tooth [10]. Mastication also promotes wear at the contact points of the teeth, which is called interproximal (interstitial) wear. The continuous progression of both occlusal and interstitial wear reduces the contact surfaces between the teeth [76]. As a result, the interdental spaces are better flushed with saliva, which protects the teeth from approximal caries (e.g., anterior teeth Figure 3a). However, if the wear continues, there is a high probability that the pulp cavity will be exposed. In the past, this could lead to the death and subsequent loss of the tooth [6]. Compared to current industrialized nations, dental wear was well developed in Neolithic populations, as shown in Figure 3c,d. The main reason for this was mechanical abrasion induced by dietary habits and can be explained by the higher proportion of rough, fiber-rich food as well as naturally occurring sand and grit in processed food [10,77,78]. Flour is a perfect example, as it was much more coarsely ground in ancient times and contained grit due to the use of grinding stones [79]. A total of 74 adult individuals from the sites investigated were subjected to an analysis of the degree of dental wear [80]. The results showed that the degree of wear of the occlusal surfaces continuously increased with age and reached its maximum level in mature and senile individuals. A comparison between the anterior and posterior regions showed that the mean degree of dental wear was higher in anterior teeth than in post-canines. Slightly more wear was observed in the upper jaw, especially in the anterior teeth. Differences between the upper and lower jaw were attributed to a higher load on the upper teeth due to occupational activities and the use of teeth as a third hand [81,82].

4.5. Comparative Data from Other Neolithic Sites

Comparing the prevalence of caries in different populations from the same or from neighboring geographic regions can provide information about the living conditions and subsistence strategies (Table 7). Comparative data from early farming populations (LBK/BK) from central Germany show a similar range of CE values for adults [83,84], with a considerably higher CE at Wandersleben [85]. If AMTL is included in the calculations, the frequencies increase and align with those from Wandersleben and Sondershausen. The low variability within the CE values does not indicate any significant nutritional differences within early farming populations in the MES. Data from the LBK site at Aiterhofen (southern Bavaria) show a similar CE value for adults, but the CF differs significantly [86]. In contrast, a lower CE was observed in adults from the Early Neolithic site of Kleinhadersdorf in Lower Austria [87]. In the subadults, the CE ranged between 1 and 3%; at Aiterhofen [88] and Kleinhadersdorf [87] the proportion of affected deciduous teeth was higher. The CF showed a greater range of variation in both adults and subadults. Different environmental conditions and subsistence strategies must be expected in different geographic regions. Isotope analyses from southern Germany, for example, show higher $\delta^{15}N$ values (mean: 9.7‰) than in the MES, which is interpreted as evidence of a higher proportion of animal protein in the diet [89]. In addition, sample size and differences in the age structure of the investigated populations may also contribute to the variations.

Table 7. Caries frequency (CF) and caries experience (CE) amongst adult and subadult individuals compared to other Neolithic and Early Bronze Age datasets from the MES region, Germany.

Period/Site	CF %		CE %		References
	Subadult	Adult	Subadult	Adult	
DEB	26.7	64.3/69.9 **	1.6	8.8/9.8 **	this study
HBS	12.5	70.6/70.6 **	1.4	12.0/15.9 **	this study
KAR	30.0	72.2/77.8 **	2.9	10.9/14.5 **	this study
All sites	18.4	68.3/71.4 **	1.2/2.9 *	10.3/13.0 **	this study
BK/Wandersleben (MES)	---	63.8	---	14.4	[85] **
BK/Wandersleben (MES)	12.5	---	3.2/0.0 *	---	[88]
BK/Sondershausen (MES)	---	69.0	---	11.8	[83] **
BK/collection	---	58.1	---	11.3	[84]
LBK/Aiterhofen (SB)	36.8	---	5.4/2.8 *	---	[88]
LBK/Aiterhofen (SB)	---	37.0	---	9.2	[86]
LBK/Kleinhadersdorf (LA)	---	60.7	4.9/2.0 *	7.3	[87]

Nutrients **2022**, *14*, 1831

Table 7. *Cont.*

Period/Site	CF %		CE %		References
	Subadult	Adult	Subadult	Adult	
MN/collection (MES)	8.0	44.0	1.3	4.9	[17]
LN/collection (MES)	9.8	38.3	0.9	5.5	[17]
LN/collection (MES)	---	36.4	---	6.0	[90] **
EBA/collection (MES)	11.4	35.6	0.9	5.8	[17]
EBA/collection (MES)	---	38.3	---	6.9	[91] **

* deciduous teeth/permanent teeth; ** ante-mortem tooth loss included; BK (Bandkeramik, c. 5700–4100 BC), MN (Middle Neolithic, 3950–3025 cal BC), LN (Late Neolithic, 2800–2050 cal BC), EBA (Early Bronze Age, 2200–1575 cal BC); SB (Southern Bavaria, Germany), LA (Lower Austria).

Lower CF and CE values were observed for the later periods of the Neolithic (MN, LN) and for the Early Bronze Age (EBA) [17,90,91]. This indicates a change in subsistence and dietary patterns. The results of C/N analyses from the Middle and Late Neolithic and the Early Bronze Age suggest that the amount of animal protein in the diet increased [92]. The higher proportion of meat and dairy products might have had a positive effect not only on dental health but also on the general wellbeing. The diachronic comparison suggests that the early farmers' diet was characterized by a higher proportion of carbohydrates, which can be attributed primarily to the cultivation of cereals [17,25].

5. Conclusions

The aim of this bioarcheological study was to provide insights into the relationship of dental caries and diet in c. 7000-year-old Early Neolithic farmers from central Germany. The results show that, although consuming a diet lower in sugar content compared to modern populations, carious lesions were not uncommon among early farmers. We found no significant differences between the sexes or between burial communities but, as anticipated, a strong effect of age on the presence of dental caries. A diet rich in carbohydrates can be blamed for this, with grain consumption playing an important part. Single cases illustrate the painful fate of some older individuals. It is evident that caries acquired symptomatic significance with increasing age, while carious lesions did not yet play a role in infants still relying strongly on mother's milk. The absence of a sex effect is supportive of the notion of a comparatively egalitarian lifestyle, in which both sexes have equivalent access to plant and animal-based foods.

Author Contributions: Conceptualization, N.N. and V.M.O.; methodology, N.N. and V.M.O.; formal analysis, N.N. and V.M.O.; investigation, N.N. and V.M.O.; data curation, N.N. and V.M.O.; writing—original draft preparation, N.N., V.M.O. and K.W.A.; writing—review and editing, N.N., V.M.O., K.W.A., O.S. and H.M.; visualization, N.N., V.M.O. and O.S.; supervision, K.W.A. and H.M.; project administration, K.W.A. and H.M.; funding acquisition, K.W.A. and H.M. All authors have read and agreed to the published version of the manuscript.

Funding: This research was supported by the German Research Foundation, grant number Al 287/7-1 and 7-3, Me 3245/1-1 and 1-3.

Institutional Review Board Statement: Not applicable.

Informed Consent Statement: Not applicable.

Data Availability Statement: All relevant data are contained in the article.

Acknowledgments: We would like to thank Sandy Hämmerle (prehistrans.com (accessed on 15 February 2022)) for her support.

Conflicts of Interest: The authors declare no conflict of interest.

Appendix A

Table A1. Number of individuals, permanent teeth, deciduous teeth and teeth lost ante-mortem (AMTL) of the three burial sites by age groups.

Age (Years)	Individuals	Permanent Teeth	Deciduous Teeth	AMTL
		Derenburg		
0–6	6	54	50	0
7–14	4	84	23	0
15–20	2	44	0	0
21–40	18	390	0	4
41–60	10	204	0	5
>61	0	0	0	0
total	40	776	73	9
		Halberstadt		
0–6	8	40	83	0
7–14	5	65	33	0
15–20	3	58	2	0
21–40	10	231	0	9
41–60	7	178	0	14
>61	0	0	0	0
total	33	572	118	23
		Karsdorf		
0–6	5	11	55	0
7–14	4	45	31	0
15–20	1	29	0	0
21–40	9	252	0	0
41–60	8	204	0	18
>61	1	21	0	5
total	28	562	86	23

References

1. Marcenes, W.; Kassebaum, N.J.; Bernabé, E.; Flaxman, A.; Naghavi, M.; Lopez, A.; Murray, C.J. Global burden of oral conditions in 1990–2010: A systematic analysis. *J. Dent. Res.* **2013**, *92*, 592–597. [CrossRef] [PubMed]
2. Pitts, N.B.; Zero, D.T.; Marsh, P.D.; Ekstrand, K.; Weintraub, J.A.; Ramos-Gomez, F.; Tagami, J.; Twetman, S.; Tsakos, G.; Ismail, A. Dental caries. *Nat. Rev. Dis. Primers* **2017**, *3*, 17030. [CrossRef] [PubMed]
3. Peres, M.A.; Macpherson, L.; Weyant, R.J.; Daly, B.; Venturelli, R.; Mathur, M.R.; Listl, S.; Celeste, R.K.; Guarnizo-Herreño, C.C.; Kearns, C.; et al. Oral diseases: A global public health challenge. *Lancet* **2019**, *394*, 249–260. [CrossRef]
4. Werneck, R.I.; Mira, M.T.; Trevilatto, P.C. A critical review: An overview of genetic influence on dental caries. *Oral Dis.* **2010**, *16*, 613–623. [CrossRef]
5. Strużycka, I. The Oral Microbiome in Dental Caries. *Pol. J. Microbiol.* **2014**, *63*, 127–135. [CrossRef]
6. Alt, K.W.; Türp, J.C.; Wächter, R. Periapical Lesions–Clinical and Anthropological Aspects. In *Dental Anthropology. Fundamentals, Limits, and Prospects*; Alt, K.W., Rösing, F.W., Teschler-Nicola, M., Eds.; Springer: New York, NY, USA; Vienna, Austria, 1998; pp. 247–276.
7. Selwitz, R.H.; Ismail, A.I.; Pitts, N.B. Dental caries. *Lancet* **2007**, *369*, 51–59. [CrossRef]
8. Lukacs, J.R. Dental paleopathology: Methods for reconstructing dietary patterns. In *Reconstruction of Life from the Skeleton*; Kennedy, M.Y.I., Kennedy, K.A.R., Eds.; Wiley: New York, NY, USA, 1989; pp. 261–286.
9. Larsen, C.S. *Bioarchaeology: Interpreting Behavior from the Human Skeleton*, 2nd ed.; Cambridge University Press: Cambridge, UK, 2015; pp. 67–86.
10. Caselitz, P. Caries–ancient plague of humankind. In *Dental Anthropology. Fundamentals, Limits, and Prospects*; Alt, K.W., Rösing, F.W., Teschler-Nicola, M., Eds.; Springer: New York, NY, USA; Vienna, Austria, 1998; pp. 203–226.
11. Petersen, P.E.; Bourgeois, D.; Ogawa, H.; Estupinan-Day, S.; Ndiaye, C. The global burden of oral diseases and risks to oral health. *Bull. World Health Organ.* **2005**, *83*, 661–669.
12. Hillson, S. *Dental Anthropology*; Cambridge University Press: Cambridge, UK, 2002.
13. Bailey, S.E.; Hublin, J.J. *Dental Perspectives on Human Evolution*; Springer: Dordrecht, The Netherlands, 2007.

14. Maixner, F.; Turaev, D.; Cazenave-Gassiot, A.; Janko, M.; Krause-Kyora, B.; Hoopmann, M.R.; Kusebauch, U.; Sartain, M.; Guerriero, G.; O'Sullivan, N.; et al. The Iceman's Last Meal Consisted of Fat, Wild Meat, and Cereals. *Curr. Biol.* **2018**, *28*, 2348–2355.e9. [CrossRef]
15. Koruyucu, M.; Erdal, Y.S. Reconstruction of dietary habits in the Early Bronze Age of Anatolia through the analysis of dental caries and wear. *Int. J. Osteoarchaeol.* **2021**, *31*, 902–915. [CrossRef]
16. Larsen, C.S.; Shavit, R.; Griffin, M.C. Dental caries evidence for dietary change: An archaeological context. In *Advances in Dental Anthropology*; Kelley, M.A., Larsen, C.S., Eds.; Wiley-Liss: New York, NY, USA, 1991; pp. 179–202.
17. Nicklisch, N.; Ganslmeier, R.; Siebert, A.; Friederich, S.; Meller, H.; Alt, K.W. Holes in teeth-Dental caries in Neolithic and Early Bronze Age populations in Central Germany. *Ann. Anat.* **2016**, *203*, 90–99. [CrossRef]
18. Haak, W.; Balanovsky, O.; Sanchez, J.J.; Koshel, S.; Zaporozhchenko, V.; Adler, C.J.; Der Sarkissian, C.S.; Brandt, G.; Schwarz, C.; Nicklisch, N.; et al. Ancient DNA from European early neolithic farmers reveals their near eastern affinities. *PLoS Biol.* **2010**, *8*, e1000536. [CrossRef] [PubMed]
19. Brandt, G.; Haak, W.; Adler, C.J.; Roth, C.; Szécsényi-Nagy, A.; Karimnia, S.; Möller-Rieker, S.; Meller, H.; Ganslmeier, R.; Friederich, S.; et al. Ancient DNA reveals key stages in the formation of Central European mitochondrial genetic diversity. *Science* **2013**, *342*, 257–261. [CrossRef] [PubMed]
20. Oelze, V.M.; Siebert, A.; Nicklisch, N.; Meller, H.; Dresely, V.; Alt, K.W. Early Neolithic diet and animal husbandry. Stable isotope evidence from three Linearbandkeramik (LBK) sites in Central Germany. *J. Archaeol. Sci.* **2011**, *38*, 270–279. [CrossRef]
21. DeNiro, M.; Epstein, S. Influence of the Diet on the Distribution of Nitrogen Isotopes in Animals. *Geoch. Cosmochim. Acta* **1981**, *48*, 341–351. [CrossRef]
22. Katzenberg, M.A. Stable Isotope Analysis: A Tool for Studying Past Diet, Demography, and Life History. In *Biological Anthropology of the Human Skeleton*; Katzenberg, M.A., Saunders, S.R., Eds.; Wiley: Hoboken, NJ, USA, 2008; pp. 411–414.
23. Masclans, A.; Bickle, P.; Hamon, C. Sexual inequalities in the Early Neolithic? Exploring relationships between sexes/genders at the cemetery of Vedrovice using use-wear analysis, diet and mobility. *J. Archaeol. Method Theory* **2021**, *28*, 232–273. [CrossRef]
24. Friederich, S. Frühneolithikum: Linienbandkeramik bis Gatersleben. In *Früh-und Mittelneolithikum*; Meller, H., Ed.; Landesamt für Denkmalpflege und Archäologie Sachsen-Anhalt: Halle (Saale), Germany, 2021; pp. 87–98.
25. Ostritz, S. Naturräumliche Grundlagen der neolithischen Besiedlung im Mittelelbe-Saale-Gebiet (MESG). In *Das Neolithikum im Mittelelbe-Saale-Gebiet und der Altmark*; Beier, H.-J., Einicke, R., Eds.; Beier & Beran: Wilkau-Haßlau, Germany, 1994; pp. 3–6.
26. Litt, T. Naturraum Mitteldeutschland im Neolithikum. In *Früh-und Mittelneolithikum*; Meller, H., Ed.; Landesamt für Denkmalpflege und Archäologie Sachsen-Anhalt: Halle (Saale), Germany, 2021; pp. 119–124.
27. Nicklisch, N. Spurensuche an Skeletten. Paläodemografische und epidemiologische Untersuchungen an neolithischen und frühbronzezeitlichen Bestattungen aus dem Mittelelbe-Saale-Gebiet im Kontext populationsdynamischer Prozesse. In *Forschungsberichte des Landesmuseums für Vorgeschichte Halle*; Landesamt für Denkmalpflege und Archäologie Sachsen-Anhalt: Halle (Saale), Germany, 2017.
28. Fritsch, B.; Claßen, E.; Müller, U.; Dresely, V. Die linienbandkeramischen Gräberfelder von Derenburg "Meerenstieg II" und Halberstadt "Sonntagsfeld", Lkr. Harz. *Jahresschr. Mitteldt. Vorgesch.* **2011**, *92*, 25–229.
29. Behnke, H.J. Erste Siedler der Linienbandkeramik in der Karsdorfer Feldflur. Ergebnisse der Grabungen im Jahr 2005. *Arch. Sachsen-Anhalt* **2007**, *5*, 18–33.
30. White, T.D.; Folkens, P.A. *Human Osteology*, 2nd ed.; Academic Press: San Diego, CA, USA, 2000.
31. Buikstra, J.E.; Ubelaker, D.H. Standards for Data Collection from Human Skeletal Remains. In *Proceedings of a Seminar at the Field Museum of Natural History*; Arkansas Archeological Survey: Fayetteville, NC, USA, 1994.
32. Meindl, R.S.; Lovejoy, C.O. Ectocranial suture closure: A revised method for determination of skeletal age at death based on the lateral-anterior sutures. *Am. J. Phys. Anthropol.* **1985**, *68*, 57–66. [CrossRef]
33. Lovejoy, C.O.; Meindel, R.S.; Pryzbeck, T.R.; Mensforth, R.P. Chronological metamorphosis of the auricular surface of the ilium: A new method for the determination of adult skeletal age and death. *Am. J. Phys. Anthropol.* **1985**, *68*, 15–28. [CrossRef]
34. Buckberry, J.L.; Chamberlain, A.T. Age estimation from the auricular surface of the Ilium: A Revised Method. *Am. J. Phys. Anthropol.* **2002**, *119*, 231–239. [CrossRef]
35. Brooks, S.T.; Suchey, J.M. Skeletal age determination based on the os pubis: A comparison of the Acsádi-Nemeskéri and Suchey-Brooks methods. *J. Hum. Evol.* **1990**, *5*, 227–238. [CrossRef]
36. Ubelaker, D.H. *Human Skeletal Remains: Excavation, Analysis, Interpretation*, 2nd ed.; Taraxacum: Washington, DC, USA, 1998.
37. Stloukal, M.; Hanáková, H. Die Länge der Längsknochen altslavischer Bevölkerungen unter besonderer Berücksichtigung von Wachstumsfragen. *HOMO* **1978**, *29*, 53–69.
38. Ferembach, D.; Schwidetzky, I.; Stloukal, M. Recommendations for age and sex diagnoses of skeletons. *J. Hum. Evol.* **1980**, *9*, 517–549. [CrossRef]
39. Phenice, T.W. A newly developed visual method of sexing the os pubis. *Am. J. Phys. Anthropol.* **1969**, *30*, 297–302. [CrossRef] [PubMed]
40. Murail, P.; Bruzek, J.; Houët, F.; Cunha, E. DSP: A tool for probabilistic sexdiagnosis using worldwide variability in hip-bone measurements. *Bull. Mem. Soc. Anthropol. Paris* **2005**, *17*, 167–176. [CrossRef]
41. Knussmann, R. Vergleichende Biologie des Menschen. In *Lehrbuch der Anthropologie und Humangenetik*; Fischer: Stuttgart, Germany, 1996; p. 169.

42. Alt, K.W.; Türp, J.C. Roll call: Thirty-two white horses on a red field. The advantages of the FDI two-digit system of designating teeth. In *Dental Anthropology. Fundamentals, Limits, and Prospects*; Alt, K.W., Rösing, F.W., Teschler-Nicola, M., Eds.; Springer: New York, NY, USA; Vienna, Austria, 1998; pp. 41–55.

43. Alt, K.W. Karies in Vergangenheit und Gegenwart. Zur Epidemiologie einer "Volksseuche". In *Pein und Plagen. Aspekte Einer Historischen Epidemiologie*; Kemkes-Grottenthaler, A., Henke, W., Eds.; Edition Archaea: Gelsenkirchen, Germany, 2001; pp. 156–213.

44. Hillson, S. Recording dental caries in archaeological human remains. *Int. J. Osteoarchaeol.* **2001**, *11*, 249–289. [CrossRef]

45. Machiulskiene, V.; Campus, G.; Carvalho, J.C.; Dige, I.; Ekstrand, K.R.; Jablonski-Momeni, A.; Maltz, M.; Manton, D.J.; Martignon, S.; Martinez-Mier, E.A.; et al. Terminology of Dental Caries and Dental Caries Management: Consensus Report of a Workshop Organized by ORCA and Cariology Research Group of IADR. *Caries Res.* **2020**, *54*, 7–14. [CrossRef]

46. Hillson, S. *Teeth*; Cambridge University Press: Cambridge, UK, 2005; p. 295.

47. Richards, M.P.; Hedges, R.E.M. Stable Isotope Evidence for Similarities in the Types of Marine Foods Used by Late Mesolithic Humans at Sites along the Atlantic Coast of Europe. *J. Archaeol. Sci.* **1999**, *26*, 717–722. [CrossRef]

48. Ambrose, S.H. Preparation and Characterization of Bone and Tooth Collagen for Isotopic Analysis. *J. Archaeol. Sci.* **1990**, *17*, 431–451. [CrossRef]

49. R Development Core Team. *R: A Language and Environment for Statistical Computing*; R Foundation for Statistical Computing: Vienna, Austria, 2013. Available online: http://www.R-project.org/ (accessed on 11 August 2021).

50. Beug, H.-J. Vegetationsgeschichtliche Untersuchungen über die Besiedlung im Unteren Eichsfeld, Landkreis Göttingen, vom frühen Neolithikum bis zum Mittelalter. *Neue Ausgr. Forsch. Niedersachs.* **1992**, *20*, 261–339.

51. Drucker, D.G.; Bridault, A.; Hobson, K.A.; Szuma, E.; Bocherens, H. Can carbon-13 in large herbivores reflect the canopy effect in temperate and boreal ecosystems? Evidence from modern and ancient ungulates. *Palaeogeogr. Palaeoclimatol. Palaeoecol.* **2008**, *266*, 69–82. [CrossRef]

52. Burger, J.; Kirchner, M.; Bramanti, B.; Haak, W.; Thomas, M.G. Absence of the lactase-persistence-associated allele in early Neolithic Europeans. *Proc. Natl. Acad. Sci. USA* **2007**, *104*, 3736–3741. [CrossRef] [PubMed]

53. Fogel, M.L.; Tuross, N.; Owsley, D.W. Nitrogen isotope tracers of human lactation in modern and archaeological populations. In *Annual Report of the Director: Geophysical Laboratory*; Carnegie Institution: Washington, DC, USA, 1989; Volume 88, pp. 111–117.

54. Moynihan, P.; Petersen, P.E. Diet, nutrition and the prevention of dental diseases. *Public Health Nutr.* **2004**, *7*, 201–226. [CrossRef] [PubMed]

55. Halvorsrud, K.; Lewney, J.; Craig, D.; Moynihan, P.J. Effects of Starch on Oral Health: Systematic Review to Inform WHO Guideline. *J. Dent. Res.* **2019**, *98*, 46–53. [CrossRef]

56. Adler, C.J.; Dobney, K.; Weyric, L.S.; Kaidonis, J.; Walker, A.W.; Haak, H.; Corey, J.A.; Bradshaw, C.J.A.; Townsend, G.; Sołtysiak, A.; et al. Sequencing ancient calcified dental plaque shows changes in oral micro-biota with dietary shifts of the Neolithic and Industrial revolutions. *Nat. Genet.* **2013**, *45*, 450–455. [CrossRef]

57. Alt, K.W.; Nicklisch, N.; Held, P.; Meyer, C.; Rossbach, A.; Burwinkel, M. Zähne als Gesundheits- und Mortalitätsrisiko. In *Traumatologische und pathologische Veränderungen an prähistorischen und historischen Skelettreste. Diagnose, Ursachen und Kontext*; Piek, J., Terberger, T., Eds.; Verlag Marie Leidorf: Rahden/Westf., Germany, 2008; pp. 25–42.

58. Zoellner, H. Dental infection and vascular disease. *Semin. Thromb. Hemost.* **2011**, *37*, 181–192. [CrossRef] [PubMed]

59. Rustemeyer, J.; Bremerich, A. Necessity of surgical dental foci treatment prior to organ transplantation and heart valve replacement. *Clin. Oral Investig.* **2007**, *11*, 171–174. [CrossRef]

60. Pathak, J.L.; Yan, Y.; Zhang, Q.; Wang, L.; Ge, L. The role of oral microbiome in respiratory health and diseases. *Respir. Med.* **2021**, *185*, 106475. [CrossRef]

61. Bennike, P. *Palaeopathology of Danish Skeletons*; Akademisk Forlag: Copenhagen, Denmark, 1985.

62. Lukacs, J.R. Sex differences in dental caries rates with the origin of agriculture in South Asia. *Curr. Anthropol.* **1996**, *37*, 147–153. [CrossRef]

63. Lukacs, J.R.; Largaespada, L.L. Explaining sex differences in dental caries prevalence: Saliva, hormones, and "life-history" etiologies. *Am. J. Hum. Biol.* **2008**, *18*, 540–555. [CrossRef]

64. Peterson, J. Woman's Share in Neolithic Society: A View from the Southern Levant. *Near East. Archaeol.* **2016**, *79*, 132–139. [CrossRef]

65. Vacca-Smith, A.M.; van Wuyckhouuse, B.C.; Tabak, L.A.; Bowen, W.H. The effect of milk and casein proteins on the adherence of streptococcus mutans to saliva-coated hydroxyapatite. *Arch. Oral Biol.* **1994**, *39*, 1063–1069. [CrossRef]

66. Kashket, S.; DePaola, D.P. Cheese consumption and the development and progression of dental caries. *Nutr. Rev.* **2002**, *60*, 97–103. [CrossRef] [PubMed]

67. Aimutis, W.R. Bioactive properties of milk proteins with particular focus on anticariogenesis. *J. Nutr.* **2004**, *134*, S989–S995. [CrossRef]

68. Lukacs, J.R. Sex differences in dental caries experience: Clinical evidence, complex etiology. *Clin. Oral Investig.* **2011**, *15*, 649–656. [CrossRef] [PubMed]

69. Bergdahl, M. Salivary flow and oral complaints in adult dental patients. *Community Dent. Oral Epidemiol.* **2000**, *28*, 59–66. [CrossRef]

70. Dodds, M.W.J.; Johnson, D.; Yeh, C.-K. Health benefits of saliva: A review. *J. Dent.* **2005**, *33*, 223–233. [CrossRef]

71. Laine, M.; Tenovuo, J.; Lehtonen, O.P.; Ojanotko-Harri, A.; Vilja, P.; Tuohimaa, P. Pregnancy-related changes in human whole saliva. *Arch. Oral Biol.* **1988**, *33*, 913–917. [CrossRef]
72. Salvolini, E.; Di Giorgio, R.; Curatola, A.; Mazzanti, L.; Fratto, G. Biochemical modifications of human whole saliva induced by pregnancy. *Br. J. Obstet. Gynaecol.* **1998**, *195*, 656–660. [CrossRef]
73. Christensen, K.; Gaist, D.; Jeune, B.; Vaupel, J.W. A tooth per child? *Lancet* **1998**, *352*, 204–210. [CrossRef]
74. Laine, M.A. Effect of pregnancy on periodontal and dental health. *Acta Odontol. Scand.* **2002**, *60*, 257–264. [CrossRef] [PubMed]
75. Russell, S.L.; Ickovics, J.R.; Yaffee, R.A. Parity and untreated dental caries in US women. *J. Dent. Res.* **2010**, *89*, 1091–1096. [CrossRef] [PubMed]
76. Rose, J.C.; Ungar, P.S. Gross dental wear and dental microwear in historical perspective. In *Dental Anthropology. Fundamentals, Limits, and Prospects*; Alt, K.W., Rösing, F.W., Teschler-Nicola, M., Eds.; Springer: New York, NY, USA; Vienna, Austria, 1998; pp. 349–386.
77. Alt, K.W.; Rossbach, A. Nothing in Nature Is as Consistent as Change. In *Comparative Dental Morphology*; Koppe, T., Meyer, G., Alt, K.W., Eds.; Karger: Basel, Switzerland, 2009; Volume 3, pp. 190–196.
78. Sperber, G.H. Dental Wear: Attrition, Erosion, and Abrasion-A Palaeo-Odontological Approach. *Dent. J.* **2017**, *5*, 19. [CrossRef] [PubMed]
79. Mays, S. *The Archaeology of Human Bones*; Routledge: London, UK; New York, NY, USA, 1998.
80. Nasse, D. Betrachtung Abnormaler Abrasionsmuster Prähistorischer Bevölkerungen aus Sachsen-Anhalt. Master's Thesis, Johannes-Gutenberg-University, Mainz, Germany, 2011.
81. Alt, K.W.; Pichler, S.L. Artificial modifications of human teeth. In *Dental Anthropology. Fundamentals, Limits, and Prospects*; Alt, K.W., Rösing, F.W., Teschler-Nicola, M., Eds.; Springer: New York, NY, USA; Vienna, Austria, 1998; pp. 387–415.
82. Molnar, P. Dental wear and oral pathology: Possible evidence and consequences of habitual use of teeth in a Swedish Neolithic sample. *Am. J. Phys. Anthropol.* **2008**, *136*, 423–431. [CrossRef]
83. Bach, A. *Neolithische Populationen im Mittelelbe-Saale-Gebiet. Zur Anthropologie des Neolithikums unter Besonderer Berücksichtigung der Bandkeramiker*; Weimarer Monographien zur Ur- und Frühgeschichte: Weimar, Germany, 1978.
84. Penser, E. Stomatologische Untersuchungen an Erwachsenen Neolithikern aus Dem Mittelelbe-Saale-Gebiet. Ph.D. Thesis, Ludwig-Maximilians-University, Munich, Germany, 1985.
85. Haschen, S. Stomatologische Untersuchungen an der Linienbandkeramischen Bevölkerung von Wandersleben, Kreis Gotha. Ph.D. Thesis, Friedrich-Schiller-University, Jena, Germany, 1991.
86. Baum, N. Aiterhofen-Ödmühle. Paläodontologie eines bandkeramischen Gräberfeldes in Niederbayern. *Prähist. Zeitschr.* **1989**, *65*, 157–202.
87. Tiefenböck, B.; Teschler-Nicola, M. Teil II: Anthropologie. In *Das Linearbandkeramische Gräberfeld von Kleinhadersdorf*; Horjes, B., Ed.; Mitteilungen der Prähistorischen Kommission, Österreichische Akademie der Wissenschaften: Wien, Austria, 2013; Volume 82, pp. 382–392.
88. Carli-Thiele, P. *Spuren von Mangelerkrankungen An Steinzeitlichen Kinderskeletten*; Fortschritte in der Palaeopathologie und Osteoarchaeologie; Erich Goltze: Göttingen, Germany, 1996.
89. Knipper, C. Kohlenstoff-und Stickstoffanalysen an bandkeramischen Bestattungen vom "Viesenhäuser Hof" bei Stuttgart-Mühlhausen: Implikationen zur Ernährungsrekonstruktion, Geschlechtsspezifik und Siedlungsdynamik. In *Der Zahn der Zeit*; Meyer, C., Held, P., Knipper, C., Nicklisch, N., Eds.; Landesamt für Denkmalpflege und Archäologie Sachsen-Anhalt: Halle (Saale), Germany, 2020; pp. 211–225.
90. Bach, A.; Bach, H. Zur Anthropologie der Schnurkeramiker. In *Beiträge zur Kultur und Anthropologie der Mitteldeutschen Schnurkeramiker II*; Bach, A., Bach, H., Gall, W., Feustel, R., Teichert, M., Eds.; Alt-Thüringen: Weimar, Germany, 1975; Volume 13, pp. 43–107.
91. Holtfreter, J. Zur Anthropologie der Aunjetitzer des Mittelelbe-Saale-Gebietes. In *Paläanthropologie im Mittelelbe-Saale-Werra-Gebiet*; Feustel, R., Ed.; Weimarer Monographien zur Ur-und Frühgeschichte: Weimar, Germany, 1989; Volume 23, pp. 105–132.
92. Münster, A.; Knipper, C.; Oelze, V.M.; Nicklisch, N.; Stecher, M.; Schlenker, B.; Ganslmeier, R.; Fragata, M.; Friederich, S.; Dresely, V.; et al. 4000 years of human dietary evolution in central Germany, from the first farmers to the first elites. *PLoS ONE* **2018**, *13*, e0194862. [CrossRef]

MDPI

St. Alban-Anlage 66

4052 Basel

Switzerland

Tel. +41 61 683 77 34

Fax +41 61 302 89 18

www.mdpi.com

Nutrients Editorial Office

E-mail: nutrients@mdpi.com

www.mdpi.com/journal/nutrients

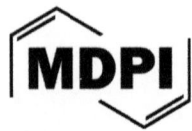